Contents

Pathways in Surgery

Third Edition

Edited by

Michael Hobsley TD MChir DSc PhD FRCS
Emeritus Professor of Surgery
Department of Surgery
Academic Division of Surgical Specialties
Royal Free and University College Medical School
London

Paul B Boulos MS FRCS FRCSEd FCS HK(Hon)
Professor of Surgery
Department of Surgery
Academic Division of Surgical Specialties
Royal Free and University College Medical School
London

ARNOLD

A member of the Hodder Headline Group
LONDON

First published in Great Britain in 1979 by
Edward Arnold

Second edition 1986

This edition published in 2002 by
Arnold, a member of the Hodder Headline Group,
338 Euston Road, London NW1 3BH

http://www.arnoldpublishers.com

Distributed in the United States of America by
Oxford University Press Inc., 198 Madison Avenue, New York, NY10016
Oxford is a registered trademark of Oxford University Press

Whilst the advice and information in this book are believed to be
true and accurate at the date of going to press, neither the authors
nor the publisher can accept any legal responsibility or liability for
any errors or omissions that may be made. In particular (but
without limiting the generality of the preceding disclaimer) every
effort has been made to check drug dosages; however, it is still
possible that errors have been missed. Furthermore, dosage
schedules are constantly being revised and new side-effects
recognized. For these reasons the reader is strongly urged to
consult the drug companies' printed instructions before
administering any of the drugs recommended in this book.

British Library Cataloguing in Publication Data
A catalogue record for this book is available from the British Library

Library of Congress Cataloging-in-Publication Data
A catalog record for this book is available from the Library of Congress

ISBN 0 340 63186 4

1 2 3 4 5 6 7 8 9 10

Publisher: Nick Dunton
Development Editor: Michael Lax
Production Editor: Rada Radojicic
Production Controller: Martin Kerans
Cover Design: Terry Griffiths

Typeset in 10/12 Minion by Charon Tec Pvt. Ltd, Chennai, India
Printed and bound in Malta by Gutenberg Press

What do you think about this book? Or any other Arnold title?
Please send your comments to feedback.arnold@hodder.co.uk

Contributors

M Adiseshiah MS FRCP FRCS
Consultant Surgeon
University College London Hospitals
London

George Bentley ChM FRCS
Director and Professor of Orthopaedic Surgery
Institute of Orthopaedics
Royal National Orthopaedic Hospital
Stanmore

Paul B Boulos MS FRCS FRCSEd FCS HK(Hon)
Professor of Surgery, Department of Surgery
Academic Division of Surgical Specialties
Royal Free and University College Medical School
London

D John Brazier FRCS FRCOphth
Consultant Ophthalmologist
Royal Free and University College London Hospitals
London

Martin J Burton MA DM FRCS
Consultant Otolaryngologist and
Honorary Senior Clinical Lecturer
Department of Otolaryngology
Radcliffe Infirmary
Oxford

Lydia Chang FRCOphth
Specialist Registrar
Royal Free and University College London Hospitals
London

Philip Coleridge Smith DM FRCS
Reader in Surgery and Consultant Surgeon
Department of Surgery
Academic Division of Surgical Specialties
Royal Free and University College Medical School
London

Tim Davidson ChM MRCP FRCS
Senior Lecturer and Consultant Surgeon
Department of Surgery
Royal Free Hospital
London

Rebecca Grant BSc
Research Associate
Department of Cardiothoracic Surgery
University College London Hospitals
London

Michael Hobsley TD MChir DSc PhD FRCS
Emeritus Professor of Surgery
Department of Surgery
Academic Division of Surgical Specialties
Royal Free and University College Medical School
London

Jasmin Hussein FACS
Research Fellow
National Hospital for Neurology and Neurosurgery
London

Celia L Ingham Clark MChir FRCS
Consultant Surgeon
Department of Surgery
The Whittington Hospital
London

Christopher BD Lavy
Honorary Consultant Orthopaedic Surgeon
University College London Hospitals
London

DA McGrouther MD FRCS
Professor of Plastic and Reconstructive Surgery
Department of Surgery
Academic Division of Surgical Specialties
Royal Free and University College Medical School
London

Anthony R Mundy MD FRCS
Director
Institute of Urology and Nephrology
University College London
London

Wilfred Pugsley BA FRCS
Department of Cardiothoracic Surgery
Royal Sussex County Hospital
Brighton

RCG Russell MS FRCS
Consultant Surgeon
University College London Hospitals
London

Julian Shah FRCS
Senior Lecturer and Honorary Consultant Urologist
Institute of Urology and Nephrology
University College London
London

Mervyn Singer MD FRCP
Professor in Intensive Care Medicine
Bloomsbury Institute of Intensive Care Medicine
Royal Free and University College Medical School
London

Dishan Singh FRCS(Orth)
Consultant Orthopaedic Surgeon
Royal National Orthopaedic Hospital
Stanmore
and Honorary Senior Lecturer
Institute of Orthopaedics
London

Irving Taylor MD ChM FRCS
Chairman of Division and
David Patey Professor of Surgery
Department of Surgery
Academic Division of Surgical Specialties
Royal Free and University College Medical School
London

Vanessa M Wright FRCS FRACS
Consultant Paediatric Surgeon
The Royal Hospitals
London

John H Wyllie BSc MD FRCS
Emeritus Professor of Surgery
Department of Surgery
Royal Free and University College Medical School
London

Preface to the first edition

The arrangement of this book is unorthodox. Its relationship to a conventional textbook of surgery is comparable with that of a thesaurus to a dictionary.

A dictionary lists words, many of which have more than one meaning, and defines these various meanings. A thesaurus, on the other hand, starts with an idea and then lists all the words and phrases which in general express that idea, although with wide differences in emphasis and specialization.

Similarly, a conventional textbook of surgery lists surgical diseases and describes the symptoms and signs to which they might give rise: most of these symptoms and signs may occur in more than one disease. On the other hand, this volume starts with some common combinations of symptoms and signs such as the surgeon is likely to meet every day, and works backwards to show how one can identify which of several possible diseases produced that clinical picture.

Since the aim of surgical teaching is to make the student competent to deal with patients, and since these present with clinical pictures rather than with diseases, the author hopes that this book may prove helpful both to students of surgery and to their teachers.

MH

Preface to the second edition

The aims and methods of this book remain as described in the preface to the first edition.

The major changes in this edition are a first chapter on physical signs with reference to lumps, ulcers and tenderness, and increased emphasis on the role of the general practitioner. Many surgical decisions are now easier to make because of the availability of improved investigations such as ultrasound. Factors like these have enabled the text of several chapters, for example that on Jaundice, to be considerably simplified.

MH

Preface to the third edition

This edition differs from the previous two in that it covers not only general surgery but also the other surgical specialties. Of necessity, it is now multi-authored and twin-edited. It remains devoted to a pathways approach, concentrating not so much on narrative descriptions of diseases, but on how the surgeon approaches the management of commonly encountered clinical situations and problems. The flow-diagrams that follow each chapter distinguish **surgical actions** from other material with **bold type**.

Inevitably there is overlap between chapters and contributors and it follows that diverging views on the same subject are sometimes expressed. The editors have not tried to iron out these inconsistencies; there is much in surgery which remains controversial. This allows the student to be familiar with contrary views and be able to make a decision on the line of management based on logical grounds.

The standard is aimed at covering the learning needs of the medical student, although it is also adequate for those preparing for the Membership of the Royal Colleges of Surgeons in the United Kingdom.

MH
PBB

Acknowledgments

All the authors are members of the staff of University College London and its associated hospitals, or they were at the time they were invited to contribute. Many other colleagues helped with advice and criticism.

We thank Emma Collins for co-ordinating the work on the manuscripts, and the Publishers, particularly Nick Dunton, Michael Lax, Rada Radojicic, Anke Ueberberg and Martin Kerans, for their support and patience during the lengthy gestation period of this edition.

We are also grateful for the forbearance and support of our families.

MH
PBB

Non-emergencies

1

Lumps; tenderness

MICHAEL HOBSLEY

AIMS

1 Determine whether a 'lump' is normal or abnormal
2 In the history, concentrate particularly on temporal relationships
3 Describe the physical signs, especially site, shape, consistency, layer, lymph nodes
4 Recognize the characteristic features of common skin lumps
5 Determine the management

INTRODUCTION

The most common situations in which patients present are a *lump*, or else pain; of these, pain is a subjective complaint, but it is frequently associated with *tenderness*. This chapter therefore presents some introductory remarks about the assessment of a lump and of tenderness.

LUMPS

A lump may be defined as a feature which is distinguishable from its surroundings by sight and/or touch, *and is abnormal*. The question of abnormality is important: a frequent error for the unwary is to fail to appreciate that the 'lump' may be a normal structure. Normal anatomical structures vary in their sizes, and bilateral pairs are often asymmetrically developed. Some individuals have particularly large hands or feet, or have one ear or breast that is larger than the other. It is by examining patients from top to toe that we become aware of normal variation.

The words *swelling* and *lump* are often used as though they were synonymous. Some use the word *swelling* to indicate a normal structure that has become abnormal by growing larger, others for lumps whose borders are diffuse rather than well-demarcated. To avoid confusion, it is best to avoid the word *swelling*.

Another source of confusion is that the palpability of a lump depends upon its consistency being firmer than that of its surroundings. The mere presence of a structure does not necessarily mean that it is palpable: the parotid covers a large area of the face and neck, yet it is not palpable, whereas the normal submandibular salivary gland is firmer than the surrounding subcutaneous tissues, and therefore in most individuals is readily palpable.

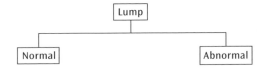

When the lump is a normal structure, the patient is suitably reassured. Having decided that a lump is abnormal, the symptoms and physical signs are reviewed. The most important aspect of the history is the dynamic relationship of the size of the lump with time which, although subjective and possibly imprecise, reflects on the underlying pathology. The physical signs include *size*, which is more precisely measured in a lump with defined borders that can be outlined by palpation rather than inspection. Size can influence management and the technique of surgical excision, and is a measure of the response to medical therapy. Of the many other signs that are described, five are especially helpful: *site, shape, consistency, layer* and the neighbouring *lymph nodes*.

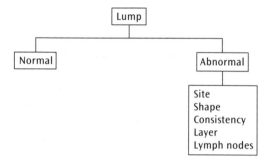

Site

The location of a lump is not in its co-ordinates but its relation to neighbouring or underlying anatomical structures. A lump described as 7.5 cm medial to the anterior superior iliac spine and 3.5 cm below it may enable someone else to find the lump; but reference to its position at the mid-inguinal point indicates that it overlies the femoral artery and therefore could be an aneurysm which is more descriptive and meaningful.

Lumps not specific to any particular site are considered below, whereas those that are of particular relevance to a site will be discussed in the appropriate chapters.

Shape

Many lumps have shapes that do not contribute to management. However, there are four shapes of diagnostic significance.

Spherical lumps are nearly always liquid-containing cysts. As the lump grows, the pressure in the liquid is transmitted equally in all directions, and uniform growth in all directions results in the spherical shape. Although only half the lump (or maybe two-thirds, because it is usually possible to indent the neighbouring skin sufficiently to feel more than half) is smoothly spherical, it is reasonable to assume that the inaccessible aspect is similar.

Lobulation of the surface, with palpable or visible indentations between the lobules, is typical of a subcutaneous lipoma or a mammary fibroadenoma (Chapter 3).

Discoid lesions are uncommon, but sometimes sufficiently typical to establish a working diagnosis (see gynaecomastia, Chapter 3). The typical shape of the *parotid salivary gland* is considered in Chapter 2.

Consistency

There are five important aspects of consistency.

Degree of hardness. In order to avoid disparity of definition among observers, it is unnecessary to strive after several grades of consistency. It is simpler to describe a lump as *hard* when not deformable, *soft* when easily deformable and *firm* when the superficial surface of the lump yields to some extent but a hard core then becomes apparent.

There follow four signs that only apply to soft lumps, and relate to the volume of the lump when it is deformed by pressure.

Fluctuance. Pushing the lump in at one point results in its border projecting outwards elsewhere (Fig. 1.1). If the lump is mobile, mass movement of the lesion could be confused with fluctuance; it is therefore necessary that the lump is fixed. Fluctuance is demonstrable in lumps that are soft and constant in volume. The sign is often claimed to be pathognomonic of a liquid-containing cyst, but some cysts are not fluctuant (those with rigid walls or high internal pressure) and some solids, for example a subcutaneous lipoma, are soft enough to be fluctuant. Muscle, at least when relaxed, shows fluctuance but only at right angles to its axis: it cannot expand along its axis because of its fixity to bone at its origin and insertion.

Emptying or reduction. With external pressure, the volume decreases and may even disappear. This sign

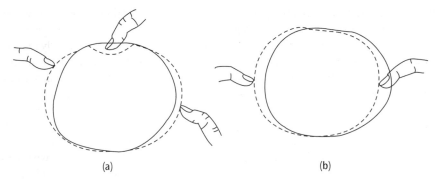

Fig. 1.1 *(a) The sign of fluctuance. When the lump is deformed by pressure in one area, its borders move outwards elsewhere because it is constant in volume; (b) Pressing from one side should be avoided because if the whole lump moves under pressure, the movement of the side opposite to the pressure may be misinterpreted by the other finger as bulging.*

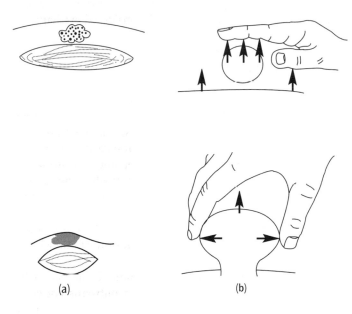

Fig. 1.2 *The sign of expansile cough impulse; (a) A soft lump superficial to the muscle may be impalpable until the muscle is contracted. An expansile cough impulse can only be diagnosed if a lump at rest becomes larger on coughing; (b) A common error is to try to diagnose an expansile cough impulse with the fingers flat. With the fingers in this position the examiner can only demonstrate an overall thrust, it needs the cupped fingers and thumb to detect expansion.*

is present in lesions which are in continuity with larger cavities; the contents of the lesion are emptied into the cavity and so they disappear from the field of examination. Examples are hernias when reducible and haemangiomas that empty into the circulation.

Expansile cough impulse. The lump becomes larger when the patient coughs or performs any other act, such as straining, that raises the pressure in the subjacent body cavity. This is a valuable sign of abdominal hernias (Chapter 10), but Fig. 1.2 indicates some common errors. An expansile impulse can only be demonstrated if there is already an existing lump at rest, and if the observer gently grasps the lump with fingers and thumb rather than placing the palm of the hand over it, he will be able to appreciate that the lump is getting larger rather than being pushed outwards by the thrust of the abdominal wall on coughing.

Pulsation. A lump that throbs in time with the pulse is an *aneurysm* if the pulsation is *expansile*, but is some other lesion that is overlying an artery when the pulsation is *directly outward at all points and is therefore transmitted* (Fig. 1.3). The distinction is often difficult.

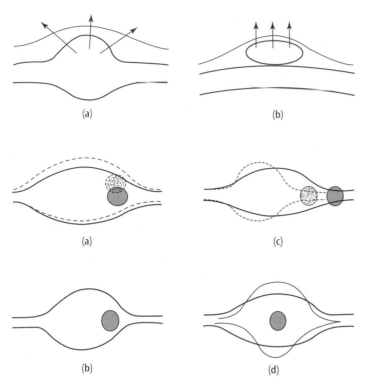

(a)

(b)

Fig. 1.3 *(a) True expansile pulsation in a lesion in direct communication with an artery; (b) Transmitted pulsation from a lump overlying an artery.*

(a)

(c)

(b)

(d)

Fig. 1.4 *Attachment to muscle; (a) At rest the muscle is flaccid and the palpable lump moves from side to side with the muscle when the examiner tests mobility at right angles to the muscle fibres; (b) On contraction of the muscle the lump is no longer mobile from side to side; (c) The alternative test when the lump moves proximally with the muscle when it contracts works satisfactorily in this case if the lump is in the region of the tendon; (d) The test illustrated in (c) does not work when the lump is near the centre point of the muscle mass.*

Layer

In general, there are four layers to consider: *skin, subcutaneous tissue, muscle* and *bone*. In the abdominal wall, it must also be determined whether the lesion is *in the abdominal wall itself* or *within the abdominal cavity*.

Bone. It is usually obvious that a lesion is in, or attached to, bone when the lump and the bone cannot be moved independently of each other.

Muscle. The evidence that a lesion is attached to a muscle is that the mobility of the lump in a direction at right angles to the line of the muscle when at rest is reduced when the muscle is contracted (Fig. 1.4 (a), (b)). Less valuable is movement of the lump in the line of its pull when the muscle contracts: for example, a muscle producing movement equally at its points of origin and insertion would not move at its mid-point (Fig. 1.4 (c), (d)).

A lesion within or deep to a muscle, becomes less palpable, or disappears completely when the muscle contracts, unless its consistency is firmer than that of the contracted muscle. A lump lying on the superficial

aspect of a muscle becomes more prominent and feels harder when it is thrust forward by the expansion outwards of the shortened, thickened, muscle belly (see Fig. 1.2 (a) above).

Skin. Whether a lump is in the most superficial layer, the skin, is not always easy to decide. There is no problem if the skin can be pinched up over the lesion and lifted away from it (Fig. 1.5 (a)). However, the sign may not be obvious if the skin is naturally tight across the surface of the lump or if the lesion lies mainly in the subcutaneous layer but is attached to skin at one small area. Fig. 1.5 (b) and (c) demonstrates two useful techniques. If there is still doubt, it usually turns out that the lump is, indeed, attached to skin.

Subcutaneous tissue. By exclusion, lumps that are not attached to skin and not attached to muscle or bone lie in the subcutaneous tissue.

Abdomen: wall or cavity? Since the firmest structure of the anterior abdominal wall is muscle, lumps within the abdominal cavity become less prominent or disappear, lumps in the muscles become fixed and lumps superficial to the muscles become harder and

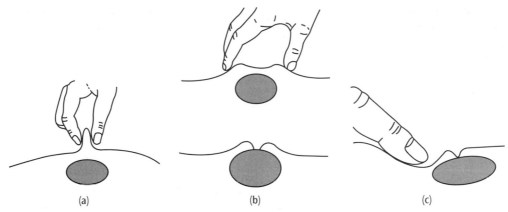

Fig. 1.5 *Attachment to the skin. (a) A lump not attached to the skin. The skin can be picked up easily over the lump; (b) If the skin is tight in the region of the lump and therefore difficult to pick up, excess skin can be brought in from the periphery as shown (two separate hands can be used if necessary) and it then becomes obvious if the skin is free from or bound down to it. The pit that appears when the skin is bound down to the lump is called 'skin-dimpling'; (c) In the author's experience it is not as reliable as that shown in (b).*

more prominent on contracting the abdominal wall muscles.

Cautionary notes

First, the decision that the lump is attached to a particular layer does not exclude its attachment to other layers. For example, a tumour of bone may grow out through the muscles and subcutaneous tissue, finally to involve the skin and then it is attached to all the layers.

Second, the significance of attachment of a lump mainly in one area to another layer needs to be considered carefully. It may imply a pathological extension, commonly neoplastic infiltration; less commonly, inflammatory. However, the attachment may be anatomical rather than pathological. A lump at the lower pole of the parotid salivary gland lies deep to the sternomastoid muscle; when the muscle is contracted the bowstring effect across the surface of the lump reduces its mobility and gives the impression that it is fixed to the muscle.

Regional lymph nodes

The regional lymph nodes should always be examined, as their enlargement or induration may provide evidence of spread from a primary inflammatory or malignant lesion and thereby influence management.

Other signs

Many other features of a lump may, in certain instances, help clinicians in their assessments: for example, the black colour of a malignant melanoma or redness of inflammation, the warmth of an abscess, the papillary surface of a wart. However, the five features described above are generally the most helpful.

Physical signs

- *Site*: in relation to underlying anatomy
- *Shape*: spherical, discoid, lobulated; all others are non-contributory
- *Layer*: skin, subcutaneous tissue, muscle, bone, intra-abdominal
- *Consistency*: soft, firm, hard
  with soft lumps,
    fluctuance – volume constant
    emptying/reduction – volume ↓
    expansile cough impulse – volume ↑
    pulsation ↑↓ – true or false

DIAGNOSTIC APPROACH

After history and examination, either a confident diagnosis is reached or the nature of a lump remains unknown.

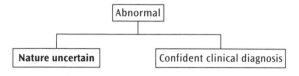

Nature uncertain

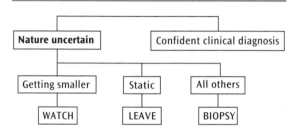

In the second situation, management is dictated by the history of the duration and change in size of the lump. If the lump is rapidly diminishing in size, there is no indication for treatment apart from surveillance to ensure that, ultimately, it disappears. If the lump remains the same size and has been present for years then unless it is symptomatic or unsightly, it is reasonable to advise leaving it alone. The argument here is that if the lump has not caused trouble over many years then it is unlikely to do so in the future. However, if the lump has appeared recently, and does not show recognizable features, then biopsy is necessary to exclude malignancy.

All lumps *deep to the deep fascia* are impossible to diagnose on clinical grounds and must be subjected to histological examination. A common lesion is an intramuscular lipoma, whose typical lobulation is masked by the tough, dense unyielding deep fascia overlying it.

Confident clinical diagnosis

An *epidermal cyst* or *sebaceous cyst* is a spherical, soft, fluctuant lesion which lies mostly in the subcutaneous tissue, but can always be demonstrated to have an attachment to the skin at its summit. The point of tethering is often called a *punctum* and said to be a blocked sebaceous gland duct but this interpretation may be inaccurate. These cysts are frequently multiple and are common in the scalp and the scrotum, but they can occur almost anywhere. In light-coloured people the waxy content, which is keratin rather than sebaceous material as originally believed, gives the cyst a distinctive colour.

Excision is advised when the cyst is large, unsightly, interfering with clothing or combing the hair, or because of repeated infections. When infected, the cyst is tender and the overlying skin is inflamed. Infection is treated with antibiotics or, if it has developed into an abscess, by incision and drainage. After its contents have been drained, the cyst may not recur because of healing by fibrosis.

A *lipoma* is a benign multi-lobular mass of fatty tissue. When a lipoma lies in the subcutaneous region it is possible to be sure of the features that characterize the lesion: the softness in consistency usually with fluctuation; the lack of attachment to underlying muscle; and the lobulated outline when the overlying skin is stretched. Attachment to skin is unusual, but may occur especially on the back. Lipomas are occasionally tender, particularly if multiple. If symptomless, a lipoma need not be excised unless it is large and unsightly. The lipoma is dissected off the skin and its deeper attachment without breaching the delicate investing fibrous membrane or else some of its fatty tissue is mistaken for surrounding subcutaneous fat and is not excised, a mistake that leads to recurrence.

A *ganglion* is a spherical, fluctuant cyst-like lesion derived from the lining of synovial joints and tendon sheaths, and occurs in relation to the sheaths of extensor tendons and the extensor aspects of small joints in the neighbourhood of the wrist and ankle. A fluctuant cyst in these regions with a demonstrable attachment to the underlying tendon is diagnostic of the condition, but an attachment to the joint is usually difficult to demonstrate, since the communication with the joint is narrow and the contents of the ganglion, although fluid, are glairy in consistency so they are not readily emptied into the joint. A common complaint is pain and tenderness because of repeated friction or impact with solid surfaces, and is usually the main indication for excision.

The operation is preferably performed under a general anaesthetic, under tourniquet control to provide a bloodless field, and with full aseptic precautions to avoid infection of the underlying tendon sheath or joint, ensuring complete excision without disrupting the capsule or else it recurs.

Dermoid cysts are spherical, fluctuant and subcutaneous. They are formed by the inclusion of epithelial remnants beneath the surface at lines of embryological fusion of skin during pre-natal development, and are therefore lined by squamous epithelium and contain keratin, hair and other ectodermal structures. They are usually found at the mid-line of the scalp, neck and lower jaw and the outer angle of the eyebrow (external angular dermoid). A communication with an intra-cranial dermoid, if large, is demonstrated by a cough impulse and a defect with a sclerotic margin in a skull X-ray. This should be taken into consideration before excising a dermoid cyst.

Implantation dermoids arise from epidermal fragments implanted in the dermis or subcutaneous tissue following puncture wounds, commonly of the fingers. Like epidermal cysts they are lined by squamous epithelium and filled with keratin but also contain foreign material.

Skin lumps

Histiocytoma or *dermatofibroma* are common, well-circumscribed benign nodules about 1 cm in diameter, brownish in colour and regular in outline. They usually occur on the limbs and are of clinical significance in that they can be mistaken for malignant melanoma. When in doubt, they are better excised. Histologically they contain numerous lipid-filled macrophages (histiocytes).

The *common wart* presents rather different appearances according to whether the lesion is in the sole of the foot (plantar wart) or elsewhere, commonly in the genital and perineal regions. Warts are benign papillomas which are a result of viral infection and are diagnosed with confidence from their appearance. Except in the soles of the feet, they are domed hemispherical lesions of a brown colour and with a papilliform surface. In the sole of the foot a wart becomes buried under a thick layer of keratin and presents as a pale yellow or light tan, characteristically translucent nodule that may be exquisitely tender. Warts are usually treated with various caustic chemicals to destroy them, or with liquid nitrogen or cryosurgery, but persistent or recurrent lesions are better excised.

Keratoses are roughened brown areas with a papilliform surface which commonly occur in elderly people (*seborrhoeic keratoses/warts*) usually on the face or the back, and are of no particular significance. However, when they present in younger people, or in the scars of old burns, radiation burns, etc., they should be watched closely because of the risk of malignant change to squamous cell carcinoma. Excision is unnecessary as they are easily shaved off the skin with a sharp blade.

A *neurofibroma* arises from the fibroblasts of peripheral nerves. When solitary, it is a firm and usually rounded nodule in the subcutaneous region which may have no distinguishing characteristics and so may not be diagnosable, but should be suspected if tender. In von Recklinghausen's disease, which is an autosomal-dominant inherited syndrome, the lesions are multiple and are often associated with coffee-coloured skin patches, called 'café-au-lait' spots, as well as freckling in the axillary skin and thickening of the subcutaneous tissues and skin folds. The full clinical picture is so classical that a diagnostic biopsy is unnecessary. There is some tendency for neurofibromas to undergo malignant transformation into fibrosarcomas. Therefore, any change in size or tenderness of a nodule requires histological examination.

Pigmented skin lumps. Everyone's skin displays a host of pigmented lesions that vary in colour from pink to dark brown. The histological nature of most of these lesions is either angiomatous or naevus cell in origin. Some of these pigmented lesions are not lumps but merely areas of discoloration of the skin, such as the port wine stain of a cavernous haemangioma or the café-au-lait stain in neurofibromatosis. It would not be practicable, even if it were thought desirable, to biopsy all these lesions and the important principle is to recognize that small, pigmented lesions which have remained entirely static in their physical appearance for a long period can safely be left alone. If a particular lesion is large enough to embarrass the patient or to produce symptoms by, for example, rubbing with the clothing, it should be excised and the opportunity taken for histological confirmation of its benign nature. The question of what constitutes an overstepping of the clinical dividing line between these lesions and a possible malignant melanoma is considered later.

The preceding list, although not exhaustive, covers most of the common conditions which can be confidently diagnosed as requiring no treatment or simple local treatment. To these can be added swellings that are obviously inflammatory in nature, such as boils, styes (infected hair follicles of the eyelids) or carbuncles (multiple confluent boils).

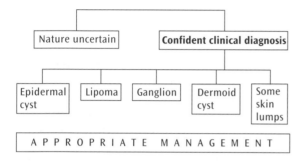

Malignant skin lesions

There are three serious neoplastic lesions: basal cell carcinoma; squamous cell carcinoma; and malignant melanoma. These can usually be diagnosed accurately on clinical grounds alone, but must be biopsied because they can be confused with benign conditions.

Excisional biopsy under local anaesthesia removes the lesion and allows histological examination. This is the approach provided that the size of the excision needed to achieve clearance does not compromise skin closure. Otherwise, an incisional biopsy from the edge of the lesion and the adjacent normal skin is initially required to justify a wider excision which may require a reconstructive procedure.

Basal cell carcinoma is often called a *rodent ulcer*, although ulceration may only appear late during the genesis of the lesion. In the earliest stage, the lesion is a slightly raised pinkish nodule without specific features so that the diagnosis cannot be made with confidence, although the site of the lesion (they may occur anywhere, but in particular on the skin of the head and neck, especially around the eyes and in the naso-labial fold) raises suspicion. Later on a characteristic raised rolled edge is manifest, the skin becomes

translucent (pearly) and at some time it breaks down to produce an ulcer. This lesion is locally invasive and if left untreated it erodes cartilage and bone. Metastasis is very rare and adequate local treatment is usually curative. Excision and radiotherapy are equally effective, but radiotherapy is inadvisable where the lesion overlies bone or cartilage because of the risk of radionecrosis of these tissues. Surgical excision involves a margin of 5 mm all round the visible and palpable limits of the growth. This may be combined with the biopsy if facilities are available for the examination of frozen sections, which is particularly helpful in infiltrative or multi-centric disease to ensure clearance.

Squamous cell carcinoma is also common on the head and neck, but occurs at sites where basal carcinoma is rare, for example the pinna, lip, genitalia and perineum. It also develops in skin damaged by solar or X-irradiation, chemicals or longstanding sepsis. Induration and fixity of skin, exophytic growth and ulceration are indications of malignant change. Dissemination to the regional lymph nodes may occur early in the course of the disease, although enlarged lymph nodes may be due to secondary infection. Once the diagnosis is confirmed by biopsy the primary lesion is treated either by surgery or by radiotherapy, but again, the latter is contraindicated by the risk of radionecrosis where cartilage or bone lies close to the lesion. However, radiotherapy may be employed in the unfit patient for palliation of disseminated disease.

Surgical clearance requires a margin of at least 1 cm or more in infiltrative lesions. Prophylactic regional lymph node dissection is not justifiable as the risk of metastasis is not high and dissection does not offer a survival benefit. However, if the regional lymph nodes are enlarged, lymph node biopsy must be avoided as it will increase the morbidity and recurrence rate after formal lymph node dissection. The diagnosis should be confirmed by fine needle aspiration (FNA) cytology or frozen section at the time of node dissection. It is wise to wait a few weeks after the primary has been excised before proceeding to block dissection, to allow the inflammatory rather than neoplastic involvement of the lymph nodes to subside.

A *keratoacanthoma* is a particularly confusing lesion because it can be difficult to distinguish clinically and histologically from a squamous cell carcinoma. Although benign, it grows rapidly and may be disfiguring. Around a core of keratinous material, which may later become ulcerated, a spherical lesion develops with a smooth and shiny pink surface. Diagnosis and treatment is by curettage and coagulation of the base or by local excision with primary closure, unless the lesion is showing spontaneous resolution which occurs in weeks or months. Excision or biopsy is preferable if the diagnosis is in doubt. Radiotherapy can be used if surgery is refused.

Malignant melanoma must be borne in mind whenever a pigmented lesion changes in its physical characteristics. The change may be a lightening or a darkening in colour, an increase in size, bleeding or ulceration, or the onset of a subjective sensation, such as burning or itching. It is crucial that the observer decides whether the lesion is superficial, spreading or nodular, and estimates the level of invasion and thickness of the lesion by palpation, as these factors influence the surgical treatment. Advanced malignant melanoma has a very poor prognosis, among the worst of all types of malignant disease, and once this possibility is raised urgent biopsy is necessary. The traditional advice has been that a full excisional biopsy should be performed, on the grounds that cutting into the tumour rather than completely removing it worsens the prognosis by promoting metastatic spread. There is little evidence to support this hypothesis. Incisional biopsy has not been shown to be detrimental, but disrupts the lesion and makes the measurement of thickness difficult.

A wide margin of excision is required, but less than the 5 cm previously believed. Subcutaneous fat, but not underlying fascia or muscle, is included with the skin. The clearance margin is based on the thickness of the lesion on histological examination (Breslow), which correlates well with the likelihood of regional and distant metastases and consequently long-term survival. For thin melanomas of less than 1 mm, a clear margin of 1 cm is adequate; for thicker, just-palpable melanomas (1–4 mm), a wider excision of 2 cm clearance; and for lesions thicker than 4 mm, that is, nodular, a 3-cm margin is required. If there is any doubt about the diagnosis or the clearance, the scar is excised with whatever margin is necessary depending on the Breslow measurement of the paraffin-fixed sections.

Elective prophylactic block dissection is recommended when the primary lesion is 1–4 mm thick because of a high incidence of regional metastases, when the primary lesion is close to the lymph nodes so that both the lesion and the lymph nodes are readily removed in a monoblock excision, when the regional lymph nodes are clinically involved or if the lesion is rapidly advancing and histological examination shows invasion of the dermal lymphatic channels.

A large variety of red, brown or even blue pigmented lesions may be mistaken for a malignant melanoma. The best mimic is the *juvenile melanoma* which may, for a time, grow quite fast and histologically can be indistinguishable from a malignant melanoma; nevertheless, before puberty such lesions are nearly always benign in their ultimate behaviour.

Seborrhoeic keratosis and some haemangiomas are brown and may cause confusion, although the haemangiomas often blanch on pressure with a transparent plate such as a microscope slide. Among the reddish lesions an important one is the *pyogenic granuloma* which results from minor penetrating foreign bodies, such as splinters or a thorn, and forms a rapidly growing pink nodule which attains its full size within a few weeks and then remains static. Excision with curettage or cauterization of the base to prevent recurrence is the treatment.

Haemangiomata may be pink, and benign naevi may be pink or brown (the hairy mole falls into the category of benign naevi).

Bowen's disease is an intradermal squamous cell carcinoma that presents as a pink, thickened plaque growing slowly in the skin, with scaling and crusting of its surface mimicking eczema. When it occurs on the glans penis or on the foreskin it is called *erythroplasia of Queyrat*. This is a pre-malignant condition and when diagnosed histologically it should be treated by excision, or cryotherapy. Patients with Queyrat's erythroplasia should be circumcised.

With regard to skin lumps which are clinically undiagnosable, the management is inevitably some form of biopsy or excision biopsy so that a histological diagnosis can be made, after which any treatment appropriate to the condition can be carried out.

TENDERNESS

Definition

Tenderness, as a clinical sign, means the complaint of pain in response to local external pressure. This definition corresponds with one of the everyday meanings of the word, but is inadequate in one respect. If the sign is to be of any value in management, it must indicate the presence of an abnormality. Everyone experiences pain if the examiner presses hard enough in a certain area and the question is whether an individual's sensation of pain for the degree of pressure applied is within normal limits or outside those limits.

The problem is complicated by the wide range of the normal response, influenced by individual variation in pain threshold, anxiety, nervousness, the severity of illness and other psychic factors apart from malingering. The assessment of this sign, which is a measure of the degree of pain the patient is experiencing, is dependent on the patient's description of his complaint and his reaction (e.g., wincing) and requires considerable experience. *Distraction* and *reproducibility* are often valuable aids. In children, in particular, success in directing the patient's attention elsewhere may reduce apparent tenderness to the level of the normal range. The child's suspect right

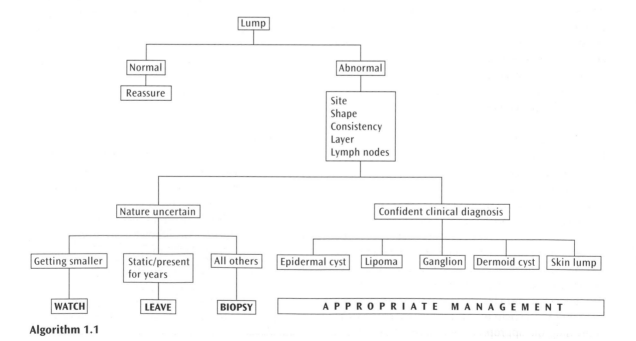

Algorithm 1.1

lower abdominal quadrant can be re-tested with the clinician's elbow whilst the fingers press the left upper quadrant! And pain which is not reproducible with the same degree of pressure at the same site is unlikely to be significant.

Site

The precise zone of tenderness, and the point of maximal tenderness if present, are usually crucial to the diagnosis. The tenderness may be an area either of an abnormality in an anatomical structure that is larger or harder than normal or of a pathological change in the tissues, such as infection (e.g., an abscess), trauma or neoplasm. In such cases the tenderness itself is not critically important without an overall assessment of the lesion. However, when there are no obvious signs of pathological change then the precise site becomes critical in the assessment.

In everyday practice, a complaint of tenderness at a specific anatomical site is frequently associated with a history of trauma to the musculoskeletal system. Apart from an obvious wound, common sites of tenderness are at the points of insertion of a muscle, tendon or ligament into bone which are the points that take the main mechanical strain of distracting forces. With tenderness there is usually swelling due to traumatic oedema, and sometimes bruising due to bleeding into the tissues from the torn fibres. In the absence of these signs, the diagnosis is based on the history of the mechanism of injury, and reproducibility of the pain on straining the muscle, tendon or ligament by movement. Such lesions, torn muscles or tendons, 'sprained' ligaments, are not always acute: they may become chronic, like the torn fibres of the brachioradialis muscle at the head of the radius and the consequent *tennis elbow*.

Other than the site, it is important to define the layer of tenderness, especially when it is abdominal. It is a common error to assume that if digital pressure on the anterior abdominal wall elicits pain, the tenderness arises in an intra-abdominal structure. Often, the tender area lies in the abdominal wall muscles: in such a case, when the patient contracts the abdominal muscles by raising the head from the bed without the help of the arms while the clinician is pressing the appropriate spot sufficiently hard to produce mild pain, the contraction greatly increases the pain. Conversely, if the tenderness arises within the abdomen, the firmly contracted muscles prevent the deformation of the abdominal wall that is necessary to reach the diseased structure and so the patient experiences less rather than more pain (Carnet's sign). The aetiology of these tender spots in the anterior abdominal wall is unknown, but probably traumatic. A careful history usually demonstrates that the pain is related to turning over in bed, bending forwards, carrying heavy shopping or similar activities.

A common site is at the lateral margin of the right rectus abdominis, at the junction of its lower and middle thirds. The syndrome of chronic pain and tenderness at this site has given rise to the myth of the 'grumbling appendix' and the removal of countless normal appendices. Similarly, in the right upper quadrant there may be confusion with chronic cholelithiasis.

Treatment

Treatment, which when effective proves the diagnosis, is by infiltrating the area of tenderness with a mixture of 1 ml 1% lignocaine and 1 ml (25 mg) hydrocortisone acetate. After piercing the skin, the point of the needle is moved around until the pain is reproduced before injecting. Further injections may be needed at four-weekly intervals until permanent relief is gained, but the patient should be warned with each injection that when the effect of the local anaesthetic wears off (in 2–3 hours) the pain can be worse for a few days before it gets better.

HIGHLIGHTS

- True tenderness is recognized by reproducibility despite distraction and by a magnitude outside normal limits
- Common sites of traumatic tenderness are the insertions of muscle tendons and ligaments
- With regard to the abdomen, the tissue layer in which the tender spot exists, whether within the abdomen or in the abdominal wall, is crucial to diagnosis of the cause
- Local infiltration with steroid/local anaesthetic is helpful in relieving abdominal wall tender spots

Neck and parotid salivary gland

MICHAEL HOBSLEY AND TIM DAVIDSON

AIMS

1 Recognize and understand life-threatening situations; be able to delineate the territories of the neck
2 Learn the clinical characteristics of certain neck swellings

INTRODUCTION

Note whether or not the swelling moves vertically upwards during the act of swallowing, returning to the resting position as the act is completed. *This test should always be applied, even if the lump appears to be far from the anterior mid-line of the neck.*

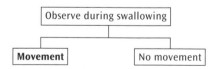

MOVEMENT ON SWALLOWING

Movement on swallowing indicates that the lump is either in the thyroid gland, is attached to the thyroid gland by direct continuity of tissue or is pressed against the gland so tightly by the pre-tracheal fascia that it cannot help but move with the gland. There is no clinical method of distinguishing between the first and third possibilities. The only example of the second possibility which can sometimes be diagnosed on clinical grounds is the thyroglossal cyst.

Thyroglossal cyst

If the lump lies above the level of the thyroid isthmus (i.e., at or above the level of the second ring of the trachea) and moves vertically upwards when the patient protrudes the tongue, it is probably a thyroglossal cyst. If the lump seems to be solid, a radio-iodine scan may rarely reveal that the lump is an ectopic thyroid gland which has not completed its embryological journey from the tuberculum impar at the root of the tongue to the usual post-natal position. Removal of the swelling would then result in myxoedema and a life-long dependence on exogenous thyroxine.

The thyroglossal cyst is a remnant of the embryological tract (Fig. 2.1) and when the cyst presents itself as a cervical swelling it lies symmetrically about the mid-line, or near it. When removing the cyst, all remnants of the tract must be excised to prevent recurrence. The tract consists of a well-defined band of fibrous tissue: a part lies in immediate relationship to the back of the centre of the hyoid cartilage, so it is essential to excise this central segment of the cartilage as part of the operation.

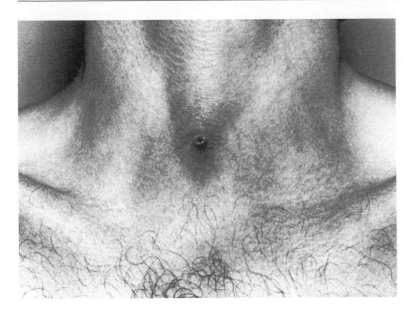

Fig. 2.1 *Thyroglossal fistula. When the thyroglossal tract remains patent at its lower end, presenting with an external opening in the skin of the lower part of the neck near the mid-line, there is usually no cystic lesion (thyroglossal cyst). In the case of the young man shown, the tract extended upwards behind the hyoid bone, but there was no extension to the base of the tongue.*

Goitre

The clinical definition of a goitre is a swelling in the neck that moves on swallowing but not on movements of the tongue. A goitre is classified according to both its morphology and its functional activity.

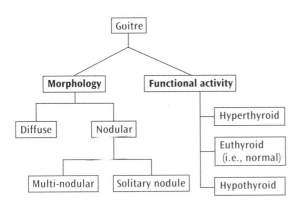

Most goitres present as a chronic neck swelling; presentation acutely as pressure on the airway is rare, but important because it can rapidly be fatal.

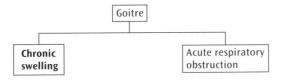

CLASSIFICATION OF CHRONIC SWELLINGS

Diffuse or nodular?

By careful and gentle palpation with the pulps of the fingers, best done standing behind the seated patient, the thyroid is examined for its size, shape and consistency in order to decide whether it is diffusely enlarged or is nodular, and if the latter, whether it is a single nodule or a multi-nodular swelling.

The normal thyroid gland is not visible or palpable, even when pushed towards the examining finger from the opposite side. If a smooth enlargement of one side only of the thyroid is felt, the goitre is regarded as a single nodule. The overlying strap muscles render the gland impalpable and make the sign of fluctuance unreliable. Examination should include identifying the lower edge of the thyroid gland to exclude retrosternal extension, feeling for cervical lymph nodes and auscultating over the gland for increased vascularity.

Thyroid status

This is suggested by clinical features (Table 2.1 and Table 2.2) and quantified by measurements of thyroid activity. Most patients presenting with a

Table 2.1 *Hyperthyroidism*

Symptoms
Nervousness, emotional lability, insomnia, tiredness, heat intolerance, excessive sweating
Palpitations
Increased appetite with weight loss, diarrhoea, oligomenorrhoea

Signs
Eye-signs are exophthalmos, lid retraction, weakness on convergence
Hyperkinaesia, warm moist hands, tremor
Tachycardia even while asleep, collapsing pulse, atrial fibrillation
Proximal myopathy with increased muscle tone, increased limb reflexes
Pre-tibial myxoedema

Table 2.2 *Hypothyroidism*

Symptoms
Apathy, decreased energy, tiredness, intolerance of cold, dryness of the skin, weight gain and constipation

Signs
Slow pulse
Loss of hair from scalp and lateral ends of eyebrows
Thickness and dryness of the skin
Non-pitting oedema, especially of the shins
Reduced muscle tone and limb reflexes

goitre are euthyroid, some are hyperthyroid, and a few are hypothyroid. Hyper- and hypothyroidism are both dangerous conditions whose presence modifies management.

Many of the symptoms and signs of thyrotoxicosis are present in anxiety state. The most useful feature supporting the diagnosis of thyrotoxicosis is weight loss without decrease in food intake.

Special tests

Estimation of serum thyroxine (T_4) or free thyroxine (fT_4) and of thyroid stimulating hormone (TSH) is standard in all cases. The metabolic activity of thyroxine is proportional to the small proportion carried free in plasma; the remaining thyroxine is bound to plasma proteins and is metabolically inactive,

although in dynamic equilibrium with the free fraction. In pregnancy and at puberty the thyroid binding of globulin is elevated and the level of free thyroxine provides a better measurement for discriminating physiological from pathological thyroid activity. The free thyroxine index is a measurement related to the concentration of free thyroxine. The tri-iodothyronine (T_3) concentration is measured if the patient is clinically hyperthyroid but the serum thyroxine is normal. The TSH concentration is low in hyperthyroidism and elevated in hypothyroidism. The presence of long-acting thyroid stimulating factor is diagnostic of Graves's disease. Long-acting thyroid stimulating factor is an immunoglobulin which reacts with TSH receptors in the thyroid but has a much longer half-life in the circulation. Hence a patient with a goitre can be identified as euthyroid or hypo- or hyperthyroid. However, hypo- or hyperthyroidism can be the primary presentation without any apparent thyroid swelling.

Diffuse goitre

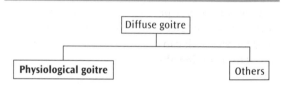

'*Physiological' goitre* occurs in females when there is an excessive demand for thyroid hormones at pregnancy, lactation and the menopause. The gland is diffusely enlarged and soft, and may not regress in size after the period of physiological stress has ceased. No treatment is required. This is a valid diagnosis based purely on the history and physical signs, but any unusual circumstance must lead to further investigation.

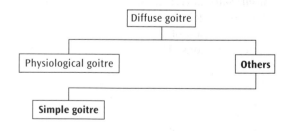

Other diffuse goitres all share a consistency firmer than the softness of a physiological goitre. Several distinct pathological conditions can be encountered: in many, the associated clinical features suggest a clinical diagnosis, but all patients should be subjected at least to an ultrasound examination and to measurement of thyroid metabolic activity, and most require fine needle aspiration (FNA) cytology.

Simple goitre is endemic in certain areas remote from the sea, where the soil is deficient in iodine and sea-food as another source is scarce. Goitrogenic agents (e.g., in cabbage) or drugs, such as carbimazole, aminoglutethamide, or rarely, dyshormonogenesis due to a genetic deficiency of thyroid enzymes, interfere with the synthesis of thyroid hormones. The thyroid gland is subjected to increased stimulation by TSH, which results in follicular hyperplasia and diffuse thyroid swelling which may later become multi-nodular. The patient is euthyroid and is asymptomatic unless the gland compresses adjacent structures.

Treatment is by iodine or by thyroxine; thyroxine is more likely to be successful. When iodine is administered it must be started in small doses as an iodine-starved gland, hypertrophied under TSH-stimulation, may, if presented with a large dose of iodine, produce excess thyroxine before negative pituitary feedback can damp down thyroxine secretion. The resulting thyrotoxicosis is known as the Jod–Basedow phenomenon.

The medical treatment of simple goitre is often disappointing, and for cosmetic reasons, and especially if complicated by compression symptoms, surgical intervention is required.

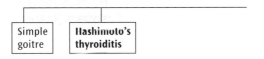

Hashimoto's disease must be considered in any female with a goitre who has a family history of thyroid antibodies, of thyroiditis or of other autoimmune conditions. The enlarged gland is usually firmer than a physiological goitre, initially tender and there may be mild features of hyperthyroidism, but most patients remain euthyroid before they develop hypothyroidism when the gland becomes atrophic and fibrosed. The diagnosis is made by demonstrating high titres of antithyroid autoantibodies, and on a needle biopsy, follicular atrophy and fibrosis with diffuse lymphocytic infiltration. Treatment is with thyroxine to maintain the euthyroid state.

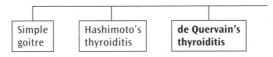

Sub-acute or de Quervain's thyroiditis, probably due to a viral infection, can in the typical case be distinguished from Hashimoto's thyroiditis and other causes of thyroid swellings by its presentation as an acutely painful and tender diffuse enlargement of the thyroid gland. It is often accompanied by fever, general malaise and weight loss. The patient may develop transient, mild hyperthyroidism. This condition resolves spontaneously but may recur. Treatment with analgesics and steroids may also be required for pain relief.

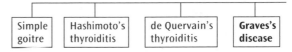

Graves's disease presents with a diffuse thyroid enlargement and thyrotoxicosis as a result of thyroid overactivity due to a circulating immunoglobulin, the long-acting thyroid stimulating hormone. Examination reveals a diffuse smooth enlargement of the thyroid, and there are sometimes a palpable thrill and an audible bruit due to increased vascularity. Medical treatment includes carbimazole, propranolol and radioactive iodine; when unsuccessful, thyroidectomy is indicated.

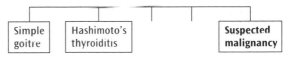

Suggestion of malignancy

The most obvious and common feature to give rise to a suspicion of malignancy in a patient with a diffuse goitre is the hardness of the gland, but the box below shows several other items.

An underlying pre-existing disease of the thyroid helps to distinguish clinically between two groups, but the definitive diagnosis depends upon FNA cytology or open biopsy.

A rapid and asymmetrical change in consistency in a goitre can be due to bleeding into a cyst or to

Evidence suggesting malignancy

- Rapid enlargement; hard consistency
- Hoarseness: laryngoscopy = poorly moving vocal cord(s)
- Fixity: reduced movement on swallowing
- Metastases: hard cervical lymph nodes distant

malignant change. Lymphomas can arise in pre-existing autoimmune (Hashimoto's) thyroiditis and tend to occur in the fifth decade. Treatment is with radiotherapy. The five-year survival is 85% when the disease is confined within the capsule, but falls to 40% when local spread has occurred.

In the absence of previous thyroid disease, the most likely diagnosis is a malignancy. Thyroid tumours are considered later as most present problems in nodular goitres. However, there is a very rare condition called Riedl's thyroiditis or struma that gives rise to a hard, 'woody' goitre, often asymmetrical. It behaves like a malignancy and produces pressure symptoms. Despite the dense fibrosis the patient remains euthyroid. Excision is considered.

If malignancy is suspected because of metastases, the usual reason is that a pulsating mass has presented in a bone. Such a metastasis can also arise from the kidneys; investigations of the thyroid and iodine metabolism should be completed before asking for an intravenous pyelogram using an iodine compound to opacify the kidney!

If diffuse carcinoma of the thyroid is suspected because of metastasis, biopsy of the metastasis may confirm the diagnosis. In any case, the neck must be explored and as much of the goitre removed as possible. The management with regard to biopsy, frozen section and subsequent procedures is the same as in dealing with a solid solitary nodule, except that one has to accept a far lesser chance of being able to remove the whole lesion. Ultimately, threatened respiratory obstruction may demand tracheotomy.

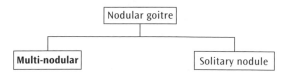

Multi-nodular goitre

The aetiological factors already described in a simple goitre cause follicular hyperplasia with diffuse or nodular enlargement of the thyroid gland. A multi-nodular goitre is composed of adenomatous and colloid nodules with cystic degeneration. The patient is usually euthyroid. Multi-nodular goitre is unlikely to improve with treatment with iodine or thyroxine. Treatment is surgical, and is indicated for cosmesis, stridor from tracheal compression caused by retrosternal extension, or dysphagia from pressure on the oesophagus. Secondary hyperthyroidism with predominantly cardiovascular manifestations can develop in predominantly middle-aged patients with longstanding multi-nodular goitre, whereas in Graves's disease a goitre and hyperthyroidism present simultaneously in young patients and metabolic features are prominent. There is no place for medical treatment in a toxic multi-nodular goitre and surgery is essential.

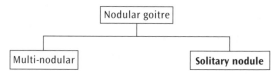

Apparently solitary nodule

A common presentation is a clinically solitary thyroid nodule, but half prove to be part of a multi-nodular goitre and 10% of true solitary nodules are malignant. Ultrasonography reliably identifies those patients in whom an apparently solitary nodule is a dominant nodule in a multi-nodular goitre, or those in whom the lump is a discrete nodule, and also distinguishes a solid nodule from a cyst. The majority of thyroid nodules can be categorized by FNA cytology.

The solitary nodule

If the patient has a *multi-nodular goitre*, management is as already described. If the lesion is a *solitary cyst*, which is a large follicle filled with colloid, this excludes malignancy. When the history is short, it is reasonable to allow time for spontaneous resolution. With a long history, or if the cyst is large or increases in size, surgical treatment involves exploration of the thyroid gland and enucleation of the cyst. Alternatively, ultrasound-guided needle aspiration is a simpler initial option, reserving excision, provided that the aspirated fluid contains no abnormal cells, should the cyst recur.

In a *solitary solid* nodule, FNA cytology is performed. If the aspirate shows normal epithelial cells it may be appropriate to observe the patient unless this would be cosmetically unacceptable; however, follicular carcinomas cannot reliably be distinguished from benign follicular adenomas. When neoplastic cells are obtained, exploration is necessary. When the report on the aspirate is equivocal, some clinicians request radioisotopic scans of the thyroid using ^{123}I to identify the distribution of isotope activity in the gland and differentiate between a cold, hot or warm nodule.

A *cold nodule* shows an isolated area devoid of isotope uptake and indicates non-secreting tissue: it might be a cyst or a benign adenoma, or in 15% of cases, a carcinoma.

The *hot nodule* concentrates the radioactive iodine because it is an autonomous focus of excess secretion of thyroxine, whereas the rest of the gland shows no uptake because pituitary-mediated stimulation of TSH production is diminished by high serum thyroxine levels. The patient is usually euthyroid, but can be hyperthyroid – the 'toxic nodule'. The autonomous toxic nodule is never malignant.

The term 'hot nodule' is sometimes confused with the 'warm nodule' where the radioactive iodine uptake is the same as in the rest of the gland due to a functioning adenoma; nevertheless there is a 1–5% chance that the lesion is a carcinoma.

Treatment policies

The *cold nodule* must be explored because of the fairly high risk of carcinoma.

The risk of carcinoma in the *warm nodule* is smaller, but most clinicians recommend excision.

The *hot nodule*, in a euthyroid patient, can be observed even if the FNA cytology result is inconclusive, but requires treatment in a thyrotoxic patient by hemithyroidectomy. In other words, hemithyroidectomy is usually advised both for hot and warm nodules, and only in euthyroid patients with a hot nodule can radioactive scanning avoid hemithyroidectomy. Since hot nodules constitute only 1% of all solitary nodules, many clinicians do not use radioactive scanning.

Exploration of a solitary nodule

The neck is explored through the usual collar incision and both lobes of the thyroid gland exposed, but not mobilized.

A solitary cyst (this can only be deduced if it is lying at the surface of the gland) is enucleated and sent for histological examination, and the incision closed. A recurrent cyst that had been treated by aspiration usually contains blood and can be difficult to distinguish from solid tumours, so is better treated as a solid nodule.

A solid nodule is either an *adenoma* or a *carcinoma*; the latter is more likely to be a *papillary* or *follicular*, rather than an *anaplastic* or a *medullary* carcinoma. There is a marked propensity to implantation recurrence, similar to salivary gland, urinary bladder and large bowel tumours, if tumour is spilled during dissection. It is therefore preferable to remove the nodule with a wide margin of normal tissue or excise the whole lobe, rather than to enucleate the nodule. After excision, if frozen section does not definitely exclude malignancy, the wound is closed until a definite diagnosis is established by examination of paraffin sections, when further treatment is planned. A carcinoma proven at the time of exploration or later is managed as described below.

Behaviour of thyroid carcinomas

Thyroid malignancy is only about 1% of all malignancies. Nearly all thyroid carcinomas arise from thyroid epithelial cells.

Papillary adenocarcinoma constitutes 60% of thyroid malignancies in adults and nearly all thyroid malignancies in children. It affects females in particular and the peak incidence is in the second and third decades. The tumour is multi-focal with satellite microscopic deposits in the same lobe (one in three) or in the opposite (one in seven) and metastasizes to the regional lymph nodes. It usually presents as a solitary thyroid nodule. Occasionally, a palpable cervical lymph node is the sole presenting feature, which histologically has the appearances of normal thyroid tissue and was once known as the 'lateral aberrant thyroid'. The diagnosis is made on FNA cytology, and if an isotope scan is performed, it usually shows no uptake. The standard treatment is total thyroidectomy and l-thyroxine is given to suppress TSH in order to minimize the risk of stimulating any malignant cells. Thyroglobulin is used as a tumour-marker. Recurrence in lymph nodes is treated by excision. External radiation can be applied to local recurrence and chemotherapy to distant metastases. The prognosis is excellent, even with distant metastases.

Follicular carcinoma comprises 20% of all thyroid carcinomas, occurs in an older age group and is more common in women. Follicular carcinoma is slow-growing, rarely multicentric and metastasizes at a late stage via the bloodstream to distant sites. It usually presents as a solitary nodule. On FNA cytology it may be indistinguishable from follicular hyperplasia or adenoma. Chest X-ray and bone scan are performed to identify any secondary deposits as they influence surgical treatment. Thyroid lobectomy is carried out when the tumour is within the thyroid capsule. A total thyroidectomy is performed when there is capsular invasion or distant spread, in order to enhance ^{131}I-uptake by metastases should this be required for diagnosis or treatment. The 10-year survival is more than 90%, but falls to 30% when there are metastases.

Anaplastic carcinoma is an undifferentiated tumour that represents 10% of all thyroid cancers. It occurs almost exclusively in elderly patients and presents as a diffuse hard thyroid swelling. It grows rapidly, giving rise to symptoms of tracheal and oesophageal obstruction and recurrent laryngeal nerve damage. Spread to the regional lymph nodes and by the haematogenous route to distant sites is also early. Resection is usually not possible, and radiotherapy and chemotherapy are ineffective. Most patients die within a year.

Medullary carcinoma is derived from the parafollicular or C-cells of the thyroid and accounts for 5% of all thyroid cancers. It is more common in women, frequently in the fifth decade. The tumour secretes calcitonin, which may be used as a marker of tumour recurrence after excision, and may also secrete other peptides and amines, such as serotonin and ACTH-like peptide. The tumour stroma contains deposits of amyloid, which makes the thyroid mass stony hard. It is slow-growing, metastasizes to the local lymph nodes and later to the lungs, liver and bones. Medullary carcinoma may be sporadic, or else familial as part of the multiple endocrine neoplasia type II (MEN II) syndrome associated with APUD cell tumours, in particular phaeochromocytoma and parathyroid adenoma.

Treatment of medullary carcinoma should be undertaken only after a phaeochromocytoma has been ruled out by computed tomography (CT) and by measuring 24-hour urinary vanillylmandelic acid (VMA). The treatment consists of total thyroidectomy and excision of regional lymph nodes. Without metastasis, thyroidectomy is curative, but when nodes are involved the 10-year survival falls to 50%. If during follow-up raised calcitonin levels are found, surgical re-exploration of the neck to remove invaded lymph nodes is considered.

Hypothyroidism

Infantile hypothyroidism or *cretinism*, is a result of a congenital defect of the thyroid which fails to develop or may lack enzymes required for the synthesis of thyroid hormones. The child may be goitrous, or goitrous and a cretin. The facial features are coarse: a broad, flat nose, thick lips and a large tongue. Other features include a prominent abdomen and an umbilical hernia. Mental deficiency or retardation is usual. If thyroid replacement treatment is started early, physical development is indistinguishable from normal but full mental development is rarely achieved and imbecility follows.

Juvenile hypothyroidism or myxoedema appears for the first time in childhood. There is no disability if it is recognized early and treated adequately.

In adults, hypothyroidism is usually the result either of Hashimoto's thyroiditis or primary thyroid atrophy. In either case the gland is small and fibrous.

Hypothyroidism is a late complication in up to 25% of patients after sub-total thyroidectomy for thyrotoxicosis, and in all patients after total thyroidectomy for cancer and following radioiodine treatment.

Apart from underlining the need for effective treatment with thyroxine to make the patient euthyroid, hypothyroidism has no influence on the management of multi-nodular goitre or a solitary nodule.

Hashimoto's disease or *autoimmune thyroiditis* typically produces a firm diffuse goitre, and ultimately hypothyroidism, but in the early stages the patient is euthyroid or occasionally even thyrotoxic. Antibodies to thyroid tissue are present in high titre in the patient's plasma. The diagnosis is confirmed by drill or needle biopsy; the histology of the tissue obtained shows the round-celled infiltration typical of immune phenomena. Treatment is with thyroxine and the gland usually shrinks to normal size.

Hypothyroidism can result from the treatment of hyperthyroidism, whether with drugs, radioactive iodine or operation.

Hyperthyroidism

The treatment options available are anti-thyroid drugs, radioactive iodine and surgery.

Thyroidectomy is not undertaken until thyrotoxicosis is controlled. Potassium iodide is given for 10 days before operation to reduce the vascularity of the gland. Before surgery, indirect laryngoscopy is performed to document that both vocal cords are moving freely. In toxic goitre, most of both lobes is removed, leaving behind an estimated 5 g of tissue on each side, preserving the parathyroid glands and taking special precautions to avoid damage to the recurrent laryngeal nerves. The isthmus of the thyroid gland must also be removed, otherwise an unsightly median enlargement may result.

A toxic nodular goitre (Plummer's disease) is best treated by surgery. In contradistinction to primary thyrotoxicosis (Graves's disease), a toxic nodular goitre tends to occur in elderly patients who are prone to develop cardiac complications, so initial rapid control with β-blockers and carbimazole is crucial. Radioactive iodine takes a few months to render the patient euthyroid, whereas the effect of anti-thyroid drugs is uncertain and often temporary.

In Graves's disease, or primary thyrotoxicosis, the treatment of choice is by anti-thyroid drugs which inhibit the synthesis of thyroid hormone and are curative in more than half of patients. Carbimazole is effective in reducing T_4 to normal levels in 4–6 weeks; thereafter a smaller maintenance dose is continued for up to 2 years. Propranolol is used to control the heart rate more effectively. The majority of patients remain euthyroid, but one-third relapse and require further treatment or referral for surgery or radioactive iodine.

Anti-thyroid drugs are contraindicated if the goitre is markedly retrosternal (because swelling may occur during therapy and obstruct the trachea or great veins in the mediastinum) or if the patient is not compliant or is judged to be psychologically or socially (perhaps because of way of life or distance from medical centres) unsuited to long-term medical treatment.

Radioactive iodine destroys most of the active thyroid tissue and its effect is progressive so that hypothyroidism is an inevitable sequel to treatment. The risk of inducing malignancy is low, but irradiation is reserved for patients over the age of 40 years who have failed to respond to medical treatment, or are unfit for, or have refused surgery. It is contraindicated in retrosternal goitres for the same reason as mentioned above.

In pregnant patients, thyrotoxicosis generally starts early in pregnancy and usually responds well and rapidly to anti-thyroid drugs which can be reduced or dispensed with in the last few weeks of pregnancy. The baby may be born hypothyroid if treatment is continued in the last trimester. Occasionally, the response to drugs is poor, when sub-total thyroidectomy can be carried out in the middle trimester with little risk to the pregnancy. Radioiodine is ruled out and surgery must be avoided in the first and final trimesters.

Urgent presentation

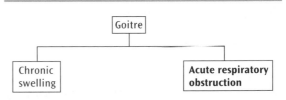

Respiratory obstruction

There is no more urgent situation in surgery than a haematoma resulting from reactionary haemorrhage following thyroidectomy, producing airways obstruction and laryngeal oedema leading to stridor, dyspnoea and hypoxia. A similar situation can result from spontaneous bleeding into a goitre, especially into a solitary nodule.

The thyroidectomy wound is reopened immediately to evacuate the haematoma, and if this does not result in immediate improvement in the patient's clinical condition, or if there has been no recent thyroidectomy, per oral endotracheal intubation or tracheostomy is required. Once the airway has been re-established, further investigation and treatment of the cause can be carried out.

Other post-thyroidectomy problems

Injury to recurrent laryngeal nerve(s)

The cords should be examined by an expert otolaryngologist *before* thyroidectomy if there has been previous surgery or a history of a change in voice, because the incidence of unsuspected unilateral palsy is not negligible. During the operation the recurrent laryngeal nerves must be identified and protected. The anaesthetist should be able to visualize the cord movement during intubation and at extubation.

Permanent damage to one cord probably occurs in about 2% of cases, with transient damage in a further 5%. Unilateral damage to the recurrent laryngeal nerve results in hoarseness which may be transient if the damage is a neurapraxia. If the hoarseness is permanent, teflon injection of the cord improves the voice.

Bilateral damage results in the cords lying adducted, causing laryngeal obstruction after extubation, and requires immediate tracheostomy and subsequent arytenoidectomy.

Hypoparathyroidism

Hypoparathyroidism is defined as a plasma calcium concentration below 2 mmol/l (8 mg/100 ml). Its presence should be suspected if after the operation the patient experiences a tingling sensation and carpopedal spasm. Tetany may be *latent* and made manifest by tapping a motor nerve (*Chvostek's sign*: when the facial nerve is tapped the facial muscles twitch) or by reducing the blood supply to an area (*Trousseau's sign*: a sphygmomanometer cuff inflated on an arm to a pressure above the systolic results in carpal spasm).

Treatment is by the administration of 20 ml 10% calcium gluconate intravenously for acute symptoms followed by supplements of oral calcium 2–3 g per day. Vitamin D 25,000–100,000 units per day may also be required to maintain the calcium level.

Thyrotoxic crisis

This follows surgery on a thyrotoxic patient who has not been controlled adequately before the operation. It presents with a sudden onset of agitation, confusion, hyperpyrexia, profuse sweating, tachycardia and atrial fibrillation. The mainstays of treatment are intravenous potassium iodide (to prevent any further output of thyroxine from the remnant of the gland), hydrocortisone for its anti-pyrexial effect and propranolol to block the effects of thyroxine on the heart (β-adrenergic blockade). Supportive therapy includes sedation, physical measures (such as tepid sponging to reduce the temperature), diuretics and digoxin for heart failure.

Tracheomalacia

The tracheal rings are softened by the long-standing compression of a large goitre and easily collapse, causing stridor when the thyroid is removed. This may require temporary intubation and tracheostomy.

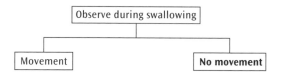

No movement on swallowing

Further classification is by region (Fig. 2.2). Swellings in the parotid region are described later (p. 28). The parotid region encroaches on both the other two main regions of the neck, the anterior and posterior triangles, separated by the anterior border of the sternomastoid muscle. The submandibular (or submental) region is the upper part of the two anterior triangles, lying above the level of the hyoid bone. *If a lump spans more than one region then the fact that it is in the parotid region takes precedence, while the anterior triangle takes precedence over the posterior triangle.*

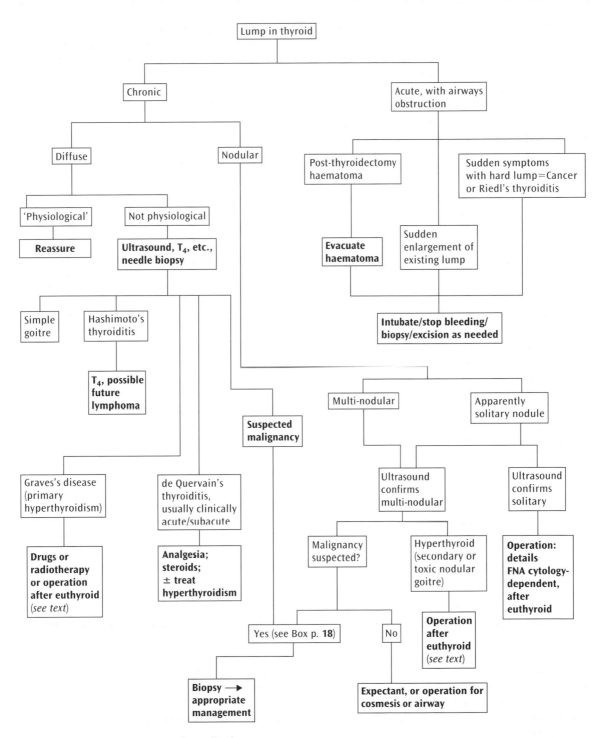

After all thyroid operations, think of complications:
thyrotoxic crisis, haematoma with airways obstruction, tracheomalacia with airways obstruction.

Algorithm 2.1

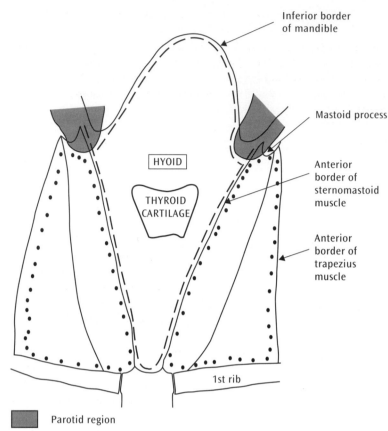

Inferior border of mandible

Mastoid process

Anterior border of sternomastoid muscle

Anterior border of trapezius muscle

HYOID

THYROID CARTILAGE

1st rib

Fig. 2.2 *Territories of the neck. Note that the parotid salivary gland encroaches on both anterior and posterior triangles, and that the demarcation between the triangles is the* anterior *border of the sternomastoid muscle.*

▓ Parotid region

— — Border of (right plus left) anterior triangles

•••• Borders of posterior triangles

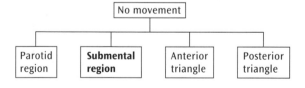

No movement

Parotid region | **Submental region** | Anterior triangle | Posterior triangle

Submental region

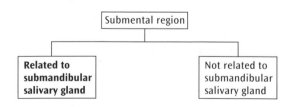

Submental region

Related to submandibular salivary gland | Not related to submandibular salivary gland

Is the lump of, or in relation to, the submandibular salivary gland? The normal submandibular salivary gland is usually (70%) palpable in the neck, and even when the lump has greatly distorted the region, the normal salivary gland on the opposite side helps in orientation.

Submandibular salivary gland

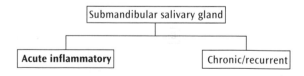

Submandibular salivary gland

Acute inflammatory | Chronic/recurrent

Acute inflammatory lumps

Such lumps usually involve the whole salivary gland and are therefore palpable in the floor of the mouth as well as in the neck.

Bilateral

Bilateral presentation of acute pain, tenderness and swelling of the submandibular salivary gland regions is unusual, but practically pathognomonic of mumps since other causes of acute inflammation are unlikely to be bilateral. Other features of mumps, such as parotitis, pancreatitis, orchitis, or circumstantial evidence, such as a history of contact or the prevalence of an epidemic, may support the diagnosis.

Unilateral

Unilateral acute inflammatory symptoms and signs may also be due to mumps, but are more likely to be due to some other cause, commonly a stone in the submandibular duct, which may be visible and palpable as a hard swelling in the floor of the mouth, lying along the course of the duct. A stone in the gland itself is unlikely to be palpable during the acute inflammatory state. Inflammation of the submandibular lymph nodes may be secondary to an infective lesion of tongue, floor of mouth, mandible, cheek or neighbouring skin. The submandibular swelling itself is treated with antibiotics but the removal of a stone in the duct is best not undertaken at this stage. Usually the inflammation subsides, and further investigation and treatment can be undertaken as considered below for chronic swellings. However, should fluctuation develop, incision to release the pus is necessary. The mandibular branch of the facial nerve is liable to damage during this procedure.

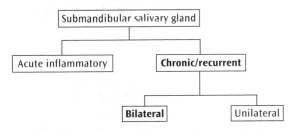

Chronic and recurrent lumps

Bilateral

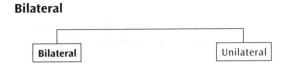

Bilateral chronic or recurrent enlargement may be part of Sjögren's syndrome or of sarcoidosis (pp. 33, 36). The diagnosis of chronic or recurrent bilateral enlargement is best made by operative removal of the whole of one submandibular salivary gland. Treatment is unsatisfactory, although corticosteroid drugs are sometimes effective. Occasionally, the histological report indicates some other disease such as tuberculosis or reticulosis.

Unilateral

A chronic mass in the submandibular region may be an enlargement and hardening of the whole gland, or a lump in the gland, or a lump superficial to the submandibular salivary gland and obscuring the latter. This salivary gland is C-shaped, with a superficial portion palpable via the neck, deep via the mouth and the concavity of the C is occupied by the posterior edge of the mylohyoid muscle. Thus, a swelling of the whole gland is bimanually palpable between a finger in the mouth and the fingers of the other hand on the neck, while any intrinsic swelling of the gland becomes fixed when the patient contracts the mylohyoid muscle by opening his mouth against resistance. By contrast, a lump superficial to the salivary gland, for example a lymph node, is not fixed by contraction of the mylohyoid. If the whole gland is involved, an *associated cause* may be demonstrable. Usually this is a *stone in the submandibular duct*. The typical history is that the patient develops pain and swelling in one submandibular region on eating, and the symptoms subside in a variable length of time after the meal, to recur with the next meal. Occasionally, such a history is complicated by an attack of sustained pain and swelling for several days, possibly with a constitutional disturbance, and the immediate management of this ascending infection is as described in the section on acute inflammatory swellings. Plain X-rays (Fig. 2.3) and sialography are useful.

In a symptomless period the stone is removed. If the stone is readily palpable in the anterior 2 cm of the submandibular duct in the floor of the mouth, it can readily be removed through the mouth. However, if the stone is further back in the hilum of the gland, it is usually not palpable in the floor of the mouth and there is always a risk of damage to the lingual nerve if one operates through the mouth: the whole

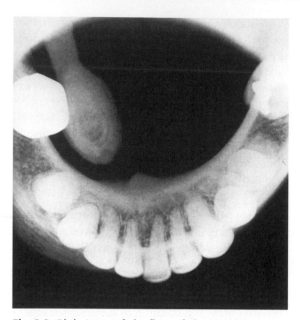

Fig. 2.3 *Plain X-ray of the floor of the mouth, showing a large submandibular calculus lying in the submandibular duct near its termination. It would appear likely that the distal oval structure was the primary calculus which, by obstructing the duct, favoured the formation of a tail of secondary calculus which extends proximally.*

gland and a portion of the proximal duct containing the stone are removed via an incision in the upper cervical skin crease.

Another possible *associated cause* in the floor of the mouth is *ranula*. The cervical swelling is fluctuant and transilluminable; the oral portion may be inconspicuous: it consists of a bluish discoloration and dome-shaped swelling of the mucosa in part of the floor of the mouth, and pressure upwards on the cervical swelling makes the oral lesion more prominent and demonstrates their continuity. A ranula is probably an extravasation cyst produced by leakage of saliva from a named or unnamed salivary gland through a small hole made by minor trauma unnoticed by the patient. The leakage of saliva provokes an intense foreign body reaction and explains why the cervical swelling is lined by granulation tissue rather than epithelium.

To cure a ranula, it is essential to remove that part of the floor of the mouth which contains the leaking duct. If the cervical part of the swelling occupies the submandibular salivary gland region, it is very likely that the duct concerned is the submandibular duct, or at least that the submandibular duct will be damaged in the course of the operation. In such cases, therefore, the submandibular salivary gland should be removed from the neck at the same operation. It is not necessary to remove the cervical swelling which subsides spontaneously when the causative lesion in the floor of the mouth has been excised.

Other *associated lesions* in the mouth, cheek, lip, neck or mandible, whether apparently inflammatory or neoplastic, may suggest that the palpable cervical swelling is a submandibular lymph node. Management is to biopsy the primary lesion so as to establish the diagnosis: cure of the primary lesion may then be possible without any necessity to treat the lymph node directly. This may be true even if the primary is neoplastic, because enlarged lymph nodes may be involved only by superadded infection and may disappear after the neoplasm has been treated.

Should the lump be near the submandibular salivary gland but not a part of it, excision-biopsy is performed. If the lump is *in* the salivary gland and no associated cause has been demonstrated then a histological diagnosis must be sought. Two situations may obtain: that the lump is *clinically benign* or that there are features of malignancy. Although malignant tumours of the parotid only constitute 10% of all parotid tumours, the corresponding incidence in the submandibular gland is over 50%. The index of suspicion should be correspondingly high.

If the lesion seems benign (long history, slow growth, no pain, no fixity to neighbouring tissues and, in particular, remoteness from the mandible) then a tissue-diagnosis is obtained by excision biopsy, that is, excision of the tumour with complete removal of the salivary gland. If the histological report confirms that the tumour is 'benign' no further treatment is needed.

If there are grounds for suspecting malignancy, it is important to achieve a tissue-diagnosis with FNA biopsy before embarking on surgical treatment. If the report is malignant, a much wider excision than for benign lesions is carried out, possibly with resection of a segment of mandible in continuity with the specimen. Opinion is divided as to whether a block dissection of the cervical nodes on the same side should be included in the procedure. Immediate repair of the mandibular defect may be carried out by prosthesis provided that radiotherapy has not been used previously. Post-operative radiotherapy is advised in all malignancies.

Not submandibular salivary gland-related

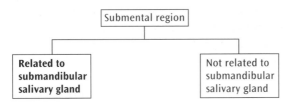

Two clinically characteristic lesions that do not move on swallowing occur in this region. One is the ranula (p. 26). The other is the median submental (or suprahyoid) dermoid, a cystic subcutaneous lesion near the mid-line that does not move on protruding the tongue. This should be removed because it may become infected.

Other lumps are usually diagnosed as lymph nodes, but their true nature may not become apparent until after biopsy or excision-biopsy.

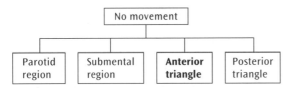

Anterior triangles

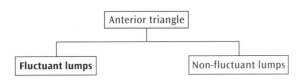

Fluctuant lumps

If the lump exhibits well-marked fluctuance there are two common possibilities: branchial cyst and 'cold' (tuberculous) abscess.

Branchial cyst

A cystic swelling emerging from deep to the anterior border of the sternomastoid muscle, in the region of the junction between upper- and mid-thirds of the muscle is likely to be a branchial cyst. The patient is usually a child or a young adult.

The cyst should be removed, both to confirm the diagnosis and because it is prone to becoming infected. The origin of these cysts from the vestigial remnants of the branchial clefts results in the frequent presence of a fibrous track of tissue leading upwards from the deep surface of the cyst. Unless this track is completely excised, recurrence is likely. The exact anatomical relations of the track depend upon which branchial cleft has given rise to the cyst. Frequently, the track may be followed upwards between the external and internal carotid arteries, to finish on the wall of the pharynx near the tonsil.

In association with a branchial cyst, there may be a fistula discharging mucus, often at some distance from the cyst, for example near the root of the neck. The *branchial fistula* may be of congenital origin or partially an acquired lesion, resulting from infection of a branchial cyst and surgical or spontaneous opening of the resultant abscess, or from incomplete removal of the branchial cyst. To excise this lesion, the fistulous opening is circumcised, the track dissected up to the cyst and then any congenital track above the cyst also dissected and removed, all in a single block of tissue.

Cold abscess

A cyst in the same region of the neck, with some mild inflammatory signs but without pain or heat in the overlying skin, and with a history that the lump was hard at first and gradually changed in consistency, is likely to be a cold abscess due to breaking down tuberculous lymph nodes. Usually, some solid parts of the lesion are still in existence. A plain radiograph of the neck may show calcification in the soft tissues. The Mantoux test is usually, but not always, positive.

Treatment is to evacuate the abscess, send scrapings from the granulation tissue of the walls for immediate microscopic examination for acidfast mycobacteria and for culture on suitable media for tubercle bacilli, and start a standard regime of triple-chemotherapy while the reports on culture and sensitivity are awaited during the next 2 months.

```
          ┌─────────────────┐
          │ Anterior triangle │
          └─────────────────┘
        ┌───────────┴───────────┐
┌───────────────┐       ┌───────────────────┐
│ Fluctuant lumps │       │ Non-fluctuant lumps │
└───────────────┘       └───────────────────┘
```

Non-fluctuant lumps

A solid lump, particularly if more than one lump is present, is likely to be diagnosed as a lymph node. However, there is one characteristic solid lesion of the anterior triangle, and it should be suspected if the lump is situated at the characteristic site of a branchial cyst, but is *pulsatile*. These circumstances suggest a carotid body tumour. A tortuous carotid artery may sometimes be confused with such a lesion.

A carotid arteriogram should be requested: splaying apart of the external and internal carotid arteries confirms the diagnosis (Fig. 2.4). The tumour

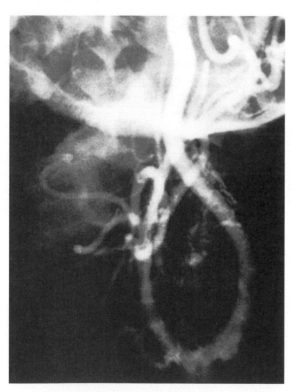

Fig. 2.4 *Carotid arteriogram: lateral view, showing the splaying apart of the external carotid artery (the vessel with branches) and the internal carotid artery by a carotid body tumour.*

should be removed. At an early stage of the operation, tapes are placed around the common, internal and external carotid arteries so that control of any severe haemorrhage during the removal is assured.

If the lump is thought to be a *lymph node*, the possible territories in which a primary source of infection or neoplasia might be present are carefully scrutinized. In particular, the ear and the nasopharynx and oropharynx should be examined by an otorhinolaryngologist, a chest radiograph obtained, and the mouth inspected. Since an enlarged lymph node may be part of a generalized disease of the reticuloendothelial system, it is important to examine the lymphatic glands elsewhere and the spleen, and to ask for a full blood count, including a white blood cell differential count. If FNA is inconclusive, excision biopsy is performed. The excised material is divided into two portions: one is sent for histological examination, the other for culture.

Posterior triangles

There is really only one lesion that is easily diagnosable on clinical grounds: *cystic hygroma*. If the lump is fluctuant, highly transilluminable and usually lying low in the neck, it is a cystic hygroma (i.e., a benign tumour of lymphatic channels), particularly common in childhood. The mass should be excised.

All other swellings in this region should be excised, and any further treatment depends upon the histology report.

SWELLINGS IN THE PAROTID REGION

AIMS

1 Distinguish between a swelling of the whole parotid gland and a lump in the parotid region
2 Appreciate the significance of this differentiation
3 Recognize the clinical features of a swelling of the whole parotid gland
4 Elicit the physical signs which indicate spread from a lump in the parotid region
5 Understand the management of a lump in the parotid region and how it is influenced by signs of spread

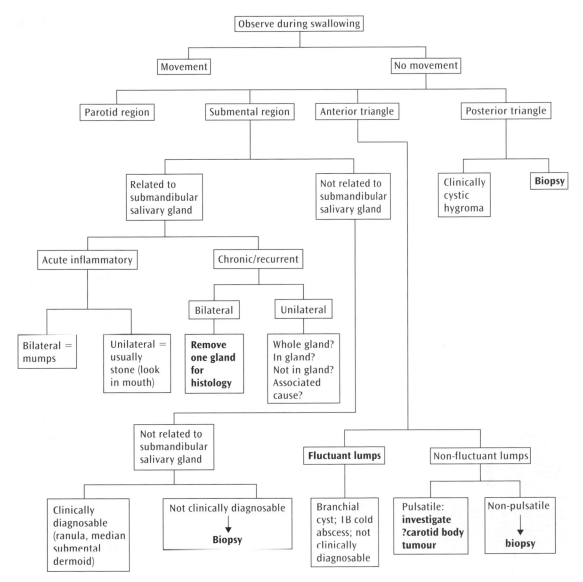

Algorithm 2.2

Parotid swellings are uncommon and pose challenging problems in management because of their variable nature and the difficulty of differentiating them from other unrelated swellings. An important aid to successful management is to distinguish between a swelling of the whole gland and a lump in the parotid salivary region. This is crucial, because an enlargement of the whole gland suggests an inflammatory process or else a mechanical obstruction of the parotid duct, whereas a lump in the parotid region, unless obviously inflammatory, raises the question of neoplasia. It is relevant therefore to be acquainted with the anatomical landmarks of the parotid salivary gland region.

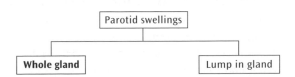

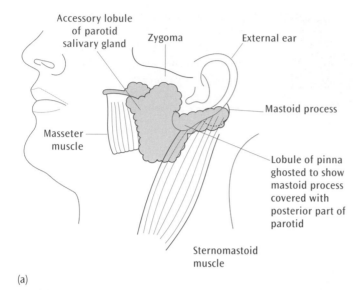

Accessory lobule
of parotid
salivary gland — Zygoma — External ear

Masseter
muscle

Mastoid process

Lobule of pinna
ghosted to show
mastoid process
covered with
posterior part of
parotid

Sternomastoid
muscle

(a)

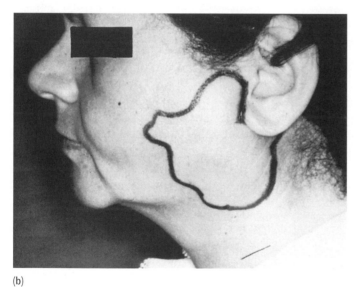

(b)

Fig. 2.5 *(a) This is a sketch of the lateral aspect of the parotid, superimposed on an outline of the face and head in profile, the external ear, the zygoma, the masseter muscle, the mastoid process and the sternomastoid muscle. Readers may wish to practise drawing this diagram and may trace the blank outline; (b) The outline of the parotid salivary gland. This woman's left parotid gland was hardened by the changes of Sjögren's syndrome and therefore easily marked out. Note particularly the extensions forwards along the parotid duct, downwards into the neck behind the submandibular salivary gland, and backwards over the mastoid process (mostly concealed by the pinna). When the whole parotid gland is hardened by inflammation or obstruction, the resultant swelling has this characteristic shape. (Reproduced from* Postgraduate Surgery Lectures, *Ed. John McFarland. London, Butterworth, by courtesy of the editor and publisher.)*

The parotid region and examination of the parotid gland

The gland (Fig. 2.5 (a)) lies in front of the external ear, filling the hollow between the ear and the angle and ascending ramus of the mandible. Above, it rises to the *zygoma*; anteriorly, it spills forwards over the posterior one-quarter to one-half of the *masseter muscle*, and a further extension (the 'accessory lobule') projects forwards in company with the parotid duct, sometimes almost to the anterior border of the masseter muscle. Posteriorly, there is a backward projection covering the *mastoid process*, hidden by the lobule of the pinna. Inferiorly, the lower pole of the gland extends down into the neck: the inferior edge of the parotid and the posterior border of the submandibular salivary gland are separated only by a thin band of fascia attached to the angle of the jaw, the *stylomandibular ligament*.

The normal gland is impalpable but when it is inflamed or obstructed becomes firmer and easier to

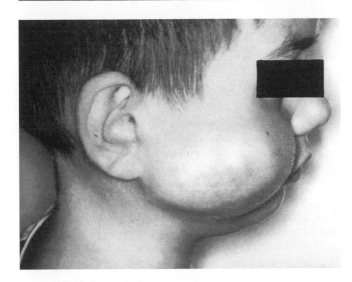

Fig. 2.6 *The boy shown had a large parotid swelling which did not extend backwards over the mastoid process and was thus not an enlargement of the whole parotid gland; ultimately, it proved to be a carcinoma. (Reproduced by courtesy of the editor,* Annals of the Royal College of Surgeons of England.*)*

palpate, although its shape remains unchanged (Fig. 2.5 (b)).

Fig. 2.6 shows a large parotid swelling that did not occupy the whole gland. *A lump within or overlapping the margins of the parotid region is likely to be of parotid origin unless a different diagnosis is clinically obvious.*

It is essential to realize that a lump near the margins of the parotid, for example overlying the mastoid process, in the vicinity of the posterior pole of the submandibular salivary gland or immediately below the zygoma is likely to be of parotid origin. Clinical examination of both parotid regions should include inspection and palpation of the duct from the cheek, as it lies on and hooks around the anterior border of the masseter muscle, one finger's breadth below the interior border of the zygomatic bone. The orifice of the duct, opposite the second upper molar tooth in the mouth, is inspected under good illumination and palpated by a finger in the mouth exerting pressure against the other hand placed on the cheek.

Swellings of the whole gland

Once it is established that there is a swelling of the whole gland, two situations must be considered: the *primary acute* and the *chronic*. In this context, the term 'chronic' also refers to *recurrent acute* parotid swelling because recurrent acute episodes may result in progressive changes in the gland and develop into a chronic swelling.

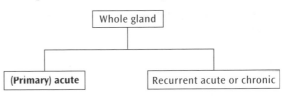

An important enquiry therefore is the history of previous similar attacks and their frequency.

Primary acute

In primary acute parotitis, the gland is diffusely enlarged, painful and tender. The possible causes are either *mumps* or *ascending parotitis*.

When *bilateral*, and especially if the submandibular salivary glands are also involved, the cause is almost certainly mumps, although this diagnosis should still be entertained with *unilateral* parotitis as both glands are not always affected simultaneously or with the same grade of severity. *It is therefore worth observing the opposite side as a unilateral parotitis progresses or resolves.*

Confirmation of mumps usually depends on circumstantial evidence of contacts, or of prevalence of an epidemic. Any of the specific complications (pancreatitis or orchitis) confirms the diagnosis. An increase in titre of mumps antibodies in the serum over the course of a week is significant.

Ascending parotitis is the more likely diagnosis in the elderly, debilitated or post-operative patient with poor oral hygiene. Enlargement of the gland is accompanied by purulent discharge at the duct orifice.

Management

Treatment of mumps is expectant and symptomatic, consisting of analgesics for pain, anti-pyretics for fever, hydration and oral care, attention to secondary infection and complications. In addition, in ascending parotitis, systemic antibiotics may be required and an obstruction at the parotid duct orifice is sought by inspection and palpation. Whilst a few drops of turbid or purulent fluid are visible exuding from the orifice of the duct, indicative of incomplete obstruction, resolution can be awaited.

Progressive pain and swelling with surrounding cellulitis and pyrexia are evidence of a parotid abscess. Fluctuation is not evident unless pus has penetrated the parotid sheath. Drainage is performed at the point of maximal tenderness in the cheek through an incision parallel to the course of the neighbouring branch of the facial nerve in order to avoid damage to the nerve.

In short:

- Bilateral: assume mumps.
- Unilateral: mumps is the most likely diagnosis if the patient is a child, has recently been exposed to mumps, the disease is epidemic in the district or if pancreatitis or orchitis occurs: TREAT AT HOME.
- Infection ascending from the mouth is the most likely if there is oral sepsis or debility, the patient is elderly and has recently undergone major surgery, oral hygiene is poor: NEEDS HOSPITAL TREATMENT.

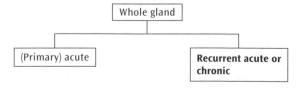

Recurrent acute or chronic

A history of recurrent parotitis without obvious physical signs should be accepted with caution. Swelling and discomfort in the parotid regions, dryness of the mouth and over-salivation are common complaints of neurotic subjects. However, if the patient's story seems reliable or there is collateral evidence, such as a convincing description of periodic swelling from a third party, it is reasonable to make a diagnosis of recurrent acute parotitis.

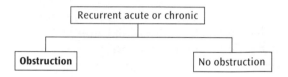

Recurrent acute or chronic parotitis requires referral for specialist opinion. The most common causes of recurrent acute or chronic parotitis are mechanical obstruction of the parotid duct, nearly always due to a stone, and Sjögren's syndrome.

Clinical features

Calculi in the parotid glands are less common than in the submandibular and present typical features described in Table 2.3.

Although these are highly suggestive features, careful examination of the duct is essential. A stone

Table 2.3 *Evidence favouring parotid duct calculus*

Age >35 years: the condition practically never occurs in younger people

Site unilateral: most unlikely to occur simultaneously on both sides

Onset during a meal: the increased flow of saliva converts a partial to a complete obstruction

Sudden onset: the stone is pushed distally and obstructs at the narrowest point of the duct

Duration short: never >7 days: sometimes only a few hours

The 'sudden gush': the patient describes a sudden spurt of saliva or foul-tasting liquid into the mouth, followed by immediate or rapid relief of pain and swelling may be visible at the orifice, or if it has passed spontaneously the orifice may appear as a gaping hole with surrounding oedema and inflammation. Prolonged obstruction causes chronic inflammation with atrophy and replacement of glandular elements with fibrous and fatty tissue. The gland remains enlarged and tender (chronic sialadenitis).

Sjögren's syndrome is common in post-menopausal women. Typical features are dryness of the mouth, eyes and vulva, associated with rheumatoid arthritis or other autoimmune disorders, for example systemic lupus erythematosus or scleroderma. The histological changes in the parotid are proliferation of the epithelial and myoepithelial cells of the ducts, causing strictures and dilatations of the ducts, and dense lymphocytic infiltration of the acini. In Sjögren's syndrome, unlike calculous obstruction, the onset and resolution of parotid swelling are gradual, the attacks last weeks rather than days and they are usually not related to meals.

It is essential at the initial assessment to determine whether the patient has unilateral or bilateral disease. Unilateral disease, particularly with unequivocal evidence of a parotid duct calculus, does not demand further attention, but bilateral disease should invariably be investigated. Although calculous obstruction and Sjögren's syndrome appear to present distinctive features, imaging provides further information.

Management

For bilateral disease, sialography is performed. The parotid duct is cannulated and 0.5 ml water-soluble contrast medium, for example Urografin (sodium diatrizoate with meglumine diatrizoate), is injected with gentle pressure until resistance is felt. Although in a few patients the sialogram may show no abnormality, the typical radiological finding is 'punctate sialectasis' (Fig. 2.7). The main duct and its branches

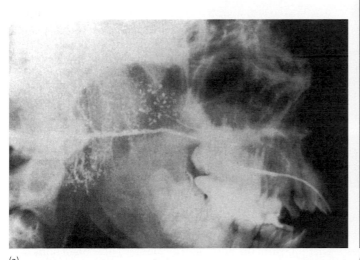

(a)

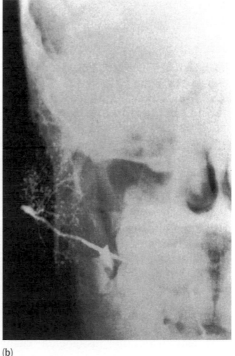

(b)

Fig. 2.7 *Punctate sialectasis; (a) Lateral view; (b) Anteroposterior (AP) view of a sialogram showing the typical picture. The appearance of saccular 'dilatations' has been produced by extravasation of the contrast material through weaknesses at the terminations of the smaller ducts. This condition is almost specific to Sjögren's syndrome.*

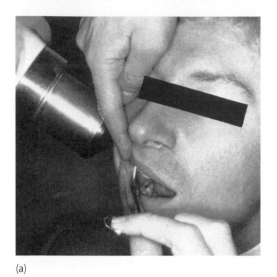

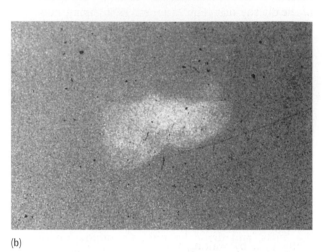

(a)   (b)

Fig. 2.8 *Plain X-rays: intra-oral view for parotid duct calculus; (a) The patient holds a small dental X-ray plate between his cheek and gums in the region of the termination of the parotid duct in the mouth, opposite the second upper molar tooth. X-rays are directed through the soft tissues of the cheek without interference from neighbouring bones; (b) An example of the results achieved. The calculus shown measured about 4 mm in length, but it had not been shown in the conventional views because it was overlain by the densities of the facial bones.*

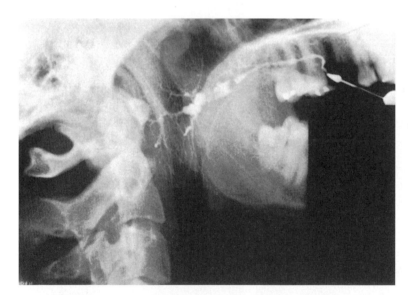

Fig. 2.9 *Parotid sialogram showing a stone in the parotid duct. In this example, the stone can be seen as a rounded filling defect in the duct near the point where dilatation of the duct commences. Frequently, no filling defect is seen, but if a parotid duct is normal in calibre at its distal (oral) end and abruptly enlarges at some point, there must be an obstruction at that point, and in practice the obstruction nearly always proves to be a stone.*

are normal, but the finer peripheral ducts terminate in spheres which are lakes of extravasated contrast, consistent with the histological changes. This appearance can be mimicked in a normal gland if the contrast is injected under pressure.

For unilateral disease, plain X-rays of the affected side are carried out in various directions, including a special intra-oral view (Fig. 2.8 (a) and (b)) which shows the oral end of the duct without interference from the neighbouring bones. These plain films may demonstrate a calculus.

A sialogram occasionally shows the stone as a filling defect, but more often a diagnosis of calculus is based on the appearance usually described by the radiologist as a 'stricture', with proximal dilatation of the duct system (Fig. 2.9). Unilateral disease may show punctate sialectasis and therefore fall into the group of Sjögren's syndrome.

Further management of unilateral disease

Patients in whom the clinical evidence suggests a stone but radiology is negative are observed: usually they settle down and it may be assumed that a small stone has been passed spontaneously. This may have already been evident on examination of the parotid duct orifice. All stones that cannot be removed via the parotid duct orifice should be treated expectantly (i.e., by waiting for them to pass spontaneously or to reach the accessible oral orifice) unless the patient's symptoms are so severe as to justify superficial parotidectomy (see below and Fig. 2.10).

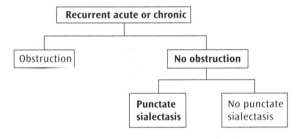

In unilateral disease, when there is no evidence of a stone and the sialogram shows punctate sialectasis, the condition is treated as Sjögren's syndrome.

Management of patients with punctate sialectasis

Most patients with punctate sialectasis show the histological changes in the parotid characteristic of Sjögren's syndrome, without necessarily other clinical manifestations. Rarely, there may be an underlying lesion, such as lymphosarcoma. When in doubt, the diagnosis of Sjögren's syndrome should be sought by biopsy. Danger to the facial nerve can be obviated by biopsy of the soft palate or the oral mucosa just below the lower lip. The small unnamed salivary glands in these regions are almost certain to show the changes of Sjögren's syndrome if that is the condition affecting

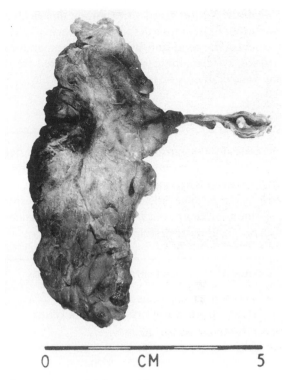

Fig. 2.10 *Superficial parotidectomy.*

the parotid. Other diagnostic tests are hypergammaglobulinaemia and autoantibodies, such as the rheumatoid factor, antinuclear factor and salivary duct antibodies.

There is no specific treatment for Sjögren's syndrome, although a minority of patients respond to corticosteroids. Should the severity and frequency of attacks of ascending infection demand symptomatic relief, the safe measure is total conservative parotidectomy.

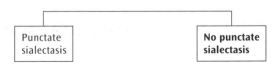

Management of patients with bilateral disease without punctate sialectasis

In some patients with a normal sialogram, the only remaining diagnostic option is a biopsy of the lower pole of the parotid gland. Occasionally, this yields a diagnosis of sarcoidosis despite the absence of other features of the condition, and it usually responds to steroids. The remaining few form an unsolved problem which can only be treated symptomatically.

Sialosis

Occasionally, the parotid is visibly enlarged, but not firmer than its surroundings. This picture is always due to fatty infiltration of the gland and is of no serious significance. Histopathologists refer to this condition as *sialosis*, but *benign lipomatous pseudo-hypertrophy* is more descriptive.

Review of chronic/recurrent acute parotitis

- Recurrent acute *unilateral* parotitis = 75% stone, 20% Sjögren's syndrome, 5% other; *bilateral* parotitis very rare.
- Chronic parotitis uni- or bilateral = 80% Sjögren's syndrome, 20% other.

Note. This whole group is rare but unilateral recurrent acute parotitis is five times more frequent than chronic. Punctate sialectasis = Sjögren's syndrome. Check Table 2.3 'Evidence favouring parotid duct calculus' on p. 32.

LUMP IN THE PAROTID REGION

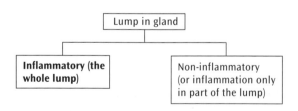

Inflammatory lumps

Inflammatory lumps are rare. An inflamed sebaceous cyst is the most likely diagnosis, identifiable by its characteristic signs (Chapter 1). This is treated by incision and drainage as an emergency, although antibiotics may suffice at the earlier stage of cellulitis.

Inflammatory parotid lumps not arising in the skin are either neoplasia- or duct calculus-associated. If the inflammatory area is only part of the lump, this is probably inflammatory degeneration in a neoplasm, a complication more likely to occur in the benign adenolymphoma than in a malignant tumour. Incision and drainage are inadvisable as the definitive treatment is wide excision. If the whole lump is inflamed, the possibility of an underlying stone is excluded by plain X-rays and sialography, as previously detailed. An abscess with a stone lying within it can be evacuated with reasonable safety by incision from the cheek (or orally if it seems to be pointing into the mouth). The resulting salivary fistula heals spontaneously provided that distal obstruction is eliminated.

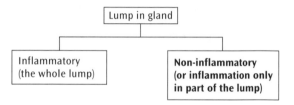

Non-inflammatory lumps

Lumps arising in the skin (usually sebaceous cysts) are easily recognized and treated. A few of the remainder have *distinctive clinical features* which allow an exact clinical diagnosis to be made. In most instances, the nature of the lump is unknown and the working diagnosis is 'lump in the parotid region'.

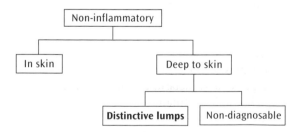

Distinctive lumps

These rarities are mentioned to be dismissed. Examples include a palpable calculus in the duct, a haemangioma changing in volume with digital pressure and with posture and confirmed by angiography, and hypertrophy of the masseter muscle, a physiological variation that becomes obvious when the patient is asked to clench the jaw. When a confident clinical diagnosis can be made, the appropriate treatment can be offered. However, the diagnostic discipline must be rigorous: a lobulated, fluctuant lump could be a lipoma, but it might also be an adenoma as described later.

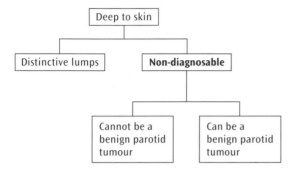

Non-diagnosable lumps

Most non-diagnosable lumps (90%) are parotid tumours and most of the tumours (85%) are benign in the sense that it is very rare for them to metastasize and the extent to which they invade the surrounding tissues is so small that it can only be demonstrated microscopically. For these reasons, benign tumours are curable by excision with a generous margin of normal surrounding tissue, care being taken to avoid damage to the facial nerve – the operation of *conservative parotidectomy*. Malignant tumours may require more radical treatment.

Clinical features do not distinguish reliably between malignant and benign tumours. Signs of malignancy are those of spread, that is, attachment to skin, muscle, bone, facial nerve (demonstrated by facial palsy) and metastases. These signs can all be mimicked in inflammation, or in the case of attachment to the sternomastoid muscle, by the fact that the lower pole of the parotid is deep to the muscle and therefore appears to be tethered to it. On the other hand, whereas most lumps with no clinical evidence of spread are benign, about 5% are malignant. Preliminary tissue diagnosis of an undiagnosable lesion therefore appears to be indicated, but this approach is disputed.

Non-diagnosable tumours – clinically benign

Opinion is divided as to how such patients should be managed. Open biopsy results in an unacceptable incidence of implantation recurrence, which can be multiple and resistant to radiotherapy or chemotherapy, rendering excision without damage to the facial nerve difficult or impossible. FNA cytology is reportedly free from this problem, but follow-up averages only about 5 years. At least half of all recurrences of benign parotid tumours eventuate 10 years or more after operation. Since at least half of malignant parotid tumours arise in a pre-existing benign parotid tumour, tissue sampling by FNA cytology or open biopsy could be misleading. Finally, the results of aspiration cytology rarely make a difference to management (see below).

The alternative approach is to embark, without any attempt at biopsy or FNA cytology, on the operation of conservative parotidectomy. At operation, the excision is extended if spread to neighbouring tissues such as the facial nerve or extra-parotid structures is evident. A successful removal with a margin of normal tissue cures the benign tumours, of which the pleomorphic adenoma is the most frequent, also other benign lesions that occasionally are found within the parotid, as well as the small proportion of malignant tumours which, in the absence of clinical signs of spread, are of intermediate malignancy and do not demand further treatment (Table 2.4). In the very rare circumstance that histology reveals an unexpected frank malignancy, further management is radical parotidectomy followed by radiotherapy if the histological evidence suggests that the tumour had been completely removed, or radiotherapy alone if it had not.

The most common benign adenoma after the pleomorphic is the *adenolymphoma*, which is strongly associated with smoking. Characteristically, it occurs in elderly males, is situated in the lower pole of the gland, is soft and fluctuant, and is frequently bilateral. However, these features cannot be relied upon in the diagnosis of the condition. A pleomorphic adenoma is occasionally soft and an adenolymphoma can occur in other parts of the parotid. When bilateral, since a pleomorphic adenoma or acinic cell tumour can be bilateral, the best policy is to carry out a parotidectomy on one side

Table 2.4 *Parotid tumour pathology*

Benign	Malignant
Pleomorphic adenoma ('mixed tumour')	Intermediate malignancy: mucoepidermoid carcinoma; acinic cell carcinoma
Monomorphic adenomas: adenolymphoma; others, e.g., oxyphilic adenomas	Pronounced malignancy: carcinoma, various types

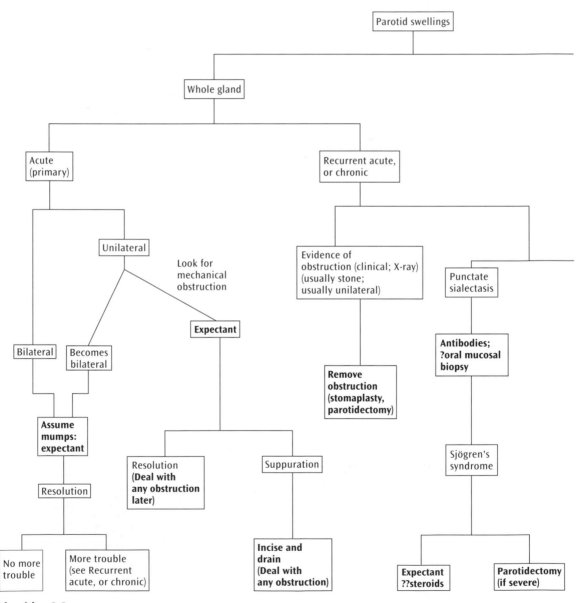

Algorithm 2.3

and if it proves to be an adenolymphoma the lump on the other side can reasonably be assumed to be another adenolymphoma and treated expectantly. Otherwise, bilateral removal will have to be performed.

Lumps showing signs of spread

Lumps that show signs of spread to neighbouring tissues are highly suspicious of malignancy. An open biopsy is indicated, although in 2% the signs of spread are due to inflammation. When malignancy is confirmed, a CT scan to outline local involvement is essential as it determines the extent of excision. Pre-operative radiotherapy improves resectability of the tumour. The operation involves extensive local excision of the gland with the facial nerve (*radical parotidectomy*), may include the mandible and is combined with *en bloc* dissection of the cervical lymph nodes.

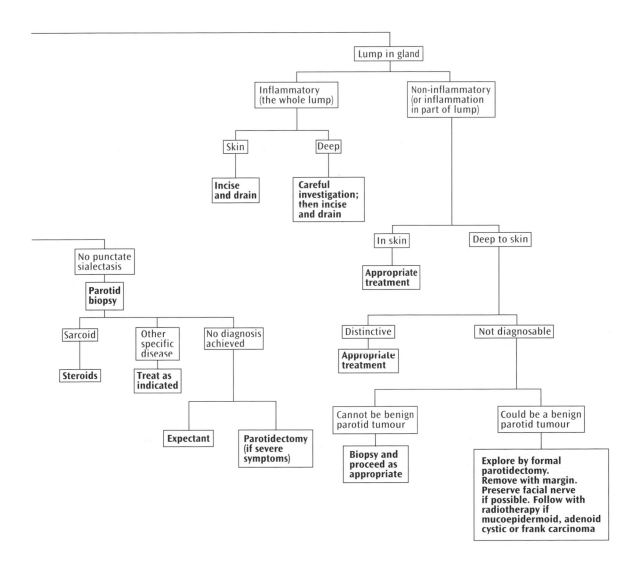

Parotidectomy

The patient with a lump which could be a benign parotid tumour has the nature of the operation explained fully, and is cautioned about the risk of a temporary or permanent facial nerve palsy. The patient is also warned about a salivary fistula, causing a leak of saliva from the duct on to the face at mealtimes, a rare condition that heals spontaneously if the policy described below is followed; and about Frey's syndrome of gustatory sweating, due to cross-regeneration of sympathetic and parasympathetic nerve fibres supplying the vessels and sweat glands of the skin. Frey's syndrome probably occurs after all parotidectomies, but is usually so mild as to be unnoticeable. Only rarely does it pose a significant clinical problem.

The facial nerve trunk is exposed and the superficial part of the parotid dissected forwards off the nerve and its branches. When the tumour is superficial to the nerve, its removal is thus accomplished as a *superficial parotidectomy*; however, when the tumour is deep to the nerve, the latter is raised off the deep parotid after superficial parotidectomy and the deep part excised with the tumour as a *total parotidectomy*. In either case, when the facial nerve trunk and its branches are preserved, the operation is called *conservative*; when one or more branches has to be excised in order to maintain an adequate margin around the tumour, the operation is *semi-conservative*, whereas when the whole nerve has to be sacrificed, the operation is *radical*.

Removal of as much parotid tissue as possible, including the main duct to the anterior border of the sternomastoid muscle, prevents fistulas.

Post-operative facial nerve palsy

After conservative parotidectomy, some facial nerve impairment can be demonstrated in nearly all patients.

Provided that the surgeon is sure that all named branches of the facial nerve were preserved intact during the operation, the patient may be reassured that post-operative weakness will resolve spontaneously. The median time for recovery is 4 months, but there is a long tail of delayed recovery with 95% achieving full recovery in 1 year and all in 2 years.

Division of a single named facial nerve branch always ends with spontaneous recovery except in the case of the mandibular branch.

Division of two or more contiguous nerve branches requires immediate repair, but can be followed by complete spontaneous recovery.

If the trunk of the nerve and its main branches are destroyed, nerve-grafting should be undertaken by an expert as soon as feasible, and preferably within a week, using cutaneous nerves such as the sural.

HIGHLIGHTS

- Diffuse swelling of the whole gland is inflammatory/obstructive
- Acute parotitis is commonly due to mumps and sometimes due to ductal stone obstruction
- Recurrent or chronic unilateral parotitis is more often due to stone-associated sialadenitis than to Sjögren's syndrome
- A lump in the parotid without evidence of spread can be treated by formal parotidectomy without preliminary biopsy
- A lump in the parotid region with evidence of spread is treated by preliminary biopsy

Lump in the breast; breast pain; nipple discharge

TIM DAVIDSON

AIMS

---

1 Be able to palpate the breast efficiently in order to determine whether a lump is present
2 Distinguish between inflammatory and non-inflammatory lumps
3 Be aware of the relevance of the triple assessment
4 Learn the principles of diagnosis and management of common benign lesions
---

INTRODUCTION

There is increasing public awareness, with accompanying anxiety, of breast cancer as the most common fatal malignancy in women. For women in the UK there is a lifetime risk of one in 12 of developing breast cancer and 15,000 women in the UK die from this disease annually. However, of those attending a breast clinic with a worrying breast symptom, only about 5% prove to have cancer; the remaining 95% are reassured once a diagnosis has been reached. The most common symptoms for which women are referred to a breast clinic (in order of frequency) are a suspected lump in the breast, breast pain and nipple discharge.

THE PATIENT COMPLAINS OF A LUMP IN THE BREAST

The initial decision

The clinician's primary decision is whether or not the patient does have a breast lump. Women are encouraged by health promotional literature to palpate their own breasts in order to achieve an earlier diagnosis of cancer, but it is often difficult to palpate one's own breasts accurately. The female breast consists of soft adipose and glandular tissue arranged between fibrous tissue septa, so that the examining finger prodded into the surface of the breast may sense a localized area of resistance which may easily be misconstrued as a lump. For this reason, clinicians should examine the breast using the pulps of the fingers, but *with the hand flat*; in the same way women are advised to carry out self-examination in the bath or shower with a flat soapy hand, and in the first part of the menstrual cycle soon after the period when hormonal nodularity in the breast is minimal.

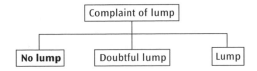

No lump

The management in this situation is simply reassurance. Although most patients are readily reassured, the occasional anxious patient may seek other, perhaps several opinions, until someone expresses doubt and unjustifiably recommends biopsy. Therefore, thorough examination and strong reassurance are crucial, with a clear explanation about the structural changes in breast tissue associated with the menstrual cycle best described to the patient as the natural granularity or lumpiness of a normal and healthy breast. A breast imaging investigation may help to allay anxiety.

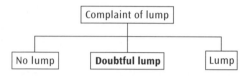

Doubtful lump (or poorly defined nodularity)

There is a wide spectrum in the degree of lumpiness and of texture of breast tissue, associated with the menstrual cycle and most noticeable during the second half and before menstruation. Cyclical proliferation and involution of breast tissue producing fibrosis, epithelial hyperplasia, adenosis and cyst formation and often referred to by a number of synonyms, including fibroadenosis (*see later*), may contribute to lumpiness, and, especially when localized, can be difficult to differentiate from a true discrete lump. The upper outer quadrant and axillary tail are most often affected. It may be necessary to repeat the examination at the beginning of the menstrual cycle and any suspicious physical signs are compared with the opposite breast. When doubt remains, more information is obtained from radiological imaging. Although mammography is the optimal examination in post-menopausal and elderly women, radiation risk from repeated examinations and the breast density in younger females make ultrasonography the favoured option, particularly in distinguishing a solid from a cystic lump. Should the uncertainty remain unresolved, fine needle aspiration

(FNA) from the area for cytology is indicated. This can be carried out with precision under ultrasound control. The needle is inserted into the lump and suction is applied by the syringe as the needle is withdrawn; the aspirate is fixed and stained. A definite decision is then made as to whether the patient has a lump, or not.

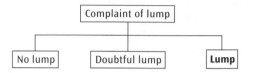

Lump confirmed

A careful clinical examination to differentiate a lump in the breast from a lump arising in the chest wall or in the overlying skin is essential. All breast lumps, whether discrete or areas of persistant localized nodularity, are investigated in outpatients by *triple assessment*. This comprises a clinical examination, imaging by ultrasonography or mammography or occasionally both, and FNA cytology. It is always preferable to arrange mammography and ultrasonography to precede aspiration under ultrasound control in order to avoid any artefactual changes created by needling that might distort the appearances on imaging. The result of FNA should be considered in conjunction with the clinical presentation and taking into account the cytologist's experience. When all three modalities *concur*, a robust diagnosis of either a benign or a malignant breast lump may be made in almost all cases. This allows counselling for the patient and facilitates the making of arrangements for elective surgery if required.

Whenever there is *discordance* within the triple assessment, a definite diagnosis cannot be made without formal histological examination. A tissue specimen is obtained by open biopsy or percutaneous core biopsy under local anaesthesia. This avoids the serious pitfall either of leaving an early carcinoma untreated or proceeding to cancer surgery, particularly if it involves mastectomy, for a suspicious lump which may prove to be benign.

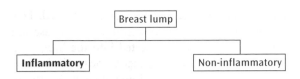

Lumps with inflammation

A patient presenting with a tense, painful, diffuse or localized swelling and induration of the breast, skin reddening and tenderness, with or without pyrexia, is likely to have a breast abscess. Most patients with a breast abscess are breast-feeding which causes an ascending duct infection, most commonly with *Staphylococcus aureus*, secondary to an excoriated or cracked nipple which is relatively common before breast-feeding is comfortably established.

A breast abscess is usually obvious but may show minimal or no signs of inflammation or fluctuation despite the presence of pus deep within the breast tissue. An ultrasound examination is particularly useful in outlining a deep abscess with needle aspiration of the pus. There is a place for a trial of conservative treatment with antibiotics, analgesics and regular expression of milk from the breast or emptying with a breast pump (to avoid engorgement) in the early cellulitic phase.

Otherwise, in most cases, incision and drainage, breaking down all loculi to produce a single cavity, is required. A specimen of the pus is collected for culture and antibiotic sensitivity, but unless there is residual cellulitis or systemic disturbance antibiotics are not required after the operation. Dressings are designed to absorb the discharge, to prevent secondary exogenous infection and to delay skin healing until the cavity fills in with granulation tissue. The patient is advised to express the affected breast manually while feeding is continued from the opposite breast and the mother is reassured that antibiotics secreted in the milk should have no adverse effect on the baby apart from occasional diarrhoea.

Occasionally, no pus is found when the breast is incised. Possible reasons are that the inflammatory process, although infective, did not progress to suppuration, particularly to be suspected in patients who had been on antibiotics; is non-pyogenic as in periductal mastitis and tuberculosis, or is neoplastic. Therefore a tissue specimen should be obtained for histological and bacteriological examination, including acid-alcohol-fast bacilli.

'*Plasma cell mastitis*' or '*periductal mastitis*' is associated with peri-areolar inflammation and may be complicated by non-lactational abscesses which discharge spontaneously through the skin, forming a *mammillary* (or *mammary*) *fistula*. The condition is due to hormonally induced changes in the breast causing ductal obstruction, dilatation (ectasia) and rupture, with extravasation of inspissated secretions that provoke a chronic inflammatory response with prominent plasma cell infiltration.

Controversy exists as to whether mammary duct ectasia and peri-ductal mastitis are two separate or related conditions. Peri-ductal mastitis often occurs in young female smokers, whereas mammary duct ectasia is not associated with smoking and is probably an age-related involutional phenomenon, common near the menopause. The clinical features of a nipple discharge, painless lumpiness in the sub-areolar region with localized reddening and tenderness, and nipple retraction may be confused with an abscess or carcinoma. The condition rapidly resolves with broad-spectrum antibiotics, although it is likely to recur in persistent smokers. Drainage is avoided as a mammary fistula will result. Mammography may show diagnostic features, but when doubt remains a biopsy is required. When the changes are extensive, subareolar excision of all the major ducts (Haagensen's operation) may be necessary.

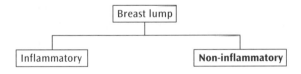

Lumps with no inflammation

The most common benign lumps in the breast are fibroadenomas and cysts. A fibroadenoma is common in women under 30 years of age, whereas carcinoma is very rare under the age of 25, fibroadenosis is more often seen between the ages of 25 and 45 years, and carcinoma occurs over the age of 35. Although the periodicity of pain, lumpiness in relation to the menstrual cycle, a history of previous breast disorders or trauma can be suggestive of benign disease, breast lumps should be assumed to be carcinoma unless proved otherwise.

Breast cysts can be multiple, although usually single. They are either isolated and discrete or within an area of irregular thickening. A cyst is smooth, and often fluctuant, although the latter is not a consistent sign because it cannot be elicited in a cyst deep in the breast substance, or tense, or with a rigid capsule. A cyst is spherical, because pressure in a liquid is transmitted equally in all directions, and since the surrounding breast tissue is homogeneously soft the cyst as it enlarges adopts a spherical shape (Chapter 1).

A breast cyst is treated by aspirating its contents with a syringe and needle until it is emptied completely. Provided that after aspiration the lump completely disappears *and* that the fluid obtained is not blood-stained, carcinoma can be excluded and the patient is reassured. Although conventionally the cyst fluid is sent for cytological examination, this investigation rarely yields a positive result and is unnecessary if the above criteria have been met; if they have not, or if the cyst recurs, the lump should be excised.

A *fibroadenoma* is a firm, almost hard, lump which is particularly mobile within the breast, hence the term 'breast mouse'. However, these features do not distinguish a fibroadenoma from other lesions. A more typical sign of a fibroadenoma is the presence in at least one region of a linear depression which is the groove between two lobulations (Fig. 3.1). A smooth, firm or hard, lobulated swelling in a woman younger than 25 years is almost certainly a fibroadenoma.

The diagnosis of fibroadenoma must be confirmed by triple assessment and under no circumstance can the patient be assured that the lump is definitely benign without a tissue diagnosis. In young women, the treatment of a confirmed fibroadenoma is optional, excisional or expectant. In patients aged over 35 years, even if FNA cytology confirms the diagnosis this result should be interpreted with caution and the patient is better advised to have excision biopsy.

Cystosarcoma phyllodes, despite its name, is a rare form of fibroadenoma and is considered by histopathologists to be benign. Phyllodes tumours can be

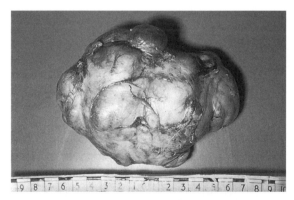

Fig. 3.1 *Fibroadenoma of the breast. This is an example of the rather unusual 'giant' variety, measuring 10 cm across. Its surface shows the typical lobulated appearance which, when palpated in a clinical lesion, allows a confident diagnosis of fibroadenoma to be made. (Specimen in the collection of the Bland Sutton Institute of Pathology.)*

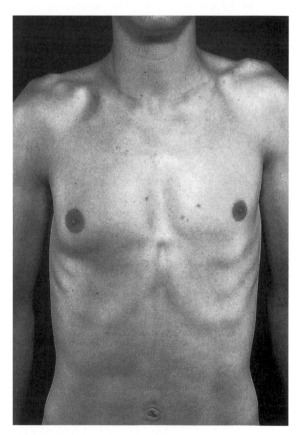

Fig. 3.2 *Gynaecomastia in a man aged 22 years. The enlargement of the right breast and enlargement plus deepened pigmentation of the right nipple and areola lasted for about 6 months and then regressed spontaneously.*

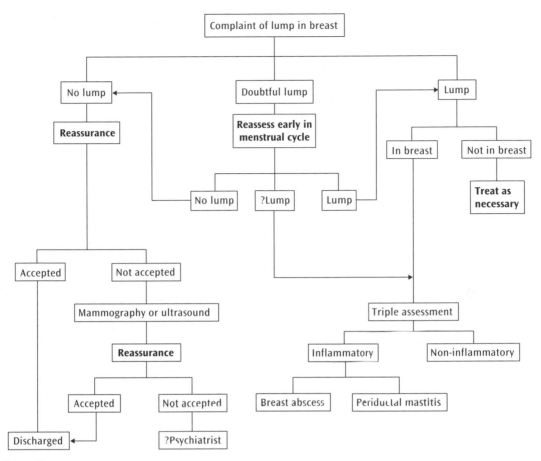

Algorithm 3.1

very large, and may be confused with a carcinoma. However, FNA or a Tru-cut biopsy fails to demonstrate carcinoma. It is treated by wide excision because it is not encapsulated, the margins are not always clearly defined and 20% metastasize, thereby belying their apparent histological innocence. A simple mastectomy may be necessary for large tumours.

Fat necrosis of the breast tissue following trauma manifests itself as a rare lump which is hard and irregular with skin dimpling and is clinically indistinguishable from carcinoma. The definitive diagnosis is only made on excision biopsy.

Breast lumps in men

Breast cancer is occasionally seen in men and accounts for approximately 0.5% of breast cancers overall. The diagnosis, as in women, requires the triple assessment described above. However, *gynaecomastia* is more frequent and presents such a typical clinical picture that a confident clinical diagnosis is easily made. The complaint is of a tender swelling deep to the nipple and areola, and on examination the affected breast is more prominent than the contralateral, due to the presence of a firm, tender, discoid mass just larger in diameter than the areola and concentric with the nipple and areola (Fig. 3.2). The mass is hypertrophied breast tissue, and in an adult male breast can reach 5 cm in diameter.

Gynaecomastia at birth, due to maternal oestrogens, and at puberty, associated with hormonal changes, is transient and resolves spontaneously. Although gynaecomastia may persist after adolescence, in older patients primary causative factors that should be considered and managed appropriately are medication with oestrogens, cimetidine, cyproterone acetate and spironolactone, liver disease, feminizing testicular neoplasms or testicular atrophy. However, in most instances the condition is idiopathic and likely to subside spontaneously over a period of a few months. Persistent gynaecomastia, particularly when uncomfortable or cosmetically embarrassing, is treated by excision of the enlarged breast disc by sub-areolar mastectomy.

HIGHLIGHTS

- Discrete breast lumps require diagnosis by 'triple assessment'
- In young women with dense glandular breast tissue, ultrasound is the appropriate imaging modality, whereas in post-menopausal women mammography is of greater benefit
- Breast abscess is often encountered in lactating women, but may complicate peri-ductal mastitis, particularly in smokers
- Ultrasound is useful for detecting deep-seated breast abscess when clinically not apparent
- Incision/drainage of peri-ductal mastitis may be complicated by a mammillary fistula and should be avoided
- A breast cyst is treated by needle aspiration, but excision biopsy if the cyst fluid is blood-stained after aspiration, there is a residual lump or the cyst recurs
- Fibroadenoma is better excised, particularly in females more than 35 years of age

---

BREAST PAIN (MASTALGIA)

AIMS

1 To distinguish cyclical from non-cyclical mastalgia
2 To appreciate that cyclical mastalgia usually responds to reassurance
3 To recognize that in most patients with non-cyclical mastalgia, the cause lies outside the breast

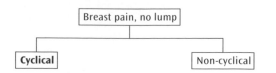

Cyclical mastalgia

Of patients presenting with persistent mastalgia (i.e., pain for over 6 months), about 60% is cyclical and 40% non-cyclical. The distinction is important and is usually determined from the relationship of pain and tenderness to the mentrual cycle, maximal in the luteal phase, especially the week or so before the onset of menses. Cyclical mastalgia where the pattern is unclear from the patient's description may become apparent with the use of a breast pain chart (Fig. 3.3). Mastalgia is considered severe when it is experienced for more than 7 days each cycle, is uncontrolled with simple analgesics and interferes with the patient's lifestyle.

The term 'mastitis' is incorrect for this condition: hormonally induced glandular activity within the breast tissue, not inflammation or infection, is the mechanism for pain, tenderness and nodularity in the female breast. A variety of other terms, fibro-adenosis, fibro-cystic disease, fibrosis, adenosis or cystic mammary dysplasia have also been used, but relate to histological appearances that may or may not be associated with symptoms. Antibiotics and diuretics are no longer considered acceptable treatment for cyclical mastalgia.

In nearly 90% of patients the pain is mild or moderate. A careful history, clinical examination and reassurance that there is no serious underlying breast condition is all that is necessary. In the remaining minority of women the pain is severe and requires medical therapy, although the placebo effect in controlled trials of treatment of cyclical mastalgia is in the region of 40%. Evening primrose oil and Efamast both contain gammalenic acid (GLA) as their active ingredient and they produce an improvement in pain score of about 50%. Bromocriptine and danazol have a slightly better response, but up to a third of patients prescribed these hormonal agents discontinue the tablets because of side-effects, and only in patients whose lifestyle is severely affected is such treatment appropriate. Other hormonal manoeuvres, such as

Daily Breast Pain Chart

Name

Please record the amount of breast pain you experience each day by shading in each box as illustrated.

	Severe pain
	Mild/moderate pain
	No pain

For example if you get severe pain on the fifth of the month then shade in completely the square under 5.

Please note the day your period starts each month with the letter 'P'

Month	1	2	3	4	5	6	7	8	9	10	11	12	13	14	15	16	17	18	19	20	21	22	23	24	25	26	27	28	29	30	31

Day of month

Please bring this chart with you on each visit

Fig. 3.3 *Patient's pain chart to assess the cyclical nature of mastalgia.*

the LHRH-agonist, goserelin, by monthly depot injection, tamoxifen and testosterone have been tried in specialist centres for those very few patients with refractory incapacitating breast pain.

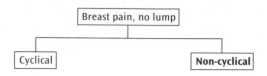

Non-cyclical mastalgia

Non-cyclical mastalgia usually presents in older patients and, rarely, may be the only symptom of breast cancer. In patients over 30 years of age with persistent localized breast pain, investigations to exclude an underlying cause are warranted. In over half the patients non-cyclical pain is not related to the breast, but is of musculoskeletal origin from the chest wall due to arthritis, rib injury or costochondritis, or from the shoulder girdle muscles.

If a localized area of chest wall tenderness can be identified, there is usually a good response to injection with a local anaesthetic–steroid combination. Where pain is diffuse across the breast and chest wall, treatment is less satisfactory, although some patients respond to non-steroidal anti-inflammatory agents (NSAIDs) given either orally or as a topical gel.

> **HIGHLIGHTS**
>
> - Most females with cyclical mastalgia and no clinical abnormality can be reassured and require no specific treatment
> - Occasionally, females with cyclical mastalgia which is refractory to gammalenic acid (GLA or evening primrose oil) may require referral for hormonal treatment
> - Non-cyclical mastalgia is frequently due to musculoskeletal pain from the chest wall referred to the breast

DISCHARGE FROM THE NIPPLE

> **AIMS**
>
> 1 Distinguish surface discharge from ductal discharge
> 2 Discriminate between discharge from a single duct and discharge from several ducts
> 3 Distinguish between physiological and pathological discharge from the nipple
> 4 Understand the management of nipple discharge

It must be realized that a woman may erroneously describe a discharge from the skin surface of or

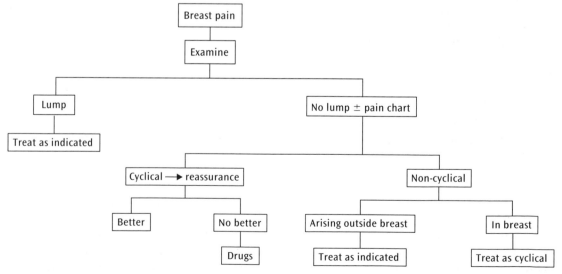

Algorithm 3.2

around the nipple as a discharge from the nipple. Careful examination should determine the precise source of the discharge and the nature of those conditions that may confuse the clinical picture. The presence of a breast lump takes precedence over discharge from the nipple and is managed accordingly, as already described.

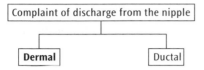

Discharge from the surface of the nipple and areola

Ulceration of the nipple is taken seriously because of the possibility of malignancy. A diagnosis of eczema is likely when there is itchy, superficial scaling involving the areola as well and when both breasts are affected. With skin excoriation there is serous or blood-stained discharge. This skin condition is expected to resolve rapidly on topical steroids, but if treatment fails, *Paget's disease of the nipple* should be excluded by a skin biopsy. In Paget's disease the external lesion is a slowly spreading scaling erosion of the skin starting on the nipple and extending onto the areola, often associated with an underlying occult duct carcinoma (Fig. 3.4).

Discharging foci include mammillary fistula and minor septic lesions due to trauma or infection of local sebaceous glands or Montgomery's tubercles in the areolar skin. The typical history of mammillary fistula is of repeated attacks of inflammation, subsiding spontaneously after the discharge of a periductal abscess. The local signs are more florid and are distinguishable from the other minor septic lesions already mentioned (Fig. 3.5).

A mammillary fistula is treated by excision of the blocked duct that is the primary cause of the fistula. A lacrimal duct dilator is passed through the skin opening and usually can be introduced to at least some extent into the offending duct, and a sector of nipple, areola and breast tissue is excised to include both the sinus track and the duct from which it arises. Alternatively, *en bloc* excision of all the major lactiferous ducts is carried out for recurrent inflammation and fistulation.

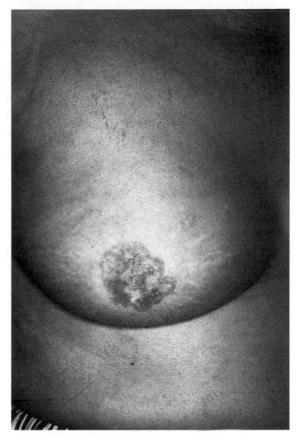

Fig. 3.4 *Paget's disease of the nipple. The small area of ulceration with a surrounding region of patchy pigmentation and scaling should arouse suspicion of the lesion. There is always a duct carcinoma in the breast nearby. (Photograph by courtesy of Mr David Rulphs.)*

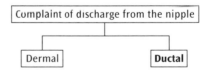

Discharge from within the nipple

Physiology

Apart from the period of lactation, the adult female breast secretes a small quantity of fluid at all times, this is discharged via the lactiferous ducts onto the surface of the nipple, where it is removed by evaporation, by contact with clothes or by washing. Normally, a woman is unaware of this secretion but

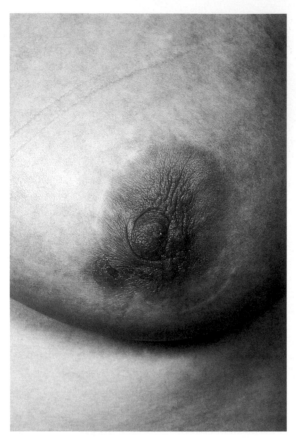

Fig. 3.5 *Mammillary fistula with opening of fistula track at the typical site on the areolar margin. Note the circumareolar scar from previous attempts at surgical excision.*

occasionally, perhaps due to hormonal changes, secretion becomes excessive and noticeable at one or both nipples and the patient may complain of it.

This is a physiological phenomenon, of no significance provided that a pathological cause is eliminated. In the search for an underlying disorder, the nature of the liquid and its site of origin are helpful.

Findings on examination

Nature of discharge

A clear, colourless or yellow discharge which is homogeneous and slightly sticky in consistency, or else white (i.e., milk) is usually but not necessarily physiological.

The most important abnormalities of the discharge are staining with frank or altered blood and turbidity, which may amount to particulate matter of a green or black colour mingled with the liquid. The discharge can be sent for cytological examination, although degenerate cells interfere with the diagnostic accuracy of carcinoma which is far poorer than with FNA cytology.

Site

It is of crucial importance to decide whether the discharge arises from many ducts or from a single duct. Often, the liquid within the duct system is scanty, and if expressed by accidental or uncontrolled pressure on the breast without focusing on its site of origin, an opportunity to establish a diagnosis is lost.

Therefore at the time of examination, under good illumination, the index finger is pressed on one area at a time at the periphery of the areola, in order to localize the breast segment from which a discharge is arising. Fingertip pressure is repeated around the whole circumference of the areola to determine whether the discharge has a diffuse or localized origin. When pressure produces a bead of discharge at the nipple, the site from which the liquid emerges and the nature of this liquid are noted. Any suspicion of blood is tested by use of urinalysis dipsticks.

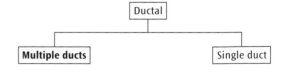

Diffuse origin

Should pressure on all or several of the points at the periphery of the areola produce discharge from the nipple, the underlying cause is clearly a generalized breast disorder.

A persistent milky discharge, *galactorrhoea*, in a non-lactating woman suggests hyperprolactinaemia due to an anterior pituitary tumour or which is drug-induced.

If the discharge is not milky, there are two possibilities: physiological secretion or duct stagnation.

Physiological nipple discharge is diagnosed if the secretion has the characteristics of physiological secretion as previously described, and if the examination of the breast is normal. The patient may be reassured, advised to ignore the discharge and, most importantly, to stop squeezing or expressing the nipples (often done repeatedly by an anxious patient to see if the discharge is still present) as this often perpetuates the symptom. As with gynaecomastia, physiological secretion is not always equally prominent in both breasts. A discharge from only one breast does not rule out physiological secretion.

Duct stagnation is associated with mammary duct ectasia, often occurring in the decade leading up to the menopause and therefore probably a manifestation of the pre-menopausal involutional changes in the breast. Nipple discharge is the result either of excessive secretion or periodic ductal obstruction with spontaneous resolution and ejection of inspissated secretion containing particulate debris. The discharge is usually green in colour because of its cholesterol content and becomes purulent or blood-stained as a result of secondary infection. With this presentation, the absence of any other abnormality on examination of the breast, both clinically and by mammography, confirms a working diagnosis of duct ectasia. Associated signs of peri-ductal

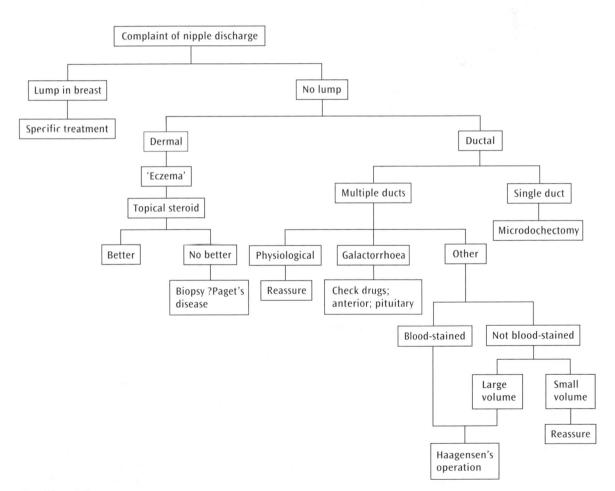

Algorithm 3.3

mastitis or mammary duct fistula make the diagnosis clearer and the condition is managed accordingly.

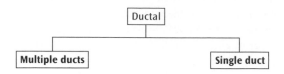

Localized origin

When a discharge is localized to a single duct, the causes are a *duct papilloma*, an *intra-duct carcinoma* (DCIS) (p. 53) or much less commonly an *invasive carcinoma*.

A duct papilloma is a benign hyperplastic lesion that is usually impalpable. The absence of a lump does not exclude an intra-duct or invasive carcinoma. Blood in the discharge discriminates poorly between benign and malignant tumours; it occurs in about 15% of the malignant and about 7% of the benign. Both cytology of the discharge and mammography are unreliable. Injection of contrast medium into the affected duct (ductogram) may confirm the presence of a ductal tumour, but gives no information about its histology. Irrespective of the appearance in the ductogram, microdochectomy is carried out by passing a probe into the duct and excising it. This operation cures the papilloma and intra-duct carcinoma. An invasive carcinoma is treated appropriately (Chapter 4).

HIGHLIGHTS

- In excoriation or ulceration of the nipple it is imperative to exclude Paget's disease
- Mammary duct ectasia is a cause of nipple discharge. When complicated with peri-ductal mastitis and mammillary fistula, the discharge is from the edge of the areola
- Single-duct nipple discharge, particularly if persistent or blood-stained, requires further investigation to exclude intra-duct papilloma or malignancy

Management of carcinoma of the breast

IRVING TAYLOR AND MICHAEL HOBSLEY

AIMS

1 Establish early diagnosis by clinical examination, imaging and cytology
2 Understand the principles of management of breast cancer
3 Prevent and treat local and regional disease in early cases
4 Understand the roles of radiotherapy, chemotherapy and hormone therapy
5 Control advanced and disseminated disease

INTRODUCTION

Cancers of the breast are predominantly adenocarcinomas, and the majority (75%) are invasive ductal carcinomas. Lobular carcinoma (10%) is multicentric and tends to be bilateral, but like the remaining variants of invasive cancer, tubular, papillary, medullary and mucous, has a better prognosis. Non-invasive carcinomas are rare and confined within the epithelial layer of duct or lobule *in situ* before infiltrating.

Management of carcinoma of the breast is both complex and controversial. The aim is detection of pre-symptomatic cancer and, when symptomatic, to make a definitive pre-operative diagnosis, determine the clinical stage of the disease and plan the appropriate management. This involves a combination of surgery, radiotherapy and systemic management, usually either chemotherapy or endocrine therapy. Clinicians should be familiar with the therapeutic options that are most likely to be effective.

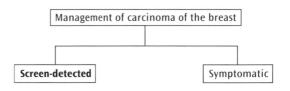

SCREENING-DETECTED BREAST CARCINOMA

Pre-invasive breast cancer, ductal carcinoma *in situ* (DCIS) or, more rarely, lobular carcinoma *in situ*, can be recognized on mammography. Accordingly, a national breast cancer screening programme has been instituted in women between the ages of 50 and 64 who are encouraged to undergo bilateral mammography every 3 years. The characteristic mammographic appearances consist of clustered micro-calcifications or a solid density. The diagnosis of cancer can be established in more than 60% of women by fine needle aspiration (FNA) cytology performed under ultrasound or X-ray stereotactic control, although there is a false positivity rate of less than 1%.

When areas of ductal carcinoma *in situ* are recognized, the treatment is excision of the abnormal area which usually requires localization since these lesions are frequently impalpable. This involves the placing of a fine guide wire, under mammographic or ultrasonographic screening, into the abnormal area. At operation the wire is traced and the adjacent abnormal area excised with a wide margin. Conservative surgery is inappropriate in the presence of multifocal lesions when more than one quadrant of the breast is affected.

Axillary surgery is not required, or is at least limited to axillary node sampling, provided the tumour is under 10 mm in diameter. The benefit of postoperative radiotherapy is now established for ductal carcinoma *in situ* when the tumour exceeds 10 mm or is invasive. The value of tamoxifen in this situation in menopausal women is uncertain. Several randomized trials of patients offered screening in this age group have demonstrated a reduction in mortality from breast cancer of approximately 30%.

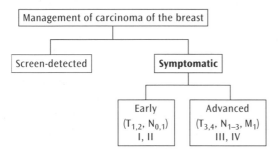

SYMPTOMATIC CARCINOMA

Clinical features

Breast carcinoma usually presents as a lump in the breast, although occasionally with discharge from the nipple. The disease should be suspected in all female patients aged above 25 years, in particular those above 40 years of age. Important risk factors are a family history in first-degree relatives, nulliparity, early menarche, late menopause, first pregnancy after the age of 35 years and a previous history of malignant breast disease. A causal link with the contraceptive pill and hormone replacement therapy is unclear.

Diagnosis

In over 95% of patients with breast cancer the diagnosis is established before operation by triple assessment: clinical examination, imaging and aspiration cytology or occasionally 'core' biopsy.

Clinical examination

The clinical features suggesting that a lump in the breast is malignant are signs of spread, either local infiltration or regional lymph node palpability, or evidence of more distant metastases.

The patient is first examined sitting up. Attachment of a lump to neighbouring tissues may produce asymmetry of the breast or of the level of the nipple relative to the opposite side. This becomes more obvious when the patient raises her arms above her head. Involvement of the skin is noted as dimpling, peau d'orange or ulceration, or by retraction or 'eczema' (injection and scaling) of the nipple. Palpation is carried out with the patient lying down (one pillow), turned 30° towards the contralateral side, and with her ipsilateral hand under her neck. This spreads the breast disc evenly over the chest wall which becomes horizontal in this position and reduces the thickness of the breast, thus facilitating the examination. Palpation is performed using the pulps of the fingers but with the clinician's hand and forearm horizontal. If a lump is found, its size and position are noted and it is tested for attachment to the skin and nipple, to pectoralis major as identified by reduction in the mobility of the mass when the patient contracts that muscle by pressing her hands on her hips, and to the chest wall in which case the lump cannot be moved relative to the chest wall. The axillae and neck are examined for lymph nodes, and evidence of metastatic spread is sought in the chest and abdomen.

A cautionary note about physical signs

- Signs of attachment do not necessarily mean that the lump is malignant. Infection can produce the same signs, both locally and in the lymph nodes
- Absence of signs of attachment does not necessarily mean that the lump is benign

---

The early case

Imaging

Imaging mammography is carried out in two planes and the opposite breast is also examined. The characteristic features of malignancy of a lump are increased opacity, irregular margins, micro-calcifications, spiculation, skin thickening and distortion. In pre-menopausal women, ultrasonography is a valuable adjunct and improves the sensitivity of the diagnosis. It is the primary investigation in women less than 35 years of age, or during pregnancy and lactation.

A chest X-ray is always required to exclude metastases. Bone radiography and isotope scanning are not performed routinely unless there is marked anaemia or leukopenia, the serum calcium or alkaline phosphatase are abnormal or the patient has symptoms suggestive of bone metastases.

Needle biopsy

Two types of needle biopsies are used pre-operatively to confirm the diagnosis of malignancy:

- *FNA cytology.* By the use of a fine needle, cells can be aspirated from a solid lump and submitted for cytological examination. This is a reliable method of diagnosis. However, the sample of cells must be sufficiently large in number for the cytologists to be able to provide an accurate diagnosis. Hence the diagnostic accuracy is graded between C_0 (insufficient cells obtained) to C_5 (definitely malignant).
- *Large needle biopsy (core biopsy).* In patients in whom there is a doubt about the diagnosis on aspiration cytology the procedure can easily be repeated, or a larger sample is obtained for histology by means of core biopsy by use of a large-bore needle such as a 'Tru-cut'.

Frozen section

This was a popular method of obtaining a diagnosis but has been superseded by the above. A biopsy is taken under general anaesthesia and is fixed by freezing. The pathologist examines the specimen while the patient is under anaesthesia and a definitive diagnosis is obtained. This enables the surgeon to proceed with the operative procedure without the need for waking the patient and therefore necessitating two operative procedures, provided that prior consent for definitive operation has been obtained.

Plan of management

Management is based on the clinical stage of the disease according to the size of the tumour (T), spread to the regional lymph nodes (N) and the presence or absence of metastases (M) as determined by triple assessment (Table 4.1). However, the accuracy of this approach is limited by difficulties in assessing axillary lymph nodes clinically.

Palpable lymph nodes

When the lymph nodes in the neck and supra-clavicular region are palpable, these are invariably involved by tumour and should be regarded as distant metastases. The possibility of a co-existent nodal disease, such as tuberculosis or lymphoma, is rare. However, lymph nodes palpable in the ipsilateral axilla do not constitute evidence of axillary node invasion by the tumour as their enlargement may be due to reactive hyperplasia. Clinical examination is inaccurate in determining axillary node involvement, with a false positive rate of 25% and a false negative rate of 30%. Therefore, palpability of axillary lymph nodes should not affect the choice of operative procedure unless the lymph nodes are large and fixed, indicative of advanced disease. Axillary sampling combined with

Table 4.1 *The UICC system*

Grade

I	A tumour 2 cm or less in size (T_1, N_0, M_0)
II	A tumour 5 cm or less in size plus mobile ipsilateral axillary nodes (T_2, N_1, M_0) or a tumour greater than 5 cm in size with no direct extension to skin or chest wall and no nodes (T_3, N_0, M_0)
III	The remainder (T_{0-4}, N_{0-3}, M_0) includes tumour of any size invading skin or chest wall (T_4) and mobile lymph nodes (N_1), fixed involved axillary lymph nodes (N_2) and supra-clavicular nodes (N_3)
IV	Supra-clavicular nodes and/or distant metastases (T_{0-4}, N_{0-3}, M_1)

excision of the primary tumour is an accurate method of determining nodal involvement and avoids the morbidity associated with axillary clearance in nearly two-thirds of patients without nodal involvement. However, axillary clearance provides a more accurate estimate of prognosis, which is related to the number of involved nodes, and obviates the need for radiotherapy of the axilla. More recently, sentinel node biopsy has been investigated. This is the first node containing lymphatic drainage from the tumours and can be recognized by injecting radioactive colloid particles around the primary tumour. Radiotherapy should be avoided after a clearance as the risk of lymphoedema of the rest of the arm is increased.

Scope of excision

The aim is to remove the primary tumour completely so that it does not recur locally and in order to prolong survival. There are two separate approaches, and the patient should be offered the choice provided certain criteria are met (Table 4.2).

Breast-conserving surgery is the treatment of choice for the majority of women presenting with Stage I and Stage II and certainly $T_{1,2}$, N_0, M_0, and removes the tumour with a margin of at least 2 cm of normal tissue (Fig. 4.1).

This procedure, known as *wide local excision* or *lumpectomy*, or *segmental resection* (or *quadrantectomy* if more extensive), needs to be followed by a course of radiotherapy to the residual breast tissue (Fig. 4.2). Without radiotherapy the local recurrence rate is unacceptably high, reaching 40%. Breast-conserving surgery is combined with axillary sampling or clearance which determines the extent of the involvement of the ipsilateral lymph nodes.

Mastectomy is particularly appropriate in patients with multiple breast cancers, large tumours in relatively small breasts and diffuse micro-calcification. This involves removing the entire breast (*simple mastectomy*) combined with removal of the ipsilateral axillary lymph nodes in continuity by full clearance of the axillary tissue up to the axillary vein (a *Patey modified radical mastectomy*), avoids the need for radiotherapy to the residual breast tissue but is mutilating and provides an unacceptable cosmetic result. In women who have had this procedure for localized early disease, breast reconstruction in the form of an

Table 4.2 *Indications for conservative surgery in breast cancer*

Tumour less than 5 cm in diameter
Lymph nodes either impalpable or mobile
No multi-focality on mammography
No extensive invasion of the overlying skin
Not involving the nipple/areola complex
The patient's choice

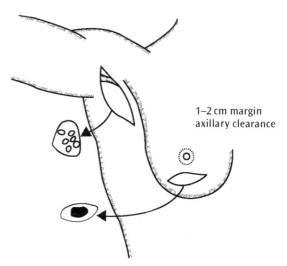

Fig. 4.1 *Operative procedure of wide local excision and axillary clearance of lymph nodes.*

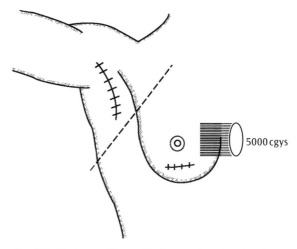

Fig. 4.2 *Post-operative radiotherapy in patients who have undergone wide excision and axillary clearance.*

implant or a myoplastic flap can be offered. This is performed either immediately or after an interval of about one year when it is apparent that the patient has not developed local recurrence.

After operation – adjuvant therapy

After adequate excision of the primary tumour there remains the possibility of micro-metastases, both locoregionally and systemically. This determines the long-term prognosis in the individual patient. Therefore, adjuvant therapy, in the form of radiotherapy, chemotherapy or hormonal therapy, is used selectively after surgery for early breast cancer in order to improve the outcome. Although there is still some controversy, the most commonly held views on adjuvant therapy following excision of the primary are summarized in the box below.

Adjuvant therapy after surgery in the individual case

- Pre-menopausal women with involved lymph nodes should receive a combination of cyclophosphamide, methotrexate and 5-fluorouracil (CMF)
- Post-menopausal women, irrespective of lymph node status are given tamoxifen for a minimum period of 2 years
- Pre-menopausal women (and all women aged under 40) whose lymph nodes are not involved, but whose primary tumours are poorly differentiated may also benefit from adjuvant chemotherapy
- Pre-menopausal women who have oestrogen receptor-positive tumours may also benefit from tamoxifen, particularly if the primary tumour is poorly differentiated
- Chemotherapy is also prescribed to post-menopausal patients with ER-negative tumours and positive axillary nodes
- Patients with positive lymph nodes after sampling of the axilla, rather than clearance, should receive radiotherapy to the axilla
- After lumpectomy or quadrantectomy and axillary clearance, whole-breast radiotherapy reduces the incidence of local recurrence

---

Follow-up

The cost-effectiveness of follow-up after treatment is debatable because between 75% and 95% of recurrences are detected by the patient. Although regular mammography is advocated after breast conservation surgery, there is no evidence that this improves outcome.

Prognosis

Seventy per cent of women presenting with breast cancer can expect to survive for 10 years. Prognosis is strongly related to the extent of spread of the tumour at presentation. Ten-year survival is about 80% in the early case, about 55% in advanced cases. The risk of a woman dying from breast cancer increases with age. In England and Wales, it is one in 2873 in the decade 25–34 years and rises steadily through one in 474, one in 136, one in 65 and one in 39 in succeeding decades to reach one in 26 in women aged 75–84 years.

ADVANCED DISEASE

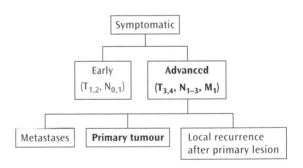

Advanced cases may be considered under three headings:

- Patients with a primary breast tumour.
- Patients with local recurrences after excision of a primary tumour.
- Patients with metastases either at presentation or after treatment of the primary tumour.

In advanced breast cancer, the objective of treatment is palliation to improve the quality of life.

The primary tumour

The disease is considered advanced either because the primary tumour is associated with lymph node or widespread metastases or because the primary tumour is bulky or fixed to skin or deeper structures, or has features suggestive of inflammation. The purpose in dealing with the breast lump is to prevent progression of the tumour with its unpleasant side-effects. When neglected, the growth ulcerates through the skin and produces a malodorous discharge. Skin infiltration results in a hard plaque of tissue, the *cancer en cuirasse*, which causes pain and even restricts breathing.

Therefore, when resectable, local excision or toilet mastectomy for palliation of symptoms is performed. Otherwise, radiotherapy in conjunction with chemotherapy or tamoxifen, in post-menopausal women in particular, can have dramatic effect, improves the chance of resectability at a later stage, and is of benefit for residual disease after local treatment. The particularly aggressive inflammatory type is treated with chemotherapy only. The lymph nodes are managed as described later.

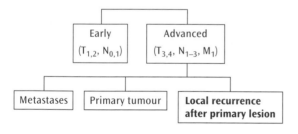

Local recurrence

The incomplete removal of a primary breast tumour may result in the appearance of one or more nodules of tumour in the skin flaps, near the scar of the incision. A solitary nodule is excised and its histological nature confirmed. If there are several nodules, histological confirmation is obtained by FNA cytology, Tru-cut or open biopsy of one of these lesions. The area of recurrence is treated with radiotherapy, or radical local excision combined with a skin graft may be feasible. Should surgery or radiotherapy fail, or when radiotherapy is not feasible because previous radiotherapy for the primary has used up skin

tolerance, or in the presence of metastases in other sites, systemic chemotherapy or tamoxifen is an option.

Although local recurrence does not necessarily imply incurability, the prognosis is adversely affected in statistical terms as many patients develop visceral metastases within 2 years.

Regional lymph nodes

Regional lymph nodes that are fixed by malignant infiltration into the surrounding tissues cause brachial plexus neuropathy and lymphoedema, which are features of advanced disease associated either with the primary breast cancer or with nodal disease presenting as a recurrence after treatment of the primary tumour.

The patient with a primary breast cancer and palpable large and fixed axillary lymph nodes requires a biopsy of the affected lymph nodes for histological confirmation, followed by radiotherapy and some form of resection of the primary depending on its stage. The same applies to patients with a primary breast tumour and supraclavicular lymph node involvement.

Occasionally a patient presents with a primary breast tumour and palpable nodes in the *opposite* axilla. Although this is usually interpreted as a sign of advanced metastatic disease, biopsy usually reveals that the enlargement of the nodes is due to reactive hyperplasia. The appearance of recurrence in the regional lymph nodes after previous treatment of the primary breast cancer is managed as already described. However, if the initial treatment did not include treatment to the axilla then axillary clearance is carried out, or else radiotherapy if the nodes are irresectable because of their size or fixity.

A rare presentation is the patient with a palpable axillary lymph node which, on biopsy, shows invasion with carcinoma which on histological grounds is likely to have originated in the breast. In the absence of physical signs in the breast, mastectomy requires great courage on the part of the surgeon and faith on the part of the patient, but this approach, together with some form of treatment to the axilla, is the conventional advice. With the advent of mammography and ultrasonography, it is most unlikely that a small primary tumour in the breast would be missed, and it is wiser, if imaging were negative, to wait and re-examine frequently.

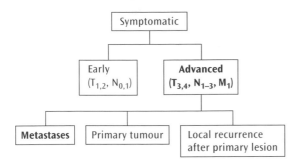

Distant metastases

It is essential to recognize the salient features that should alert the clinician to metastatic disease. Pain is commonly due to bone metastases, disease in lymph nodes, soft tissue and liver. Dyspnoea, chest pain and cough are produced by pleural effusion or lung metastases. Patients with anaemia due to bone marrow infiltration may also present with breathlessness. Nausea and vomiting can be induced by drugs or radiation, but also by hypercalcaemia, liver or brain metastases and ascites. Abdominal distension due to ascites or intestinal obstruction by tumour, a palpable liver or jaundice suggest intra-abdominal spread. Anorexia, weight loss and lethargy indicate progressive disease.

Principles

First, the management of distant metastases must not overshadow the management of the primary tumour, because the symptoms produced by an uncontrolled primary loom large in the wide spectrum of morbidity produced by the disease. Second, the presence of distant metastases does not in itself constitute an indication for treatment unless symptomatic or progressing so rapidly that death is early unless the rate of progress is reduced. Third, if the metastases requiring treatment are solitary or localized then local treatment is used in the first instance because it has a higher success rate than systemic treatment.

Local treatment

The options are varied and are influenced by symptoms and sites of metastatic disease and should take into account the patient's age and performance status, as invasive procedures may be required. These local therapeutic modalities are described under the special problems commonly seen in advanced breast cancer.

Systemic therapy

Endocrine therapy. About 30–50% of patients show a response to endocrine manipulation that may last for several years. Breast cancer, like normal tissue cells, may have binding capacity for oestrogen through protein receptor sites, which can be measured in tissue obtained from the excised tumour. The response rate for oestrogen-positive tumours is higher (60%) than the 20% rate in oestrogen receptor-negative patients.

All drugs in use interfere with the metabolism or action of oestrogen and other related steroids. The choice of drugs depends on the menopausal status of the patient. Should the patient relapse after an initial response, she is likely to respond to second-line drugs.

Tamoxifen is an anti-oestrogen which acts on the anti-oestrogen receptor and probably has a direct cytotoxic-like effect since some oestrogen receptor-negative women also benefit from the drug.

Aminoglutethimide, an aromatase inhibitor, diminishes steroid production and thyroxine synthesis, and several other similar drugs, such as anastrazole (Arimidex) are under investigation for treatment of metastatic breast cancer.

Ovarian ablation can be effected by surgery, radiotherapy or LHRH analogues. It is only an option for pre-menopausal women. Patients with mild or moderate symptoms who developed metastatic disease after a long disease-free interval and had an oestrogen receptor-positive tumour are particularly suitable for endocrine therapy.

Chemotherapy

Nearly 59% of women with metastatic breast cancer respond to chemotherapy with a median disease-free survival of 1 year and an overall median survival of 18–24 months.

Various chemotherapy regimens are now available. The most effective drugs are combinations of cyclophosphamide, methotrexate and 5-fluorouracil or mitomycin C, doxorubicin, methotrexate and mitozantrone. The cyclophosphamide/methotrexate/5-fluorouracil (CMF) regimen is widely used and well-tolerated. Response rates for different regimens are similar. The choice should therefore depend on toxicity, the side-effects and quality of life during treatment.

Chemotherapy is indicated in patients with severe symptoms who have failed to respond to endocrine therapy, who had a poorly differentiated or an oestrogen receptor-negative tumour.

Radiotherapy

This provides effective palliation of symptoms from local disease, in short courses with minimal side-effects, provided the tolerance of tissues is not exceeded. However, radiotherapy has no impact on survival. The place of radiotherapy in the spectrum of metastatic disease will be described.

Special problems

Bone metastases

Approximately 70% of patients develop bone metastases, causing pain and functional impairment, pathological fractures, spinal cord compression, hypercalcaemia and infiltration of the bone marrow. If the disease is confined to the skeleton without spread to other sites, the survival is often several years.

Local radiotherapy achieves a complete symptomatic response in nearly half of patients. For fractures or impending fractures of the long bones, which may occur after trivial injury without any preceding signs, internal fixation is indicated provided that the life expectancy is not short. Post-operative radiotherapy to the involved bone promotes healing and stabilizes the prosthesis.

Cancer-induced hypercalcaemia

This may complicate extensive skeletal metastases and should be suspected in these patients should they develop nausea, vomiting, constipation, confusion, polyuria and extra-cellular depletion which may be complicated by renal failure and coma. Blood electrolytes, creatinine and urea are therefore monitored along with calcium levels. Patients should be treated promptly with intravenous fluids, and with biphosphonates after rehydration. Alternative treatment is with calcitonin, gallium nitrate or forced diuresis with frusemide.

Chest metastases

Pulmonary metastases affect 60% of patients with metastatic disease. In most cases the disease is widespread and requires systemic therapy. A chest X-ray is adequate for demonstrating pulmonary spread, but computerized tomography (CT) is more sensitive in detecting small deposits and involvement of intestinal lymph nodes.

Pleural effusions respond well to systemic therapy. Aspiration of the fluid with instillation of sclerosing agents such as bleomycin or tetracycline may be required to control dyspnoea and pain. Pleurectomy, or pleurodesis by instillation of talc, is a better and more effective treatment but because of associated morbidity it is recommended after the failure of conventional treatment.

Malignant pericardial effusions are rare but occur more commonly in patients with bilateral pleural effusions and present with the symptoms and signs of cardiac tamponade. The chest X-ray and electrocardiogram show typical changes. Percutaneous drainage under ultrasound control is effective, but the liquid rapidly reaccumulates so pericardiectomy is justifiable if the patient is fit and the metastatic disease is not advanced or terminal.

Liver and peritoneum

Liver metastases are usually diffuse and are treated by chemotherapy. When associated with jaundice, the possibility of bile duct obstruction by affected lymph nodes should be investigated by ultrasonography or CT scanning, since endoscopic placement of a stent relieves the jaundice and improves symptoms.

Malignant ascites is treated by repeated aspiration or a permanent indwelling peritoneal catheter

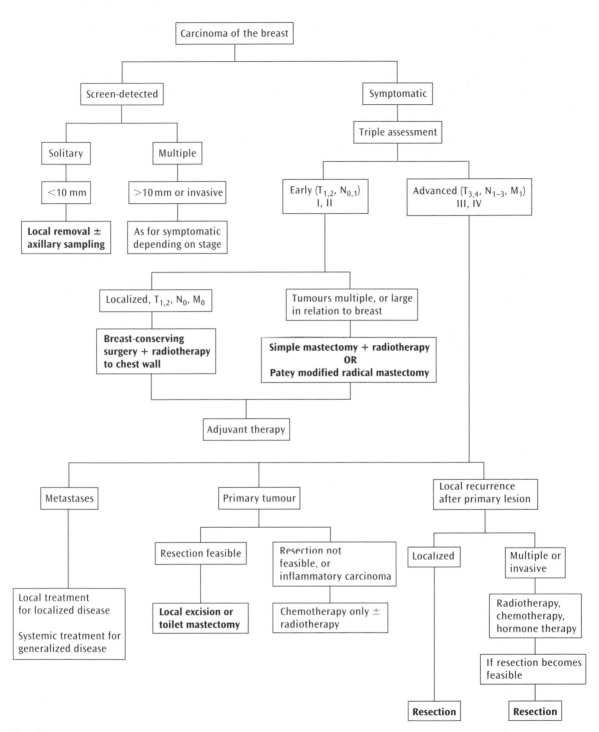

Algorithm 4.1

connected to a closed system to allow intermittent drainage. Large quantities of ascitic fluid should be drained slowly and some of the volume replaced with intravenous dextran to avoid embarrassing the circulation. In patients with limited disease but uncontrollable ascites, the fluid is drained from the peritoneal cavity into the circulation via the internal jugular vein using a specially designed shunt system (Le Veen or Denver shunts). However, a large proportion of shunts block, some patients with functioning shunts develop disseminated intravascular coagulopathy, and tumour embolism occurs in a very few.

Central nervous system

Brain metastases occur in 20% of patients with an overall median survival of 6 months. Patients with controlled systemic disease, minimal neurological symptoms or a solitary metastasis as demonstrated on a CT scan are treated with corticosteroids and local radiotherapy to the whole brain with symptomatic control in 80% of patients. Excision of a solitary deposit is considered in selected cases. Chemotherapy can be added or used instead of intensive radiotherapy, particularly in patients with systemic disease.

Breast cancer spreads to the meninges, and this should be considered in patients with neurological symptoms and signs. CSF cytology is diagnostic. CT and magnetic resonance imaging (MRI) can be normal but may show diffuse or irregular thickening of the meninges. Treatment consists of the intra-thecal administration of methotrexate or thiotepa combined with radiotherapy to areas of macroscopic tumour deposit identified by CT scan. Neurological deficits are irreversible, but survival is prolonged. The results are improved if treatment is administered before neurological defects are evident.

Spinal cord compression

Bone metastases in the spine causing a pathological fracture with pressure on the cord should be suspected in patients with backache, lower limb weakness, sensory loss and sphincter malfunction. The thoracic spine is most frequently affected. The diagnosis is confirmed by a myelogram or MRI. The latter is favoured because it is accurate and non-invasive. Treatment is by high-dose steroids and radiotherapy. Decompressive surgery is recommended for patients with an unstable spine or those whose symptoms progress despite radiotherapy. Prompt treatment before neurological deficits become manifest improves the outcome.

HIGHLIGHTS

- In metastatic breast cancer, the median survival is 18–24 months, the 3-year survival 20–30%
- The treatment is palliative, to control symptoms, improve quality of life and prolong survival
- Endocrine therapy achieves a response in 30–50% of patients
- Response to chemotherapy occurs in 50–60% of patients
- Radiotherapy provides symptomatic control for loco-regional recurrence, spinal cord compression, bone and brain metastases
- Surgery is required for pathological fractures of long bones, loco-regional recurrence, cardiac tamponade, solitary brain metastasis and spinal cord compression

Dysphagia

JOHN H WYLLIE

Dysphagia is difficulty in swallowing and is characteristic of oesophageal disease. Patients often do not understand the symptom and complain of 'vomiting' when they mean regurgitation – food sticks in the oesophagus and is finally rejected; careful history-taking is therefore essential. The causes are several (see Fig. 5.1). Initially it is important to distinguish whether the difficulty in swallowing is *pharyngeal*, that is, difficulty in getting the food to leave the mouth, or *oesophageal*, that is, food is swallowed but sticks in the oesophagus. The onset of dysphagia and other accompanying symptoms aid diagnosis and determine the urgency of investigation.

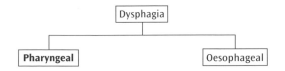

PHARYNGEAL DYSPHAGIA

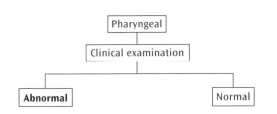

A patient with pharyngeal dysphagia has difficulty in forcing a food bolus from the mouth into the gullet. Examination, initially with a spatula, will rule out common inflammatory causes of dysphagia due to pain. *Pharyngitis* is identified and treated with antibiotics. A *peri-tonsillar abscess* presents as a bulge in the region of the fauces. Urgent drainage is needed, with care because the carotid artery, jugular vein and vagus nerve lie adjacent. Conventionally, drainage is carried out under local anaesthesia because of the risk of the abscess bursting and spilling pus into the lungs during intubation.

The 'water test' is the next simple diagnostic test. Some patients with pharyngeal dysphagia, when given water to drink, choke and cough because of spill-over into the larynx and down the trachea. (This symptom can also be caused by a tracheo-oesophageal fistula.) In contrast, patients with an obstruction in the oesophagus take a few sips before they feel uncomfortable, and regurgitate but do not cough.

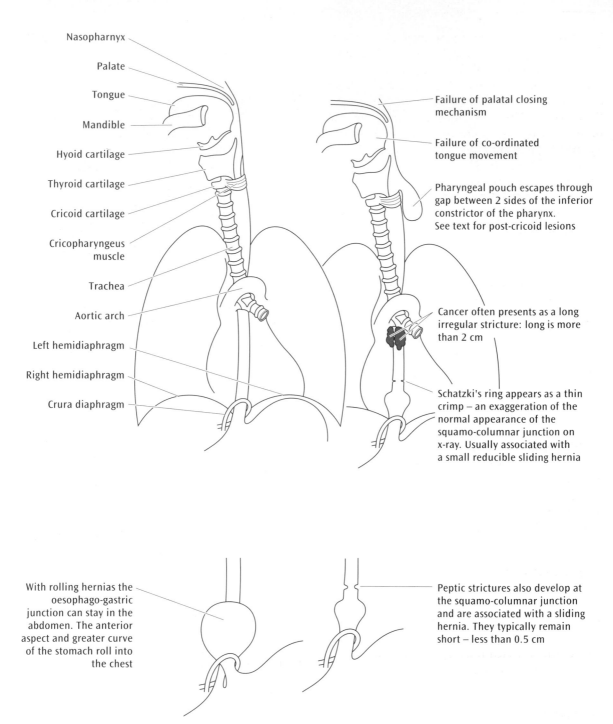

Nasopharynx

Palate

Tongue

Mandible

Hyoid cartilage

Thyroid cartilage

Cricoid cartilage

Cricopharyngeus
muscle

Trachea

Aortic arch

Left hemidiaphragm

Right hemidiaphragm

Crura diaphragm

Failure of palatal closing
mechanism

Failure of co-ordinated
tongue movement

Pharyngeal pouch escapes through
gap between 2 sides of the inferior
constrictor of the pharynx.
See text for post-cricoid lesions

Cancer often presents as a long
irregular stricture: long is more
than 2 cm

Schatzki's ring appears as a thin
crimp – an exaggeration of the
normal appearance of the
squamo-columnar junction on
x-ray. Usually associated with
a small reducible sliding hernia

With rolling hernias the
oesophago-gastric
junction can stay in the
abdomen. The anterior
aspect and greater curve
of the stomach roll into
the chest

Peptic strictures also develop at
the squamo-columnar junction
and are associated with a sliding
hernia. They typically remain
short – less than 0.5 cm

Fig. 5.1 *Causes of dysphagia: on the left, the principal anatomical landmarks; on the right, some causes of dysphagia.*

Water coming back out of the nose is diagnostic of failure of the *palatal closing mechanism*. This could be due to an anatomical abnormality, visible with a spatula, but usually there is a neuromuscular lesion such as bulbar palsy, pseudobulbar palsy or myasthenia gravis. Therefore the cranial and peripheral nerves should be examined. If there is no obvious abnormality it is important to appreciate that nasal reflux can result from impaired pharyngeal or palatal movement caused by underlying pathology, such as a tumour infiltrating the posterior pharyngeal wall, which might not be recognizable without biopsy and histology.

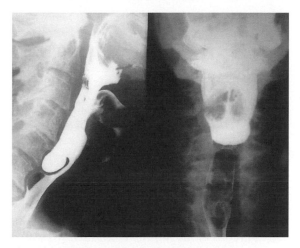

Fig. 5.2 *Barium swallow (with patient erect) showing a pharyngeal pouch. The lateral view on the left was taken during the act of swallowing. It shows how the direct path for a food bolus leads to the bottom of the pouch. The antero-posterior view shows how a half-moon shaped puddle of barium persists in the mouth after the swallow is complete.*

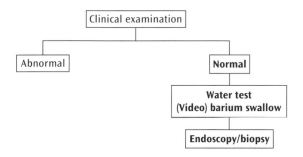

Other causes of pharyngeal dysphagia are the *tongue syndrome, pharyngeal pouch, cricopharyngeal bar, post-cricoid cancer* and *oesophageal webs*. These are diagnosed on a barium swallow, and best demonstrated on lateral views, particularly if continuous video-recording is employed.

Tongue syndrome

After a stroke patients often show this syndrome, in which repeated rapid attempts to swallow a bolus of food fail to launch it off the back of the tongue. This can be demonstrated radiologically with a piece of bread soaked in barium.

Pharyngeal pouch (Zenker's diverticulum)

The pouch appears immediately above the cricopharyngeus, through a divarication of the left and right halves of the inferior constrictor muscles.

A swallowed bolus lodges in the pouch and finds its way into the oesophagus only by overflowing. As the pouch enlarges, food is regurgitated, and during sleep, material is aspirated into the lungs causing recurrent chest infection. There is a risk of passing an endoscope into a pharyngeal pouch resulting in its perforation and mediastinitis. It is for this reason that a barium study should precede endoscopy in all cases of dysphagia (Fig. 5.2).

Pouches enlarge progressively so should be treated surgically. They are approached from the neck or through the mouth. *From the neck*, the pouch is exposed on the left side where it is usually situated and its lower margin is located, sharply demarcated by the cricopharyngeus muscle. The pouch is excised above, and the mucosa and muscle are closed by suturing or with a linear stapling instrument. It is recommended that the cricopharyngeal sphincter muscle is divided as part of the procedure, but its benefit is doubtful. *From the mouth*, in Dolmen's operation, the partition between the pouch and the proximal oesophagus is divided. This divides the cricopharyngeus, enlarges the opening from the pouch into the oesophagus, but does not remove any of the pouch.

Cricopharyngeal bar

The cricopharyngeus muscle is normally contracted except for brief relaxations during acts of swallowing. The appearance of a cricopharyngeal bar is seen in lateral view as a constant, smooth indentation into the back of the oesophagus at its junction with the pharynx (Fig. 5.3). In severe cases patients are unable to swallow solids and can only sip liquids. The pathology is a myopathy confined to the cricopharyngeus, with partial fibrosis of the muscle. When stretched with a bougie or balloon the symptoms are usually cured, but if dilatation fails, dividing the muscle is curative. This condition is probably under-diagnosed.

Post-cricoid cancer

The diagnosis is sometimes difficult and there is a danger that patients are thought to be hysterical (p. 76). The typical appearance of a ragged stricture is shown in Fig. 5.4, but barium swallow may appear normal. Fibreoptic endoscopy is unsatisfactory because contraction of the cricopharyngeus muscle prevents adequate visualization of this part of the oesophagus. A rigid oesophagoscope or pharyngoscope is preferable but can still fail to detect a submucosal cancer. Deep biopsies may be needed to prove the diagnosis. Treatment is usually with chemoradiotherapy; if this fails, pharyngolaryngectomy can be curative.

Webs

A web appears in a barium swallow as a thin shelf projecting into the lumen of the upper oesophagus (Fig. 5.5). Some are circumferential and so identifiable on anteroposterior (AP) as well as lateral X-ray films. Often, there are two or even three, spaced about a centimetre apart in the upper oesophagus. Occasionally, the mucosa between webs appears irregular and the appearance is then indistinguishable from cancer.

It is claimed that webs are associated with iron-deficiency anaemia and glossitis; the combination

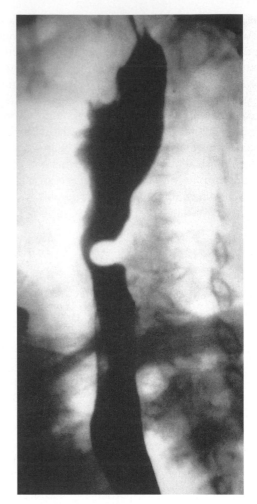

Fig. 5.3 *Cricopharyngeal bar shown on video swallow. The thumb-print impression represents the cricopharyngeus muscle; it is abnormal because this frame shows the widest channel during a swallowing sequence. Normally the muscle relaxes and the channel opens momentarily to the full bore of the oesophagus.*

is known as the Plummer–Vinson (or Patterson–Brown–Kelly) syndrome. It is doubtful whether such a syndrome exists. The comment on Vinson's original presentation in 1921 was, 'This is a very unusual picture. Outside of the Rochester Clinic, there are no other people in medicine today who have found the syndrome.' This is still true. However, webs are very common and their pathology is obscure. Instrumental dilatation relieves dysphagia. Repeated biopsies may be necessary to exclude cancer.

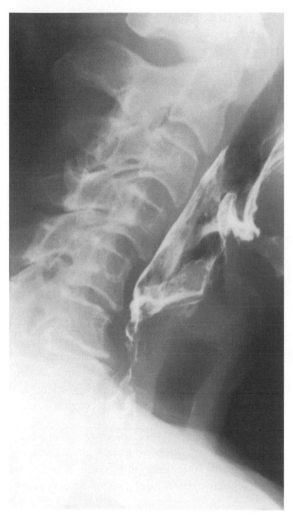

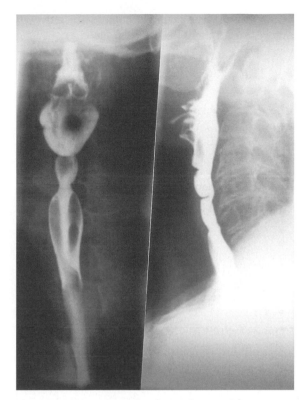

Fig. 5.5 *An oesophageal web seen in anterior-posterior and lateral views.*

Fig. 5.4 *Post-cricoid cancer. In addition to the irregular stricture, notice the soft tissue mass between the barium in the upper oesophagus and the air in the upper trachea.*

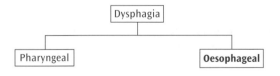

OESOPHAGEAL DYSPHAGIA

The patient with oesophageal dysphagia is able to pass food into the oesophagus, but senses that the food bolus is not progressing and is stuck. When the block is total (*complete dysphagia*) the patient can swallow neither food nor drink, and even saliva has to be spat out.

Difficulty in swallowing solids means there is physical narrowing – an organic stricture – but if liquids also go down slowly, this suggests spasm of the lower oesophageal sphincter.

Impaction of a bolus of solid food at an organic stricture also blocks the passage to liquid which is regurgitated; this requires immediate treatment because of the risk of aspiration pneumonia. Besides, swallowed objects (typically false teeth), if not promptly removed, will erode through the wall of the oesophagus.

These patients are investigated by barium swallow and fibreoptic endoscopy, supplemented by computerized tomography (CT) scans and endoluminal ultrasonography when appropriate.

Absence of demonstrable obstruction on endoscopy suggests oesophageal dysmotility, which is often studied by oesophageal manometry, although the diagnosis should be clear from video-barium swallow.

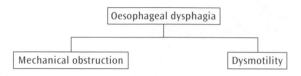

Causes of oesophageal dysphagia

Mechanical obstruction:

- Gastro-oesophageal reflux, peptic oesophagitis, peptic stricture
- Schatzki's ring
- Strictures due to pills, corrosives and nasogastric tubes
- Cancer
- Candida and herpes oesophagitis

Dysmotility:

- Achalasia
- Systemic sclerosis
- Pseudodysphagia
- Globus hystericus

GASTRO-OESOPHAGEAL REFLUX, OESOPHAGITIS AND PEPTIC STRICTURE

Oesophageal pH recording shows that, in normal people, acid in the stomach intermittently refluxes up the oesophagus, especially at night. When acid reflux is excessive, it damages the oesophageal lining causing *oesophagitis*.

At the lower end of the oesophagus there is a physiological sphincter whose activity is co-ordinated by the vagus nerve. This sphincter prevents reflux of stomach contents into the oesophagus. It is aided by anatomical mechanisms: the acute angle of entry of the oesophagus into the stomach; the presence of a length of intra-abdominal oesophagus which is occluded by the effect of the intra-abdominal pressure; and the contraction of the diaphragmatic crura.

Pathological gastro-oesophageal reflux is usually associated with *hiatal hernia* of the *sliding type*. Like other hernias, they are reducible. They may only be found on provocation by (i) barium swallow with the patient supine 15 degrees head-down and lifting the legs just clear of the table, or standing up and touching the toes, or (ii) endoscopy, when a well-inflated stomach allows a view of the gastro-oesophageal junction including the impression made by the crura of the diaphragm. About 10% of hiatal hernias are of the *para-oesophageal* or *rolling type* (Fig. 5.1). They can become very large, with half the stomach in the chest, upside down. Although they may cause dysphagia, they more often present with bizarre symptoms or anaemia.

The oesophagus is lined with squamous epithelium, apart from the last two centimetres above the stomach; the squamo-columnar junction is an abrupt change to glandular epithelium, clearly visible on endoscopy. It is the squamous, not the columnar epithelium which is damaged by extensive gastro-oesophageal reflux, and the damage is always worst near the squamo-columnar junction where exposure to gastric juice is greatest. Superficial loss of the squamous mucosa leads to bleeding, ulceration and slough formation (Fig. 5.6), submucosal oedema and eventually fibrosis and stricture formation causing dysphagia (Fig. 5.7).

Long-continued reflux produces metaplastic change of the squamous mucosa which is replaced by columnar epithelium so the squamous-columnar junction migrates up the oesophagus. This is *Barrett's columnar-lined oesophagus*. Perhaps it provides a

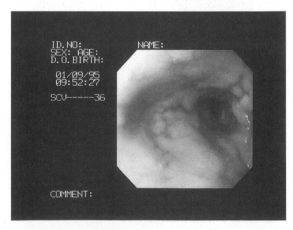

Fig. 5.6 *Severe oesophagitis.*

natural defence against reflux because columnar lining resists acid, pepsin and bile; but if it ulcerates, the ulcer is deep like a gastric ulcer. It may bleed, causing anaemia or haematemesis, and it may penetrate a lung or even the aorta. It heals by fibrosis causing a stricture. Besides, the columnar-lined oesophagus is much more prone to cancer than normal.

The patient with oesophagitis experiences a burning retro-sternal pain on drinking hot liquids, solutions with high potassium content (e.g., pineapple juice) or concentrated alcohol. Symptoms of reflux are also precipitated when bending and when lying down during sleep. When a stricture develops, the

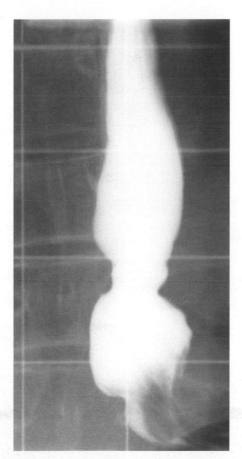

Fig. 5.7 *Stricture at the squamo-columnar junction of the oesophagus demonstrated by drinking barium while head-down. This distends the normal oesophagus and shows, by reference to the 2-cm grid behind the patient, that the stricture is about 8.5 mm bore and less than 10 mm long, favouring a benign stricture.*

patient soon finds swallowing difficult and modifies his diet, regressing to liquidized food. Pain from the oesophagus is referred like other visceral pain, to the surface of the body in a way that gives little indication of the level of the lesion. Thus, pain from the lower oesophagus may be felt at the sternal notch or it may be referred to the neck or arm and easily mistaken for angina. If the pain goes through to the back, a trans-mural lesion should be suspected.

Treatment

Many patients are successfully treated for dyspepsia by general practitioners without investigation. It may not matter whether the symptoms were due to oesophagitis or duodenal ulcer as treatment with H_2 antagonists, proton-pump inhibitors or triple therapy for *Helicobacter pylori* are equally effective for both conditions.

Oesophagitis heals and strictures resolve or improve if acid reflux is reduced to a tolerable level. Useful measures are:

- *Reducing reflux.* Losing weight and stopping smoking are valuable long-term measures.
- *Antacids, barrier agents.* Corrosion of the oesophageal mucosa can be reduced by swallowed antacids, especially when combined with surface-coating agents such as alginates.
- *Reducing acid (and pepsin) production.* Histamine H_2-receptor antagonists are effective but proton pump inhibitors are even more effective. These drugs reduce both volume and corrosiveness of gastric juice, but do not prevent reflux so the risk of aspiration pneumonia remains. Strictures improve because most, like Fig. 5.7, are inflammatory and not fibrous.
- *Improving motility.* Prokinetic agents, such as metaclopramide and cisapride, are claimed to enhance oesophageal peristalsis and gastric emptying and improve the tone of the oesophageal sphincter.
- *Surgery.* Many patients need perpetual drug treatment to keep them comfortable so there is a swing back to surgery now that a laparoscopic approach is available. Operations aim to reduce

reflux without altering the quality of the gastric juice, so medical and surgical treatments complement each other. The principle of the common Nissen operation is shown in Fig. 5.8. This can be done either at open operation or by laparoscopy. Anti-reflux procedures may limit the progression of Barrett's epithelium and reduce the risk of cancer.

- *Dilatation of strictures.* Despite full doses of a proton pump inhibitor, dysphagia may persist. Dilatation under sedation, using endoscopic balloons or bougies, is the next option. The measured effect of dilatation is modest, often only a 2 mm increase in bore of the stricture. Nevertheless, a small increase in diameter is clinically significant. If, however, gastric reflux continues, the stricture will recur, so repeated dilatations may be

required – alternatively, an anti-reflux procedure is considered in the fit patient. Rare intractable fibrotic strictures may require resection, but a safer option in elderly patients is the endoscopic placement of an indwelling tube.

SCHATZKI'S RING

The history is pathognomonic. The patient experiences sudden and total dysphagia, relieved once the food bolus is regurgitated. Such episodes of dysphagia recur at long intervals during which swallowing is completely normal and the patient is symptomless. Schatzki ascribed the symptoms to thin, web-like rings (1–2 mm) just above the oesophago-gastric junction, that can only be demonstrated when viewed perpendicular to the X-ray beam (Fig. 5.9). They are difficult to see on endoscopy. It seems that they correspond to the squamo-columnar

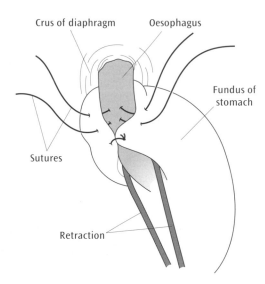

Fig. 5.8 *Nissen's fundal plication. The sliding hernia is reduced by traction. The fundus of the stomach is wrapped around the abdominal oesophagus and is held in place by stitches which pick up the oesophagus but do not penetrate the lumen. If the cuff of stomach so formed is too tight, intractable dysphagia follows; and if it is too slack, more stomach can herniate at the back causing an hour-glass constriction of the stomach. Several variations of this operation have been described, suggesting none is totally reliable.*

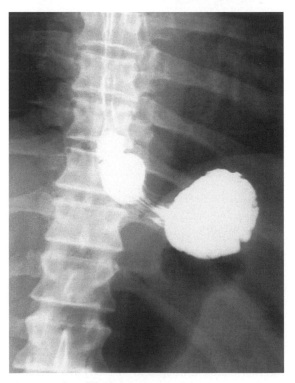

Fig. 5.9 *Schatzki's ring.*

junction which is normally just visible as a slight crimp in the outline of the oesophagus in a barium study. A small hiatal hernia is often present, so Schatzki's rings are regarded as a mild type of benign peptic stricture. Certainly some develop into typical benign strictures.

PILL STRICTURES

These are probably more common than is recognized, and can occur in patients with a normal oesophagus, but are more likely to develop if there is a pre-existing abnormality. A tablet or a sugar-coated pill lodges in the oesophagus (Fig. 5.10). Perhaps the patient is elderly and has poor peristalsis or the patient swallows the tablet while lying down in bed with insufficient water to wash it down. The sugar coating dissolves, exposing pure compound which damages the mucosa. This causes subsequent tablets to stick in the same area and repeat the injury. The result is a tight stricture. Measures recommended for other types of stricture are unnecessary and futile. The patient should be made to grind the tablets before taking them, and to wash them down with lots of water. Alternatively, a liquid formulation is prescribed instead. With this approach, these strictures resolve spontaneously.

Possible causes of pill strictures

- Several varieties of tetracyclines
- Iron salts
- Potassium chloride, and diuretics compounded with it
- Alprenolol (and possibly other β-blockers)
- Ibuprofen and other NSAIDs (including aspirin), quinidine, and zidovudine

NB. This is not an exhaustive list.

CANDIDA AND HERPES OESOPHAGITIS

Colonization of oesophageal mucosa with candida can be gross (Fig. 5.11) without involvement of the mouth. Candida is liable to overgrow other oesophageal flora when antibiotics are given. Apart from this, established mould is associated with a failure of immunity. The most common identifiable cause is local suppression by steroid insufflation for asthma. Other causes include: cancer chemotherapy; immune suppression after organ transplantation; and AIDS, and rarely, oesophageal diverticulosis, a condition in which there are numerous minute pouches in which the mould shelters. The patient complains of pain on swallowing, and the diagnosis is usually a surprise to the endoscopist. Treatment involves courses

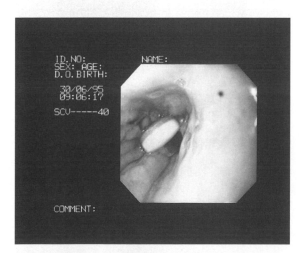

Fig. 5.10 *Endoscopic appearances of a pill arrested in the lower oesophagus.*

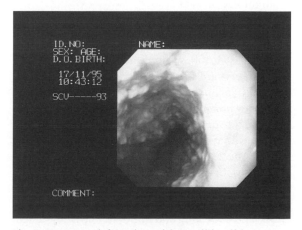

Fig. 5.11 *Severe infestation with* Candida albicans.

of topical antifungal agents, for example nystatin suspension. Recurrence is likely unless the predisposing factors are eliminated.

Herpes simplex virus infects the oesophagus under the same conditions which favour the growth of candida, and the two conditions may co-exist. Symptoms are similar. The endoscopic appearance is of clusters of tiny vesicles, punched-out ulcers with red margins or confluent erosive oesophagitis. Histology and cytology of mucosal biopsies show characteristic features. Treatment is with acyclovir.

CORROSIVE STRICTURES AND NASOGASTRIC TUBE STRICTURES

In the UK, suicide by drinking sodium or potassium hydroxide (*lye*) or other chemicals is not popular. Accidents do occur, however, as for example ingestion of a chemical descaling agent used to clean a kettle or teapot that has not been washed out before serving. Damage to the oesophagus is instant. In the immediate management:

- If the airway is compromised, establishing the airway requires endotracheal intubation or tracheostomy because of laryngeal oedema.
- Oral intake is withheld and intravenous fluids, analgesics and antibiotics, including metronidazole and nystatin or other antifungal agents, are administered.
- Steroids are also prescribed in large doses, to minimize fibrosis.
- Endoscopy is deferred for at least one week until the acute inflammation has subsided.

Nasogastric tubes, commonly placed after abdominal surgery, are usually innocuous. Rarely, after a few days (or longer) ulceration of the oesophagus occurs and a long stricture, which can be very troublesome, ensues. The cause is unknown. One suggestion is that the tube splints the cardia and allows reflux. Another is that the material of the tube is irritant to the oesophagus and causes damage in susceptible people.

Strictures caused by corrosives or nasogastric tubes tend to be long and multiple. The whole length of the oesophagus may be involved. The extent of the damage may be better shown by radio-contrast swallow (Omnipaque 300) than by endoscopy (Fig. 5.12). Managing those who survive the acute insult can be difficult. If they cannot swallow a liquid diet, they need a feeding gastrostomy. This may have to be placed by surgery rather than endoscopy because of difficulty in passing the endoscope through the stricture. Otherwise, the oesophagus is dilated regularly to improve swallowing, but 40% of such patients ultimately require oesophageal replacement by gastric or colonic transposition, although with lye the stomach may be damaged as well and may not be suitable for translocation to the chest (*see* section on cancer).

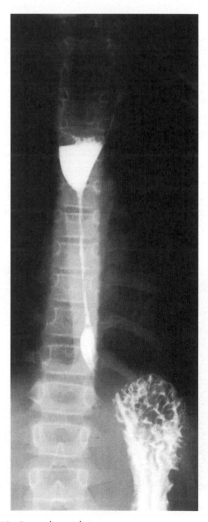

Fig. 5.12 *Corrosive stricture.*

MALIGNANT STRICTURE: SQUAMOUS CARCINOMA, ADENOCARCINOMA, EXTRINSIC PRESSURE

Squamous carcinomas arise from the squamous mucosal lining down to the squamo-columnar junction. *Adenocarcinomas* develop in columnar-lined oesophagus, especially in Barrett's columnar lining. Squamous tumours are becoming less, and adenocarcinomas more, common.

The history is often so ominous that the diagnosis is scarcely in doubt, even before investigation. The patient, who was previously asymptomatic, develops progressive dysphagia and within a few weeks can only swallow liquids. This rapid deterioration is because dysphagia is not perceptible until the bore of the oesophagus is reduced below 12 mm, and this does not occur until the tumour has encircled two-thirds of the oesophageal lumen. The patient is therefore asymptomatic until late. This is the main reason for the poor results of treatment.

Physical examination is usually unrewarding, but the neck should be examined for enlarged lymph nodes and the abdomen for an epigastric mass, a palpable liver enlarged by metastases and for ascites.

Investigations are performed to establish the diagnosis and determine the spread of the disease. Endoscopy allows a view of the lesion and biopsy for histological confirmation (Fig. 5.13).

Unless the tumour completely occludes the lumen, its full length and distal extent should be viewed, especially tumours in the lower end of the oesophagus because these may prove to arise from the stomach. When full endoscopic examination is unsatisfactory, a barium swallow is a helpful alternative (Fig. 5.14).

A chest X-ray and an ultrasound, or preferably CT scan, of the liver determine distant spread, and if clear, the extent of the local disease is examined. Some endoscopes are equipped with an ultrasound that can outline the depth of infiltration of the tumour, invasion of adjoining structures and enlargement of lymph

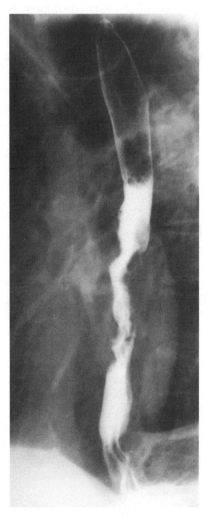

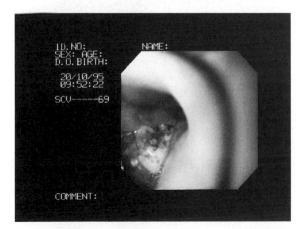

Fig. 5.13 *Endoscopic appearances of a carcinoma of the lower oesophagus.*

Fig. 5.14 *Barium swallow showing a long ragged stricture suggestive of a carcinoma.*

nodes. A spiral CT scan of the chest provides similar information. In patients with tumours of the upper oesophagus, particularly in the presence of respiratory symptoms, bronchoscopy is necessary to exclude infiltration of the airways. Laryngoscopy may be required to exclude vocal cord paralysis due to malignant infiltration of the recurrent laryngeal nerve.

Treatment

Treatment for intrinsic cancers is not standardized. The main options are surgery and chemoradiotherapy. The disease is often discovered at an advanced stage when it cannot be cured by surgery. The alternative treatment is chemo-radiotherapy, in particular for squamous cell carcinoma; in some instances, tumour regression may allow resection that previously seemed impossible.

Surgical resection is followed by reconstruction. The resected oesophagus is replaced by the mobilized stomach which is pulled into the chest and anastomosed to the proximal oesophagus. In the transhiatal approach, the stomach is mobilized in the abdomen. The dissection is continued into the chest by opening the diaphragmatic hiatus, and the intrathoracic oesophagus is dissected blindly from below and from the neck. When the oesophagus has been resected, the fundus of the stomach is pulled up to the neck where it is anastomosed to the stump of the proximal oesophagus. Alternatively, in the Ivor Lewis operation, the stomach is mobilized through an abdominal incision which is then closed. The patient is turned on the side; through a right thoracotomy, the tumour is resected under vision and the stomach is pulled into the chest and anastomosed to normal upper oesophagus.

Surgical treatment for tumours of the upper third involves a laryngectomy and a permanent tracheostomy. Surgery is considered carefully as chemoradiotherapy can be very effective and is not mutilating.

Surgery carries a mortality of 15%, with a five-year survival of only 10%, although it provides symptomatic benefit.

Palliation. For unfit patients and those with advanced disease as determined by the length of the tumours (greater than 7 cm), local invasion, or distant metastases, the aim is to restore swallowing. This is achieved temporarily by tunnelling through the tumour with a laser, or by intubating the oesophagus to hold it open with an endoscopically placed tube. Chemotherapy and radiotherapy can both be helpful in some cases.

Extrinsic pressure. When a bronchial cancer involves the oesophagus, the appearance on barium swallow is of a smooth stricture several centimetres long, associated with a soft tissue mass on a plain X-ray film or CT scan of the chest. At endoscopy the mucosa, unless infiltrated, looks normal. Swallowing can temporarily be restored by endoscopic insertion of a stent.

OESOPHAGEAL MOTILITY DISORDERS

Achalasia

After hiatal hernia (with oesophagitis and stricture) and cancer, *achalasia* is the third important cause of oesophageal dysphagia. However, it is rare, only one new case per 100,000 population being diagnosed each year. For this reason, and because the symptoms are often not understood, the diagnosis is often missed.

The basic pathology remains unknown, but there is loss of ganglion cells in the myenteric plexus of the distal oesophagus. This is associated with spasm of the lower oesophageal sphincter due to failure of relaxation, and in the distal oesophagus there is loss of normal peristaltic movements which are sometimes replaced by violent writhing movements. This striking change is called 'vigorous achalasia' or 'nutcracker oesophagus'. Perhaps it is the disordered peristalsis that causes the typical pains of achalasia. However, spasm of the lower sphincter is neither absolute nor perpetual. It may be absent in the early stages, and this is viewed by some as a separate disease – 'diffuse spasm'. Variations in the severity of sphincter spasm probably explain the periodic and inconsistent intensity of dysphagia. Most patients have spasms of retro-sternal pain that sometimes radiates down the arms like angina and may antedate the development of dysphagia by years. In time the oesophagus dilates and aspiration of retained residue results in repeated chest infections or pneumonia. Weight loss does not occur until late.

Diagnosis

Chest X-ray. In advanced achalasia there is a fluid level in the dilated oesophagus and a mottled appearance of food residue in the liquid. This prevents swallowed air from reaching the stomach so the gastric air bubble is absent, although presence of a gastric air bubble does not exclude achalasia. The main purpose of this examination is to exclude associated pulmonary complications.

A practical diagnostic test is *failure of barium to reach the stomach* with the patient supine and tilted 15° head down. In the absence of an obstructing lesion, this is evidence of failure of peristalsis. In the erect position, a spastic sphincter will support a column of barium, tapering smoothly to a point at the sphincter. When, occasionally, the sphincter opens, a thin jet of barium runs into the stomach. These two features, and the writhing peristalsis, make the diagnosis virtually certain. However, cancer at the oesophago-gastric junction infiltrates and destroys the adjacent nerve plexus and can produce a very similar radiological picture.

Endoscopy is unremarkable, and the smooth passage of the endoscope down through the oesophago-gastric junction and into the stomach is a characteristic observation. The importance of this investigation is to exclude a carcinoma of the oesophago-gastric junction and to examine the rest of the oesophagus because achalasia predisposes to carcinoma.

Manometry is considered by many to be crucial to the diagnosis, but adds nothing to the findings of properly performed *radiology*.

Treatment

It is important to explain to patients that swallowing may be improved but it can never be normal. The aim of treatment is to relieve the dysphagia caused by spasm of the lower oesophageal sphincter. Drug treatment is disappointing: calcium channel-blockers and long-acting nitrates may provide some relief but the therapeutic benefit is variable;

injecting botulinum toxin into the sphincter via the endoscope apparently gives relief, but the effect is not permanent and the muscle recovers its contractility over months.

Endoscopic dilatation of the sphincter under radiological control is effective by disrupting the sphincter fibres, although recurrence of the symptoms is common and there is the risk of perforation, especially with repeated dilatation. Therefore, in young and fit patients the optimal treatment is cardiomyotomy (*Heller's operation*) which involves division of the lower oesophageal sphincter by a longitudinal incision through the muscle layers of the lower oesophagus and upper stomach down to the mucosa. This is performed either via a thoracotomy, a thoracoscopic or a laparoscopic approach. It is crucial that the crural mechanism is not damaged, or if damaged, is repaired, because a hiatal hernia is liable to cause particularly intractable oesophagitis if the oesophagus cannot clear the refluxed juices.

Systemic sclerosis (CRST syndrome)

Systemic sclerosis. This is a generalized disease of connective tissue that, in the oesophagus, presents as a motility disorder. Peristalsis fails in the oesophagus below the aortic arch so barium swallowed in the 15° head-down position does not readily reach the stomach. However, the sphincter muscle is also weakened so the barium immediately flows into the stomach when the patient is erect. The patient may also show clinical signs of *scleroderma* – crow's foot wrinkles radiating from the mouth, Raynaud's phenomenon with calcium deposits in the skin, and rheumatoid arthritis. On endoscopy, oesophagitis and a peptic stricture may be evident. The first line of management is a proton pump inhibitor. If it is not satisfactory, an anti-reflux operation may give relief.

Pseudo-dysphagia: tender oesophagus

This condition is similar to the 'irritable bowel syndrome' (Chapter 6), but affecting the oesophagus rather than the gut. Patients present with an incoherent complaint. The history is not of difficulty in swallowing, the food never gets stuck on its way down the gullet as can be proved by drinking, but of pain that sometimes continues for hours. The oesophagus is not sensitive to heat, fruit juice or alcohol. Video-barium swallow and endoscopy are normal. Some patients also have bowel symptoms compatible with irritable bowel syndrome. Patients should be reassured. However, review after an interval is a wise precaution because mild or early achalasia can be difficult to detect.

Globus hystericus

The patient complains of 'a lump in the throat'. In the absence of any abnormality on examination or investigation it is ascribed to hysteria, but all the conditions mentioned above must be excluded before making this diagnosis. However, the existence of such a condition is disputed.

HIGHLIGHTS

- All cases of dysphagia need specialist investigation
- Physical examination is more likely to be helpful in pharyngeal than in oesophageal dysphagia
- Most cases of oesophageal dysphagia can be diagnosed accurately by a combination of history, barium swallow, oesophagoscopy and biopsy
- Radiology is a very powerful tool provided the patient is correctly positioned and all oesophageal movement is captured on video-recorder

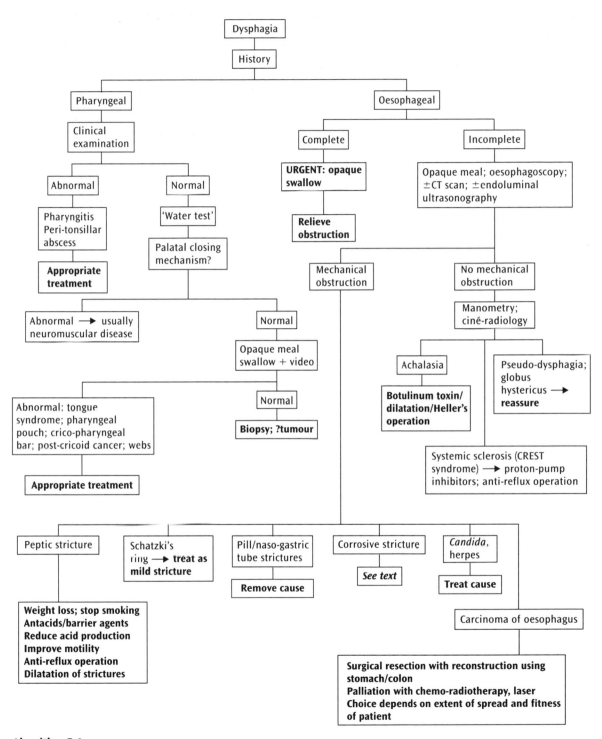

Algorithm 5.1

6

Chronic or recurrent abdominal pain

MICHAEL HOBSLEY

AIMS

1 Learn the common conditions causing upper abdominal pain and their salient clinical features
2 Understand the principles underlying management of a patient complaining of upper abdominal pain

INTRODUCTION

This chapter discusses the problem of upper abdominal pain, even when it is clearly related to food, without the use of the words *dyspepsia* or *indigestion*. The reason for this omission is that these words have no precise meaning: patients may use the terms to describe any symptom they consider to be related to the digestive tract, from headache to constipation. Acceptance by the clinician of these terms, without probing into what the patient really means, can result in serious misinterpretations and therefore misdiagnoses.

The reasons for referring a patient with chronic or recurrent upper abdominal pain for a specialist opinion are shown below:

- Unrelieved severe symptoms.
- Continuous symptoms.
- Typical pattern of symptoms.
- Patient's request.

THE INITIAL SORTING

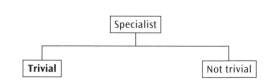

If the general practitioner has had access to special investigations, the diagnosis may have already been made. With the usual history and examination, and the benefit of time since the patient consulted the practitioner, the specialist sorts a group of patients who have trivial complaints that do not warrant further investigation, and for whom reassurance and symptomatic remedies will be adequate. Irritable bowel syndrome (IBS), *see later*, is the prominent example. However, if the symptoms recur or persist the patient should return.

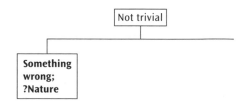

Second, there is a group of patients in whom the history and examination suggest that there is a serious underlying disease, but do not give a strong lead on its most likely nature. A good procedure is to request both an ultrasound examination and upper gastrointestinal endoscopy.

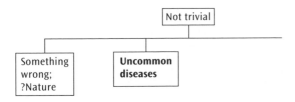

Third, in a few patients a diagnosis will be reached which is different from the main group of six diseases commonly responsible for upper abdominal pain (*see below*) and even possibly originating far from the upper abdomen. Fairly common examples follow. In the mid-line of the upper abdomen, a very localized point of tenderness that becomes more, rather than less, tender when the patient contracts his recti muscles, signifies a *herniation of extra-peritoneal fat* through a small defect in the linea alba. A routine operation to reduce the tag of fat and repair the defect cures the symptoms. Epigastric pain and tenderness may be due to an *abdominal aortic aneurysm* (Chapter 7) or to tension in the capsule of a liver enlarging rapidly due to congestive cardiac failure or inflammatory, cystic or neoplastic disease; or from retroperitoneal lymph nodes associated with lymphoma or intra-abdominal malignancy. Pain related to meals can result from organic disease of the large bowel, because eating a meal activates the gastro-colic reflex and the resultant peristaltic rushes in the colon may aggravate symptoms due to inflammation or partial obstruction (Chapter 9), or from IBS. Each condition found is managed appropriately.

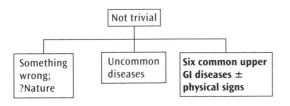

Finally, there is a group where the history alone, or taken in conjunction with abnormal physical findings, directs attention to either the gall bladder, the oesophagus, stomach and duodenum, or the pancreas.

POINTERS FROM THE HISTORY

In the UK, as seen in hospital practice, the six common *diseases* are gallstones, reflux oesophagitis, peptic ulcer, chronic pancreatitis and carcinoma of the pancreas, and carcinoma of the stomach.

Gallstones

Pain is continuous and lasts a few hours to a few days during each episode, is not related to a meal but may be associated with nausea and vomiting. Pain-free intervals last weeks or months. The pain is epigastric or in the right upper quadrant and may radiate round the (right) ribs to the back, or through to the back, or to the right shoulder-tip.

The features of acute cholecystitis (Chapter 26) facilitate the diagnosis if the patient is examined during an attack. Nevertheless, a history alone should result in a working diagnosis of gallstones, especially if there has been transient jaundice.

There is another clinical presentation which is traditionally said to suggest gallstones. The patient has mild epigastric discomfort at random times, associated with abdominal distension and eructations, and sometimes heartburn. Such a patient, especially if female, fat, fertile (the mother of several children), in her forties and complaining that fatty foods are particularly likely to bring on the symptoms, used to be considered almost certain to have gallstones. However, there is strong evidence that gallstones are as common in patients without such symptoms as in patients with them, and that true fat intolerance is rare.

Reflux oesophagitis

The cardinal feature of this condition is postural heartburn; that is, a burning sensation starting in the epigastrium and radiating upwards for a variable distance behind the sternum, brought on or aggravated by stooping or lying flat. *Odynophagia*, that is, pain on swallowing, is also a symptom, due to spasm and, in advanced disease, the result of a stricture. For further details, *see* Chapter 5.

Peptic ulcer

Although gastric ulcers tend to occur more commonly in elderly females and duodenal ulcers in younger males, most clinicians cannot reliably, on clinical grounds, distinguish the less-common gastric ulcer from the much more common duodenal variety; both types are discussed together as a *peptic ulcer*. The characteristic features are epigastric pain that comes on some time after a meal, radiation in some cases through to the back, a burning or gnawing character, relief by food or alkalis, and periodicity: symptomatic remissions or relapses, each of the order of weeks or months.

To elicit the relation of the pain to food takes skilful questioning. Some patients say they are afraid to eat because it brings on the pain, whereas others say they have to eat to avoid symptoms: the remission produced by the food lasts much longer in the second group than in the first. In both types, pain during food intake is rare. In other words, the onset of pain is related to an empty stomach, and this explains why the pain often wakes the patient in the early hours of the morning.

Complications of peptic ulcer

Complications usually occur in patients with a history of chronic upper abdominal pain, but occasionally arise *de novo*. The main ones are perforation, bleeding and pyloric outlet obstruction.

- *Perforation* results in generalized peritonitis (Chapter 25).
- *Bleeding* presents as haematemesis (vomiting of recognizable blood or altered blood – 'coffee grounds') and, if the blood loss is particularly rapid, melaena. The management of such patients is outlined in Chapter 9.
- *Pyloric obstruction* presents with vomiting, sometimes projectile, of large volumes of liquid that characteristically contains recognizable food

that has been eaten some time previously. Pyloric obstruction can also be due to carcinoma of the stomach or of the pancreas.

Carcinoma of the pancreas and chronic pancreatitis

It is best to consider these two diseases under a single heading, both because they can co-exist and because a mass in the pancreas may be due to either and the diagnosis may remain unclear even after laparotomy.

Carcinoma of the pancreas seems to be increasing in incidence. When it arises in the head of the pancreas, jaundice is an early feature (Chapter 8). With carcinoma of the body and tail, as in carcinoma of the stomach, weight loss may be a prominent feature and an insidious course may remain symptomless until the cancer is too advanced to cure. Pain, when it occurs, is typically felt in the back, worse when the patient lies down, and in a few patients it is relieved particularly by adopting a squatting position.

The pain of chronic pancreatitis is epigastric, it may be exacerbated by lying down and by the ingestion of alcohol, and radiation through to the back is common. However, these features are not constant and the severity of the pain may vary widely and without any recognizable pattern. The diagnosis is suggested by features such as a history of chronic alcohol abuse, of steatorrhoea due to reduction in pancreatic exocrine secretions (including lipase) and the consequent failure to absorb dietary fat, resulting in the passage of pale, greasy-looking stools, or of symptoms suggestive of diabetes mellitus due to reduction in the secretion of insulin.

Carcinoma of the stomach

This disease does not always produce pain; when it does, the pain may be similar to that of a peptic ulcer or it may have no recognizable pattern. A patient who complains of epigastric pain in association with marked anorexia and weight loss should be assumed to have carcinoma of the stomach and investigated urgently. Many such patients will, in the event, prove to have a benign gastric ulcer, but the distinction cannot be made clinically. Even without pain, the combination of anorexia and weight loss constitute sufficient grounds for a presumptive diagnosis of carcinoma of the stomach.

RELEVANT PHYSICAL SIGNS

Evidence pointing to the gall bladder include: jaundice (Chapter 8); a palpable gall bladder (Chapter 7); abdominal tenderness in the right upper quadrant, and (*Murphy's sign*) exacerbation of this tenderness when the subject takes a deep breath.

A palpable supra-clavicular lymph node suggests a secondary deposit from a carcinoma of the stomach or pancreas. Localized tenderness in the mid-line of the epigastrium also points to the stomach and duodenum rather than to the gall bladder. An epigastric mass may be palpable (Chapter 7).

In pyloric obstruction, copious vomiting results in depletion of the patient's extra-cellular space (Chapter 16), so the characteristic evidence of confusion, loss of skin elasticity, empty superficial veins and reduction in eyeball tension are manifest. The distended stomach is usually readily palpable, often with its lower border below the umbilicus, and gently shaking the patient elicits a succussion splash. It may be easier to hear the splash with the aid of a stethoscope. However, this sign is only valid if the patient has been starved for at least 2 hours. Peristaltic waves may be seen travelling from left to right along the greater curvature.

There are no relevant physical signs in patients with reflux oesophagitis, and few in patients with pancreatic disease, although a pancreatic mass may very occasionally be palpable. Finally, liver palpably containing secondary deposits (Chapter 7) is, in the present context, most likely to have resulted from carcinoma of the pancreas or stomach, although many other primary sites are possible.

MANAGEMENT

A jaundiced patient, one with severe vomiting and disturbance of fluid balance or significant weight loss, should be admitted soon. Ultrasound is usually the first investigation, alone or combined with endoscopy. In patients with pyloric stenosis, resuscitation is performed rapidly; in severe cases 6–8 l of physiological saline are needed. Potassium losses have also been incurred, but it is more important in the first instance to expand the extra-cellular volume so as to restore the peripheral circulation. Endoscopy at this stage would be hazardous because of the risk of the patient aspirating stomach contents into the respiratory passages. The stomach is evacuated and washed out with saline by use of a wide-bore tube, and when it is kept empty by continuous aspiration for a few days the pyloric spasm often relaxes and permits safe endoscopy to establish the diagnosis.

For the remaining patients, outpatient investigations are appropriate using the same imaging modalities.

Ultrasonography

Stones in the gall bladder, dilatation of the extrahepatic bile ducts and masses in the region, including within the stomach and pancreas, are reliably visualized. A small stone in the common bile duct is not always detectable. Liver lesions and aortic aneurysmal dilatation as well as renal pathology are demonstrated.

Oesophagogastroduodenoscopy

Examination and biopsy of the lower oesophagus to diagnose reflux oesophagitis has already been mentioned (Chapter 5). In the stomach, the endoscopist pays particular attention to the lesser curvature where most gastric ulcers and carcinomas occur. A typical gastric ulcer has a sharp vertical ('punched out') edge, whereas a carcinoma has heaped edges, although the picture is not always clear-cut. Several biopsy specimens are taken of the edge of any lesion. Although the most common diagnoses revealed are peptic ulcer and carcinoma of the stomach, others less common include lymphomas and benign connective tissue tumours of the gastric wall. The endoscopist provides information about the site and extent of tumour infiltration, which determines the plan of surgical treatment. There may be submucous spread of the tumour beyond its visible margins and a stiffness of the wall of the stomach may be apparent due to deep neoplastic infiltration (*linitis plastica* or *leather-bottle stomach*). This is recognized by the indistensibility of the stomach to air insufflation during endoscopy.

If the gastric mucosal folds are particularly coarse, Zollinger–Ellison (Z–E) syndrome is suspected (*see below*).

In the duodenum, an ulcer in its first part (the *duodenal bulb*) is almost certainly peptic – carcinoma of the duodenum is very rare. A distal site for the ulcer, that is, beyond the duodenal bulb region, or multiple ulcers also suggest Z–E syndrome. However, a pair of 'kissing' ulcers, one each on the anterior and posterior walls of the first part of the duodenum, do not have this connotation. A diverticulum from the inner border of the curve of the second part of the duodenum is only rarely of clinical significance. The papilla of Vater is inspected and any associated abnormality biopsied as carcinoma arises at this site.

Status of barium meal

Barium meal is an obsolescent investigation where facilities exist for upper gastrointestinal endoscopy. Its value lies, if the patient has previously undergone gastric resection, in elucidating the anatomy of the gastric remnant and various attached loops of the intestine elsewhere and there is inadequate information about the exact operation performed; and in the investigation of oesophageal disease.

AFTER THE INVESTIGATIONS

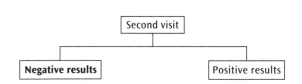

The negative results group

If the level of suspicion of serious disease was not high and the further interview yields no new information the effect of reassurance may be tried. However, it is difficult to prove a negative, and most patients will be submitted to a computerized tomography (CT) scan and magnetic resonance cholangiopancreatography (MRCP) (*see below*).

The possibility of pancreatic disease is investigated by looking for *steatorrhoea* – which may be confirmed by collecting the stools for 3 days on a normal ward diet: the upper limit for normal fat excretion is 5 g/day; and for *diabetes mellitus* by testing for glycosuria and an abnormal glucose tolerance test. Ultrasound, CT and MRCP are good at demonstrating lesions such as swelling of the whole gland, a focal mass in one area or a pseudocyst. These imaging procedures have practically superseded endoscopy, although if MRCP is not available, duodenoscopes give a direct view of the ampulla of Vater, and it is usually possible for the endoscopist to cannulate separately the common bile duct and the pancreatic duct. Radiographic contrast material can then be injected along the pancreatic duct and X-rays taken: these give an accurate diagnosis of anatomical abnormalities of the pancreas, such as strictures of the duct.

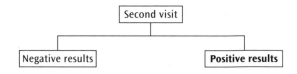

The positive results group

The positive results occasionally identify an unexpected disease as being the cause of the symptoms; for example, aneurysm of the aorta or carcinoma of the colon. In this event, management follows the lines for those conditions, as described in other chapters. It is more likely that the diagnosis will prove to be one of the six common conditions.

Gallstones

The presence of gallstones does not constitute an indication for cholecystectomy. Surveys have shown that *asymptomatic gallstones*, diagnosed by chance in the investigation of other conditions, constitute more than half of all the patients with gallstones, and the risk of developing acute biliary pain is only about 1% each year. The modern operation of laparoscopic cholecystectomy carries a mortality rate of about 0.1%, but there is a 0.3% risk of damage to the extrahepatic bile ducts and most patients will never get symptoms. For these reasons, most surgeons do not advise cholecystectomy for these patients.

There are patients who, although symptomless most of the time, have *symptomatic gallstones*: clear-cut attacks of epigastric pain lasting for several hours and requiring opiates for the relief of pain. These patients are advised to undergo elective chole-cystectomy unless they are old or frail or have a major medical contraindication. This policy protects against the possibility of painful and dangerous complications: acute cholecystitis; perforation of the gall bladder with generalized peritonitis; or migration of stones into the common duct with the consequent possibilities of obstructive jaundice and ascending cholangitis. A patient presenting with any such *complication of gallstones* requires urgent admission.

The patients who have vague, chronic symptoms of flatulence, fat intolerance and epigastric discomfort, without any obvious pattern in relation to time or to external factors, where the gallstones are probably incidental, are best managed like the symptomless patients.

Cholecystectomy is occasionally technically difficult for reasons of anatomical anomalies or the blurring of anatomy produced by fibrosis after inflammation. The approach is usually via the laparoscope – the only specific contraindications are late pregnancy and coagulopathy. The mortality of the open operation, 0.5%, is greater than the 0.1% for the laparoscopic – but the surgeon is prepared to convert to a standard laparotomy should the dissection via the laparoscope prove too difficult or should a complication arise that requires wider access. The crucial step is the demonstration of the junction of the cystic, hepatic and common ducts, so that the latter two cannot be inadvertently damaged by being mistaken for the cystic duct and therefore ligated. The cystic artery can also be awkward to secure, or the right hepatic artery mistaken for it.

The major decision is whether to explore the common bile duct. The criteria that determine the need for cholangiography, performed either before operation by the endoscopic route or by MRCP, or during the operation, are: ductal dilatation; a suspicion of a ductal stone on ultrasonography; deranged liver function tests with a high alkaline phosphatase; a high serum amylase; or a recent history of jaundice or pancreatitis.

Per-operative cholangiography, properly performed and interpreted, will confidently rule out residual stones in bile ducts and avoid unnecessary exploration. However, the laparoscopic technique is more demanding than in the open operation and expectant management is adopted by some who feel that residual stones may pass spontaneously or can be retrieved later endoscopically by sphincterotomy with the insertion of a pig-tailed stent into the common bile duct which helps with their spontaneous passage, whereas large stones can be crushed with a lithotripter. Such an approach arguably does less damage to the delicate lower end of the duct than operative removal. In the poor-risk elderly patient it might be justifiable to avoid cholecystectomy altogether, and simply to perform endoscopic sphincterotomy to extract ductal calculi, because 90% of such patients get no further symptoms.

Reflux oesophagitis

See Chapter 5.

Peptic ulcer

Peptic ulcers, whether of stomach or duodenum, never occur in the complete absence of hydrochloric acid – *achlorhydria*. Defence mechanisms protect the lining wall of the stomach and first part of the duodenum from digestion by the acid–pepsin mixture secreted by the stomach, and a peptic ulcer probably results from an imbalance between acid attack and mucosal defence, for example, an excess of hydrochloric acid secreted by the stomach.

It is generally accepted that the most important factor in the majority of patients (70–95%) is colonization of the pyloric antral mucosa with *Helicobacter pylori*. However, there are other risk factors: non-steroidal anti-inflammatory drugs (NSAIDs), which interfere with wound healing; 80–90% of patients smoke tobacco, which increases the number of parietal cells in the stomach and so enhances maximal acid secretion; there is a familial tendency; and there is evidence of aggressive as well as protective factors in various foods.

Treatment includes a combination of anti-acid medication and eradication of *H. pylori*. The

H_2-receptor antagonists, for example ranitidine, given orally, reduce maximally stimulated gastric secretion by 90%. On a regime of an H_2-antagonist once or twice daily, 80% of patients with duodenal ulcer lose their symptoms and heal their ulcer by 4–6 weeks. Unfortunately, if the antagonist is stopped, most patients have recurrent symptoms within 2 years. However, if *H. pylori* is eliminated simultaneously by appropriate therapy, healing seems to be more stable and relapses are less frequent or do not occur for many years. Claims have been made that the eradication of *H. pylori* effects a cure, and it is true that re-infection is unusual; however, there is evidence that recurrent duodenal ulcer can occur in 10–20% of patients within 1–6 years and without re-infection with *H. pylori*. Changes in this field are ongoing and rapid, but 14 days' treatment with ranitidine bismuth citrate plus clarithromycin, or clarithromycin and amoxycillin, are recommended. Antibiotic resistance sometimes develops to clarithromycin, and a good second-line regime is a proton-pump inhibitor such as omeprazole, with bismuth, tetracycline and metronidazole.

The indications for elective definitive surgical treatment are the presence of pyloric stenosis and severe symptoms unresponsive to medical measures, particularly if there is an antecedent history of perforation or bleeding.

A patient with a *gastric ulcer* is treated for 6 weeks after stopping smoking, and standard anti-acid and anti-*H. pylori* treatment, and then endoscopy is repeated. Treatment is continued if the ulcer shows signs of healing, but otherwise surgery should be advised because of the risk that a gastric ulcer is carcinomatous.

With the advent of effective medical therapy there is no indication for surgical treatment of uncomplicated duodenal ulcer, although in an underprivileged country surgery can be more cost-effective. Surgery aims at reducing acid–pepsin production when the stomach is maximally stimulated, and a variety of operations have been used.

A vagotomy, the treatment of choice for a duodenal ulcer, diminishes the stomach's response to secretory stimuli (sight and smell of food, and direct contact of food with the stomach wall) that follow the vagal pathway, and also diminishes the response of the intact parietal cell mass to chemical stimulation via the gastrin mechanism. A truncal vagotomy divides the two main trunks of the vagus nerves as they lie anterior and posterior to the abdominal oesophagus. However, this results in gastric stasis as gastric motility is also reduced. Truncal vagotomy can be combined with gastroenterostomy or pyloroplasty in order to enhance gastric emptying, but the rate of emptying is then often so large as to produce unpleasant symptoms, known as the *dumping syndrome*.

This syndrome is composed of two sets of symptoms, systemic and abdominal. Systemic symptoms include the manifestations of shock: faintness; sweating; pallor; palpitations; and dyspnoea. They are due to the osmotic attraction of the hypertonic food in the intestine for a large volume of extra-cellular fluid, thereby depleting the circulating plasma volume. Abdominal symptoms include borborygmi, bloating and sometimes watery diarrhoea, the results of the distension of the bowel with this large fluid load.

However, it is possible selectively to denervate the parietal cell mass (e.g., by *proximal gastric vagotomy*) and such procedures are much less likely to produce disturbances of gastric emptying.

A particularly intractable form of peptic ulcer diathesis, Zollinger–Ellison syndrome, results from gastric hypersecretion in response to hypergastrinaemia produced by a non-β-cell tumour of gastrin-secreting cells in the pancreas, duodenum and other rarer upper abdominal sites. This may be an individual disease or else part of the MEN 1 syndrome (Chapter 27). *Hypergastrinaemia*, that is, serum gastrin concentration greater than 100 pg/ml, can be due to other causes, in particular the use of proton pump inhibitors, and also in pernicious anaemia, renal failure and atrophic gastritis. However, patients with Zollinger–Ellison syndrome have a large parietal cell mass and therefore a large maximal acid secretion, but the most important distinction from duodenal ulcer patients without Zollinger–Ellison syndrome is that the basal acid secretion is a large fraction of maximal secretion (over 40%; more than 15 mmol/h or more than 5 mmol/h after a previous operation for duodenal ulcer). Unless the site of the tumour can be demonstrated and the lesion removed, nothing short of *total gastrectomy* prevents recurrent peptic ulceration, although operation can be deferred by the use of powerful proton-pump inhibitors. A battery of non-invasive and invasive imaging methods yields the location and extent of the tumour in four-fifths of patients. The most useful single method is *somatostatin receptor scintigraphy* (SRS), the radio-labelled somatostatin analogue attaching itself to somatostatin receptors which most gastrinomas possess.

Carcinoma of the pancreas and chronic pancreatitis

There are five main situations.

Focal pancreatic mass. A mass in the pancreas is usually demonstrated by CT scan or ERCP. Although many types of investigation are available, enthusiasm must be tempered with the knowledge that carcinoma of the pancreas has a poor prognosis; half the patients have succumbed in 6 months from diagnosis.

If there is evidence that suggests cancer with a poor prognosis, for example back pain or cachexia, the diagnosis can be achieved without operation by fine-needle aspiration (FNA) or biopsy under imaging control.

A cytological diagnosis of carcinoma is reliable, but there are many false negatives. However, because of the risk of seeding, FNA is contraindicated if the evidence suggests that radical resection might be curative. CT and MRI scans, and especially the more recent MRCP, are improving and help greatly in defining the relationship of the tumour to the superior mesenteric and portal veins (*resectability*) and lymph node metastases.

Modern experience suggests that, except in the special case of carcinomas in the region of the papilla of Vater (these tend to be diagnosed early because they draw attention to themselves by producing obstructive jaundice and are readily diagnosed by ERCP and endoscopy) carcinoma of the pancreas is unlikely to be curable by resection. Only 3% of tumours of the body and tail are resectable. Of the 70% of pancreatic tumours in the head, about 10% are suitable for resection but the five-year survival rate is only 10%. The standard 'curative' operation is *Whipple's pancreaticoduodenectomy*, but preservation of the pylorus has gained some popularity and survival rates do not seem to be any smaller (Chapter 8).

Palliative procedures for locally advanced disease include operations to prevent incipient jaundice (cholecystenterostomy, choledocho-enterostomy) or pyloric obstruction (gastroenterostomy) and procedures to relieve pain. Coeliac plexus blocks give better results in carcinoma than in chronic pancreatitis (*see later*). Radiotherapy and chemotherapy are ineffective.

Cystic pancreatic tumours are rare and usually benign. They are distinguished from pancreatic pseudocysts (*see later*) by imaging or the finding of epithelial elements in a biopsy. The best management is resection with frozen section histological examination.

For completeness, a rare class of pancreatic tumours are those of the endocrine, of which the most common are the gastrinomas and the insulinomas. Insulinomas are usually benign, the others usually malignant. They do not usually cause dyspepsia, but may be picked up by imaging. *See also* multiple endocrine neoplasia (MEN) syndromes, Chapter 27.

Strictures, dilatations of main pancreatic ducts. Ultrasound, in the best hands, can demonstrate strictures and dilatations of the pancreatic duct, otherwise MRCP or ERCP may be necessary. This picture indicates chronic pancreatitis, further characterized by atrophy of islets and acini, and fibrosis.

The main aetiological factor is alcohol abuse, although in some tropical areas the disease seems to be caused by eating cassava. The most common type, *chronic calcific pancreatitis*, is related mainly to alcohol, *chronic obstructive* to carcinoma of the pancreas and *chronic inflammatory* to autoimmune diseases such as Sjögren's syndrome.

The first and most important line of therapy is to remove the causative factor: the patient who abuses alcohol is advised to stop drinking and this is usually successful. If the symptoms continue, a conservative approach is maintained for as long as possible. The management of pain, both in acute attacks and as a persistent feature, requires NSAIDs; narcotics are avoided as long as possible because of the danger of addiction. Coeliac plexus blocks have been unreliable, but thoracoscopic splanchnicectomy is being tried. Diabetes mellitus requires careful but restrained control, whereas steatorrhoea is treated with replacements for the exocrine secretions with pancreatic enzymes preparations, such as Creon, supplied in enteric-coated microspheres to prevent inactivation by gastric acid.

A few patients are suitable for removal of pancreatic duct stones, extra-corporeal lithotripsy and placing of stents to drain strictures via the endoscopic route.

If pain cannot be relieved by more conservative measures, open operations on these patients aim at preserving as much of the normal anatomy of the gastro-pancreatico-duodenal region and the secreting parenchyma of the pancreas as possible. Most commonly preferred at present are the duodenal-preserving resection of the head of the pancreas (*Beger's operation*) or an extensive drainage of the pancreas into the jejunum (*Puestow's operation*). Perhaps 80% of patients derive some benefit from these attempts to mitigate their very severe symptoms. Beger's procedure avoids the dumping syndrome induced by Whipple's pancreatico-duodenectomy.

Occasionally, the whole pancreas seems to be totally disorganized, and if symptoms are severe one can resort to the extreme step of total pancreatectomy. The patient can thereafter be maintained in a reasonable state of nutrition by careful replacement therapy with the enzymes of pancreatic exocrine secretion, with insulin for the ensuing diabetes mellitus, but the high mortality of the operation and the problems of the aftercare are formidable.

Obstructive jaundice. This presentation is discussed in Chapter 8.

Pancreatic pseudocyst. A pancreatic pseudocyst is a mass of tissue of chronic inflammatory nature containing a cavity that communicates, at the surface of the pancreas, with the pancreatic duct system. Presumably it results from rupture of a duct through the surface of the pancreas and containment of the resultant slow leak of pancreatic exocrine secretion by reactionary tissue. It usually follows an attack of acute pancreatitis (Chapter 25) which may well resolve spontaneously; when it occurs with chronic pancreatitis, resolution is less likely but may still be expected with conservative management if symptomless. It may present clinically as a mass, or be diagnosed only by ultrasound or CT scan. A pseudocyst lacks an epithelial lining.

Percutaneous catheter drainage is suitable for very ill patients, enlarging pseudocysts which are 'immature' (have not developed a fibrous wall) or pseudocysts that are infected. If ERCP can demonstrate a connection between the pseudocyst and the ductal system of the pancreas, stenting of the pancreatic duct opening into the duodenum drains the pseudocyst into the duodenum, but this technique is demanding. A pseudocyst that is thin-walled and bulges into the stomach or duodenum can be drained endoscopically, but an open (or laparoscopic) operation is needed for cysts that have thick walls or are anatomically remote from the gut.

Carcinoma of the stomach

Tumours arise mainly at the two ends of the stomach. Distal (*antral*) tumours are becoming less common and the overall incidence of gastric carcinoma is declining, but *proximal* tumours are becoming a little more common. The only treatment that can provide a cure is surgery; neither radiation nor chemotherapy has proved useful as adjuvant therapy.

Patients present late because weight loss is often ignored and the first manifestations are often obstructive – either dysphagia with proximal tumours or vomiting with distal tumours. If technical considerations permit removal of the tumour with reasonable ease and safety, this should be done even if there is no chance of cure. The relief of symptoms such as anorexia and nausea is more likely to be achieved if an ulcerated, infected mass in the stomach can be excised. Even in a palliative resection, the lines of section should be as far as feasible from the visible and palpable borders of the growth in order to reduce the risk of recurrence at the anastomosis because the consequent obstruction produces very distressing symptoms which may be difficult to relieve. For proximal tumours, total gastrectomy is required, with reconstruction usually with a *Roux-en-Y gastrojejunostomy*; but for distal tumours distal sub-total gastrectomy is the operation of choice, with reconstruction of Billroth II type. The anastomosis should be as wide as possible.

If resection proves at operation to be feasible and there are no signs of metastases then the peri-gastric lymph nodes along the greater and lesser curvatures should be removed with the lesser or greater omentum but not the spleen or the tail of the pancreas or more remote lymph nodes as such extensive dissections

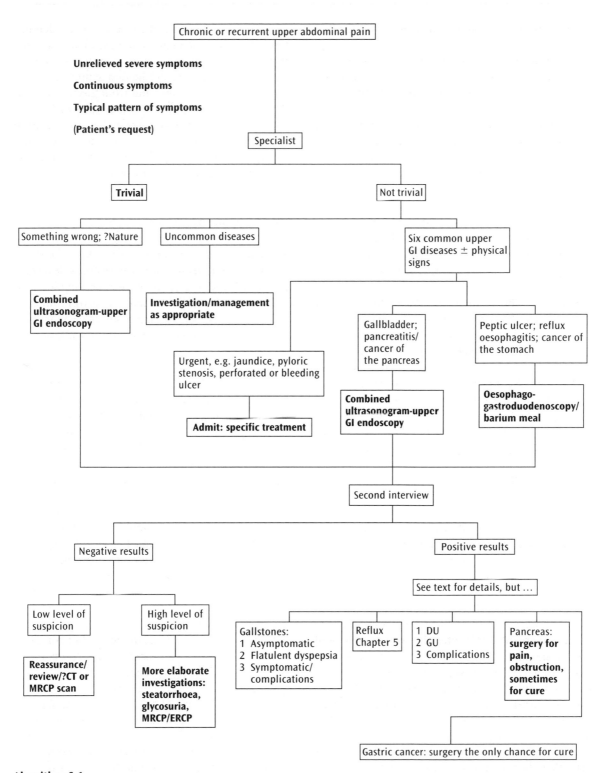

Algorithm 6.1

increase morbidity and operative mortality without conferring survival benefit – although this is disputed.

If obstruction has already occurred and the growth is irremovable then palliation may be effected by the endoscopic route. A laser can be used to cut a channel through the tumour at the oesophago-gastric junction, and an obstructed pyloric channel can be held open with a stent. Alternatively, an open bypass operation, such as gastro-jejunostomy, might be necessary.

The tendency towards spread by the lymphatics is marked, and such spread reaches at an early stage lymph glands in vital areas such as around the coeliac axis and aorta, in the pancreas and in the porta hepatis. In general, the prognosis is bad because this is a highly malignant tumour. However, in the individual case it is remarkably uncertain, and a few patients live for many years despite features that seem to herald a poor prognosis. Experience in Japan suggests that very early diagnosis resulting from endoscopic screening of the population, with radical removal of the local lymph nodes, may improve prognosis, but it has not been possible to reproduce these results in the West.

NOTE ON IRRITABLE BOWEL SYNDROME

It is doubtful whether this can be called a disease because we know virtually nothing about its aetiology or pathology. Its importance is that it is responsible for about one-tenth of all new consultations in general practice. The chief symptom is abdominal pain, often spasmodic, which may occur anywhere in the abdomen but commonly in the right or the left iliac fossa. Disturbances of bowel habit are often associated: constipation is more common than diarrhoea, and the two disturbances may alternate and be accompanied by abdominal distension so that intestinal obstruction may be mimicked (Chapter 26). However, the distinguishing feature of IBS is that the symptoms extend over many months or years,

without deterioration of the patient's general condition. The diagnosis may be difficult to make when the patient is first seen if there is no long history. It is unwise to make this diagnosis if the symptoms started for the first time after the age of 40 because other more serious causes of abdominal pain become so much more likely once middle age has been reached.

The presence of abnormal physical signs rule out the diagnosis of IBS.

A popular theory is that the symptoms are due to spasm of the bowel, and other tracts of smooth muscle are sometimes similarly affected: ask patients about irritable bladder, asthma and dysmenorrhoea.

Treatment is reassurance, plus increasing the roughage content of the diet. Bran may be appropriate for those with mainly constipation, but ispahagula husk is emollient and more likely to help whether the bowel upset is constipation or diarrhoea. Anti-spasmodic agents are helpful for severe symptoms.

Investigations, to be requested to meet patient demand or if the practitioner loses his nerve, are never positive in IBS, but a small possibility always remains that organic disease is being missed.

HIGHLIGHTS

- Six common diseases provide the majority of clinically diagnosable cases
- In patients with no strong clinical lead to the diagnosis, especially if the patient is ill, combined ultrasound and other imaging techniques and upper gastrointestinal endoscopy provide the best route to management
- The same combination of investigations is required if the clinical features suggest pancreatic disease
- If history, examination and first-order investigations fail to achieve a diagnosis but the index of suspicion is high, further investigations are required

7

Palpable abdominal mass

MICHAEL HOBSLEY

AIMS

1 Distinguish normal from abnormal masses
2 Differentiate abdominal wall from intra-abdominal masses
3 Relate abdominal masses to underlying organs
4 Discriminate between masses by certain characteristic signs
5 Employ appropriate diagnostic aids

INTRODUCTION

A palpable abdominal mass must be assumed to be due to serious abdominal disease unless the clinician is certain that the mass is a normal abdominal viscus.

The site and physical characteristics of a mass, with the patient's history of the complaint, other physical signs and derangements in the blood count and biochemistry provide some indication of the nature of a mass. Ultrasound and computerized tomography (CT) scanning are the mainstay of management in providing a precise outline of the mass in relation to other structures and access for fine needle aspiration (FNA) for biopsy, and have in most circumstances superseded other imaging procedures.

The management of lumps not considered elsewhere in this book is described in this chapter.

GENERAL CONSIDERATIONS

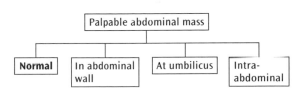

The normal bladder becomes palpable if it is sufficiently distended by retained urine. The lower pole of the right kidney is occasionally palpable, but the left kidney is impalpable unless the patient is very thin. In a thin person, the abdominal aorta is palpable in the epigastrium. In infants, for a variable period of a few weeks after birth, the normal liver is palpable in the upper abdomen. In complete health the intestines cannot be felt directly, but pressure over a loop that happens to be distended with gas and liquid gives a typical spongy sensation and a squelching noise, whereas faeces in the colon may be palpable in a thin and costive patient.

In no other circumstances (apart from pregnancy) should a palpable abdominal mass be assumed to be normal.

Status of the liver

Except in neonates, the list above does not include the normal liver. This omisson is contrary to the standard concept. It is generally understood that the normal liver is occasionally palpable, depending upon how far it projects downwards below the costal margin. However, every abdominal surgeon knows from the experience of laparotomy that, with the patient lying supine, the liver edge projects well below the costal margin in most patients. This has also been demonstrated to be true by scinti-scanning in 70% of normal conscious adults in the supine position. Failure to palpate the liver edge can be explained by basic physical science: to feel structure B through structure A, structure B must be firmer than structure A; the mere presence of structure B deep to structure A is not sufficient. The muscles of the anterior abdominal wall are firmer structures than the liver and so the latter is not palpable even when it extends below the costal margin unless diseased or distended with blood or bile, when it tends to be firmer.

Normal liver is palpable in the neonate probably because of the high proportion of firmer reticulo-endothelial tissue in the neonate compared with the adult.

Site

Most palpable abdominal swellings can be classified according to their site into one of the following categories:

- *Hernial orifices*, including the umbilicus.
- *Right and left upper quadrants.*
- *Epigastric.*
- *Right and left lower quadrants.*
- *Supra-pubic* (Fig. 7.1).

This is more practical than other regional classifications when defining abdominal masses.

Before dealing with individual sites, the significance of three important physical signs must be discussed. A fourth, the equally important sign of *cough impulse*, is discussed in Chapter 1.

Abdominal wall or intra-abdominal?

The importance of making this decision is frequently overlooked. When the patient contracts the

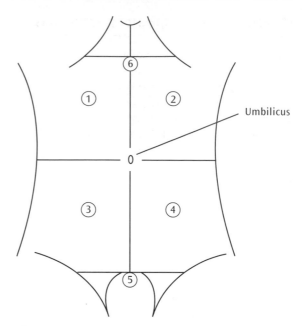

Fig. 7.1 *Territories of the abdomen. The horizontal line through the umbilicus divides the abdomen into upper and lower parts. The mid-line further divides these into four quadrants: (1) right upper; (2) left upper; (3) right lower; (4) left lower. Masses that can be demonstrated to arise strictly in the mid-line are mostly hernias. The umbilicus has distinct lesions. Above the umbilicus, and between the costal margins, the mid-line epigastric region encroaches upon both upper quadrants. Similarly, above the pubic symphysis (5) lies the supra-pubic region. The horizontal line is particularly important in that any abdominal mass which lies wholly, or partly, above the line must be tested for attachment to the diaphragm, whereas any mass below the horizontal line must be tested for whether it arises from the pelvis.*

abdominal muscles, an intra-abdominal swelling becomes less prominent or disappears, whereas a mass in the abdominal wall becomes firmer and more obvious.

For lumps straddling or abutting the mid-line, the patient is asked to lift the head off the bed without aid from the elbows: this requires maximal contraction of the recti. For more lateral masses, all the muscles of the anterior abdominal wall should be brought into play by asking the patient to strain, or to lift both lower limbs with the knees extended.

Movement with respiratory excursions

The lower margin of the swelling is observed and palpated to determine whether it moves downwards during inspiration and upwards with expiration. The interpretation of this sign is that the mass is, or arises in, some abdominal viscus that is in contact with the diaphragm, so that it is constrained to move with the excursions of the diaphragm. However, this is only conceivable if the mass is part of, or interposed by, an organ which is rigid enough to transmit the thrust. All abdominal masses which lie to some extent in the upper half of the abdomen should be tested for movement with the diaphragm.

Percussion note

The presence of gas in the intestine is responsible for the resonant note on percussion of the abdomen. The percussion note therefore helps to determine whether an abdominal mass is or is not covered with intestines. As it grows, a pelvic mass displaces the small intestine upwards, hence the mass is dull on percussion unless a loop is tethered to its surface. The small intestine and colon are pushed forwards by a mass arising from the posterior abdominal wall so that resonance is retained over the mass, although if it infiltrates into the peritoneal cavity the note may become dull. Percussion note is a helpful differentiating feature, but the exceptions mean that the findings must be interpreted with care.

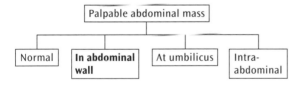

LUMPS OF THE ANTERIOR ABDOMINAL WALL

Lumps superficial to the muscles, that is, in the skin and subcutaneous tissues, may be of the same nature as lesions elsewhere, for example lipoma. Most are demonstrably free of the underlying muscle and their management has been discussed (Chapter 1).

Other lumps specific to the anterior abdominal wall which show evidence of attachment to the muscle layer are *hernias* and certain *umbilical lesions*.

Hernias

These occur when the scar of an abdominal incision is weak (*incisional hernia*) or at specific hernial orifices where the musculature of the abdominal wall is normally defective. The common *groin hernias* are discussed in Chapter 10.

The mid-line raphe of the linea alba may stretch, especially in obese elderly patients with poorly developed muscles, causing a mid-line bulge, prominent when the abdominal wall muscles are contracted and known as *divarication of the recti*. The lateral border of the rectus muscle is also a point of potential weakness, especially in the lower third of the abdomen where the posterior sheath is absent, and a hernia coming through between the rectus and the lateral abdominal muscles is called a *Spigelian hernia*. The very rare *lumbar hernia* protrudes through the space between the quadratus lumborum and the transversus abdominis muscles. The scar of a surgical incision, commonly in the mid-line, is also a point of weakness, and a hernia may occur through the scar tissue.

The umbilicus is a site of weakness, and two different kinds of hernia occur. One is a persistence of the fetal prolongation of the peritoneum through the umbilical scar. This *true umbilical hernia* is common in infants at birth as a relatively small bulge, and requires no treatment because it is a self-limiting condition that usually undergoes spontaneous cure, often by the age of 2 years and certainly by 5 years of age, but failure to heal requires repair. Although rare in adults, weakness at the umbilicus from long-term intra-abdominal distension, as occurs in ascites, may develop into a hernia. A severe form of umbilical defect is *exomphalos*, in which the neonate's whole abdominal contents may lie outside the umbilicus and is associated with other congenital anomalies. This rare situation demands complicated surgery to achieve skin cover for the viscera. The second form of hernia at the umbilicus appears through a defect in the linea alba close to, but not actually through, the umbilical scar. This is the *para-umbilical hernia*, common in the elderly obese subject, and it requires formal repair.

When not strangulated, these hernias are easy to diagnose by their expansile cough impulse. Those with a narrow neck, that is, admitting only a finger or two, such as the para-umbilical hernia, are much more likely to become strangulated than those with a broad neck, that is, several fingers sink into the gap, such as a divarication of the recti or many incisional hernias which have broad necks because they occur in large incisions. In some incisional hernias, however, the defect is only a small portion of the scar and strangulation is a serious risk.

All these hernias are best managed by surgical repair, but an abdominal supportive belt may be reasonable treatment for a broad-necked hernia in a patient in whom there are medical contraindications to operation.

Fatty hernia of the linea alba presents in the midline of the upper abdomen, a very localized point of tenderness that becomes more, rather than less tender when the recti are contracted, signifies a herniation of extra-peritoneal fat through a small defect in the linea alba. Sometimes the protrusion is so small that no lump is palpable. However, with these symptoms and signs it is worth exploring the region surgically. A routine operation that can be performed under local anaesthesia to reduce the tag of fat and repair the defect readily cures the symptoms.

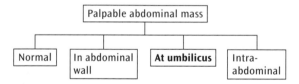

Umbilical nodules

These include a *granuloma*, resulting in the neonate from low-grade infection of the stump of the umbilical cord, in adults in association with a persistent urachus, or an intestinal fistula, either after abdominal surgery or complicating Crohn's disease. A primary tumour, or secondary deposit from an intra-abdominal neoplasm, are very rare presentations. Poor hygiene may result in encrustation of foreign material and exfoliated skin epithelium and debris which should be recognized and not confused as pathological. The *caput medusae* is a system of engorged veins radiating from the umbilicus. It

shows the classical signs of a vascular structure in its bluish tinge, ease of emptying under pressure and refilling when pressure is released. This lesion signifies obstruction of the portal venous circulation and the spleen and liver are palpable.

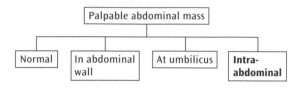

INTRA-ABDOMINAL MASSES

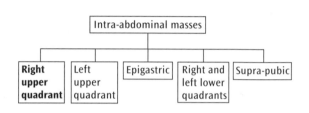

Right upper quadrant

If the mass moves with ventilation, the likely possibilities are liver, kidney and gall bladder. The liver and kidney are rigid organs in contact with the diaphragm. The gall bladder is normally soft and remote from the anterior abdominal wall, but when obstructed it becomes sufficiently distended to reach the wall, sufficiently hard to be palpable and moves downwards during inspiration. A mass in the region of the gastric antrum and pylorus or the porta hepatis may, if in contact with the under-surface of the liver, also show similar signs.

The characteristic feature of the liver is its thin, sharp, inferior border, where its anterior and infero-posterior surfaces meet; this margin may be blurred by disease affecting the liver, but it is nearly always sufficiently distinct to aid the diagnosis. By contrast, when palpable, the gall bladder and the lower pole of the kidney have a smooth hemispherical inferior aspect without an edge. A palpable kidney always presents in the loin and can be palpated between two hands, one on the anterior abdominal wall and the other in the loin. The gall bladder is an anterior structure and therefore not palpable in the loin. The liver and gall bladder are dull to percussion because resonance is lost as they displace the small bowel, but the kidney is resonant because of the gas in the overlying colon. A mass in the gastric antrum or nearby is rarely recognized on physical examination because it mimics a secondary neoplastic deposit in the lower border of the liver which is the usual interpretation of these physical findings.

Masses in the right upper quadrant that do not move with respiration may arise in the hepatic flexure and neighbouring segments of the large bowel, and are frequently malignant, but if they arise in the small bowel are usually inflammatory due to Crohn's disease, or rarely, lymphomatous. Masses arising in the small bowel and mesentery are likely to be mobile. A feature frequently quoted of a mass in the mesentery of the small bowel is that it moves in a plane from the right hypochondrium to the left iliac fossa, but not in the direction at right angles. However, this is not readily demonstrated in most cases because of pathological adhesions. Masses arising from retro-peritoneal structures that are bound down to the posterior abdominal wall are fixed. It should be realized that fixity is not always related to the anatomical site of the lesion, but inflammatory or neoplastic infiltration to adjacent viscera may equally limit the mobility of structures that are normally mobile. Another feature of a retro-peritoneal mass is that it is resonant on percussion, as already explained.

Liver

A smooth and uniformly palpable liver suggests that it is engorged with blood or bile, or diffusely infiltrated with new growth. An increased content of blood may arise from congestive cardiac failure, in which case other features of that condition, including a raised jugular venous pressure and peripheral oedema, should be identifiable. Engorgement with bile occurs in intra- and extra-hepatic obstruction. Infiltrations include reticuloses and some unusual diseases of unknown aetiology, such as *Hand–Schuller–Christian disease* in which granulomatous lesions develop with a proliferation of histiocytes, or rare metabolic disorders, as in *haemochromatosis*, or a glycogen storage disease. The diagnosis of these conditions depends upon a liver needle biopsy.

A finely nodular liver suggests primary biliary cirrhosis, and the patient is usually jaundiced or, if not, then skin marks from scratching are present. A coarsely nodular liver suggests *Laennec's cirrhosis* (*hobnail liver*; *alcoholic cirrhosis*) or multiple secondary deposits. A history of chronic alcoholism or the stigmata of liver failure point to the former, as patients with malignant deposits are likely to die before hepatic failure results. If secondaries are suspected, a search is made for a primary in the common areas: breast in women; bronchus in men; and colon in both sexes.

A palpable solitary hepatic mass, when tender and associated with signs of sepsis, is an abscess, either pyogenic or amoebic. *Pyogenic abscesses* are usually associated with biliary sepsis or portal pyaemia secondary to visceral inflammation such as appendicitis or divertivulitis and are common in diabetic patients. *Amoebic abscesses* should be considered in those visiting or living in endemic areas. Otherwise, most masses in the liver, which include a primary or secondary carcinoma and hydatid cysts, are not necessarily associated with constitutional symptoms.

Liver palpability, its consistency and the presence of tenderness are easily recognized, but the surface marking can be subtle and not always so easily discernible as to enable diagnosis with the precision suggested above. The liver abnormality is best shown on ultrasound examination which differentiates between a cystic and a solid mass, and if not clearly outlined, a CT scan provides detailed information on the nature and extent of the liver lesion and its relation to the adjacent structures. Imaging guides precise access for needle aspiration biopsy as well as drainage.

Gall bladder

A palpable tender gall bladder with its domed fundus below the costal margin is suggestive of an empyema due to stone obstruction of the cystic duct. However, the configuration of the gall bladder may not be easily definable when it is wrapped in omentum to form an inflammatory mass. This should be distinguished clinically from an empyema as the management is different. A non-tender gall bladder in a patient showing no sign of sepsis or jaundice is more likely to be a *mucocele* with incomplete obstruction of the cystic duct. However, if the patient is jaundiced, the gall bladder distension is part of the biliary dilatation caused by obstruction at the lower end of the common bile duct, usually by pancreatic or peri-ampullary carcinoma.

Ultrasound is a satisfactory initial investigation of the biliary system in most instances and detects stones better than CT scanning which is, however, superior in defining lesions obstructing the biliary tree. These are being superseded by magnetic resonance (MR) cholangiography which combines all the benefits of the current imaging modalities.

Kidney

The normal right kidney is occasionally palpable, but when it is enlarged, ballotment and movement with respiration are easier to elicit. The possible causes can be classified as obstructive, neoplastic or congenital. Considerable help may be derived from whether or not the other kidney is also palpable. *Bilateral abnormalities* suggest congenital anomalies, such as *polycystic kidneys* or *horseshoe kidney*, or else *obstruction of the lower urinary tract* (bladder and below) where a single site of obstruction produces back-pressure in both upper renal tracts causing hydronephrosis. Rectal and/or vaginal examination are essential to exclude pelvic pathology in this situation. If the abnormality is confined to one side, it is either due to an obstructive lesion in the upper tract on that side, or neoplasia. Imaging is the determinant investigation in most cases. Ultrasound examination outlines the size and shape of the kidneys, demonstrates dilatation of the renal pelves and the presence of stones, differentiates solid from cystic lesions, and identifies abnormalities of the bladder and prostate. CT scan is crucial in distinguishing a renal carcinoma from haematoma or other benign disease. These informative techniques have superseded the conventional intravenous urogram in this situation, although the latter is still important in the diagnosis of renal colic.

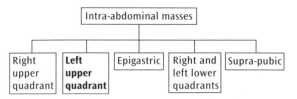

Left upper quadrant

In this quadrant, a mass that moves with breathing arises from liver, kidney or spleen, whereas one that does not probably arises from colon, small bowel, mesentery or retro-peritoneal lymph nodes.

Compared with the characteristics of the liver and kidney, the spleen has a fairly sharp inferior border, is dull to percussion and is not bi-manually palpable or ballotable so that it is unlikely to be confused with the kidney. More difficulty may arise in distinguishing spleen from liver. If the liver is palpable in the right upper quadrant as well, its lower border can usually be followed across the mid-line of the abdomen to demonstrate that what is palpable to the left of the mid-line is one and the same. Occasionally, a mass in the left lobe of the liver projects downwards and is palpable only to the left of the mid-line, whilst the right upper quadrant feels normal, and then the liver may easily be mistaken for the spleen. The spleen is said to move downwards and to the right on deep inspiration, rather than just downwards, and if the characteristic notch halfway along the inferior border is palpable, there can be no doubt but that the mass is the spleen. Particular difficulty may be experienced when the spleen and liver are simultaneously palpable, a not uncommon event in reticuloses and in portal hypertension.

Clinical signs of chronic liver disease, portal hypertension and palpable lymph nodes associated with reticuloses, should supplement the examination if the spleen is enlarged.

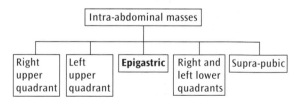

Epigastric

Masses around the mid-line of the epigastrium that move with respiration are either spleen or liver, and have already been discussed. Although occasionally a carcinoma in the distal region of the stomach or in the transverse colon is confused with a liver mass, the clinical presentation is usually suggestive. In doubt, ultrasound examination is a less invasive procedure than, and should precede, endoscopy. A *carcinoma of the body of the pancreas*, although rarely palpable, and a *pancreatic cyst*, are masses that do not move with respiration and should be differentiated from an *aortic aneurysm* which exhibits characteristic signs.

An aortic aneurysm presents as a vertical longitudinal mass extending downwards from the costal margin to about the region of the umbilicus, exhibiting a pulsation in time with the pulse beat elsewhere. It is essential to appreciate that the pulsation must be demonstrably expansile. Both aortic pulsation and the aorta itself are palpable in thin subjects. The dividing line between a normally palpable aorta and an aneurysm is usually set at a width of 2.5 cm, but physical measurement by palpation is inexact.

An aneurysm of the abdominal aorta is always visible in a lateral view plain abdominal X-ray as the calcified shadow of its anterior and posterior walls (Fig. 7.2). Ultrasound and CT scanning are reliable methods of establishing the presence and size of an aneurysm. A CT scan is more precise in showing the relationship of the aneurysm to the renal arteries, which is important information when planning treatment. Aortography is never necessary, and may be misleading because much of the lumen may be obliterated by clot, but is useful if there is evidence of lower limb ischaemia to outline the peripheral circulation.

The natural history of an aneurysm of the abdominal aorta is that it gradually grows, with an increasing threat of rupture, so that there is a good case for operation. Between 2.5 and 5.5 cm in size (as determined by imaging), the aneurysm is regarded as small and it is not absolutely necessary to perform prophylactic surgery to prevent rupture. Above 5.5 cm, the operation is required urgently.

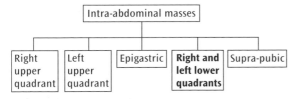

Both lower quadrants

Masses in the right and left lower quadrants are considered in Chapters 25 and 27.

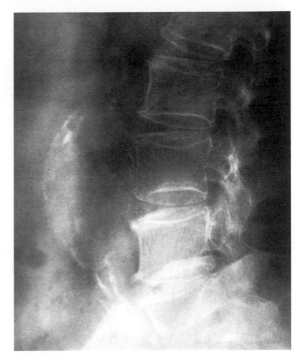

Fig. 7.2 *A lateral plain radiograph of the abdomen showing calcification in the wall of an aneurysm of the abdominal aorta, anterior to the lumbar vertebrae. (Radiograph kindly provided by Mr Adrian Marston.)*

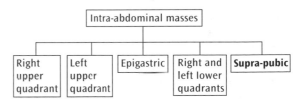

Supra-pubic

A mass in this region is arising either from the pubic bone or from the pelvic viscera. One arising from the pubic bone is hard and fixed. Radiology followed by biopsy determines its nature, which is likely to be neoplastic, although a non-specific inflammatory condition called *osteitis pubis* may occasionally present in this way. A mass arising from the pelvis lies against the pubic crest, so that one cannot feel its lower edge, and it is usually dull to percussion because the bowel is displaced. The bladder should be recognized by its typical domed shape, and by arousing in the patient the desire to micturate when the examiner presses gently on the overlying anterior abdominal

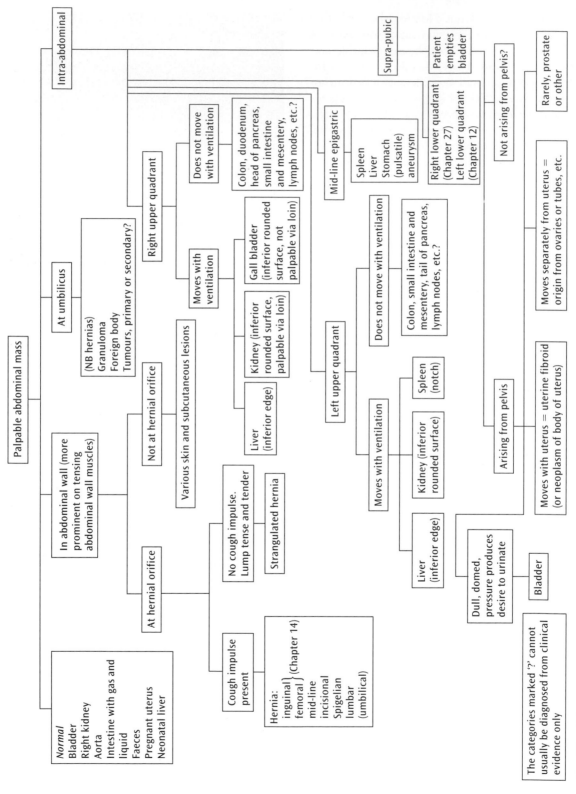

Algorithm 7.1

The categories marked '?' cannot usually be diagnosed from clinical evidence only

wall. As it is structurally part of the abdominal wall, when the patient raises the head off the bed the mass becomes fixed and can no longer be moved from side to side. It is important to try to ensure that the bladder is empty when examining a mass in this region. Asking the patient to void, in the absence of retention, distinguishes between bladder and other pelvic masses, although a diverticulum of the bladder may remain palpable or become more prominent, because it is deficient in muscle and fills with urine when the bladder contracts during micturition.

Digital examination of the rectum and vagina differentiates a rectal carcinoma and sigmoid carcinoma or inflammatory mass usually palpable in the recto-vesical or recto-uterine pouch, from a uterine fibroid, an ovarian cyst or tubo-ovarian mass in females, an invasive prostatic carcinoma in males, and also determines the degree of mobility of a pelvic mass. Bi-manual palpation demonstrates movement of the cervix with uterine or ovarian masses and may permit discrimination of a uterine from an adnexal lesion. An ovarian cyst appears to lie centrally, although the ovaries lie laterally. This is because it emerges through the brim of the pelvis which lies symmetrically about the mid-line.

An ovarian cyst may grow so large as to fill the abdomen. The physical signs of such a cyst are a dull percussion note, shifting dullness and a fluid thrill, indistinguishable from ascites, and it may be so soft in consistency that its physical signs can be confused with the fluid thrill and shifting dullness of ascites. An abdominal X-ray may show some distinguishing features, but these are better demonstrated by an ultrasound examination.

An ultrasonogram of the pelvis is fairly precise in outlining the pelvic viscera and identifying the nature of a pelvic mass, and further information is derived from endo-vaginal ultrasound. A CT or MR scan provides clear demarcation in the difficult case and is useful in assessing resectability.

Cautionary note

It is essential that the scrotum is examined for undescended testes whenever an abdominal mass is diagnosed in a male patient, in case the mass is a neoplasm of an undescended testis.

HIGHLIGHTS

- Contracting the abdominal wall muscles differentiates an intra-abdominal from an extra-abdominal mass
- Wide-necked abdominal wall hernias are unlikely to strangulate and do not require repair
- Fixity of an abdominal mass is related both to its anatomical site and its pathological nature
- Rectal and vaginal examination are essential when assessing a supra-pubic mass
- Ultrasound and CT scans are the mainstay of management of an abdominal mass

8

Jaundice

RCG RUSSELL

AIMS

1 Differentiate between acholuric and cholestatic jaundice
2 In cholestatic jaundice, distinguish extra-hepatic from intra-hepatic obstruction
3 Understand the principles of management of patients with obstructive jaundice
4 Appreciate the risks of interventional procedures in jaundiced patients

DEFINITION

Jaundice is a yellow discoloration of the skin and mucous membranes due to staining with bilirubin when the plasma concentration exceeds 18 mmol/l (1 mg per 100 ml).

In the early stages, the yellow colour is often seen most clearly in the sclerae. The primary sub-division of jaundice into pre-hepatic or acholuric and post-hepatic or cholestatic is readily made by observing whether there is any bile in the urine. The distinction between these two kinds of jaundice is related to the metabolism of bilirubin.

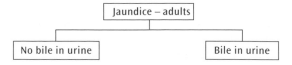

BILIRUBIN METABOLISM – 1

Bilirubin is formed, mainly in the spleen, by the breakdown of haem, 80% of which is derived from senescent erythrocytes, the remainder from other sources such as myoglobin and tissue cytochromes. The microsomal enzyme haem oxygenase converts haem to biliverdin which is then converted to bilirubin by biliverdin reductase. This *unconjugated* bilirubin is insoluble and is transported in the plasma, bound to albumin. It cannot pass the glomerular filter in the kidney and therefore does not appear in the urine. Unconjugated bilirubin is avidly taken up by the liver where it is converted in the hepatocytes into a water-soluble form by conjugation as a diglucuronide. This process, mediated by the microsomal enzyme bilirubin UDP-glucuronyl transferase, facilitates its excretion in the bile.

Unconjugated hyperbilirubinaemia results from increased production, impaired hepatic intake or impaired conjugation of bilirubin.

Acholuric jaundice

Haematological investigations are the key to management. Excessive haemolysis increases the concentration of free haem in the plasma and shortens the lifespan of the erythrocytes. These refinements are usually unnecessary: anaemia and an increased reticulocyte count are sufficient if a reason for increased haemolysis is apparent. Such conditions include abnormal red cells, as in congenital spherocytic jaundice, or red cells containing abnormal haemoglobin, as in the megaloblasts of pernicious anaemia, and the antibody-coated cells of acquired haemolytic anaemia demonstrated by the Coombs' test. If there is no obvious cause for haemolysis, red cell fragility can be tested by exposing the patient's cells to varying concentrations of sodium chloride and the limits of concentration outside which haemolysis occurs are compared with normal cells.

If the erythrocytes are normal, the haemolysis may be due to over-activity of the spleen (*hypersplenism*) that occurs in a group of conditions. However, unless the spleen is palpable, it is more likely that the fault lies with the processes of uptake or conjugation in the liver cells. The most common possibility in the adult is *Gilbert's syndrome*, due partly to a defect in uptake, partly to a reduced concentration of bilirubin UDP-glucuronyl transferase. This condition is genetically determined and is one of the causes of neonatal jaundice, but it is so mild and intermittent that a young adult usually presents without a clear history of jaundice since birth. If the story is typical there is no need for further investigation, but the diagnosis can be confirmed with a needle biopsy of the liver.

Hepatic uptake is also impaired in conditions such as congestive heart failure or porto-systemic shunting because the reduction in hepatic blood flow impairs the delivery of bilirubin to the hepatocytes.

Treatment of acholuric jaundice is usually medical, although splenectomy may be necessary to reduce haemolysis or cholecystectomy for symptomatic pigment stones that result from excess bilirubin excretion in the bile.

BILIRUBIN METABOLISM – 2

Within the liver cells, the conjugated bilirubin is a constituent of bile, with water, inorganic electrolytes and other organic solutes such as phospholipids, cholesterol and bile acids. Impaired formation and excretion of bile is termed *cholestasis*: it may be a defect in formation in the hepatocyte or of passage along the intra-hepatic bile canaliculi (*intra-hepatic cholestasis*) or a mechanical impairment (*extra-hepatic cholestasis*). Cholestasis produces disproportionate elevation in serum alkaline phosphatase activity and bilirubin concentration relative to the serum aminotransferase elevation.

Moreover, although hepatic bilirubin uptake and conjugating activity are preserved in most forms of hepatic disease, canalicular excretion of bile is the rate-limiting step in overall bilirubin metabolism. Therefore, conjugated hyperbilirubinaemia due to back-pressure from cholestasis can occur in a wide spectrum of diseases, including acute and/or chronic hepatocellular damage, specific abnormalities of bilirubin excretion such as the Dubin–Johnson and Rotor syndromes, as well as extra-hepatic biliary obstruction. Since the conjugated bilirubin is water-soluble, when its blood level rises because of outflow obstruction it appears in the urine in excess (*choluria*).

Cholestatic jaundice

The site of obstruction is critical. If it is in the intra-hepatic canaliculi, the sites are multiple and not amenable to surgical relief. For mechanical problems to cause significant jaundice, the obstruction must be in the common hepatic duct or below. If an obstructive process in the left or right hepatic duct develops slowly, compensatory hypertrophy of one lobe and atrophy of the other takes place, leaving the patient unaware of these changes. Only if the obstruction is in the extra-hepatic ducts can interventional procedures help.

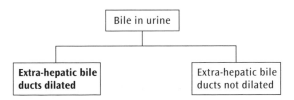

Thus, cholestatic jaundice is sub-divided into pericellular obstruction (*intra-hepatic*), which occurs with hepatocellular damage, and large duct obstruction (*extra-hepatic*). The immediate test to demonstrate large-duct obstruction is an ultrasound examination. This will show whether the intra-hepatic and extra-hepatic bile ducts are dilated, it may detect gallstones, but is unlikely to determine confidently whether the obstruction is due to stone, tumour or any other cause. It also demonstrates any gross change in the liver architecture.

If the extra-hepatic ducts are not dilated, the patient requires screening for infective hepatitis, serological testing and liver biopsy. If the ducts are dilated, management lies in the province of the endoscopist, radiologist or surgeon.

The treatment of patients with extra-hepatic jaundice must be considered urgent because obstruction to the outflow tract damages hepatocytes. The initial investigations are liver function tests of which the most useful are the alkaline phosphatase (20–85 iu/l; 3–13 King–Armstrong units/100 ml) and aspartate and alanine transaminases (both with normal levels of 50–100 iu/l), with albumin (30–49 g/l).

Alkaline phosphatase is excreted by the liver cells into the bile and obstruction to the flow of bile results in an increased rate of formation of the enzyme for reasons unknown, and a consequent early and large backflow into the plasma. Surgical jaundice tends to be associated with high plasma concentrations of this enzyme even before the hepatocytes are sufficiently damaged to become porous to the transaminases. Later, they are also unable to maintain the rate of synthesis of albumin.

Another useful test for the completeness of obstruction is to examine the urine for urobilinogen, easily estimated by dipstick testing. If bilirubin does not reach the intestine then no urobilinogen is formed in the intestine, so that there is none to be re-absorbed into the plasma and ultimately excreted by the kidney. Diminished bile excretion results in less urobilin to darken the stool and less bile acids, resulting in defective fat absorption (*steatorrhoea*). After prolonged obstruction, this gives the stool a characteristic putty colour.

REFINEMENT OF THE DIAGNOSIS OF EXTRA-HEPATIC OBSTRUCTIVE JAUNDICE

Clinical

History-taking should include enquiry about episodes of pain typical of gallstone disease, previous attacks of jaundice, blood transfusion and drug abuse, suggestive of liver disease. A history of anorexia, weight loss and non-specific upper gastrointestinal symptoms is suggestive of pancreatic or other malignant disease.

The patient is examined, with particular reference to possible metastatic spread, palpable lymph nodes, skin nodules, weight loss and loss of muscle mass. In the abdomen, the important features to look for are abdominal distension, visible veins, thickening around the umbilicus, fullness, palpable liver or spleen and ascites. The gall bladder is distended and palpable in 60% of patients with obstructive jaundice when the obstruction is at the lower end of the bile duct, but not when due to gallstones (*Courvoisier's dictum*) because with associated cholecystitis the gall bladder is thickened and fibrosed and is unlikely to be distensible.

Any other mass in the abdomen raises the possibility of a neoplasm which has given rise to secondary deposits in the liver, or in lymph nodes in the porta hepatis.

Investigations

Once the ultrasound scan determines the approximate site of the obstruction, the normality of the gall bladder and the presence of gallstones (Fig. 8.1; Fig. 8.2) the definitive and superior investigation, in centres where this method is available, is a magnetic resonance (MR) cholangiogram (Fig. 8.3). It is

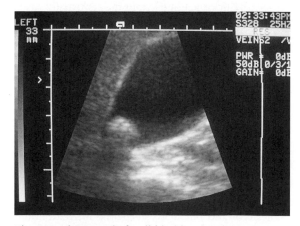

Fig. 8.1 *Ultrasound of gall bladder showing a stone obstructing the cystic duct causing distension of the gall bladder.*

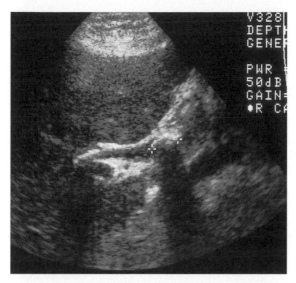

Fig. 8.2 *Ultrasound showing a stone in the common bile duct (note the 'acoustic shadow').*

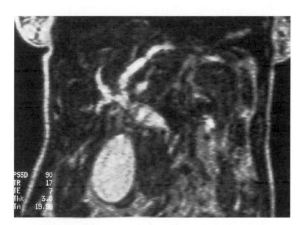

Fig. 8.3 *A magnetic resonance image (MRI) showing the gall bladder and bile ducts. The pancreatic duct is just visible.*

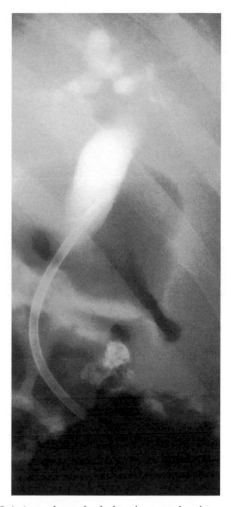

Fig. 8.4 *An endoscopic cholangiogram showing a stent placed to relieve obstruction of the bile duct by a tumour.*

non-invasive and accurately defines the size of the bile ducts, the presence and site of any obstruction, and delineates any obstructing lesion.

The hitherto standard endoscopic retrograde cholangiopancreatography (ERCP) defines the obstruction but invariably allows contrast and infection to leak into the sterile bile above the obstruction, giving rise to a cholangitis. Without the ability immediately to relieve the obstruction by placing a stent, this method is to be deprecated (Fig. 8.4).

If there is no stone, and a tumour has not been clearly defined, then spiral computed tomography (CT) with contrast-enhancement is a powerful tool for outlining a tumour mass, the extent of local invasion into the retroperitoneal tissues and portal vein, and metastatic deposits in the porta hepatis or the liver (Fig. 8.5).

Treatment of common causes

There is increasing evidence that if there is a tumour and it is operable, surgery should not be delayed until jaundice has been relieved. Placing a stent to

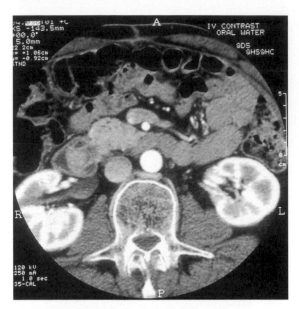

Fig. 8.5 *A contrast-enhanced helical computed tomographic (spiral CT) scan of the duodenum showing an ampullary tumour filling the duodenal lumen and obstructing the bile duct.*

drain the bile ducts increases the risk of infection, whereas in fit adults the resection of a pancreatic or low bile duct tumour is no more hazardous in the *icteric* (jaundiced) than in the non-icteric patient. The absence of infection outweighs the relief of jaundice.

Carcinoma of the head of the pancreas

In about 70% of cases, carcinoma of the pancreas arises in the head of the organ. It is histologically an adenocarcinoma and has a poor prognosis, with a five-year survival rate of 5%. Only 10% of sufferers have localized disease with a potential for cure by *Whipple's operation* (pancreatoduodenectomy), which is the standard procedure. The majority who are inoperable because of age, infirmity or local or widespread advanced disease are treated by placing a stent (endoprosthesis) across the obstruction. This can be performed by the endoscopist passing, via an endoscope positioned opposite the ampulla of Vater, a guide wire into the bile duct under radiological control and then a stent over the guide wire. Alternatively, the radiologist passes percutaneously

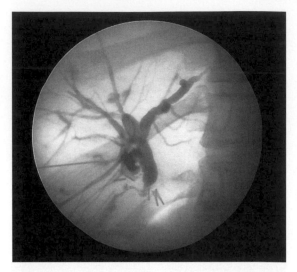

Fig. 8.6 *A percutaneous trans-hepatic cholangiogram (PTC) showing obstruction of the bile duct by surgical clips. Some contrast is seen leaking out of the duct just above the clips.*

a fine needle into the liver, until a bile duct is entered which is defined by injecting contrast (*percutaneous trans-hepatic cholangiogram*, PTC, Fig. 8.6). Then a guidewire is passed through the needle into the duct and under radiological control a stent is placed over the guidewire and positioned through the tumour to relieve the jaundice.

When neither method is feasible or the patient shows signs of duodenal obstruction, a choledochoduodenostomy and gastrojejunostomy is the alternative option.

Carcinoma of ampulla of Vater and lower third of the common bile duct

Adenocarcinoma sometimes arises at the ampulla of Vater or in the duodenal mucosa, forming friable polypoid lesions seen during ERCP (*see* Fig. 8.5 above). Even if invasive, resection is usually the preferred option and a 36% five-year survival is achievable.

Adenocarcinomas in the bile ducts (*cholangiocarcinomas*) are slow-growing and metastasize late so resection is often possible unless locally advanced. The diagnosis is made at ERCP by passing a cannula into the bile duct via the ampulla and injecting contrast medium. The appearances are usually of a stricture with failure to outline the biliary tree. Tissue diagnosis is made by brushings from the stricture and cytological examination, or by CT-guided percutaneous needle biopsy.

Whipple's resection is the procedure of choice for these lesions, but when contraindicated by advanced disease or associated medical conditions, jaundice is relieved by placing a stent as described above.

Choledocholithiasis

Stones in the bile duct usually result from passage of gallstones down the cystic duct, although in the far east patients commonly develop stones in the common duct as well as in the intra-hepatic ducts secondary to the liver fluke *Clonorchis sinensis*. Stones in the bile ducts are preferentially treated endoscopically, followed by laparoscopic cholecystectomy. Endoscopic clearance is performed via ERCP with diathermy sphincterotomy, disrupting the sphincter of Oddi with a wire loop attached to a cautery to allow a stone to fall out or enable a basket to be passed into the duct and around the stone in order to extract it. If these manoeuvres fail, a stent is placed with its tip above the obstruction to allow free drainage pending further intervention.

Alternatively, for those with particular experience, exploration and clearance of the common bile duct is combined with cholecystectomy at laparoscopy, but the technical back-up required outweighs the possible advantages of this surgical approach.

Benign biliary stricture

Solitary benign strictures of the bile ducts invariably follow trauma during operations, in particular cholecystectomy, in the right upper quadrant of the abdomen. During the introduction of laparoscopic cholecystectomy, the incidence of post-operative stricture rose to six per 1000 (Fig. 8.6). Surgical repair usually involves the inter-position of a jejunal loop (*Roux-en-Y*), but infection is common and 20% recur.

Diffuse strictures within the intra- and extra-hepatic biliary tree occur with *sclerosing cholangitis*, a condition of unknown aetiology but probably of autoimmune origin and an extra-intestinal manifestation of inflammatory bowel disease. In patients with AIDS it is associated with infection in the biliary tree with *Cytomegalovirus* and *Cryptosporidium*. These patients run a protracted course and require repeated endoscopic dilatations of the strictures. The appearances on an ERCP can be difficult to distinguish from a cholangiocarcinoma. Surgery plays no role, and colectomy for inflammatory bowel disease does not prevent its progression. In a select group of patients liver transplantation is indicated.

INTRA-HEPATIC OBSTRUCTIVE JAUNDICE

For most patients with cholestatic jaundice, in whom the extra-hepatic bile ducts are not dilated, there are no surgical implications. Occasionally, sepsis may present as intra-hepatic obstructive jaundice in association with cholangitis or portal pyaemia secondary to an intra-abdominal abscess, as occurs with abscesses complicating appendicitis or diverticulitis. Multiple small abscesses develop in the liver in the early stage before they coalesce to form a large intra-hepatic abscess. They may not show on ultrasound and a CT scan is more likely to establish the diagnosis. The treatment is to drain the abscess percutaneously under radiological control and give the appropriate antibiotic (Fig. 8.7).

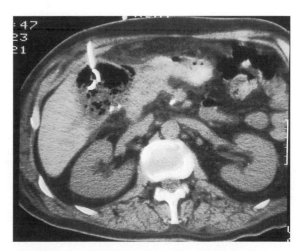

Fig. 8.7 *A spiral CT scan of the liver showing an abscess in the liver. A percutaneous drain inserted under radiological control is sited correctly.*

Occasionally, an hepatic abscess due to *Entamoeba histolytica* may present with jaundice. The serological tests for amoebiasis are likely to be positive. The lesions are readily demonstrable by ultrasound and the diagnosis is confirmed by microscopic examination of needle aspirates unless the parasites are seen in a fresh stool specimen or in rectal mucosal scrapings. The management is aspiration of the abscess and

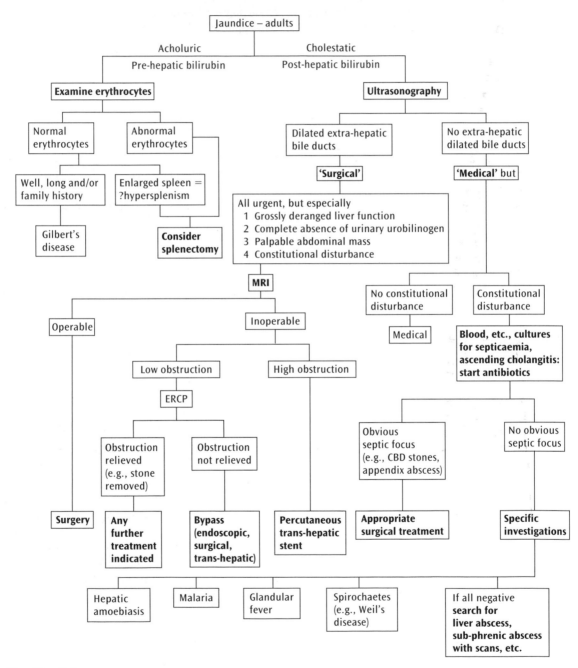

Algorithm 8.1

metronidazole given orally or parenterally depending on the severity of the illness.

Far more common are the various forms of hepatitis, which can be diagnosed by the appropriate serological tests. However, in the early stages the liver function tests are often equivocal and fail to distinguish clearly between intra- and extra-hepatic obstruction. Hence, some patients mistakenly presumed to have hepatitis are often asked to wait weeks for the jaundice to resolve spontaneously. Rather, is it safer that all jaundiced patients in whom there is the slightest possibility of an extra-hepatic cause should have an ultrasound examination. Delay is not defensible.

Hepatocellular carcinoma complicates pre-existing infection with hepatitis B and C, alcoholic cirrhosis and chronic active hepatitis; and secondary liver tumours do not usually present with jaundice until the terminal stage of the illness. Jaundice results from progressive loss of liver parenchyma and obstruction of the intra-hepatic biliary tree. An early diagnosis can be reached with ultrasonography, although a liver biopsy for tissue diagnosis may be required to justify a passive approach if the evidence is not conclusive.

DANGERS OF INTERVENTIONAL PROCEDURES IN JAUNDICED PATIENTS

Any intervention, including endoscopic procedures, in a jaundiced patient constitutes a risk because of the likelihood of developing bleeding from a coagulopathy, or renal failure (*hepato-renal syndrome*) due to a combination of sepsis and a direct effect of high bilirubin levels on the kidney. The coagulopathy is due to impaired absorption of fat-soluble vitamin K in the absence of the solubilizing effects of bile acids. Intramuscular vitamin K1, which is the substrate for prothrombin synthesis, several days before the procedure improves the prothrombin ratio, and if necessary, fresh frozen plasma is given pre-operatively. Renal function is maintained before the operation, when oral intake is restricted, and during the per- and post-operative periods by ensuring that the patient is not 'dehydrated', that is, does not lack sodium chloride and water, by administering isotonic infusions with careful monitoring of the urine output. Diuretics such as mannitol are unnecessary.

Jaundiced patients are relatively immunosuppressed so the absence of sepsis is critical to their smooth recovery and therefore antibiotics are given. An indwelling catheter provides a more accurate measure of urine output and fluid balance, but may introduce infection and its use may be counterproductive. Strict aseptic technique should be adopted when placing a catheter, which is better removed once the patient shows stable signs.

HIGHLIGHTS

- Jaundice is an emergency; diagnosis and treatment should not be delayed
- Ultrasound is the determinant examination distinguishing between extra-hepatic and intra-hepatic jaundice
- ERCP can precipitate cholangitis in obstructive jaundice unless adequate drainage is secured
- Definitive operations aimed at cure should be performed without preliminary procedures to relieve the jaundice
- In patients with extra-hepatic biliary obstruction due to stone, the common duct should be cleared endoscopically before treating the gall bladder

Change in bowel habit; 'piles'

PAUL B BOULOS

INTRODUCTION

These two presentations are described in the same chapter because they frequently overlap.

Alteration in bowel habit is frequently disregarded unless severe or persistent. Benign and malignant ano-rectal disorders present with varied symptoms that are often attributed to 'piles'. Although patients are uncomfortable and distressed they are embarrassed and tolerate their symptoms for a long time before seeking advice. Readily available commercial preparations make self-treatment easy and this delays consultation.

ACUTE PRESENTATIONS

Major rectal bleeding, diarrhoea and acute anal pain are common emergency presentations. 'Absolute' constipation, that is, the inability to pass flatus, resulting from large bowel obstruction can gradually develop over a period of days or weeks until obstruction is complete (*acute-on-chronic obstruction*, Chapter 26).

Major rectal bleeding

This refers to fresh or altered blood passed per rectum, as distinct from bloody diarrhoea. Acute lower gastrointestinal haemorrhage accounts for approximately 1.5% of all surgical emergencies, and in about 10% is severe and requires hospitalization. Gastrointestinal bleeding is major or severe if the circulation is compromised or the haemoglobin level reduced sufficiently to require blood transfusion. However, many patients are hospitalized because of anxiety that progression of bleeding may threaten life. The identified source of bleeding is from the lower gastrointestinal tract, the colon in 85% and the small intestine in 5%; and in 10% is from the upper gastrointestinal tract (i.e., proximal to the ligament of Treitz or duodeno-jejunal flexure). However, the source of gastrointestinal bleeding is not identified in 10% of all cases.

Colonic causes are the most common source; of these, *angiodysplasia* and *colonic diverticula* account for more than 60% of all the cases of major bleeding. Although colonic polyps and carcinoma are common causes of bleeding, only 5% bleed massively. Rare causes include vasculitis due to connective tissue disease causing ischaemia and ulceration, small bowel lesions (such as diverticula including Meckel's diverticulum containing heterotopic gastric mucosa) and tumours and diseases that also affect the colon (such as radiation enteritis, angiodysplasia and haemangiomas).

Initial resuscitation

It is essential to obtain a full blood count, urea and electrolytes, clotting screen, liver function tests and to cross-match and group blood for transfusion if required. ECG and chest X-rays are necessary in patients aged over 65 years or with cardio-respiratory disease. Patients who are at high risk of re-bleeding and death are those over 60 years, with a systolic blood pressure of less than 100 mmHg, a haemoglobin of less than 10 g/dl and with associated cardiovascular, respiratory, liver or renal disease. They demand vigilant resuscitation and monitoring: the rate and volume of intravenous fluid or blood replacement is adjusted according to the responses of the pulse rate, blood pressure, central venous pressure and hourly urine output. Blood products may be necessary if there is a disturbance of coagulation.

Initial assessment

Usually, the passage of fresh blood indicates bleeding from the colon, since blood originating from the upper gastrointestinal tract or small intestine is, in transit through the intestinal tract, altered by digestion to a black or plum-coloured tarry liquid, *melaena*. However, massive and rapid bleeding at any level, including upper gastrointestinal, can result in the passage of fresh blood per rectum that may be indistinguishable from a lower gastrointestinal source. Therefore, the colour of the blood in the stool does not reliably discriminate between bleeding from the upper or the lower gastrointestinal tract.

Once the patient is stable, a comprehensive history is taken: *haematemesis* indicates bleeding from the oesophagus, stomach or duodenum, but in an initial presentation the pattern of vomiting prior to bleeding may suggest Mallory–Weiss tears. Other

details of relevance are intake of non-steroidal anti-inflammatory drugs (NSAIDs), alcohol consumption, previous peptic ulceration or gastric surgery, cirrhosis and variceal haemorrhage, altered bowel habit or previous episodes of rectal bleeding. Previous aortic surgery is relevant because of the rare and frequently overlooked risk of a fistula between the prosthetic graft and the duodenum.

General and abdominal examination is usually unremarkable but may contribute signs of chronic liver disease, a palpable abdominal mass or an aortic aneurysm. A rectal examination may reveal melaena or detect a tumour. Proctosigmoidoscopy can be laborious because of a rectum loaded with blood and stool, but the diagnostic yield can be improved if preceded by an enema. This is essential as it provides an instant diagnosis and avoids extensive investigations and delay in treatment. Ano-rectal conditions such as haemorrhoids and fissure, proctitis or telangiectasias following radiotherapy and rectal cancer can cause active, although not usually life-threatening haemorrhage.

Subsequent investigation and management

Before subjecting patients to elaborate investigations, a *bleeding diathesis* should be excluded. Drugs such as anticoagulants, NSAIDs, steroids and enteric-coated potassium chloride can cause gastrointestinal haemorrhage. Nearly 90% will stop bleeding and the source of bleeding can then be determined by conventional diagnostic endoscopy and radiology. The remaining patients are investigated as rapidly as necessary and as completely as their physical state permits.

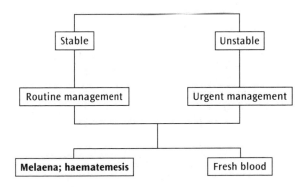

Bleeding from the upper gastrointestinal tract may be obvious. A rise in blood urea, unless the creatinine is also elevated due to renal impairment, is the result of absorption of nitrogenous products of blood digestion in the small intestine, and suggests a non-colonic source of bleeding. The absence of blood in a naso-gastric aspirate probably rules out upper gastrointestinal bleeding, although endoscopy is preferable. Endoscopy should be performed promptly in high-risk patients, otherwise deferred until the next convenient session. Endoscopy allows injection of bleeding lesions with sclerosant/adrenaline mixture and rubber band ligation of varices, it also identifies those patients with an active spurting vessel or a visible vessel, an adherent clot or gastro-oesophageal varices who are considered to be at risk of re-bleeding.

| Melaena; haematemesis | **Fresh blood** |

Lower gastrointestinal haemorrhage is investigated by use of colonoscopy, selective visceral angiography and radio-isotope scintigraphy, once bleeding from the upper gastrointestinal tract has been excluded. There is no place for a barium enema as it does not outline vascular malformations and residual barium interferes with the other diagnostic modalities and loads the colon, making emergency resection laborious and hazardous.

Colonoscopy is used more frequently now that it appears that colonic cleansing does not dislodge adherent clots and precipitate re-bleeding. Saline or sulphate purgation or whole-gut irrigation is used, but cautiously in elderly patients, as it may precipitate fluid and electrolyte disturbance. Colonoscopy has the best diagnostic yield as it allows observing the source of bleeding: patients with diverticular disease at one site may be bleeding from a vascular lesion elsewhere. The presence of fresh blood in a segment without blood proximal to it, and an adherent clot are regarded as signs of bleeding from this segment. Colonoscopy also allows treatment of colonic angiomata with sclerotherapy, electrocoagulation or laser therapy.

Selective visceral angiography, cannulating sequentially the superior and inferior mesenteric arteries and the coeliac axis using a modified Seldinger technique, successfully localizes the bleeding. The accuracy of diagnostic angiography depends on a rate of ongoing bleeding of more than 0.5–1.0 ml/min. It can be difficult to determine the optimal timing for angiography: the passage of a large amount of bloody stool may be the result of an earlier episode rather than of ongoing bleeding. Systemic heparinization, selective intra-arterial tolazoline vasodilatation and thrombolytic agents such as streptokinase or urokinase have been used to precipitate or exacerbate bleeding in order to improve the diagnostic yield of angiography (*pharmaco-angiography*).

Nuclear medicine techniques include technetium (^{99m}Tc) sulphur colloid scintigraphy and technetium red blood cell scintigraphy. ^{99m}Tc sulphur colloid is rapidly cleared by the liver and spleen, therefore the patient must be actively bleeding at the time of the study. In contrast, ^{99m}Tc-labelled red blood cells remain in the circulation longer and may produce a positive result on repeat scanning over 48 hours, making the method particularly suitable in patients with intermittent bleeding but with low transfusion requirements.

The choice of investigation after resuscitation depends on the magnitude and progression of the bleeding. The patient who is stable with minor or intermittent bleeding is prepared for colonoscopy and if a lesion is found it is treated either endoscopically or by open surgery. If colonoscopy fails to identify a lesion, the patient who is bleeding intermittently is then investigated by radio-isotope scanning or, if the bleeding is ongoing and rapid, emergency angiography is performed employing pharmaco-angiography if necessary. If a bleeding site is identified, trans-catheter therapy with intra-arterial vasopressin or embolization should be considered.

Surgical treatment

In the patient who continues to bleed from an identified site, segmental resection is carried out. If the bleeding point has not been identified, intra-operative colonoscopy and enteroscopy is undertaken. Pre-operative bowel preparation is performed in patients in whom bleeding is inactive, but if the bleeding is ongoing, rapid on-table lavage is necessary. An appendicectomy is performed and a Foley catheter is inserted into the appendix stump. Normal saline is infused while a proctoscope or suction tubing is placed in the anus to facilitate drainage. A colonoscope is passed until the bleeding point is found. If a lesion in the small bowel is suspected, push-enteroscopy is carried out by passing a paediatric colonoscope or an enteroscope orally, advanced with the help of the abdominal operator.

If all the pre-operative and intra-operative investigations have failed to identify the bleeding site or could not be performed because the bleeding is massive and the patient unstable, a sub-total colectomy with ileo-rectal anastomosis is the only active option but carries the risk of diarrhoea and incontinence in elderly patients. This is still the recommended procedure, even if left-sided diverticular disease is found at laparotomy, because there is a 30% re-bleeding rate from a non-diverticular source after blind resection of the diseased segment.

Diarrhoea

Diarrhoea can be either watery or, when associated with colitis, bloody. Diarrhoea threatens life by loss of fluid from the extra-cellular compartment. When the loss exceeds the ability to replace it orally, dehydration occurs and hospitalization is essential. Diarrhoea related to irritable bowel syndrome (IBS), infection with *Giardiasis*, malabsorption due to coeliac disease, sprue or chronic pancreatitis, post-surgical following vagotomy, gastric surgery or small bowel resection and colo-rectal cancer or diverticular disease does not usually pose such a problem.

Initial management

The initial management consists of replacing the fluid and electrolyte losses, blood transfusion if required and hyperalimentation if the patient is under-nourished. The patient is examined regularly for signs of anaemia, dehydration, abdominal distension and tenderness due to toxic megacolon that can complicate severe invasive infection of the colon and acute inflammatory bowel disease. The temperature, pulse, blood pressure and urine output are monitored. The stool frequency, its consistency and presence of blood are recorded daily.

Other investigations that measure the systemic effects of the diarrhoeal illness and its response to treatment and therefore repeated regularly during the course of the disease include the haemoglobin level and the white cell count, erythrocyte sedimentation rate (ESR), C-reactive protein (CRP), urea and creatinine, plasma sodium and potassium, plasma proteins and liver enzymes. An abdominal X-ray is repeated daily if toxic megacolon is suspected.

The few conditions that present with severe diarrhoea are intestinal infections, inflammatory bowel disease and, rarely, ischaemic colitis.

The diagnostic dilemma

Besides diarrhoea, clinical features include colicky abdominal pain, nausea, vomiting, fever, tachycardia, anaemia and signs of dehydration, abdominal tenderness and distension. It is essential to distinguish infections from inflammatory bowel disease and, rarely, ischaemic colitis in the elderly because inappropriate use of corticosteroids or delay in administering an antibiotic is undesirable and has serious consequences. This cannot be achieved by clinical assessment, although certain aspects of the history and examination may give direction to the diagnostic process.

A rapid onset of symptoms, pyrexia and severe abdominal pain favour colonic infection rather than inflammatory bowel disease. The possible geographic origins of an infection should be sought, although travel to tropical or sub-tropical regions is not necessary for the acquisition of intestinal infection. Enquiries should be made about other risk factors, such as antibiotic or chemotherapy, immunodeficiency, food recently ingested and contact with sufferers or potential carriers. Patients with inflammatory bowel disease are also at risk of superadded infection so an apparent relapse, whether they have travelled abroad or not, could be due to infection. In 10% of patients a severe attack may be the first manifestation of the disease.

Helpful clinical features include peri-anal stigmata of Crohn's disease, evidence of HIV infection (*Kaposi's sarcoma*, *hairy leukoplakia* or *oropharyngeal candidiasis*) the cutaneous signs of typhoid (*rose patch*) or extra-intestinal manifestations of inflammatory bowel disease, although joint symptoms may accompany intestinal infections, particularly

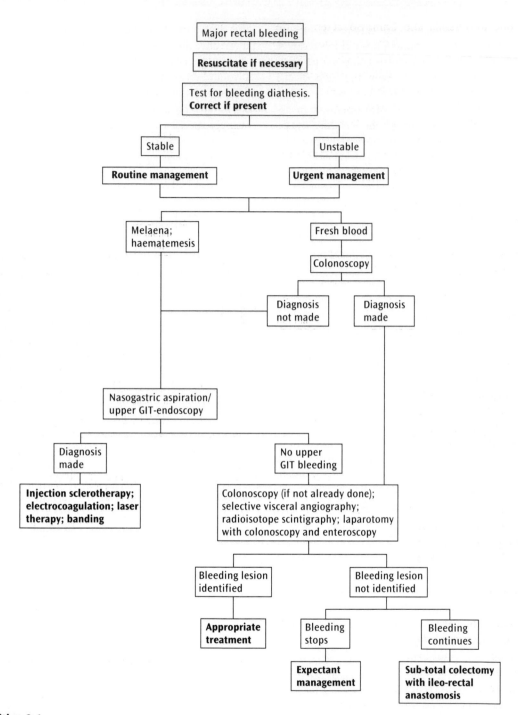

Algorithm 9.1

those due to Yersinia and Campylobacter. In the elderly patient with cardiac failure, hypertension or diabetes and following cardiac or aortic surgery, ischaemic colitis is the more likely diagnosis but infective diarrhoea is nevertheless possible.

Rigid sigmoidoscopy is an important part of the examination, although the findings may not be diagnostic. A normal rectum does not exclude proximal infective or inflammatory bowel disease or ischaemia. Even when the rectum is macroscopically inflamed it is not possible to make a specific diagnosis; bacterial infection can produce appearances identical to ulcerative colitis. The presence of pseudomembrane strongly suggests *Clostridium difficile* infection but also occurs in intestinal ischaemia. Therefore biopsies and histological and bacteriological examination are crucial.

Biopsies should be taken from the rectum at proctosigmoidoscopy, irrespective of the appearances of the rectal mucosa. *E. coli* trophozoites, *C. parvum* can sometimes be detected in mucosal biopsies. The only reliable method of confirming cytomegalovirus infection is finding the typical owl's eye inclusion bodies usually present in the sub-mucosa. Although histological appearances of inflammatory bowel disease are diagnostic, the acute inflammatory changes make the distinction between ulcerative and Crohn's colitis difficult, but this is not detrimental to acute management.

At least three fresh faecal specimens collected on separate days should be submitted to light microscopy and culture. Although many pathogens, including *E. coli*, *C. jejuni*, *E. histolytica*, Shigella spp and Salmonella spp synthesize toxins that are responsible for the secretory diarrhoea and epithelial damage, the only toxin that is routinely sought is *C. difficile,* as isolation of the organism on culture in the absence of toxin is inconclusive since healthy adults may excrete *C. difficile*.

Serology is of value in patients with invasive amoebic colitis in whom 85–95% have anti-*E. histolytica* IgG antibodies in serum, and should be performed in patients suspected of amoebiasis, although a negative test does not exclude amoebiasis. Similarly, positive rates are found in patients with amoebic liver abscess. Serology can also be of value in the diagnosis of yersiniosis when a rise in titre can usually be demonstrated within 10–14 days after presentation.

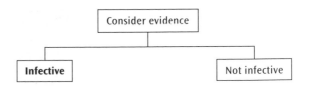

Treatment of intestinal infection

Most acute intestinal infections resolve without specific antimicrobial chemotherapy, although it is appropriate to use antibiotics for enteropathogens producing dysentery and persistent diarrhoea. Pseudomembranous colitis due to *C. difficile* is treated with metronidazole or vancomycin. Amoebic colitis is treated with oral metronidazole or another nitroimidazole for 10 days followed by a second agent, such as diloxanide furoate, to clear the encysted forms of the parasite. Shigella dysentery is best treated with 4-fluoroquinolone or nalidixic acid because of resistance to standard drugs such as ampicillin and trimethoprim-sulphamethoxazole. Salmonella enteritis usually resolves spontaneously but ciprofloxacin reduces the duration of diarrhoea. *Campylobacter jejuni* is treated with erythromycin as first choice. *Yersinia enterocolitica* infection requires antibiotics such as tetracycline, trimethoprim-sulphamethoxazole, aminoglycosides, chloramphenicol or a third-generation cephalosporin. Uncomplicated enteritis or mesenteric adenitis due to *Y. enterocolitica* does not usually require antibiotic therapy. Cytomegalovirus is treated with ganciclovir.

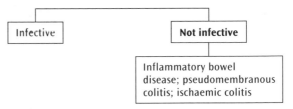

Treatment of acute inflammatory bowel disease

Acute colitis is defined as fulminant colitis when there is evidence of any two of the following:

- Tachycardia (>100/min).
- Fever (>38.6°C).
- Leukocytosis (>10.5 × 10^9).
- Hypoalbuminaemia (<3.0 g/dl).

Medical therapy is started using high doses of intravenous corticosteroids, bowel rest with nasogastric decompression, broad-spectrum antibiotics against gut flora to minimize the risk of sepsis from trans-mural inflammation or microperforation. Anticholinergic, antidiarrhoeal and narcotic agents are avoided in order not to impair colonic motility or conceal ominous symptoms. Intravenous cyclosporin is an effective alternative in patients not responding to steroids. The main ensuing complications are toxic dilatation, perforation and massive haemorrhage.

The clinical signs and investigations already mentioned are useful indices for monitoring the patient's progress. Deterioration over the ensuing 24–72 hours or failure to improve after 5–7 days of intensive medical therapy demands urgent laparotomy.

Toxic megacolon is diagnosed when pain, fever, toxicity, abrupt cessation of bowel movement, abdominal tenderness and distension are accompanied by dilatation of the transverse colon that exceeds 7 cm on abdominal X-ray. Toxic megacolon may lead to perforation that is associated with an appreciable mortality (20–40% with perforation as compared to 4% with no perforation) and therefore urgent surgery is recommended. Free perforation, massive haemorrhage, peritonitis and septic shock are indications for emergent operation.

Sub-total colectomy with end-ileostomy, retaining the rectum and the distal sigmoid colon as a mucous fistula, is the most widely practised operation for acute fulminating colitis and its complications, deferring any definitive treatment of the rectal stump until the patient's fitness allows.

Treatment of ischaemic colitis

This should be suspected in elderly patients with hypertension, cardiac insufficiency or diabetes. It presents with colicky lower abdominal pain of sudden onset, associated with diarrhoea and sometimes bleeding which is not excessive. Nausea, vomiting and anorexia may be present suggesting the presence of ileus. Physical signs, such as fever, localized tenderness and altered blood mixed with stool, may be absent. The pulse rate and blood pressure are usually normal. There is mild leucocytosis. Sigmoidoscopy

can be normal as ischaemia usually is more proximal. Colonoscopy is the investigation of choice: the mucosa is hyperaemic and oedematous, nodular, friable and ulcerated and biopsies confirm the diagnosis. Transient ischaemic colitis (*non-gangrenous colitis*) is treated expectantly with nasogastric suction to rest the bowel, intravenous fluid and antibiotics. Symptoms of abdominal pain and diarrhoea resolve within a few days. A repeat colonoscopy should be deferred until 3–6 weeks when the mucosal abnormality would have resolved completely.

If symptoms progress to manifest signs of transmural infarction (*gangrenous colitis*), such as fever, tachycardia and peritonism, urgent surgery under antibiotic cover and fluid and electrolyte replacement is performed. The extent of colonic resection is dependent on the extent of ischaemia. An anastomosis is avoided because of the underlying ischaemia. Instead, the ends of the distal and proximal viable bowel are exteriorized so that they are accessible for regular examination as further resection may be necessary if any of the exteriorized ends becomes gangrenous. Bowel continuity is restored when the patient has fully recovered. Ischaemic colitis has a high mortality.

Perspective

Although 30–60% of acute diarrhoeal episodes are due to rotavirus, Shigella spp, *E. coli*, *Staphylococcus aureus* and *E. histolytica* infections occur through a vehicle such as water, food or by direct human contact. Salmonella spp and *C. jejuni* are acquired from inadequately cooked chicken carcasses. Salmonellae infect not only the intestinal tract of chickens but also the genital tract; thus, the organism exists in eggs and outbreaks occur in foods in which eggs are used raw or only partially cooked. The most clinically important infections in immunodeficient patients are due to the intracellular protozoa (*C. parvum*, Microsporidia, *Cyclospora cayatenensis*), *Mycobacterium avium*-complex and the other invasive dysenteric enteropathogens including cytomegalovirus. *C. difficile* infection is a side-effect of antibiotic treatment and is a result of selective overgrowth, resulting in pseudomembranous colitis.

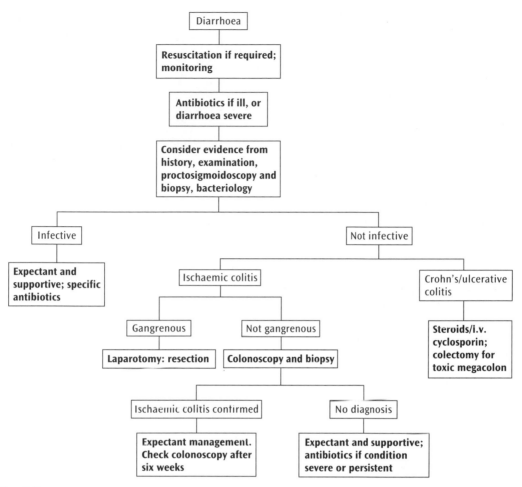

Algorithm 9.2

Acute 'piles'

Ano-rectal pain can be disabling and is commonly described as a 'severe attack of piles'. It is important to distinguish true pain from the sensation of burning and irritation of the skin caused by peri-anal skin disorders. Traumatic laceration of the ano-rectal region is painful and should be recognized from the patient's acute history. Most commonly, acute ano-rectal pain is caused by an abscess, a fissure, a thrombosed external haemorrhoid or a thrombosed internal haemorrhoid. The patient's description should help differentiate these causes. An abscess or a fissure may not show visible physical signs on inspection but digital examination can be uncomfortable, whereas a thrombosed external or internal haemorrhoid shows a peri-anal swelling.

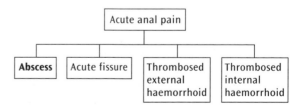

Anal abscesses

Pain often precedes the appearance of an abscess. It is a continuous throbbing pain and the patient may complain of fever. The pain increases with intensity

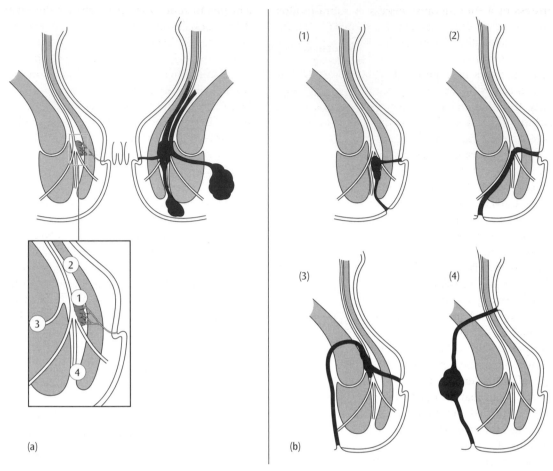

Fig. 9.1 *Ano-rectal sepsis and anal fistulae; (a) The spread of anal gland infection. The anal gland lies in the inter-sphincteric space: infection may cause an abscess (1) in the inter-sphincteric space or (2) upwards into the supra-levator or extra-rectal space, or (3) laterally through the external anal sphincter into the ischio-rectal fossa, or (4) downwards through the inter-sphincteric plane to form a peri-anal abscess; (b) (1) Inter-sphincteric fistula extending from the dentate line to the anal verge; (2) trans-sphincteric fistula; (3) supra-sphincteric fistula; (4) extra-sphincteric fistula.*

when the patient coughs or sneezes. Severe cases may be associated with urinary retention. There may be a localized area of tenderness and induration at the anal verge or the buttocks, but redness or swelling may not manifest until later; rectal examination, under anaesthesia if necessary, reveals a tender mass at the tip of the finger (*supra-levator*), lateral to the rectum (*ischio-rectal*), or a tender boggy swelling in the anal canal (*inter-sphincteric*) (Fig. 9.1).

Acute ano-rectal sepsis arises as an area of cutaneous sepsis close to the anus or as a result of cryptoglandular infection. The anal glands lie between the internal and external sphincters and drain via ducts into tiny pits at the anal crypts near the dentate line. Purulent infection in the glands may remain confined between the sphincters forming an inter-sphincteric abscess. Cephalad extension in the inter-sphincteric space will result in a high inter-muscular abscess or a supra-levator abscess. A supra-levator abscess may also originate from pelvic disease (appendiceal, diverticular, Crohn's disease, gynaecologic or malignant). Caudal spread towards the anal verge presents as a peri-anal abscess, and lateral spread across the external sphincter into the fibro-fatty tissue of the ischio-rectal fossa leads to an ischio-rectal abscess. Besides horizontal and vertical spread, sepsis may spread circumferentially in any of the three spaces: inter-sphincteric; ischio-rectal and para-rectal. Cryptoglandular infection creates an abscess which if not treated adequately in its early stages leads to a fistula between the skin surface and a point deep in the anal canal (see Fig. 9.1 (b)).

Treatment is by drainage under general anaesthesia by an internal sphincterotomy if the abscess is inter-sphincteric and by skin incision over the most fluctuant part of the abscess if peri-anal or ischio-rectal, leaving a loose pack or a drain to keep the cavity open. A supra-levator abscess is drained through an incision in the rectum via the anal canal. The pus should be sent for bacteriological analysis as growth of gut but not skin organisms can be suggestive of an underlying fistula. At the time, or when further examination under anaesthesia after a few days is carried out in order to ensure complete drainage, the anal canal is inspected for an internal opening of a fistula which may not be easily detectable because of tissue oedema. The search should not be pursued actively as such manipulation may create a false track or damage the sphincters. Instead, the wound is allowed to heal. Half the cases develop a fistula, which should be suspected if there is persistent discharge through the area of the skin incision or induration and tenderness in the area even after the incision scar has healed.

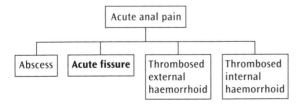

Acute anal fissure

This is a cut or crack in the anal canal that results from the trauma of a hard stool and is suggested by a history of sudden severe sharp pain during or after defaecation, lasting for few seconds to several hours. Gently separating the buttocks to look for signs of a tear in the anal verge may itself provoke pain. Digital examination may fail because of pain and sphincter spasm, when an inter-sphincteric abscess cannot be ruled out, but may elicit localized tenderness or spasm suggestive of a fissure. Proctoscopy and sigmoidoscopy to eliminate an underlying rectal disease are deferred until the fissure has healed, or performed under anaesthesia if there is uncertainty about the cause of the pain.

Management consists of warm sitz baths that are beneficial in relieving the spasm associated with a fissure, and a bulk-forming agent or bran to soften the stool. Local application of anaesthetic ointment applied directly to the fissure may provide some symptomatic relief. Topical nitroglycerine, diltiazem and nifedipine promote internal sphincter relaxation and have been successfully used in the treatment of anal fissures.

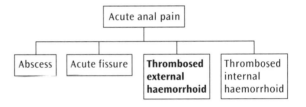

Peri-anal haematoma or thrombosed external haemorrhoid

This is the probable diagnosis when the patient presents with continuous pain not related to defaecation and associated with a tender lump. Both its names are misnomers: the thrombosis seems to be intravascular, the clot having an endothelial lining; and it is unrelated to haemorrhoids. In some but not in all patients, the condition is due to back pressure on an anal venule consequent upon straining at stool, coughing, or lifting a heavy weight. A tense, painful and tender swelling with a bluish tinge appears suddenly at the anal margin. When the patient presents soon after onset, pain is relieved by evacuating the clot through a radial skin incision under local anaesthesia. The skin edges are trimmed to avoid a true haematoma collecting. Without treatment, acute

less than twice per week or the need to strain at defaecation more than 25% of the time. For patients, the term may also mean that the stool is hard or incompletely evacuated or it may encompass a range of functional symptoms, including bloating and pain. The causes of constipation are numerous but an obstructing colonic lesion is the one of concern. *Diarrhoea* is the passage of a liquid or semi-formed stool with an increase in the number of motions. *Tenesmus* is a sensation of incomplete evacuation and a frequent urge to defaecate with poor result; it is associated with proctitis or rectal neoplasms and is frequently described by patients as diarrhoea, although it is spurious.

The examination

Inflammatory bowel disease, diverticular disease and large bowel cancer are the most common conditions to consider when patients present with a change in bowel habit with or without anal symptoms. The signs to be sought are:

- Anaemia (blood loss or malabsorption).
- Oral aphthous ulcers and gingivitis (inflammatory bowel disease).
- Jaundice, cervical lymphadenopathy, pleural effusion or lung consolidation, hepatomegaly and ascites (metastatic colorectal cancer).
- Abdominal tenderness or a palpable mass (Crohn's disease, diverticular disease or cancer).

Physical signs due to extra-intestinal manifestations associated with inflammatory bowel disease include eye disorder (uveitis, iritis and iridocyclitis), skin lesions (erythema nodosum and pyoderma gangrenosum) and arthropathy (sacroileitis, ankylosing spondylitis or rheumatoid-like arthritis, especially of large joints).

Examination of the ano-rectal region starts with careful inspection of: the peri-anal skin for erythema, discoloration, exudate and thickening; of the anal verge, observing the closure of the anal opening on voluntary contraction; any lump, external openings of anal fistulas seen as small buds of granulation tissue or scars from previous surgery; and perineal descent or rectal mucosal or full-thickness prolapse while the patient performs a Valsalva manoeuvre.

Palpation detects induration and tenderness along a fistula track and gentle external pressure may demonstrate purulent material exuding from either the internal or external fistula opening. Digital examination is only performed with informed consent, and is abandoned if the patient finds it uncomfortable or painful. Once the finger is in the anal canal, the resting sphincter tone is noted and the patient is next asked to squeeze the sphincter muscle to establish the function of the puborectalis and the external sphincter muscle. Puborectalis contraction is appreciated as a strong anterior pull of the posteriorly based muscle sling. The finger next palpates the anal canal circumferentially for induration, scarring or swelling; anteriorly the prostate gland is assessed in men, the cervix and uterus in women. An anterior sphincter defect in women can often be detected by bi-digital examination of the perineal body with the index finger in the anal canal and the thumb in the posterior fourchette. If a neoplasm is detected, the distance of its distal margin to the anal verge, its texture (hard, nodular, soft or velvety), approximate size, mobility and its position within the anal canal (anterior versus posterior or lateral) are determined. Rigid sigmoidoscopy is then carried out and the mucosa is visualized for signs of inflammation or ulceration and for the presence of a polyp or a neoplasm.

Proctoscopy demonstrates internal haemorrhoids and rectal mucosal prolapse that can easily be seen bulging into the proctoscope when the patient is instructed to strain. Instrumentation in the presence of a fissure is unnecessary and is contraindicated.

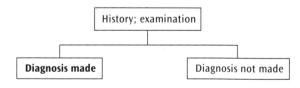

Diagnosis made

Minor anorectal disorders identified by history and examination as described hereunder can be treated without further investigations. When fungal infection is suspected a scraping of the skin is placed on a glass slide. A drop of 10–20% potassium hydroxide is placed on the scraping followed by a coverslip.

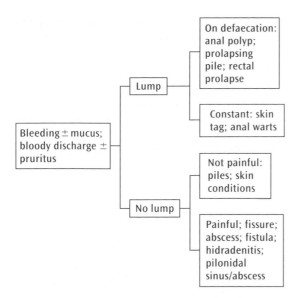

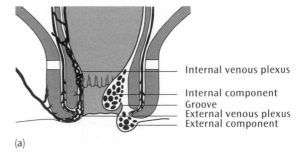

Internal venous plexus

Internal component
Groove
External venous plexus
External component

(a)

The slide is gently heated and then examined under the microscope. The diagnosis can also be confirmed by culturing the affected area for fungal organisms.

Haemorrhoids (piles)

The anal cushions contain a rich plexus of veins. They normally lie beneath the columnar epithelium in the upper anal canal, within the anal orifice. Haemorrhoids or piles are due to congestion and hypertrophy of the cushions by impeded venous drainage and engorgement of the internal venous plexus as a result of compression by faeces (*internal haemorrhoids*). The anal cushions are displaced distally, with progressive loss of their supporting connective tissue, by the forces of defaecation and extend beneath the stratified squamous epithelium to lie outside the anal orifice (*external haemorrhoids*), with engorgement of the external venous plexus because of its communication with the internal venous plexus (Fig. 9.2 (a) and (b)). They receive a rich blood supply from the rectal arteries and communicate not only through the capillaries but by direct arterio-venous shunts (*corpora cavernosa recta*), and hence they bleed bright arterial blood. Internal haemorrhoids are frequently arranged in three groups at 3, 7 and 11 o'clock with the patient in

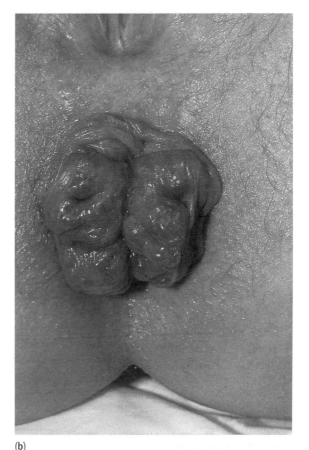

(b)

Fig. 9.2 *(a) Pathological anatomy and (b) clinical appearance of haemorrhoids.*

the lithotomy position. This distribution is ascribed to the termination of the right and left branches of the superior haemorrhoidal artery. The right one subdivides into anterior and posterior branches and the left remains single.

Bleeding with mucous discharge and pruritus are characteristic features of haemorrhoids of all degrees of severity. Bright blood, related to defaecation or spontaneous, but without an external lump constitutes the *first-degree*; a protrusion of a lump during defaecation but reducing spontaneously is the *second-degree*; lumps requiring to be manually reduced are *third-degree*; but prolapse after replacement or permanent prolapse constitutes the *fourth-degree*. The diagnosis is established by proctoscopy with normal findings at sigmoidoscopy.

Conservative management as an outpatient includes:

- A high-fibre diet.
- Injection sclerotherapy.
- 3–5 ml of 5% phenol in oil or 5% quinine and urea hydrochloride is injected into the submucosa above the haemorrhoid, inducing fibrosis in order to obliterate the vessels and fix the cushions to the underlying muscle.
- Rubber band ligation, particularly for prolapsing haemorrhoids. A special applicator is used to apply a rubber ring tightly around the neck of a tongue of mucosa at the base of the haemorrhoid, causing ischaemic necrosis of the tissues and ulceration and therefore fixation of the mucosa by fibrosis.

Haemorrhoidectomy is indicated when conservative measures fail, and for prolapsing haemorrhoids with a large external component. The operation most commonly performed is the Milligan and Morgan, in which each haemorrhoid is dissected off the internal sphincter and is excised after transfixing and ligating its base, leaving a bridge of skin and mucosa between each wound to prevent stenosis.

Skin tags

These are frequently misinterpreted by the patient as prolapsed irreducible piles but they probably represent redundant residual skin left after spontaneous resolution of thrombosed internal or external haemorrhoids or a healed chronic anal fissure (Fig. 9.3). Patients often complain that the tags make anal hygiene difficult, and that they are itchy and unsightly. Improvement in anal hygiene may itself diminish large oedematous skin tags. Excision is

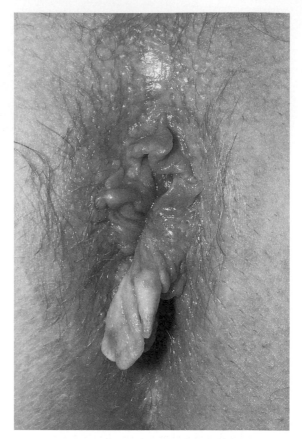

Fig. 9.3 *Skin tag.*

unnecessary and should be avoided unless the tags are large or remain symptomatic with conservative treatment. Excision, when necessary, is performed across the base rather than radially to avoid creating a skin furrow which fails to heal and develops into a painful fissure.

Anal warts (Condyloma accuminatum)

Examination reveals single, filiform, pinkish-white warts that may coalesce to form a large mass with a foul odour. They are caused by the human papilloma virus (HPV) of which four types are usually sexually transmitted. Types 6 and 11 are usually benign, but types 16 and 18 are associated with the development of dysplasia and invasive carcinoma. Warts occur in both sexes. They are commonly due to ano-receptive intercourse, but can occur by direct extension from the genital area.

Pruritus ani, bleeding, discharge, persistent dampness and pain with the presence of a lump are the usual symptoms. Giant condylomata (*Busche–Lowenstein's disease*) is a rare lesion that has the shape of a cauliflower and progressively enlarges forming a locally invasive but not metastasizing growth that may obliterate the anal canal. Dysplastic change may occur with progression to malignancy in a few cases.

Anal warts must be distinguished from *condylomata lata*, which are broad, smooth-surfaced and moist, and from hypertrophied anal papillae that are less friable. Proctoscopy is imperative as both peri-anal and intra-anal condylomata are common and some symptomatic patients have only intra-anal lesions. Vaginal or penile examination should also be performed. The diagnosis is confirmed on histology.

Treatment is by application of 25% podophyllin, which is cytotoxic to condylomata but cannot be used on intra-anal warts because of the risks of stenosis and fistula formation. Bichloroacctic acid can be used to destroy peri-anal and intra-anal condylomata. When local treatment fails or when warts are extensive surgical excision or electrocautery is effective but requires local, regional or general anaesthesia. Carbon dioxide lasers are expensive and there is concern about transmission of viable virus particles in the resulting vapour. All methods carry a high risk of recurrence. Intra-muscular or intra-lesional interferon is of value for treating recurrent warts.

Fibrosed anal polyp

This is another condition that a patient may confuse with a prolapsing pile. It is hypertrophy with elongation and fibrosis of one of the anal papillae that lie at the upper end of the anal canal skin at the mucocutaneous junction. They may remain asymptomatic and are found in nearly 50% of patients examined, but when large and pedunculated an anal polyp may prolapse (Fig. 9.4). The diagnosis is made on digital examination and on proctoscopy. It is fleshy and has a whitish smooth appearance. When symptomatic it is transfixed and excised under local anaesthetic through a bivalve speculum.

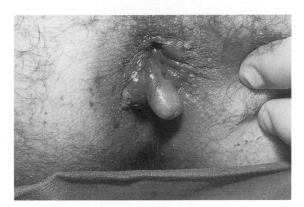

Fig. 9.4 *Prolapsed fibro-epithelial polyp.*

Rectal prolapse

This condition particularly affects women over the age of 70 years. Multipara, particularly those with a history of obstetric trauma or anal dilatation, have a high incidence of rectal prolapse with incontinence. Weakness of the pelvic floor and sphincter muscles, an anatomically mobile rectum that allows intussusception, and abnormal peritoneal reflections of the rectum with a deep pouch of Douglas and often a mobile mesorectum are aetiological factors. Neuropathy that occurs after childbirth and long-standing constipation or following spinal lesions progresses with age and gradually weakens the pelvic floor.

Typical associated features include bleeding from trauma, incontinence, excessive mucous discharge leading to pruritus and either diarrhoea or severe constipation. The diagnosis is made on inspection. The anal sphincter is patulous and there is marked perineal descent at rest or during straining. Usually, the prolapse is obvious but sometimes not, unless the patient is asked to strain forcibly. It may be necessary to ask the patient to bear down in the squatting position or even on the lavatory in order to demonstrate the prolapse. On rectal examination, there is loss of the ano-rectal angle due to a lax puborectalis. Vaginal examination may reveal complete procidentia, cystocele or rectocele. Sigmoidoscopy may show proctitis, although the examination may fail due to a lax anal sphincter preventing the retention of air; barium enema or colonoscopy, if there is

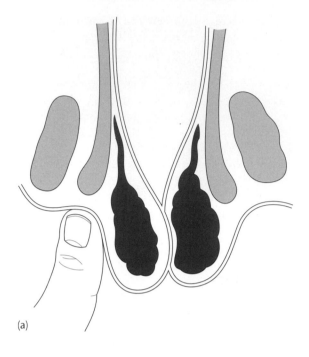

(a)

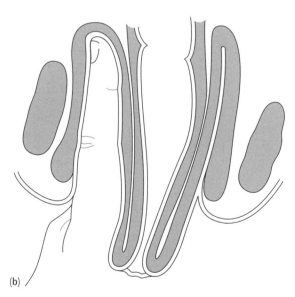

(b)

Fig. 9.5 *Differentiation of (a) haemorrhoidal from (b) rectal prolapse: the presence of a sulcus between the prolapse and the edge of the anal verge differentiates between the two.*

doubt about co-existing colorectal pathology, may be difficult to perform for the same reason.

It is important to distinguish haemorrhoidal from rectal prolapse. The former is limited to a few centimetres and there is no palpable sulcus between the lateral aspect of the prolapse and the anal verge, whereas rectal prolapse is larger and there is a sulcus between the prolapse and the edge of the anal canal (Fig. 9.5).

Management consists of correction of any associated functional bowel disturbance and surgical treatment of the prolapse. Some procedures attempt to support the sphincters and pelvic floor and others aim to reduce rectal mobility. The former include anal canal encircling devices using silver wire, silastic, silicone implantable collars or muscle. The latter include plication (Delorme's) or excision of redundant rectum (rectosigmoidectomy) that are carried out via a perineal approach, and rectal mobilization and fixation with sutures or implantable material, with or without sigmoid resection, carried out by an abdominal approach, either by open or laparoscopic surgery.

Chronic anal fissure

This is perpetuated by increased internal sphincter tone and elevated anal resting pressures that impede perfusion causing ischaemia of the anoderm.

The majority of fissures are *idiopathic* rather than secondary to underlying disease, and are encountered in younger and middle-aged adults.

Pain, bright blood – usually on the toilet paper, although occasionally it may drip into the toilet bowl – with bowel movement, and pruritus are usual symptoms. The triad of features that distinguish a chronic from an acute fissure are a sentinel pile distally, a linear ulcer with indurated and undermined edges and pale circular fibres of the internal sphincter visible in its depth, and a hypertrophied anal papilla at the apex of the fissure (Fig. 9.6). The fissure is visible on parting the buttocks. Digital examination and proctoscopy should be avoided if gentle palpation of the fissure invokes pain. Most idiopathic fissures are located posteriorly but women are more likely than men to develop an anterior fissure. A lateral fissure raises the suspicion of underlying inflammatory or

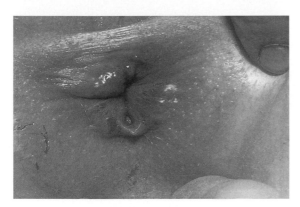

Fig. 9.6 *Chronic anal fissure showing a sentinel pile, skin indurated edges and visible circular fibres of the internal sphincter.*

sexually transmitted disease, AIDS, tuberculosis or leukaemia. Caution is needed in making the distinction of a fissure from an anal carcinoma.

Treatment is aimed at relaxing the internal sphincter and reducing anal canal pressure to improve vascular perfusion and promote healing. Chemical sphincterotomy with topical nitroglycerine, diltiazem and nifedipine, neuromodulators that relax the internal sphincter, successfully heal fissures in 75% of patients. Injection of botulinum toxin into the sphincters on either side of the fissure produces temporary chemical denervation of the internal sphincter and allows fissures to heal. Patients who heal with medical management are maintained on bulk agents. The outmoded lateral internal sphincterotomy, dividing the internal sphincter to the level of the dentate line or to the length of the fissure in females, is still used if medical treatment fails. Anal dilatation is mentioned to be condemned because of the risk of significant incontinence and a high recurrence rate.

Anal fistula

This complicates ano-rectal sepsis (*see* Fig. 9.1). A fistula consists of a chronically infected track lined with granulation tissue that extends from an internal opening at the level of the dentate line (the anal gland ductal opening) and passes through the site of the previous abscess to an external opening on the skin

surface where the abscess had drained spontaneously or surgically. The relations of the track to the external sphincter determines the type of fistula and management. *Inter-sphincteric fistulae* (45%) may or may not transgress the lowermost fibres of the subcutaneous portion of the external sphincter. In *trans-sphincteric fistulae* (40%), the primary track passes through the external sphincter into the ischio-rectal fossa. In a *supra-sphincteric fistula*, the track extends cephalad and transgresses the levators and the ischio-rectal fossa. It is rare to encounter a supra-sphincteric fistula that has not been operated on previously and it is more likely that it is an iatrogenic false track. *Extra-sphincteric fistulae* (1–2%) run directly from a pelvic septic source through the levators to the perineum or vagina with a track lying outside the sphincters.

The patient typically complains of intermittent seropurulent discharge that irritates the skin in the peri-anal region; the fistula seldom if ever closes permanently because of constant reinfection from the anal canal or rectum. Pain is not a symptom unless the external opening is occluded when pus accumulates and an abscess reforms until it discharges through the same or a new opening. On examination, an external opening presents as a small elevation with granulation tissue pouting from its mouth. Occasionally, openings are multiple on one side of the mid-line or on either side (*horse-shoe*), usually a few centimetres from the anus. There is palpable induration of the skin and within the anal canal in the direction of the track (Fig. 9.7). The greater the distance of the external opening from the anal verge the greater the likelihood of a trans-sphinteric fistula or a complex cephalad extension. An external opening in the anterior half of the anus (in front of an imaginary transverse line across the anus) has a direct track, whereas one in the posterior half of the anus (behind the transverse line) has a track that curves and may be of the horse-shoe variety but always connects to a solitary internal orifice in the mid-line (*Goodsall's rule*). Exceptions to the rule are horse-shoe fistulae or fistulae associated with Crohn's disease or cancer. The internal opening is likely to be located at the level of the dentate line; sometimes it is felt as a nodule and there is often an enlarged papilla nearby. Probing is avoided until the patient is under anaesthetic as it is painful and does

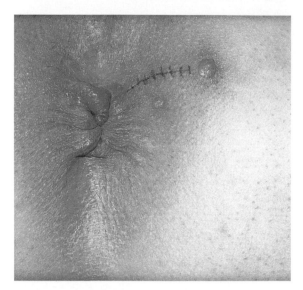

Fig. 9.7 *External opening of a fistula* in ano. *Induration of the skin along the track is marked.*

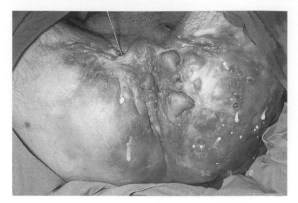

Fig. 9.8 *Hidradenitis suppurativa showing pitted scars, subcutaneous sinus tracts and multiple sinuses with purulent discharge.*

not provide more information. Previous surgery or severe acute sepsis makes assessment extremely difficult, when pre-operative imaging is employed by use of fistulography (injecting contrast material through the external orifice), although endo-anal ultrasound and, in particular, magnetic resonance imaging (MRI) are more informative.

Successful treatment depends on accurate assessment, including a full medical history and proctosigmoidoscopy in order to exclude underlying colonic disease. Management is surgical and starts with examination under anaesthesia. The internal orifice is identified by the release of pus on massaging the track, injecting saline, hydrogen peroxide or dyes, such as methylene blue and indigo carmine, via the external opening and careful probing via each opening to delineate the primary track.

The aim of treatment is to abolish the primary track and drain secondary tracks or abscesses without compromising continence by damaging the sphincters. *Fistulotomy* is the classical operation. The fistula is defined with a probe and the track divided along its whole length. In *fistulectomy* the track is dissected and excised rather than laid open. A seton (*L. seta*: bristle) is used when the position of the fistula track in relation the external sphincter is unclear or much of the sphincter lies below the level

of the primary track. Having identified the primary track, a seton is passed through it and tied using a braided or monofilament non-absorbable suture or silastic. A seton can facilitate drainage and resolution of inflammation to permit safer subsequent fistula surgery, having identified sufficient muscle above the level of the seton by determining the proportion of muscle above and below the track when the patient is not anaesthetized (*staged fistulotomy*). Alternatively, the seton is left and gradually tightened at two-weekly intervals until it cuts through the muscle, achieving a staged fistulotomy. In the presence of recurrent sepsis, as in Crohn's disease, a seton may be left indefinitely to relieve symptoms. Other more demanding procedures are reserved for complex fistulas.

Hidradenitis suppurativa

This is characterized by chronic recurrent suppurative infections which manifest after puberty in the apocrine gland-bearing skin areas, primarily in the axillae, groin and ano-rectal regions. It starts as a localized, firm, tender swelling, progressively increases in size, becomes erythematous and painful and eventually drains spontaneously. This becomes a chronic and recurrent process. The involved area has the typical appearance of pitted scars, subcutaneous sinus tracts and multiple sinuses with offensive discharge (Fig. 9.8). In the perineum, the most common organisms isolated are staphylococcus and streptococcus species. When early it can be difficult to distinguish from an anal abscess or a fistula or peri-anal Crohn's disease; the latter and hidradenitis may co-exist.

Treatment is surgical by wide local excision or by 'de-roofing' the sinus tracts; they are delineated with a probe, the overlying skin is excised and areas of granulation tissue curetted, leaving in place the base of the tract which is epithelialized. This is combined with antibiotics that include minocycline, ciprofloxacin, cephalosporin or clindamycin, the choice being directed by the results of cultures.

Pilonidal sinus and abscess

This is a chronic disease that does not manifest until puberty, has a natural regression and seldom occurs after the third decade. In the upper end of the natal cleft between the buttocks there is often a congenital dimple or pit. Shed hairs from the back, head or perineum accumulate in this nidus and gradually penetrate the skin. Once in the subcutaneous tissues, an abscess develops which cannot point in the mid-line because of pre-sacral fibrous septa and thus lateral secondary tracts are formed. The primary opening in the mid-line is tiny and usually not infected. The subcutaneous track extends for a variable distance to an abscess cavity and branching tracks may come off the primary track. The secondary openings have a different appearance from the primary in that they pout granulation tissue and discharge seropurulent material. Hairs are sometimes seen protruding from the secondary openings.

The average patient with pilonidal disease is a hirsute, moderately obese man in his second or third decade, although females can be affected. Pilonidal disease may present as acute abscess in the sacro-coccygeal area which frequently ruptures spontaneously leaving an unhealed sinus with chronic discharge.

Treatment of a pilonidal abscess is incision and drainage and strict hygiene. The chronic form is treated either by laying open the sinus tracks or by wide excision extending down to the sacral fascia to include the sinus tracks and a margin of normal tissue, with or without primary closure. However,

the failure of healing of mid-line wounds is high. Other procedures avoid a mid-line wound by employing a lateral incision to excise the infected tissue, and the wound is either closed or left open. Skin and gluteus maximus myocutaneous flaps may have to be used to obliterate the natal cleft after radical excision in chronic pilonidal sinus disease when simpler measures have failed.

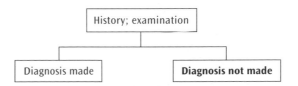

Diagnosis not made

Conditions undiagnosed or only suspected after history and examination, including rectal examination and/or proctosigmoidoscopy, demand further investigations before treatment can be planned.

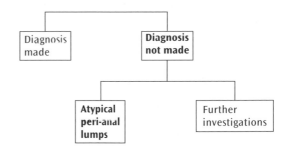

Anal carcinoma

The symptoms are varied and include pain, bleeding, pruritus, mucus discharge, the sensation of a lump in the anus, incontinence and a change in bowel habit. The findings are variable as the lesion may take the form of an ulcer, stricture or a proliferative lesion when it can be difficult to distinguish from a rectal carcinoma (Fig. 9.9). An early lesion is easily confused with an anal fissure; examination under anaesthesia allows assessment of the extent

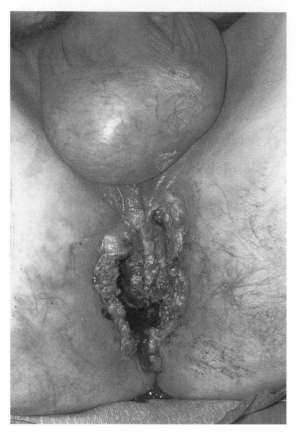

Fig. 9.9 *A proliferative anal canal carcinoma.*

of local infiltration and involvement of the anal sphincters, features relevant to the plan of treatment. Biopsy confirms the diagnosis.

A variety of cancers affect the anal canal and anus. Epidermoid carcinoma is the most common: squamous cell, basaloid and muco-epidermoid carcinomas can be differentiated histologically but appear to have the same prognosis. Endo-anal ultrasonography is particularly useful in defining deep invasion into the sphincters. A chest X-ray and CT scan of the pelvis and abdomen determine spread beyond the anal canal and lymphatic involvement. In a third of patients the inguinal lymph nodes are enlarged, but biopsy or fine needle cytology demonstrates that in half of these the swelling is due to inflammation alone. Chemoradiotherapy (45 Gy in combination with 5-fluorouracil and mitomycin C) is the standard treatment and offers a 70% five-year survival.

Surgery by local excision is only suitable for a small lesion at the anal margin, provided the sphincters are not involved, and offers an 80% five-year survival. Abdomino-perineal excision is reserved for residual or recurrent tumour after chemoradiotherapy. Inguinal lymphatic disease is treated by radiotherapy or radical excision.

Anal intra-epithelial neoplasia

This is a better term for 'Bowen's disease of the anus' and 'leukoplakia', terms which are confusing and non-specific. Pruritus and peri-anal hyperkeratotic lesions, flat, raised or ulcerated, especially in homosexuals or HIV-positive patients should be treated with suspicion. Ano-genital HPV-associated lesions are identified by examination with an operating microscope (colposcope) after the application of acetic acid on the skin surface, allowing targeted biopsy of the discoloured areas. When this microscope is not available, random incision biopsies or, provided the lesion is not extensive, excision biopsy can be therapeutic and diagnostic. Intra-epithelial neoplasia is graded from I to III, depending on the proportion of the epithelial thickness involved; thus in grade III the full thickness of the epithelium is dysplastic, an appearance referred to as carcinoma *in situ*, and complete excision should be ensured at the circumferential edges and the deeper layers. These patients should be followed-up closely.

Paget's disease

The most common symptom is pruritus, usually associated with bleeding and a lump at the anal verge. It is exceedingly rare, but least so in elderly patients. On examination, there may be a raised lesion or well-demarcated rash that may be erythematous, oozing or scaling (Fig. 9.10). The diagnosis is made by biopsy under general anaesthesia. The characteristic feature is the finding in the peri-anal squamous epithelium of large rounded cells with abundant, pale cytoplasm and a large nucleus, often situated peripherally. In 50–80% of cases there is an underlying adenocarcinoma, usually of the rectum, but rarely in a distant organ, thus a careful search for such a lesion is required. If the lesion appears isolated,

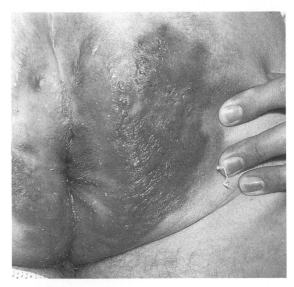

Fig. 9.10 *Paget's disease.*

wide local excision with or without a skin graft is required. When there is extensive spread within the anus or if rectal cancer is present, abdomino-perineal excision is indicated. In patients with widespread or recurrent disease chemotherapy and radiotherapy are effective. Long-term follow-up is required as local recurrence after many years also carries the risk of metastatic spread.

In local disease, long-term disease-free survival is usual. In those with associated adenocarcinoma without evidence of metastasis at the time of primary surgery, the five-year survival rate is 50%.

Melanoma

This is very rare. The lesion may mimic a thrombosed external pile due to its colour, although amelanotic tumours also occur. The most common symptom is bleeding. At presentation, at least one-third of cases have involved lymph nodes and a similar proportion have manifest distant spread.

The prognosis is very poor, with a five-year survival of less than 5%. Hence, radical treatment is considered with trepidation. Adjuvant chemotherapy or radiotherapy offers little benefit. Colostomy or palliative abdomino-perineal excision may become necessary in some cases.

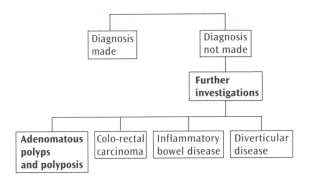

Adenomatous polyps

The adenomatous polyp (Fig. 9.11) has a pre-malignant potential that is dependent on its morphology, size and histological differentiation; it is distinguished from other polyps (Table 9.1) by the microscopic appearances. Adenomas are frequently asymptomatic and are detected by chance on a barium enema or at sigmoidoscopy or colonoscopy performed for unrelated reasons. However, excessive mucous secretion and bleeding from a sizeable polyp are clinically evident when it is in the distal colon or the rectum, or may present as anaemia. A large polyp in the recto-sigmoid region can produce tenesmus, and when pedunculated it may prolapse into the anal canal. In the proximal colon, a large adenoma may intussuscept and cause intestinal obstruction.

Treatment requires complete excision and histological examination of the polyp. Therefore, if detected at a routine sigmoidoscopy, unless it is small enough to allow complete removal with the biopsy forceps, it is excised by snare polypectomy at subsequent

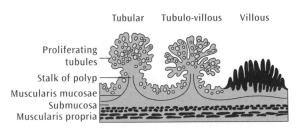

Fig. 9.11 *The morphological features of adenomatous polyps.*

Table 9.1 *Classification of polyps of the large intestine*

Type	Single or isolated Multiple polyps	Polyposis syndromes
Neoplastic	Tubular adenoma Tubulo-villous adenoma Villous adenoma	Familial adenomatous polyposis
Hamartomatous	Juvenile polyp Peutz–Jeghers polyps	Juvenile polyposis Peutz–Jeghers syndrome
Inflammatory	Benign lymphoid polyps Inflammatory pseudopolyps	Benign lymphoid polyposis Inflammatory polyposis
Miscellaneous	Metaplastic (hyperplastic polyps) Lipoma, neurofibroma, etc.	Metaplastic polyposis

colonoscopy, when total examination of the colon is performed to exclude synchronous neoplasms.

In about 5% of polyps, safe polypectomy may not be feasible because of size or because the base of the polyp is too broad. Invariably these are sessile villous adenomas with a potential for malignancy which increases from 1% when an adenoma is 10 mm in diameter to 50% when it is 25 mm or more. However, malignancy is not ascertainable until the whole specimen is examined histologically. A pre-operative biopsy is unreliable as it is likely to miss the area of invasion. Sessile villous adenomas are common in the rectum and digital examination may not be sufficiently sensitive to detect malignant change. Endo-anal ultrasonography or, when the lesion is not within the reach of the endo-anal probe, endoscopic ultrasonography outlines the layers of the bowel wall and defines any evidence of malignant infiltration into the muscularis propria. This pre-operative information determines the extent of excision required.

Neoplasms within 10 cm of the anal verge (lower and mid-rectum) too large for snare polypectomy are suitable for endo-anal sub-mucosal excision. Alternatively, trans-anal endoscopic microsurgery (TEM) is employed and for lesions at higher levels it avoids an abdominal approach but this demands special equipment and expertise. Large and circumferential villous adenomas require abdominal excision, usually by anterior resection and when in the colon a standard radical resection with lymphovascular clearance is recommended because of the high probability of malignancy.

Once an adenoma is diagnosed and treated the patient requires regular colonoscopy every 5 years; it takes about 5 years to develop an adenoma and about another 5 years to develop invasive cancer.

Polyposis syndromes

These present with abdominal colic, diarrhoea and rectal bleeding, and mucous discharge. The diagnosis is based on finding multiple polyps at colonoscopy and on histological features, although in adolescent and young adulthood specific syndromes show some characteristic features.

In *Peutz–Jeghers syndrome* the polyps are predominantly in the small intestine. Investigations include gastroscopy and colonoscopy and, if the presence of polyps with representative histology is confirmed, a small bowel meal to delineate polyps in the small intestine. *Management* involves clearing the polyps from the gastroduodenum and colon by endoscopy, from the small intestine by intra-operative enteroscopy. There is a high risk of gastrointestinal, breast and genital cancer in these patients, therefore follow-up surveillance includes regular colonoscopy, gastroduodenoscopy and small bowel meal, cervical biopsy and pelvic ultrasound in females, testicular ultrasound in males. Unaffected parents and siblings of patients are recommended to have one-time colonoscopy and gastroscopy as the syndrome is an autosomal-dominant disorder that occurs in patients with and without a family history.

Juvenile polyposis, unlike solitary juvenile polyps or mucus retention polyps common in children particularly in the rectum, is often diagnosed in adolescence or early adulthood, based on the presence of at least five gastrointestinal polyps in the colon and stomach. When in large numbers, it can be confused with familial adenomatous polyposis (FAP), but associated anomalies: heart defect, hydrocephalus, malrotation of the gut, cleft palate and polydactyly, make the distinction easier. Although there is a high risk of developing cancer by the age of 60 in these patients, prophylactic colectomy is not justified unless the number and rate of growth of polyps are beyond endoscopic treatment. Therefore these patients require regular follow-up by endoscopy and colonoscopy. In the absence of a family history a one-time examination is recommended for parents and siblings of affected patients.

Cronkhite–Canada syndrome and *Ruvakaba–Myhre–Smith syndrome* are associated with hamartomatous polyps, respectively, of the stomach and colon, and of the colon and ileum, with ectodermal changes that include hair loss, nail atrophy and skin pigmentation. Adenomas and carcinomas have been reported in Cronkhite–Canada syndrome. These syndromes are regarded as variants of juvenile polyposis and are managed similarly.

Familial adenomatous polyposis (FAP) is the most common of the polyposis syndromes and is an inherited non-sex-linked autosomal dominant condition characterized by the progressive development of hundreds of polyps. The adenomas develop at about the age of puberty and symptoms manifest at the average age of 20 years. Alternatively, patients may present with extra-intestinal lesions originally described as *Gardner's syndrome*, such as cutaneous cysts, osteomata classically in the mandible and maxilla, fibromata, pilar cysts or desmoid tumours. This is now regarded as part of the spectrum of FAP. Many patients are asymptomatic and the diagnosis is made during screening of family members of an affected patient. Since the rectum is rarely spared, digital examination, sigmoidoscopy and biopsy of the polyps provide an early clue. A barium enema or colonoscopy showing at least 50 polyps histologically categorized as adenomas is diagnostic. This is usually followed by an upper gastrointestinal endoscopy to exclude extra-colonic neoplasms: in the stomach they are usually fundic gland polyps with no malignant potential, whereas in the duodenum polyps are commonly adenomas and demand post-operative surveillance because of the risk of malignancy.

Management is aimed at treating the patient before carcinoma develops, and identifying family members at risk. Treatment should not be delayed beyond 20–25 years as by this age many are symptomatic and, if untreated, all develop carcinoma by the age of 35 years. The available options are proctocolectomy, colectomy and ileo-rectal anastomosis or restorative proctocolectomy. Proctocolectomy eliminates all polyps and therefore the risk of cancer but entails an ileostomy, whereas pelvic dissection to excise the rectum risks pelvic nerve damage resulting in urinary and sexual dysfunction. In young patients, therefore, sphincter-saving procedures are favoured. Colectomy and ileo-rectal anastomosis maintains gastrointestinal continuity with reasonable bowel function and has been the conventional treatment. However, patients require regular examination of the rectal stump for life. Restorative proctocolectomy with excision of the rectal mucosa above the retained anal canal and an ileal pouch–anal anastomosis eradicates the disease. Gastrointestinal continuity is restored while bowel function and continence are maintained. It is particularly indicated in patients deemed unlikely to comply with the strict surveillance required after an ileo-rectal anastomosis. Although morbidity and mortality are low, the pelvic dissection necessary to excise the rectum risks damage to the pelvic nerves.

Post-operatively, all patients with ileo-rectal anastomosis require biennial sigmoidoscopy and fulguration of the polyps in the rectal stump. A 3–4-monthly follow-up is necessary when the polyp density is high and in patients 50 years old because of the increased risk of cancer. In these patients a restorative proctocolectomy may have to be considered as it obviates anxiety. Patients should also undergo gastroduodenoscopy at the time of colonic surgery or at 25 years. If normal or only fundic gland polyps are identified on biopsy five-yearly follow-up is adequate, but the presence of duodenal polyps demands yearly endoscopy and diathermy excision of these polyps as there is a 12% incidence of periampullary carcinoma developing in pre-existent adenomas.

Desmoid tumours are fibrous masses that occur prior to or after colectomy in 4–12% of patients and require precise definition by CT scanning. Desmoids in the abdominal wall are removed if progressively enlarging or symptomatic, or cosmetically unacceptable. Intra-abdominal desmoids cause intestinal obstruction or hydronephrosis, are generally inoperable and attempted excision is associated with high morbidity. Alternative treatment has included radiotherapy, indomethacin, ascorbic acid and sulindac, since 40% of desmoids are oestrogen receptor-positive, tamoxifen has also been tried but the overall results have been disappointing. Chemotherapy using adriamycin and vincristine has been of variable success.

Family members of an affected patient are screened by flexible sigmoidoscopy in preference to rigid sigmoidoscopy commencing at puberty. Colonoscopy is reserved for suspected diagnosis of FAP. Adenomatous polyposis coli (APC) gene mutation and ophthalmoscopy for congenital hypertrophy of the retinal pigment epithelium (CHRPE) which is invariably present in FAP and in family members have been used to identify individuals at high risk. These individuals require annual flexible sigmoidoscopy. Low-risk individuals are followed-up every 3–5 years up to the age of 60 years.

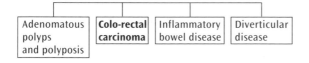

Colo-rectal cancer

In colon cancer both sexes are equally affected, whereas in rectal cancer there is male predominance; only 5% of colo-rectal carcinomas occur in patients younger than 40 years of age. Nearly 60% occur in the sigmoid colon and the rectum. The most common presentation is an insidious onset of chronic symptoms (77–92%), followed by obstruction (6–16%) and perforation with local or diffuse peritonitis (2–7%).

Diagnosis. Rectal bleeding, change in bowel habit and abdominal pain are the common symptoms. Bleeding is intermittent and the blood is passed mixed with the stool in left-sided colonic and rectal cancer, whereas blood loss from caecal and right-sided cancer is occult and presents with anaemia or melaena. A change in bowel habit is a common symptom; constipation is more often associated with left-sided lesions because the diameter of the colon is smaller and the stool is firmer. Carcinomas of the right side of the colon do not typically present with changes in bowel habit, and excessive mucus produced by a tumour may cause diarrhoea while 'spurious' diarrhoea and tenesmus, due to the sensations of incomplete evacuation and the desire to strain with poor result and sometimes with only the passage of blood and mucus, are suggestive of a lesion in the distal sigmoid or rectum. Abdominal pain is pronounced when obstruction is developing. On the left side there is cramping pain, associated with nausea and vomiting and relieved with bowel movement, whereas right sided-cancer, especially when involving the ileo-caecal valve, is accompanied by flatulent distension and audible borborygmi precipitated by meals. Pelvic pain is usually associated with advanced disease when the tumour has involved the sacrum or the major pelvic nerves.

Less common symptoms include weight loss, malaise, fever, abdominal mass and urinary symptoms (frequency, pneumaturia and faecaluria) when the bladder is involved. Bacteraemia with *Streptococcus bovis* is highly suggestive of colo-rectal malignancy.

Assessment. Patients more than 50 years old and those with a family background of large bowel cancer, especially in more than one generation, suggestive of *hereditary non-polyposis coli* cancer (HNPCC), and those with a history of ulcerative colitis, adenomatous polyps or familial polyposis are at high risk.

The patient's nutritional, cardiovascular and respiratory status are assessed. Clinical staging includes inspection for jaundice, palpation for cervical lymphadenopathy, and examination of the chest for pleural effusion or consolidation and the abdomen for gaseous distension, active bowel sounds, a palpable mass, an enlarged liver and ascites. A caecal cancer is more often palpable than tumours elsewhere in the colon. Digital examination of the rectum detects lesion within the reach of the finger and combined with vaginal examination in females allows assessment of its local extent. Sigmoidoscopy with the 25 cm instrument identifies lesions as far as the distal sigmoid colon and allows tissue biopsy. Streaks of blood on the finger cot or sigmoidoscope with no obvious lesion strengthens the probability that a lesion lies beyond reach.

It is essential that the full length of the colon is visualized by colonoscopy or a barium enema, even when a lesion is detected on digital examination or sigmoidoscopy, as a synchronous cancer occurs in 5% of patients. An ultrasound or CT scan of the liver and a chest X-ray are required to seek metastatic disease. When there is luminal narrowing by tumour, colonoscopy or a barium enema may fail to outline the proximal colon; CT colonography, a technique using dynamic intravenous contrast-enhanced thin section helical CT of the air-insufflated colon with the aid of smooth muscle relaxants, allows complete examination of the colon and the abdominal viscera and provides clinical staging of the extent of the disease in a single examination (Fig. 9.12). A pre-operative carcinoembryonic antigen (CEA) level is a useful baseline measurement for reference during follow-up. Routine haematological and biochemical tests are also performed.

The treatment of *rectal cancer* depends critically on the extent of the disease. The size of the tumour, the distance of its lower margin from the anal verge measured by sigmoidoscopy, its depth of invasion,

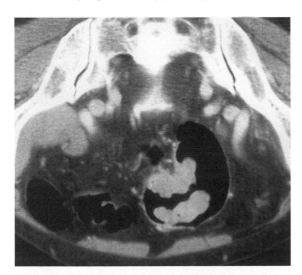

Fig. 9.12 *CT colonography showing a tumour in the transverse colon. This examination allows full visualization of the colon, and outlines the extent of local invasion of the tumour and extra-abdominal and liver involvement.*

the involvement of adjacent viscera and fixity, if not easily defined in the conscious patient, are determined under anaesthesia, when cystoscopy can be combined if bladder invasion is suspected. Endo-rectal ultrasonography defines the layers of the rectal wall and discriminates between cancers within the submucosa (T_1), those extending into the muscularis propria but confined to the rectal wall (T_2, T_3) and those invading the para-rectal fat (T_4). Although CT and MRI are less reliable in determining the extent of rectal wall invasion of an early cancer, they delineate extra-rectal invasion and visceral involvement.

Surgical management aims at cure or symptomatic palliation, with restoration of bowel continuity whenever conceivable at minimal operative risk. Surgical intervention is unjustified in the asymptomatic patient with limited life expectancy because of metastatic disease. The presence of liver secondaries does not preclude treatment since resection of the primary lesion provides symptomatic palliation and in a select group resection of the diseased liver improves survival.

Whenever a temporary or permanent stoma is planned the implications are discussed with the patient and the stoma site is selected and marked on the abdominal skin pre-operatively. Bowel cleansing facilitates bowel mobilization and reduces the incidence of septic complications. Methods of mechanical preparation include cathartics, such as magnesium sulphate, castor oil, mannitol and whole-gut irrigation. A broad-spectrum cephalosporin combined with metronidazole to cover anaerobic organisms is maintained for no longer than 24 hours peri-operatively, starting immediately before surgery. Thrombo-embolism prophylaxis is essential.

The principles of radical resection for cancer are removal of the lymphovascular tissue and *en bloc* resection of involved tissues with clear proximal and distal resection margins. The primary regional lymph nodes are in the vicinity of the named arteries and veins related to the site of the primary tumour, and therefore the arteries and veins are divided at their origins. Thus, curative resection encompasses all regional avenues of lymphatic spread and the length of bowel resected corresponds to the extent of vascular and mesenteric lymphadenectomy. A hemicolectomy with primary anastomosis is performed according to the site of the tumour (Fig. 9.13).

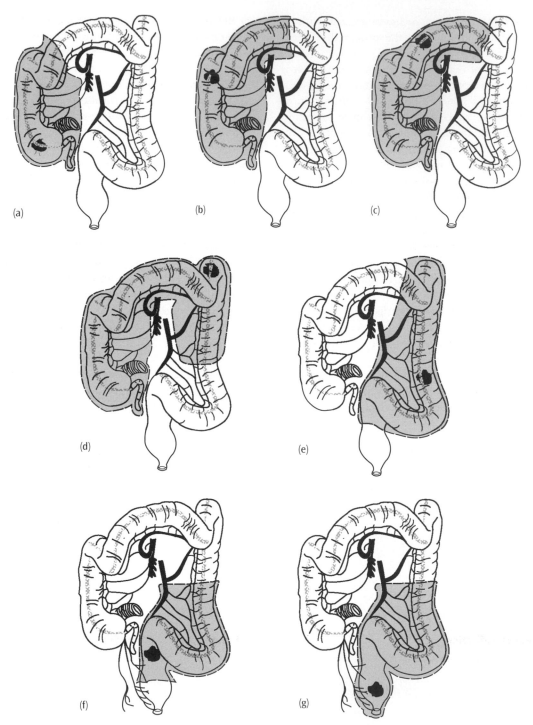

Fig. 9.13 *(a)–(g) Extent of resection for colo-rectal cancers and the levels at which major blood vessels are ligated. Source: Boulos PB, Colorectal Cancer, in I Irving, TG Cooke and P Guilliou (eds),* Essential General Surgical Oncology, *London: Churchill Livingston, 1996. Reproduced with permission.*

In *rectal cancer*, prior assessment defines those patients suitable for local excision (T_1), those with advanced but resectable cancers (T_2 and T_3) who will benefit from pre-operative adjuvant radiotherapy, and those with locally advanced cancers with extra-rectal fixity and adjacent organ invasion (T_4) where pre-operative chemo- or radiotherapy may improve resectability. In 10% of patients with a favourable tumour, local excision or endocavity irradiation can be curative and is most appropriate in elderly patients who are unfit for a major procedure and those who refuse a colostomy. The criteria for this approach are a lesion that is smaller than 5 cm, mobile on digital examination, histologically well or moderately differentiated and T_1 or T_2 on endo-rectal ultrasound. Trans-anal endoscopic micro-surgery (TEM) facilitates excision, particularly when the lesion is high in the mid- or upper rectum. Surgery for T_3 and T_4 rectal cancer aims at clearance at the several sites of tumour spread: the lymph nodes, cephalad in the bowel mesentery, the para-rectal tissue laterally and the mesorectum distally. A 2-cm clearance margin below the tumour edge is adequate since distal intra-mural spread does not exceed a few millimetres, unless the tumour is poorly differentiated when a 5-cm distal clearance is required. The anal canal is 3–4 cm long, hence a restorative resection for a well- or moderately differentiated tumour can be performed when a lesion is 7 cm from the anal verge (*anterior resection*); when greater length of clearance is required or the tumour is within 7 cm of the anal verge, rectal excision is necessary (*abdomino-perineal excision*).

Tumour staging. Staging systems are important for predicting outcomes, selecting patients for various therapies and comparing therapies for like patients across institutions. Dukes's and the TNM (tumour/node/metastasis) classifications are the most popular (Table 9.2). Classification of histological grade, cell type, lymphatic, venous or peri-neural invasion, tumour ploidy, CEA level, bowel perforation and distal and tangential margins allow for further sub-classification of the tumour and improved prognostication. Ultimately, 50% of patients who undergo curative resection develop local, regional or widespread recurrence as a result of progression of micrometastases present at the time of initial operation. Adjuvant therapy is aimed at those patients.

Adjuvant therapy: colon cancer. The use of adjuvant chemotherapy is recommended in all patients with Dukes's C/stage 3 disease (any T, $N_{1,2}$). A combination of intravenous 5-fluorouracil (5-FU) and folinic acid reduces the risk of recurrences and mortality. Portal vein infusion for 1 week as with systemic infusion for 6–12 months achieves similar results. This supports the hypothesis that chemotherapy inhibits occult hepatic micrometastases. The role of radiotherapy is limited to cases where radical clearance has not been achieved because of gross tissue infiltration.

Adjuvant therapy: rectal cancer. Radiation therapy may be delivered with or without chemotherapy, pre-operatively or post-operatively, usually reserved for stage 3/Dukes's C.

The benefits of pre-operative radiation are:

- Large tumours may shrink allowing their resectability.

Table 9.2 *Comparison of TNM system to Dukes's classification*

Dukes's classification	Tumour	Nodes	Metastasis
A (lesion confined to bowel wall)	T_1, T_2, T_3	N_0	M_0
B (penetration through full thickness of bowel wall)	T_4	N_0	M_0
C_1 (local lymph node involvement)	T_1, T_2, T_3	N_1, N_2, N_3	M_0
C_2 (regional lymph node involvement)	T_4	N_1, N_2, N_3	M_0
D (distant spread)	Any T	Any N	M_1

T_1: tumour invasion into sub-mucosa; T_2: invasion into muscularis propria; T_3: invasion through muscularis propria; N_0: no regional lymph nodes; N_1: one to three regional lymph nodes; N_2: more than three regional lymph nodes; N_3: regional lymph nodes along a vascular trunk; M_0: no distant metastases; M_1: distant metastases.

Table 9.3 *TNM stage-dependent overall five-year survival*

Stage	Depth	Nodal status	Metastasis	Survival (%)
1	T_1, T_2	N_0	M_0	76
2	T_3, T_4	N_0	M_0	65
3	Any T	Any N (except N_0)	M_0	42
4	Any T	Any N (except N_0)	M_1	16

- Tumour cells within the lymphatics may be destroyed decreasing seeding of viable tumour cells at the time of surgery.
- Radiation therapy is optimal in well-oxygenated tissues, whereas the post-operative tissue may be relatively hypoxic.
- Surgical complications may delay therapy.
- Pre-operative radiotherapy minimizes the risk of radiating small bowel that may be fixed in the pelvis after surgery.

The disadvantages of pre-operative radiotherapy are possible over-treatment of stage 1/Dukes's A and 2/Dukes's B lesions assumed to be stage 3/Dukes's C on pre-operative evaluation, and the risk of increased operative complications secondary to radiation injury. Regardless of whether it is delivered pre-operatively or post-operatively, radiation therapy reduces local recurrence and possibly increases survival. The addition of chemotherapy to radiation may further improve local control and survival (Table 9.3) but is yet to be widely recommended.

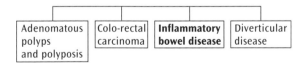

Inflammatory bowel disease

This comprises *Crohn's disease* and *ulcerative colitis* and should be suspected in young patients, although there is a bimodal distribution with the first peak at age 15–30 years and the second at 55–80 years. Clinical manifestations vary with the severity of the disease, from occasional blood and mucus with a moderate number of stools to frequent, explosive diarrhoea with significant bleeding or discharge of mucus and pus. About 20% of patients present with acute fulminant colitis. Physical examination may be normal; in severe cases there may be pyrexia, anaemia, dehydration, abdominal distension and tenderness or localized peritoneal signs. Common features outside the gastrointestinal tract involve the skin, eyes and joints and if present strongly support the diagnosis. *Erythema nodosum* describes multiple tender, red subcutaneous nodules; *pyoderma gangrenosum* develops from an erythematous lesion into a tender necrotizing ulcer. They can occur anywhere, but mostly in the pre-tibial area. *Ocular manifestations* include uveitis, iritis, episcleritis, vasculitis and conjunctivitis and infrequently precede intestinal symptoms. *Arthropathy* includes arthritis and synovitis usually of large joints, ankylosing spondylitis and sacroilitis. Digital rectal examination may reveal tenderness and blood, mucus or pus in the rectal vault. Sigmoidoscopy may show loss of the sub-mucosal vascular pattern and oedema, a granular, hyperaemic and friable mucosa, or a deep velvety appearance with ulceration and mucopurulent exudate depending on the severity of the inflammation.

Investigations. A low haemoglobin, leukocytosis, raised ESR and CRP are indices of disease activity. Stool cultures are essential to rule infectious enterocolitis. Colonoscopy or barium enema is performed to determine the extent of the disease. In most cases the distinction between ulcerative colitis and Crohn's disease can be made from the endoscopic and microscopic pathology; however, a giant cell granuloma which is diagnostic of Crohn's disease is seen in only 15–36% of patients.

Although medical therapy is similar for Crohn's disease and ulcerative colitis, surgical therapies for each differ radically, and it is imperative that a clear diagnosis is made. Nonetheless, the microscopic features of both diseases co-exist in about 15% of patients, for whom the diagnostic term used is *indeterminate colitis*.

Crohn's or ulcerative colitis? Crohn's disease affects the whole digestive tract from mouth to anus and is not limited to the colon (15–40%), but occurs in the ileo-colic region (30–40%) and in isolated small bowel (16–40%). Oral aphthous ulcers and peri-anal lesions – skin tags, fissures, abscesses and fistulae – usually signify Crohn's disease. Five per cent of patients present with peri-anal disease with no evidence of disease elsewhere. Symptoms of small bowel disease – central cramping abdominal pain, nausea, vomiting, diarrhoea and weight loss – can predominate. In Crohn's disease, unlike ulcerative colitis, the inflammation is not confined to the mucosa but is trans-mural, and serosal involvement and microperforation, inflammatory adhesions and suppuration involve adjacent viscera and result in fever and a palpable abdominal mass as well as fistulation into adjacent viscera or to the skin surface. Thus, although the initial work-up may be targeted to the presumed focus of disease activity, assessment of the entire gastrointestinal tract is necessary. An upper and lower endoscopy with biopsies and barium studies are essential to identify lesions of the stomach, duodenum or small intestine. Colonoscopy reveals patchy 'skip' lesions with spared segments rather than a diffuse distribution of inflammation as in ulcerative colitis; terminal ileal involvement and rectal sparing, with mucosal oedema and erythema, aphthous or linear ulcerations are highly suggestive of Crohn's disease. If the terminal ileum is not visualized at colonoscopy it may be evaluated with a barium enema. However, in 10% of patients with ulcerative pancolitis the distal ileum may appear inflamed and ulcerated secondary to reflux of colonic contents through the ileo-caecal valve – *backwash ileitis*. In ulcerative colitis, unlike Crohn's disease, the rectum is always involved but it may appear less diseased or even normal if the patient has been treated with topical suppositories or enemas.

Medical management. The primary treatment of inflammatory bowel disease is medical and includes aminosalicylates, commonly Sulphasalazine (sulphapyridine linked to 5-ASA), Mesalazine (unbound 5-ASA), Asacol (slow-release 5-ASA bound with resin) and Pentasa (slow-release microspheres regulated by pH); corticosteroids and budesonide which is a synthetic steroid that has better mucosal absorption and fewer systemic side-effects; antibiotics, the most effective for infectious complications of Crohn's disease, including peri-anal sepsis, being metronidazole and ciprofloxacin; and immunomodulators, such as azathioprine, 6-mercaptopurine and cyclosporine. Infliximab, a chimeric monoclonal antibody to tumour necrosis factor-alpha (TNF-α) which is increased in Crohn's disease is the latest drug being used. The aminosalicylates and corticosteroids, administered orally and topically, are the standard first line of treatment, whereas parenteral corticosteroids and the immunomodulators are reserved for severe cases. Supplementary treatment includes anti-diarrhoeals, haematinics and hyperalimentation.

Patients may have active disease with intervening periods of quiescence, and medical therapy is maintained to keep the disease in remission. Patients are followed-up to monitor the response and side-effects. Liver function tests are measured regularly as hepatobiliary complications – primary sclerosing cholangitis (PSC), liver cirrhosis or fatty infiltration – are extra intestinal manifestations particularly common in ulcerative colitis. Asymptomatic patients with biochemical abnormalities require an ERCP and liver biopsy. Treatment is symptomatic with antibiotics for cholangitis and cholestyramine for pruritus; ursodeoxycholic acid and methotrexate can also be effective. Treatment of the colonic disease with total proctocolectomy does not affect the clinical course of PSC and the only cure is liver transplantation.

Surveillance by colonoscopy in ulcerative colitis every 1–2 years after the eighth year of symptoms is important because of the increased risk of colorectal carcinoma. Patients at higher risk are those with early onset in childhood, colitis extending beyond the splenic flexure, long-standing disease for at least 8 years, and PSC. Multiple biopsies are histologically examined for dysplasia, and when associated with a lesion or mass (DALM), half have colorectal cancer.

Surgical therapy cures ulcerative colitis but not Crohn's disease. The natural course of Crohn's disease varies between patients, but in time most have exacerbations that lead to progressive disease requiring surgery. Once that occurs these patients will continue to be at increased risk for re-operative surgery of 10% per year. Surgical treatment for inflammatory bowel disease is indicated in patients with debilitating symptoms, poor nutrition and an impaired quality of life despite adequate medical therapy; for drug-related side-effects, in particular due to corticosteroids, such as psychosis, diabetes, hypertension and osteoporosis; and in children with delayed growth and maturation secondary to medical therapy and malnutrition. Severe dysplasia and DALM are strict indications for surgery.

Total proctocolectomy removes all the diseased colon but the patient is left with an incontinent end-ileostomy. This is remedied with various continence-restoring procedures, but reserved only for ulcerative colitis. A Kock continent ileostomy allows patients to control evacuation with a valvular nipple from a pouch fashioned intra-abdominally (Fig. 9.14). The patient empties the pouch with a catheter and is not required to wear an appliance. The Park's ileal pouch–anal anastomosis (*restorative proctocolectomy*) has become the standard operation for ulcerative colitis. The anal canal is retained so that the patient is able to void per anum while a conventional proctocolectomy is performed to eliminate the disease. Contraindications are pre-operative faecal incontinence and inadequate anal sphincters.

Cutaneous, ocular and peripheral articular manifestations may improve, but ankylosing spondylitis does not regress, and sclerosing cholangitis may progress to cirrhosis or cholangiocarcinoma after surgery. Hepatobiliary and thromboembolic extraintestinal manifestations of colitis increase the risk of post-operative complications.

In the 25–50% of patients with Crohn's disease who have rectal sparing an ileo-rectal anastomosis is performed, avoiding an ileostomy. However, 70% of these patients eventually develop significant disease in the residual rectum and half will require completion proctectomy.

Small intestinal or ileo-colic stenotic disease causing obstructive symptoms is treated by resection with primary anastomosis minimizing the amount of healthy small bowel and colon resected, as the recurrence rate for re-operation approaches

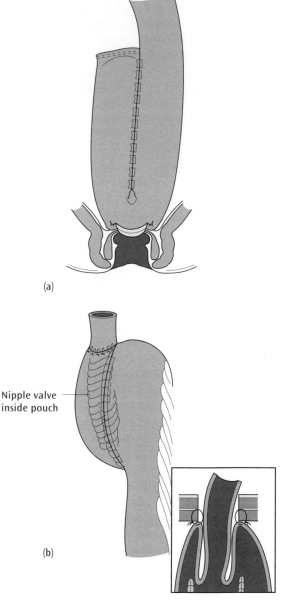

(a)

Nipple valve inside pouch

(b)

Fig. 9.14 *(a) A J-pouch ileo-anal anastomosis – modification of the original Park's S-pouch; (b) A Kock pouch with continent ileostomy.*

50% at 10 years and these patients are therefore at risk of short gut syndrome if repeated operations with resection are required. For the same reason the Kock ileostomy and ileal pouch–anal anastomosis are avoided in Crohn's disease. In order to preserve length of bowel, and particularly when multiple previous bowel resections have been performed, stricturoplasty should be considered for strictures widely separated by normal bowel.

Peri-anal complications of Crohn's disease demand cautious surgery: drainage of focal sepsis, liberal use of drainage catheters and non-cutting setons, and maximal medical therapy with antibiotics and immunomodulators. A diverting stoma can be effective, although it is regarded as a staging procedure that prepares the patient psychologically for proctectomy should it become necessary.

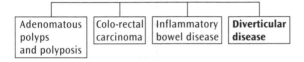

| Adenomatous polyps and polyposis | Colo-rectal carcinoma | Inflammatory bowel disease | **Diverticular disease** |

Diverticular disease

Diverticular disease is usually asymptomatic, although patients may complain of vague left-sided abdominal discomfort, anorexia, flatulence and constipation or diarrhoea. Rectal bleeding is uncommon, and when present can be due to other lesions. Patients may present with symptoms of recurrent cystitis – dysuria, frequency, haematuria, lower abdominal pain, pneumaturia and rarely faecaluria or vaginal discharge of pus, stool or flatus – without systemic symptoms or an antecedent history of diverticulitis (Chapter 25). Physical examination, usually unremarkable, sometimes elicits tenderness or a mass in the left iliac fossa. Digital examination may demonstrate a mass in the recto-vesical or recto-uterine pouch and induration or an opening or a mass in the vaginal vault if there is a fistula. Rigid sigmoidoscopy is frequently unhelpful as it is often not possible to examine beyond the recto-sigmoid junction. The diagnosis of diverticular disease is established by barium enema, which can also demonstrate a colo-vaginal fistula in about half the cases but is unreliable for demonstrating a colo-vesical fistula. Diverticula may be distributed throughout the entire colon but are commonly localized in the sigmoid colon. Flexible sigmoidoscopy or colonoscopy depending on the extent of the disease is required to differentiate diverticular disease from carcinoma

and especially if the patient has had rectal bleeding. Cystoscopy or a cystogram are diagnostic investigations for a colo-vesical fistula, although a plain abdominal X-ray may demonstrate an air–fluid level in the bladder and a CT scan is more sensitive and will also outline the degree of peri-colic inflammation.

Management. Uncomplicated diverticular disease is treated with a high-bulk diet, 20–30 g of bran daily, to reduce colonic pressure. Many patients find a high-fibre diet unpalatable and bulk-forming agents are a substitute. Based on the hypermotility of the sigmoid colon in many symptomatic patients, anticholinergic agents have been recommended.

Elective surgery, a left hemicolectomy, is indicated in patients with persistent discomfort in the left lower quadrant provided there is no other explanation. A narrowed or marked deformity of the sigmoid on barium enema with inability to exclude

---

HIGHLIGHTS

- Sub-total colectomy is the only option for life-threatrening unidentified rectal bleeding
- The distinction between infective diarrhoea and inflammatory bowel disease is crucial to management
- It is essential to differentiate between gangrenous and non-gangrenous colitis as this influences management
- The presence of an obvious ano-rectal condition does not preclude underlying colonic pathology
- It is imperative to distinguish Crohn's disease from ulcerative colitis as this influences treatment and prognosis
- Skin changes in the peri-anal region should be treated with suspicion
- In the presence of liver metastases, resection of the primary tumour provides symptomatic palliation, and in a select group resection of the diseased liver improves survival
- Assessment of the local extent in rectal cancer is essential as this determines management options
- Elective resection after acute diverticulitis should be considered in immunocompromised patients

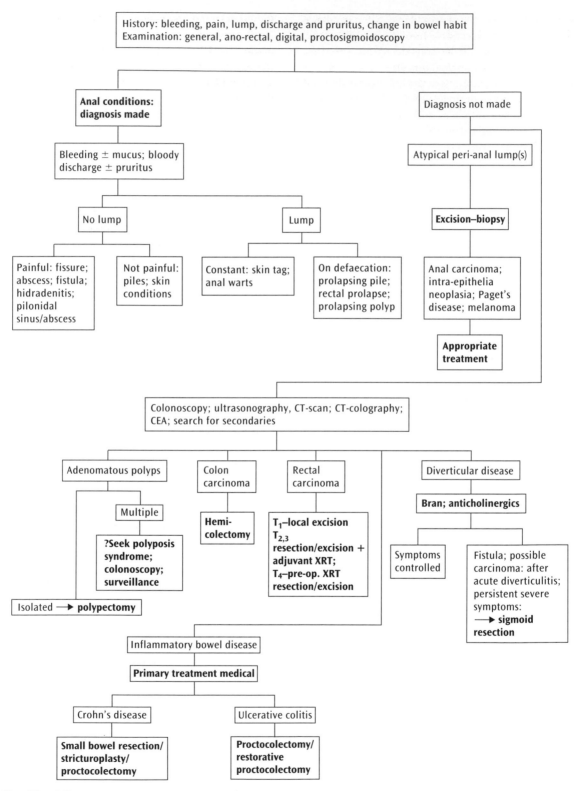

History: bleeding, pain, lump, discharge and pruritus, change in bowel habit
Examination: general, ano-rectal, digital, proctosigmoidoscopy

Anal conditions: diagnosis made

Diagnosis not made

Bleeding ± mucus; bloody discharge ± pruritus

Atypical peri-anal lump(s)

No lump

Lump

Excision–biopsy

Painful: fissure; abscess; fistula; hidradenitis; pilonidal sinus/abscess

Not painful: piles; skin conditions

Constant: skin tag; anal warts

On defaecation: prolapsing pile; rectal prolapse; prolapsing polyp

Anal carcinoma; intra-epithelia neoplasia; Paget's disease; melanoma

Appropriate treatment

Colonoscopy; ultrasonography, CT-scan; CT-colography; CEA; search for secondaries

Adenomatous polyps

Colon carcinoma

Rectal carcinoma

Diverticular disease

Multiple

Hemi-colectomy

T_1–local excision $T_{2,3}$ resection/excision + adjuvant XRT; T_4–pre-op. XRT resection/excision

Bran; anticholinergics

?Seek polyposis syndrome; colonoscopy; surveillance

Symptoms controlled

Fistula; possible carcinoma: after acute diverticulitis; persistent severe symptoms: → **sigmoid resection**

Isolated → **polypectomy**

Inflammatory bowel disease

Primary treatment medical

Crohn's disease

Ulcerative colitis

Small bowel resection/ stricturoplasty/ proctocolectomy

Proctocolectomy/ restorative proctocolectomy

Algorithm 9.3

co-existing carcinoma because of difficulty in passing the colonoscope through the narrowed segment is a valid indication. Patients with colo-vesical or colo-vaginal fistulae certainly require surgery: the offending sigmoid segment is resected and omentum placed between the bladder or vagina and the bowel anastomosis. Elective resection is also indicated after acute diverticulitis, especially in immunocompromised patients, those undergoing organ transplantation and patients younger than 30 years.

Lump in the groin

MICHAEL HOBSLEY

THE GROIN: DEFINITION

For precision, the groin is here arbitrarily defined as the region between the upper end of the symphysis pubis and the anterior superior iliac spine, bounded distally by the crest of the pubis and the skin crease separating groin from thigh, and extending upwards from this level for 5 cm above the line of the inguinal ligament.

Most lumps lie in the medial end of the groin, around the region of the pubic tubercle. This point is an important landmark that the clinician must be able to identify accurately, even in an overweight or unco-operative patient (Fig. 10.1 (a)). The examiner's hand is placed on the patient's ipsilateral anterior superior iliac spine, with the middle finger on the spine and the fingers straight and side by side, pointing medially and downwards at 30° to the horizontal. The hand is then moved medially and downwards along the direction it is pointing until the middle finger encounters the first bony point; this is the pubic tubercle. There are alternative methods. However, palpating outwards from the pubic symphysis along the pubic crest until the prominence of the tubercle is reached fails if the crest is shaped as in Fig. 10.1 (b); following the tendon of the adductor longus muscle upwards requires the co-operation of the patient in adducting the straight lower limb against the examiner's resistance; and invaginating the scrotal skin above the testis until the pubic tubercle is felt on the upper border of the pubic bone is uncomfortable for the patient.

LUMP IN THE GROIN

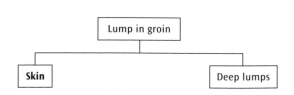

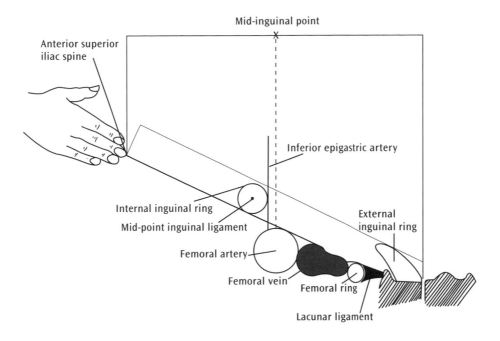

(a)

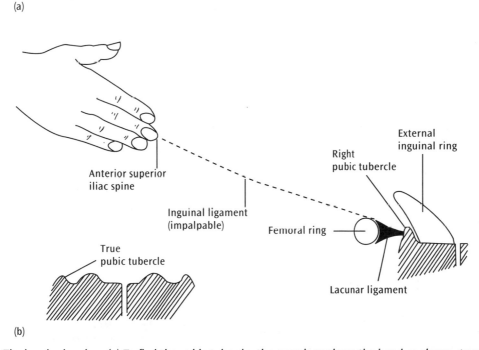

(b)

Fig. 10.1 *The inguinal region; (a) To find the pubic tubercle, the examiner places the hand as shown, touching the anterior superior iliac spine with the middle finger, and then moves the hand medially and downwards at 30° to the horizontal until bone is met: this point is the pubic tubercle; (b) The approach from lateral to medial rather than from the mid-line laterally prevents the examiner being misled by the bump occasionally present on the superior border of the pubis. Note the difference between the mid-inguinal point (landmark for the femoral artery) and the mid-point of the inguinal ligament (an approximate landmark for the internal inguinal ring).*

Lumps in the skin should be considered as elsewhere. When clinically diagnosable, the appropriate treatment is offered, but when not, excision and histological examination are advisable unless the lump is not easily resectable or is large, when a Tru-cut or incision biopsy is carried out. Further treatment depends on the histological findings. Lumps deep to the skin need separate consideration according to their relationship to the hernial orifices.

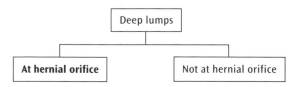

The external hernial orifices

An external hernial orifice is the opening through which the hernia reaches the subcutaneous tissue and becomes readily palpable. There are four recognized orifices in each groin: inguinal, femoral, Spigelian and obturator.

The *obturator* hernia is most unlikely to be clinically distinguishable from a femoral hernia because the *obturator hernial orifice* is the obturator foramen which is deep in the thigh, remote from the examiner's reach, and by the time the hernia comes to lie superficially in the subcutaneous tissue it occupies more or less the position of a femoral hernia.

The *orifice of a Spigelian hernia* is a fascial defect in the aponeurosis of the internal oblique and transversus abdominis muscles of the anterior abdominal wall at the lateral edge of the rectus sheath, below the linea semilunaris, where the posterior rectus sheath is absent. The hernial sac expands deep to the external oblique muscle. The defect is usually quite small and lies higher than the external ring.

The Spigelian and obturator hernias are not as common as the inguinal and femoral hernias which receive most attention in the following description.

Inguinal hernial orifice

The external orifice of an inguinal hernia is the superficial inguinal ring. This is an obtuse-angled triangular defect in the aponeurosis of the external oblique muscle, based on the pubic crest with its apex pointing upwards and laterally. The pubic tubercle is the essential landmark. Since the tubercle is at the lateral end of the pubic crest, it follows that the external ring, *at the horizontal level of the pubic tubercle*, is immediately medial to the pubic tubercle. The direction of slope of the apex of the ring, particularly as the fibres of the external oblique aponeurosis or muscle are split further upwards and laterally by an expanding bulk of hernia, may result in the uppermost part of the palpable hernia being lateral to the vertical line drawn through the pubic tubercle. Nevertheless, the hernia lies medial to the tubercle at the horizontal level of the tubercle.

Femoral hernial orifice

The external orifice of a femoral hernia is bounded medially by the *lacunar (Gimbernat's) ligament*, anteriorly by the inguinal ligament, posteriorly by the superior pubic ramus and laterally by the femoral vein. The lacunar ligament separates the orifice from the pubic tubercle, but because of its flimsy structure the immediate medial relationship of the orifice is therefore the pubic tubercle (*see* Fig. 10.1 above). Once a femoral hernia reaches the groin it may enlarge considerably in size, expanding in all directions so that various parts of the lump may have quite different relations to the pubic tubercle. However, at the neck of the hernial sac, at the horizontal level of the pubic tubercle, the hernia lies immediately *lateral* to the tubercle.

Position of the inguinal ligament

At either end of the inguinal ligament are the pubic tubercle and the anterior superior iliac spine, but between these two bony points the ligament is invisible and impalpable. The common teaching that an inguinal hernia lies above the inguinal ligament and that this fact distinguishes it from a femoral hernia, which lies below the inguinal ligament, can be confusing. An inguinal hernia within the inguinal canal lies above the medial half of the inguinal ligament, at the same level at the pubic tubercle, but is below this level if it extends into the scrotum. A femoral hernia lies originally below the inguinal ligament but, as it enlarges, it extends upwards to lie above it.

Lump at a hernial orifice

A lump that lies at one of the hernial orifices must be assumed to be a hernia unless there are features in favour of some other lesion. The critical point is for the clinician to demonstrate that the lump is not emerging from the hernial orifice by making the fingers of the two hands meet (apart from a double layer of skin and subcutaneous tissue) on the deep aspect of the lump. A physical sign in favour of the diagnosis of hernia is a cough impulse.

Expansile cough impulse

A lump is said to have a cough impulse if it expands, visibly or palpably, when the intra-abdominal pressure is raised by coughing. However, a cough produces only a momentary rise in intra-abdominal pressure, and therefore imparts only a transient expansile thrust to any lump in the groin that has free communication with the abdominal cavity. It is better to ask the patient to contract the abdominal muscles by sustained voluntary effort. This results in a sustained expansile thrust in the lump, easier for the clinician to appreciate.

A hernia is the most common type of lump in the groin to exhibit an expansile cough impulse, but other lumps may do so and some hernias do not. These points receive emphasis in the following sections.

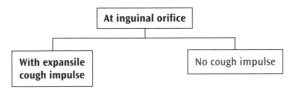

At inguinal orifice, with cough impulse

This is the most common situation encountered when the diagnosis of inguinal hernia is made. The presence of an expansile cough impulse indicates that the hernia is not strangulated. The converse is not necessarily true. A hernia when large, and of long-standing, or often after prolonged treatment with a truss, develops adhesions within the sac and between the thickened hernial sac and the walls of its canal, which prevents the sac from sliding within its surroundings to allow the hernia to enlarge when the patient coughs. In other words, some non-strangulated irreducible inguinal hernias lack a cough impulse.

Reducibility

When an attempt is made to reduce the contents of the sac back into the abdominal cavity, the obliquity of the inguinal canal should be remembered; the hernia is manipulated upwards and laterally, but not before reducing the volume of the hernia by a gentle squeeze to empty any loops of bowel that may happen to be in the sac.

Direct or indirect?

The oblique sac is probably a remnant of the processus vaginalis. It leaves the abdominal cavity at the internal inguinal ring, lateral to the inferior epigastric artery, traverses the inguinal canal within the coverings of the spermatic cord and may extend with the cord into the scrotum. The direct hernia leaves the abdominal cavity via a defect in the fascia transversalis below the arch of the conjoint tendon, and medial to the inferior epigastric artery. It does not lie within the coverings of the cord and therefore shows less tendency to follow the cord into the scrotum.

Some clinicians believe that it is important, and possible, to distinguish between the oblique (*indirect*) and the *direct inguinal hernia* on clinical grounds. The argument is that a direct hernia is not likely to strangulate because the defect is a diffuse area without defined edges and that it is therefore safe not to treat it. The criteria employed to make the distinction possible are that an inguino-scrotal hernia must be indirect and that a hernia which, after reduction, can be prevented from reappearing when the patient coughs by pressure over the internal inguinal ring, must be indirect.

However, it is neither possible with certainty to distinguish between these two types of hernia clinically, nor is it important to do so. A direct hernia may extend into the scrotum, although this is not common, and the internal ring has no immediate bony relationships, so its position and extent cannot be defined accurately. The landmark usually described is that the internal ring lies 2 cm above the surface marking of the femoral artery between the mid-inguinal point and the mid-point of the inguinal ligament, and is not more than two finger-tips in width. The true position of the ring might be more medial than the clinician realizes, in which case pressure on the wrong spot fails to control an indirect hernia which is mistaken for a direct hernia. This also happens when the internal ring is expanded medially by a large and long-standing oblique hernia. The converse error can also occur: a lateral defect of the posterior wall of the canal, close to the internal ring, may be controllable by digital pressure at a point mistakenly thought to be the internal ring, in which case the direct hernia will be diagnosed as indirect. It is irrelevant, however, to make the distinction as a direct hernia carries a small but definite risk of strangulation and operation should be advised for all inguinal hernias unless strongly contraindicated.

Management

The *irreducible* inguinal hernia should be viewed with suspicion, as one that is likely to strangulate. Therefore, the patient should be advised that surgery is essential.

The *reducible* inguinal hernia can only be cured by operation and the patient should be advised accordingly. If there is any contraindication to surgical treatment (e.g., severe cardiac or respiratory disease) or if the patient refuses operation, a *truss* is fitted.

Management by a truss does not cure a hernia. The objective is to prevent the hernia enlarging or strangulating. This is achieved by keeping the hernia reduced at all times; that is why a truss is ineffective for an irreducible hernia. The patient is informed of the signs and dangers of strangulation and instructed that the hernia must be reduced (usually the recumbent position facilitates reduction) and the truss applied before rising in the morning. The same procedure is followed whenever the truss slips and the hernia escapes, and apart from bathing the truss must not be removed until retiring to bed at night. Even in the case of those patients who are most anxious about a surgical operation, a few weeks of life with a truss often persuades them to appreciate the advantages of an operation.

Inguinal hernia repair

An advantage of not attempting to distinguish between direct and indirect hernias is that the surgeon approaches the operation with an open mind and is less likely to miss a direct bulge in a patient with an obvious indirect sac, or a small congenital sac in a patient with a large direct hernia. A direct sac is reduced, and an indirect sac is excised at its neck at the internal inguinal ring (*herniotomy*). The internal ring is narrowed to fit snugly aound the cord by plicating the transversalis fascia, and the posterior wall is repaired by approximating the conjoint tendon and the inguinal ligament (*Bassini*) or the pectineal ligament (*Shouldice*) by use of non-absorbable sutures. The *Lichtenstein* technique employs non-absorbable mesh for the repair, rather than sutures. The operation is usually performed under general, spinal or epidural anaesthesia, although local anaesthesia is becoming more popular. Laparoscopic repair of inguinal hernias by a trans-peritoneal or retro-peritoneal approach is of particular value in recurrent or bilateral hernias, but is technically demanding and can only be carried out under general anaesthesia.

In *infants* the inguinal canal runs straight backwards through the abdominal wall, therefore the internal ring lies directly behind the external. All inguinal hernias in infants are indirect and herniotomy alone is adequate. In young adults with an oblique sac and good musculature, herniotomy alone may be sufficient. As age increases, however, so does the likelihood that *herniorrhaphy* is needed.

At inguinal orifice, no cough impulse

Two situations may be distinguished: either the lump is tense and tender, or it is not.

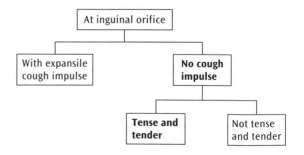

No cough impulse; tense and tender

At any hernial orifice, a tense, tender lump without a cough impulse is diagnosed as a strangulated hernia unless there is evidence to the contrary.

Strangulation develops when constriction at the neck of the sac impedes venous drainage because the pressure in the veins is lower than that in the arteries, which remain patent. With rise in the venous pressure, the capillaries leak protein-rich transudate into the interstitial space, causing tissue congestion and the *tenseness* of a strangulated hernia. *Tenderness* is produced by the accumulation of metabolites and pain substances as a result of stagnant anoxia and anaerobic metabolism. The moistness of the tissues predisposes to infection and the onset of an early, wet type of gangrene.

Although strangulation of a loop of bowel, usually small intestine, within an external hernia is a cause of intestinal obstruction, a strangulated external hernia does not necessarily contain bowel; the strangulated tissue may be omentum, or some other viscus. Conversely, only part of the circumference of the bowel may be trapped in the hernial sac (*Richter's hernia*), leaving the rest of the lumen unoccluded. It is a common error that strangulation and obstruction are referred to as synonymous. This should be avoided unless there are definite associated features of intestinal obstruction.

The search for a strangulated external hernia in a patient with intestinal obstruction needs to be extremely thorough and careful because a strangulated hernia can be small and not painful, and may well not have been noticed by the patient who is likely to be preoccupied with abdominal symptoms.

The only alternative diagnoses to strangulated inguinal hernia that are at all common are inflamed lymph nodes (*lymphadenitis*), although these usually lie below the ligament, and torsion of an undescended or a retractile testis. Therefore, if there is no definite clinical evidence that the lump is an infected lymph node, exploration should be undertaken.

Lymphadenitis is associated with signs of *lymphangitis*, showing as pink streaks in the subcutaneous tissues, converging towards the groin. A less consistent associated finding is an infected, or healing, primary lesion in the skin and subcutaneous tissues of the external genitalia or the perineum,

the anal canal, the lower limb or the ipsilateral half of the trunk up to about the umbilicus. If the diagnosis of lymphadenitis can be substantiated there is justification for not operating in order to avoid disruption of the tissue planes, spread of infection and septicaemia. Instead, antibiotics are administered and the site of the primary infection, if any, is dealt with appropriately, antibiotics are prescribed and operation deferred. However, if doubt remains, it is far safer to explore immediately; failure to operate on a patient with a strangulated inguinal hernia that contains bowel will result in peritonitis with a high morbidity and mortality that exceeds the risk of spreading infection.

Torsion of an undescended or retractile testis is suggested by the absence of the testis from the hemiscrotum on the affected side. In any case, this requires urgent exploration because unless the testis is untwisted within 6 hours of the onset of symptoms, it is unlikely to be viable.

Management

A modest incision that can be extended is made and the lump exposed. If it proves to be an inflamed lymph node, no attempt should be made to dissect or excise it. An incisional biopsy is made and tissue sent for microbiological and histological examination. If it is a twisted testis, the cord is untwisted and if the testis looks viable it is fixed in that region. At a subsequent operation, when the inflammation has subsided, an attempt is made to lengthen the cord sufficiently to permit the testis to be placed in the scrotum. If the testis is not viable, it is excised.

Much more often, the lump proves to be a strangulated inguinal hernia. The sac is opened, the blood-stained exudate aspirated and the strangulated tissues held gently but firmly by an assistant. Only then does the surgeon free the constriction at the neck of the sac by dividing the external ring with an incision that is extended along the external oblique fibres. In this way, strangulated tissue is prevented from falling back into the peritoneal cavity before its viability can be assessed. Should the strangulated tissue be of minor importance (e.g., omentum) it is excised. In the case of small bowel, time is allowed until viability is confidently established. The anaesthetist is asked to ensure a high blood oxygenation and warm packs are applied locally to encourage vasodilatation. At the end of the period, viability is judged by the sheen of the peritoneal surface, the pinkness of the bowel serosa, the presence of peristalsis and pulsation in the mesenteric arteries, with special reference to the constriction rings at either end of the loop, where the bowel entered and left the neck of the sac. Viable bowel is returned to the peritoneal cavity, non-viable bowel is resected and (in the usual circumstance that the bowel is small intestine) an end-to-end anastomosis is performed. The hernia is repaired and the wound closed.

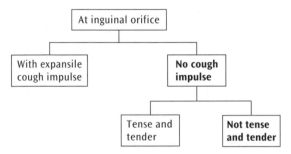

No cough impulse; not tense and tender

The usual diagnosis is an irreducible non-strangulated hernia. A few other conditions give rise to lumps in this category at the external inguinal ring.

Encysted hydrocele of the cord is a patent, isolated segment of the processus vaginalis that is obliterated at either end. It contains fluid, and is therefore a smooth, spherical or oval, transilluminable swelling that can be moved downwards by traction on the ipsilateral testis.

A *retractile testis or an undescended testis* is suspected when the ipsilateral hemiscrotum is empty, but the retractile testis can be coaxed down into the scrotum by gentle pressure on the inguinal region in warm surroundings, whereas the undescended testis cannot be so manipulated. An ultrasound examination distinguishes between the cystic nature of a hydrocele and the solid structure of a testis.

Management

An encysted hydrocele of the cord is likely to recur after aspiration and unless operation is

contraindicated it is better excised. A retractile testis needs no treatment, whereas the undescended testis should be brought down into the scrotum and fixed by surgery (*orchidopexy*), otherwise spermatogenesis is impaired. Orchidopexy past puberty is advised for cosmetic reasons, but assuming that a normal testis is present on the other side the surgeon is more likely to sacrifice the testis should orchidopexy prove difficult or the testis is atrophied. The undescended testis should not be left where it is because, although the tendency to malignant change remains high, in its natural position it is accessible for regular examination.

Other rare lumps in this category will probably not be diagnosable on clinical grounds. The general principle that an undiagnosed lump should be excised and submitted to histological scrutiny is followed.

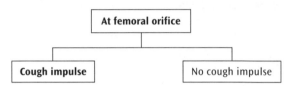

At femoral orifice, with cough impulse

The likely diagnosis is femoral hernia, although as explained later a cough impulse is frequently not detectable. Two alternative possibilities demonstrate some similar features and should therefore be considered.

Saphena varix is a varicosity of the upper end of the long saphenous vein, as it dips through the deep fascia to join the femoral vein, and lies within 3 cm below and lateral to the pubic tubercle. The degree of dilatation does not need to be great before the varix overlies the femoral canal.

The diagnosis is suggested by the blue colour of the venous blood in the varix shining through the patient's skin. The diagnostic features are that it empties on pressure and fills on release, disappears on lying down and that a fluid thrill is experienced by the examiner's hand when the patient coughs. This fluid thrill is a prolonged vibration, quite unlike the sharp impact in a hernial sac. Almost always, it is possible to trace a connection between the varix and varicosities of the superficial saphenous system further down the limb.

Management is a part of the treatment of the varicose veins in the limb (Chapter 14).

Abscess of the psoas sheath is a rare condition produced by a tuberculous caseating focus in the lumbar vertebrae or a pyogenic abscess associated with an intra-abdominal abscess complicating Crohn's disease. The abscess tracks down the sheath of the psoas muscle and presents as a swelling in the groin below the inguinal ligament. The patient is usually ill, there may be evidence of tuberculosis elsewhere, or intestinal symptoms. The lump may show cross-fluctuance with a mass above the inguinal ligament since the abscess may be large enough to appear in the right iliac fossa as well.

Clearly, the florid example of this condition is unlikely to be confused with a femoral hernia, but the safe rule to adopt is that *the spine should be examined clinically and radiologically in any patient with an apparent femoral hernia who displays unusual clinical manifestations.* An X-ray of the spine and the chest shows the bone lesion and possibly a primary pulmonary focus. An ultrasound scan, or more precisely a CT scan, will outline the abscess. Barium studies may have to be considered if there is no evidence of tuberculosis, or if there is a suggestion of intestinal disease.

Management of the abscess of the psoas sheath involves drainage and systemic anti-tuberculous therapy or specific treatment for Crohn's disease.

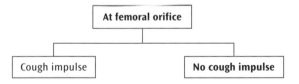

At femoral orifice; no cough impulse

Two situations may be distinguished: that the lump is tense and tender, or that it is not.

No cough impulse; not tense and tender

The usual situation is that the lump feels like a lipoma, a soft, fluctuant, lobulated subcutaneous swelling. This suggests almost certainly a femoral hernia. Because of its extra-peritoneal fatty layer when it reaches the thigh, the sac is usually only a portion of the whole mass, at the root of the swelling. The fat pad masks the cough impulse and also prevents reduction of the hernia. Irreducibility and absence of the cough impulse neither necessarily exclude a femoral hernia nor suggest strangulation.

Management

Early operation is advised for a femoral hernia. Treatment by a truss is not possible, even if the hernia is fully reducible. Because of its anatomical position, it is impossible to design a satisfactory truss that will maintain reduction.

The tendency towards strangulation is much higher for a femoral than for an inguinal hernia, therefore repair should be undertaken sooner than for an inguinal hernia.

Very occasionally, the mass turns out to be a lipoma; usually, it is a femoral hernia, whereupon the fat and sac are excised and the femoral canal closed with non-absorbable sutures between the ileopectineal ligament and inguinal ligament through a femoral or low approach (*Lockwood*), or between the conjoint tendon and the ileopectineal ligament via the inguinal canal (*Lotheissen*) or the para-rectus extra-peritoneal approach (*McEvedy*).

Other than a femoral hernia, only a few lumps in this category are diagnosable clinically. An ectopic testis (hemiscrotum empty) is an example.

Whenever the nature of the lump cannot be established, exploration for incisional biopsy is advisable.

No cough impulse; tense and tender

The possible diagnoses are: strangulated femoral hernia; lymphadenitis; or torsion of an ectopic testis.

A *strangulated femoral hernia* does not usually manifest local symptoms or signs, and the classic presenting features are those of small bowel obstruction. Except in undoubted cases of lymphadenitis, exploration is undertaken and the procedure is as described previously. The incision is planned along a high McEvedy or inguinal Lotheissen approach as these provide better access to the lacunar ligament. To release the constriction at the neck of the sac, it is usually necessary to incise the lacunar ligament. This approach also allows examination of the strangulated sac contents and resection of the bowel should that become necessary.

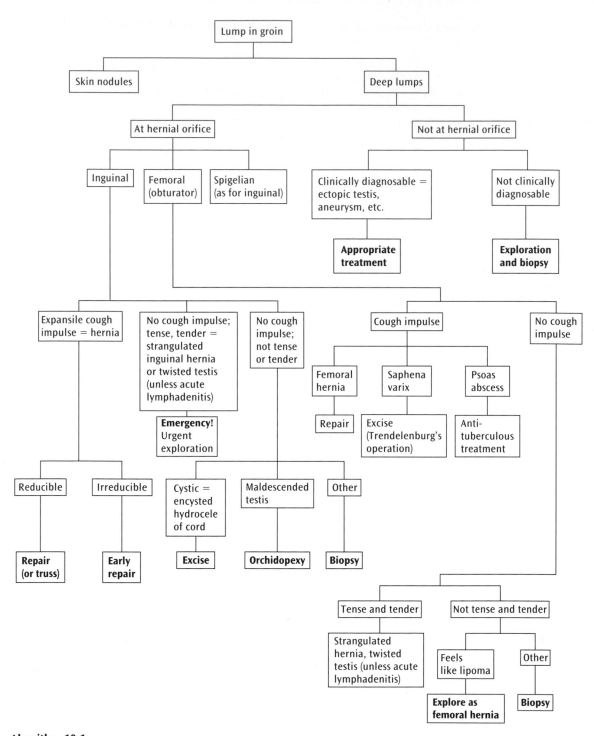

Algorithm 10.1

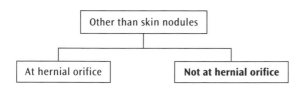

Lump not at a hernial orifice

As in other areas, the lump arises in subcutaneous tissue, or deep fascia, or muscle or bone, or from artery, vein or nerve. Characteristic signs (Chapter 1) may differentiate between these possibilities but it is unlikely that the diagnosis will be achieved without exploration and biopsy, although ultrasound examination can be helpful. Lymph nodes are frequently palpable in the groin, particularly in thin patients. Although they may be of no significance, the clinician should look for evidence that they are part of a generalized illness, such as glandular fever, lymphoma or AIDS, or secondary to inflammatory or neoplastic disease in the drainage field. Fine needle aspiration (FNA) cytology or Tru-cut biopsy is worth an attempt in the first instance, depending on the size of the lump, before an open biopsy is considered.

Femoral artery aneurysm is an uncommon lump in the groin. It lies below the mid-inguinal point (half-way between the anterior superior iliac spine and the top of the symphysis pubis) and has an expansile pulsation. Signs of atherosclerosis or other aneurysmal disease may be evident. One should be aware of this diagnosis whenever a biopsy exploration is planned.

Minimal criteria for diagnosis of hernia

This is a common and perplexing problem. The patient may attribute pain in the groin to a hernia or may describe without much certainty a swelling in the groin.

Although a general practitioner may, and should, promptly refer for a specialist opinion a patient with a story sufficiently suggestive of a hernia, he should realize that it is equally important to state whether he had seen a hernia, and must describe the findings in support of the diagnosis. This becomes invaluable information to the specialist since not infrequently a hernia may not be obvious, and the line of treatment is based on the general practitioner's statement.

However, it is more complex when the general practitioner has not found the lump and the patient is elderly and describes a swelling in the groin. Examining the patient standing up is particularly useful in demonstrating a hernia. Otherwise, the specialist might have to act on the history, from a patient who seems a reliable witness, that the swelling appears on standing and disappears on lying down, or is absent in the morning but pronounced by the end of the day. Alternatively, the patient is seen periodically until more convincing symptoms or signs are apparent. In cases of particular difficulty, *herniography* is available.

HIGHLIGHTS

- The key to management is the pubic tubercle
- A lump at a hernial orifice that one cannot get deep to and either has an expansile cough impulse or is tense and tender is a hernia
- A hernia that is tense and tender and lacks a cough impulse is strangulated
- A strangulated hernia requires urgent operation
- Irreducibility is not necessarily a sign of strangulation and vice versa
- Strangulated hernia is not always complicated by intestinal obstruction

11

Scrotal lumps: the empty scrotum

ANTHONY R MUNDY AND JULIAN SHAH

AIMS

1 Distinguish true scrotal from inguino-scrotal lumps
2 Understand the significance of an expansile cough impulse in an inguino-scrotal lump
3 Recognize the value of transillumination in differentiating between scrotal lumps
4 Appreciate the relevance of distinguishing between acute and chronic scrotal lumps for their management
5 Learn the principles of management of testicular maldescent

SCROTAL LUMPS

These usually are noticed accidentally, but the few associated with underlying inflammatory or neoplastic disease may show systemic manifestations.

Lumps *in the skin* of the scrotum are commonly sebaceous cysts which are frequently multiple (Chapter 1). Excision is unnecessary unless large, painful because of recurrent infection or cosmetically unacceptable to the patient.

Lumps *within the scrotum* are either confined within the scrotum, in which case they are true scrotal lumps, or are also palpable in the inguinal region, in which case the lump is *inguino-scrotal*. If the fingers and thumb of one hand can meet above the swelling, with the cord as the only interposed tissue apart from skin, the lump is scrotal; if not, it is inguino-scrotal. Examination with the patient standing up may help in making this decision as it increases the intra-abdominal pressure, especially on coughing, and makes the features of some lumps more prominent.

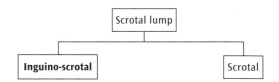

Inguino-scrotal lumps

A cough impulse and transillumination are helpful signs in determining the nature of an inguino-scrotal lump.

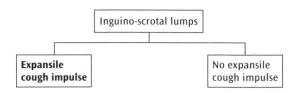

An *expansile cough impulse* indicates that the lump communicates with the peritoneal cavity and is therefore a patent processus vaginalis, which is the pre-formed sac in an inguinal hernia. The processus is not palpable, and only becomes so because of contained intra-abdominal structures, that is, an *inguinal hernia*, or liquid. In the latter case, the whole processus has usually remained patent and at its lower extremity it enfolds the testis (*tunica vaginalis*) and renders it impalpable. The condition is known as a *congenital hydrocele* (Fig. 11.1 (a)). Usually, but not always, the communicating orifice with the peritoneal cavity is too small for the development of a hernia. When the patient is supine at night the fluid drains into the abdominal cavity, but re-accumulates when erect so the swelling becomes obvious by the end of the day.

An inguinal hernia is not transilluminable when a torch is applied to one aspect of the swelling through the scrotal skin, whereas a hydrocele is. These two conditions may co-exist, when the testis appears to lie within the lower part of the hernia (*complete or scrotal hernia*), but pose no clinical problem because the management of either separately, and also of both lesions combined, is reduction of the hernial contents or drainage of the liquid

and excision of the patent processus without disturbing the tunica vaginalis. A herniorrhaphy might be necessary in the adult patient, but not in children.

Absence of an expansile cough impulse means that either there is no communication with the peritoneal cavity or that there is a communication but the processus is not free to move at the neck of the sac, the internal inguinal ring, due to adhesions within and around the sac or because strangulation has occurred.

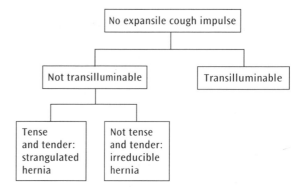

If the lump is not tense and tender then the absence of an expansile cough impulse means that

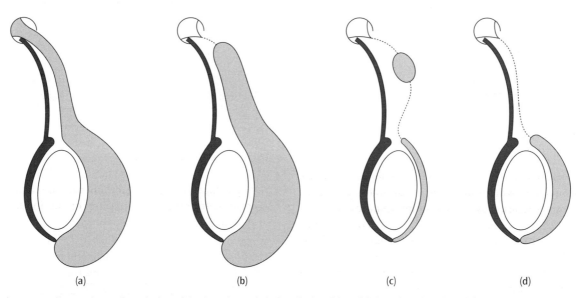

Fig. 11.1 *Illustrations of varieties of hydrocele and their relationship with inguinal hernias; (a) Congenital hydrocele; (b) Infantile hydrocele, which sometimes contains a hernia; (c) Encysted hydrocele; (d) Vaginal hydrocele, the commonest adult abnormality.*

the hernia is likely to be irreducible (Chapter 10), and if the lump is tense and tender then the hernia is strangulated. Otherwise, other lumps that occur in the groin should be considered.

Transilluminable lumps are liquid collections in the patent portion of a processus vaginalis that extend from the internal inguinal ring into the scrotum but do not communicate with the peritoneal cavity. If the lump extends downwards to the tunica vaginalis which enfolds the testis then the testis is usually impalpable and the lump is an *infantile hydrocele* (Fig. 11.1 (b)), although it does not only occur in infants. Should the lump not reach the testis so that the transilluminable swelling and the testis can be palpated separately, the lesion is an *encysted hydrocele of the cord* (Fig. 11.1 (c)). These lumps are better excised to establish the diagnosis and save the patient from the discomfort and possible embarrassment of future enlargement of the swelling.

Scrotal ultrasonography is an important and useful adjunct to clinical examination and should be used whenever there is doubt, or to confirm a clinical diagnosis because many patients need the reassurance provided by the investigation, particularly when excision is not being considered.

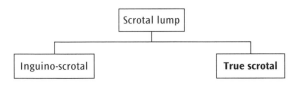

True scrotal lumps

The question of a cough impulse does not arise, and the important subdivision is based upon whether or not the testis is palpable. The distinction is not always easy, especially if the scrotal lump is very large. When examining the scrotum, the testis is held in the right hand, the cord in the left, and palpation conducted gently, bearing in mind the characteristic size, shape and consistency of the testis and its sensibility to pressure that evokes local pain. The testis usually lies in front of the epididymis and cord, although the relations of these structures are occasionally reversed. Each testis is examined independently.

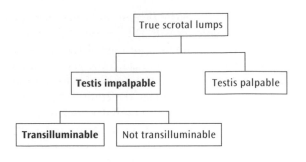

Testis impalpable

The presence or absence of transillumination may differentiate between the lumps in this situation. The most common *transilluminable* swelling that obscures the testis is a *vaginal hydrocele* or *hydrocele*, a collection of liquid in the tunica vaginalis, which is the part of the processus vaginalis that invests the testis (Fig. 11.1 (d)). Most hydroceles are idiopathic, but a minority are secondary to an associated disease of the testis, either inflammatory or neoplastic. When, as is usual, the testis is impalpable, ultrasonography is obligatory; if it is normal on palpation or ultrasonography, the diagnosis is a primary hydrocele.

Tapping of a primary hydrocele under sterile precautions is no longer required for diagnostic purposes since the advent of routine scrotal ultrasonography, but is performed to relieve the discomfort of its size. The liquid aspirated is typically straw-coloured. Occasionally, the liquid is blood-stained, a finding that is sinister until a diagnosis is confirmed, but should be distinguished from blood in the fluid at the end of aspiration as a consequence of the minor trauma involved.

A primary hydrocele occasionally will not reaccumulate after the first tapping. Should it recur, the choice of management lies between repetitive tapping (usually 6-monthly in order to keep the patient comfortable) and an operation. The choice depends on the patient's decision and fitness. The tunica vaginalis is opened through a scrotal incision, the liquid drained and the tunica plicated (*Lord's operation*) or turned inside out with excision of redundant tunica if necessary and sutured behind the cord and epididymis (*Jaboulay's operation*).

Management of a *secondary hydrocele* is treatment of the underlying testicular pathology.

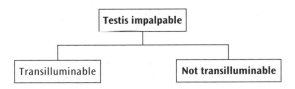

When *not transilluminable*, examination by ultrasound is necessary to define the scrotal contents and outline the testis. The testis may be obscured by material within the tunica vaginalis that is not transilluminable, either blood or pus. Pus is more likely when other signs of inflammation are present, but rarely complicates epididymo-orchitis.

Treatment is by draining the scrotum and administering antibiotics according to the bacteriological sensitivity of the drained material. A haematoma or *haematocele* may have been preceded by a history of trauma and it is reasonable to wait 2 weeks for spontaneous resolution unless the scrotal swelling is tense and painful, when exploration allows evacuation of the blood and examination of the testis for any damage. When neglected, an organized clotted haematoma forms which may damage the testis by pressure atrophy. Occasionally, the bleeding seems to have been spontaneous, because of either antecedent unnoticed minor trauma or an abnormal bleeding tendency. If a coagulopathy is confirmed, again it is reasonable to wait 2 weeks, otherwise the working diagnosis of neoplasm of the testis is made and surgical exploration undertaken.

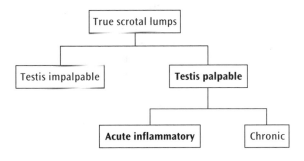

Testis palpable

Acute painful scrotal lumps

Acute pain with swelling and tenderness of the intra-scrotal contents, and redness and heat in the overlying scrotal skin may be due to acute epididymo-orchitis or torsion of the testis. The distinction can be difficult and is crucial because of the difference in the treatment of these conditions.

Acute epididymo-orchitis is a painful condition of sudden onset, occurring after puberty. Inflammation may affect the epididymis (*epididymitis*), the testis (*orchitis*) or both (*epididymo-orchitis*). It is usually secondary to urethral infection spreading via the vas deferens. Predisposing factors include a sexually transmitted infection with Chlamydia or *Neisseria gonorrhoea*, acute urinary tract infection, retention of urine, recent surgical operation on the urinary tract, neurological disease with urinary tract dysfunction, bladder stones and indwelling urethral catheters.

Fever, headache, rigors and a painful testis are the usual symptoms. On examination, the testis and epididymis are swollen and very tender to touch. In acute epididymo-orchitis it may be difficult to palpate the epididymis and testis separately. In early presentation, it is sometimes possible to detect epididymitis before it extends to involve the testis.

Treatment is with the appropriate broad-spectrum antibiotics. The infecting organism may be identified by urine culture or cultures of urethral discharge after prostatic massage. Even with antibiotics and bedrest, the swollen testis often takes many weeks to resolve. Inadequate treatment may result in chronic epididymitis and scrotal tenderness.

Acute epididymo-orchitis rarely complicates mumps; it usually presents a few days after the onset of parotitis and the treatment is symptomatic.

Torsion of the testis is not uncommon, affecting one in 160 males less than 25 years old. It usually, but not always, has a sudden onset. There may be an antecedent history of mild trauma, and the patient is usually between 12 and 16 years old. Nausea and vomiting are strongly associated with this diagnosis. On examination, the painful testis and epididymis are acutely swollen and tender, and characteristically the affected testis lies high in the scrotum with its long axis horizontal rather than vertical. The possibility of twisting seems to be associated with high investment of the tunica vaginalis extending up along the lower end of the cord.

Urgent scrotal ultrasonography, preferably with Doppler studies of testicular blood flow, may establish the diagnosis, and when equivocal, the scrotum should be explored urgently if torsion is suspected.

Recovery of the testis becomes less likely the longer the duration of torsion. The aim is to explore the testis within 6 hours of the onset of symptoms.

The explored testis is untwisted and observed for return of its vascularity for a few minutes. If the testis is black and fails to recover its colour, it is removed. Whether the tesis is or is not saved, the other testis should be explored and fixed, since predisposition to torsion is bilateral. This is unnecessary if the explored testis is found to be normal.

Fixation is either by eversion of the tunica vaginalis as for a hydrocele, with additional sutures placed between the internal aspect of the scrotum and the dartos muscle, or by placing the testis in a dartos pouch. When a testis is incorrectly explored for epididymo-orchitis, culture swabs are taken from the intra-scrotal contents and antibiotic treatment commenced.

A testicular prosthesis should be offered to post-pubertal patients: the scrotum is too small before puberty to acccept a prosthesis.

A cyst of an appendix of the testis (*hydatid of Morgagni*) forms a swelling at the upper pole of the testis; it is sometimes not clinically recognizable unless it twists, producing a clinical picture indistinguishable from a testicular torsion.

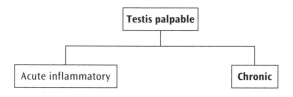

Chronic scrotal lumps

Diagnosis depends on anatomical site, testis or epididymis; and on whether the lump is transilluminable.

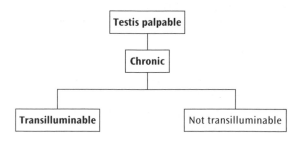

Transilluminable lumps at or near the upper pole of the testis are a *spermatocele* in the head of the epididymis, containing milky liquid, and the more common *epididymal cyst* situated behind the body of the testis and containing straw-coloured liquid. They are thought to arise from persistence of vestigial embryonic structures, and are therefore often bilateral.

These cysts are usually small and can be ignored once their nature is confirmed by aspirating fluid. Large cysts, if causing discomfort or are noticeable, are excised, although repetitive aspiration keeps the patient comfortable if operation is contraindicated. It is important to realize that excision will invariably cause infertility from blockage.

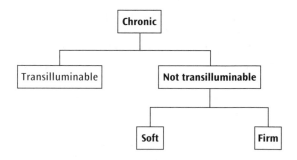

When *not transilluminable*, the consistency of the lump can be a discriminating sign.

A *varicocele* is dilatation and tortuosity of the pampiniform plexus of the spermatic vein. The majority (95%) are left-sided, possibly because the left testicular vein drains into the high pressure renal vein, whereas the right drains directly into the inferior vena cava. On examination with the patient standing, a varicocele feels like a bag of worms. A varicocele of recent onset which does not empty on lying down may be due to a renal or retro-peritoneal tumour and is investigated by renal ultrasound. Surgical treatment for a varicocele is only necessary if it is associated with pain, or if the patient is infertile as a varicocele raises the temperature around the testis, decreasing the sperm count and motility. The testicular vein is ligated at the deep inguinal ring, either by exploring the inguinal canal or laparoscopically.

Sperm granuloma is a palpable lump at the site of vasal division that follows vasectomy. One-quarter of men complain of testicular discomfort for up to 3 months, and a few for much longer. Local excision may relieve the symptoms.

An irregularly enlarged, hard and non-tender epididymis with a thickened, beaded cord is strongly suggestive of *tuberculous epididymitis*. With evidence of tuberculosis on a chest X-ray or a positive culture from sputum or an early morning specimen of urine, it is reasonable to accept this diagnosis and treat with anti-tuberculous chemotherapy. Only if the lesion enlarges or forms a cold abscess is the affected tissue excised. However, should the diagnosis be in doubt, it is safer to explore and excise the thickened area for histological and bacteriological investigation.

Other solid lesions in the cord are rare, but should be excised as these are possibly malignant.

A *solid, diffuse or discrete mass in the testis*, although rare, is usually a tumour. Other possibilities are tuberculoma, syphilitic gumma and foreign-body granuloma. A chest X-ray provides indirect evidence by ruling out a tuberculous focus or hilar lymph node involvement, and pulmonary secondaries indicate a malignancy. When a tumour of the testis is suspected, blood tests are taken for tumour markers; α-fetoprotein and β-human chorionic gonadatrophin are essential in the staging and follow-up of patients with non-seminomatous germ-cell tumours. Ultrasonography does help in the diagnosis, but when there is any doubt a working diagnosis of tumour should be made and the scrotum explored.

Exploration is performed via the inguinal canal, which is opened. The cord is cross-clamped at the internal ring with a soft clamp prior to delivery of the testis, in order to prevent vascular and lymphatic dissemination of the tumour. The testis, epididymis, cord and their coverings are excised up to the internal ring, since the high probability of a tumour will already have been demonstrated by ultrasonography. A scrotal approach to the testes by needle aspiration or incision is avoided because of the risk of involving the lymphatics which drain to the inguinal lymph nodes.

Germ cell tumours

Germ cell tumours are the most common tumours of the testis, and are divided into seminomas and non-seminomatous varieties, the majority of the latter being teratomas (Table 11.1). Teratoma affects a

Table 11.1 *Classification of tumours of the testis*

Germ cell tumours
Seminoma
Non-seminomatous germ cell tumours:
   embryonal carcinoma
   teratocarcinoma
   choriocarcinoma

Stromal tumours
Leydig cell
Sertoli cell
Granulosa cell

Table 11.2 *Staging of tumours of the testis*

Stage I	Disease confined to testis
Stage II	Retro-peritoneal lymph node involvement
IIa	nodes <2 cm
IIb	nodes 2–5 cm
IIc	nodes >5 cm
Stage III	Nodal disease above the diaphragm
Stage IV	Visceral metastases

younger age group, 20–40 years, seminoma an older age group, 30–50 years. When the diagnosis is confirmed, CT scanning is requested to determine the sites and involvement of thoracic, abdominal and pelvic lymph nodes as well as pulmonary and other metastases. A standard method of staging is shown in Table 11.2. Surgery is adequate for stage 1 disease, whereas radiotherapy and chemotherapy for more advanced disease yields a much improved cure rate. Tumour markers and sequential CT scans are used to monitor treatment. The five-year survival with a seminoma averages 95%, with a teratoma 60%.

THE EMPTY SCROTUM

See also Chapter 29.

If the testis does not lie in the scrotum, it may be *retractile*, *undescended* or *ectopic* (*maldescended*). Retractile testis is suspected when the scrotum is normal; in incomplete descent, the corresponding side of the scrotum is under-developed.

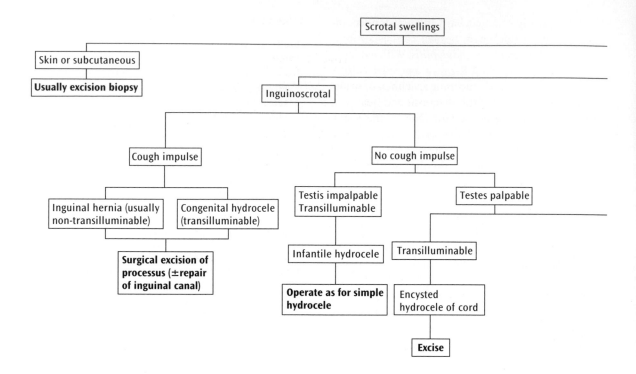

Algorithm 11.1

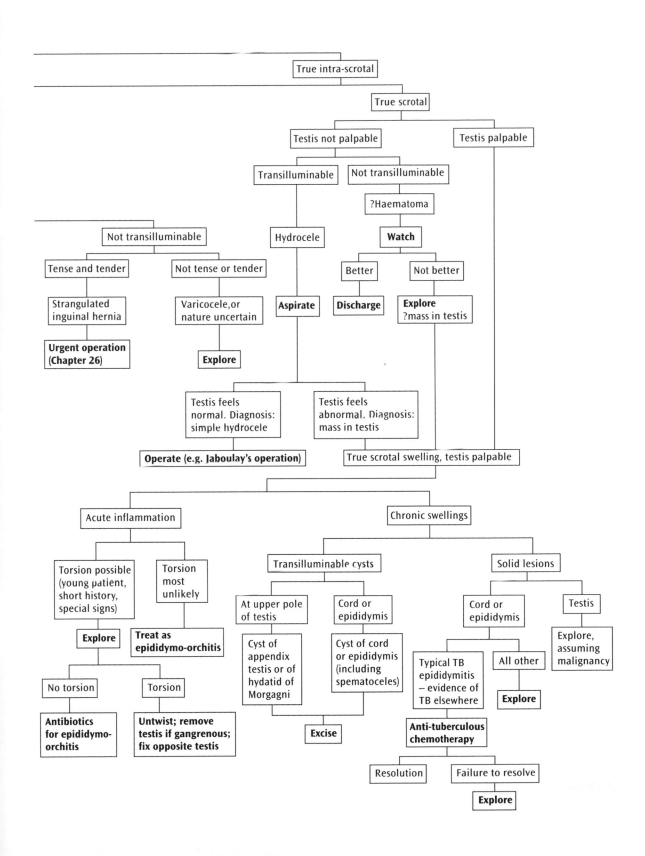

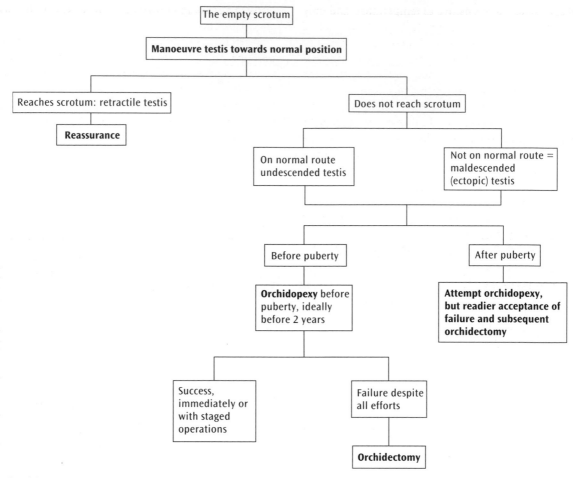

Algorithm 11.2

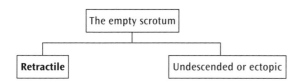

The *retractile testis* occurs only before puberty. The powerful contraction of the cremaster muscle pulls the testis up into the inguinal canal, but in a warm room, the clinician may, by gentle pressure on the inguinal canal, coax the testis downwards to occupy its normal scrotal position. No treatment except reassurance of the parents is needed: the testis settles in the scrotum at puberty. Follow-up is recommended to ensure that this happens. If the testis remains in the inguinal canal during a year or two of observation,

a course of human chorionic gonadotrophin is given, and if that fails, the testis should be brought down and fixed in the scrotum.

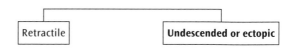

The *undescended testis* may be intra-abdominal and therefore impalpable, or it may be palpable in the inguinal canal or at the external ring, on its normal embryological route to the scrotum. It may be possible to manipulate such a testis for some distance towards the scrotum, but not to get it into its normal position. A testicular maldescent should be detected within the first year of life. The production of spermatozoa is sensitive to temperature, and only the relatively cool scrotum (2°C lower than core temperature) permits normal spermatogenesis. The longer after puberty a testis remains above the scrotum, the less likely is spermatogenesis to occur when the testis is placed in its normal position.

Management depends upon whether the condition is uni- or bilateral and on whether the patient is pre- or post-pubertal. When bilateral, the aim is to get one, preferably both testes, into the scrotum between the ages of 2 and 5 years, as there is a risk of damage to the testis with earlier intervention, otherwise spermatic dysfunction will develop. When one testis is in the normal position, the other side could be explored before the age of 2 years.

The inguinal approach is used only if the testis is palpable in the inguinal canal. Otherwise, laparoscopy is performed to identify the testis and its vessels. The cord is mobilized sufficiently for the testis to reach the base of the scrotum without tension, and is placed in a dartos pouch.

After puberty, orchidopexy is performed for cosmetic reasons, but if it is not possible, the testis should be removed because neoplasia is 30 times more likely than in the normally descended testis.

When bilateral, and a sufficient length of cord cannot be obtained, a staged operation involving a lesser degree of lengthening at each step is attempted. The *Fowler–Stephens procedure*, in which the testicular vessels are ligated at laparoscopy, may enable the testis to be brought down upon the artery of the vas after 6 months.

High bilateral abdominal testes which cannot be brought down in two stages should be removed because of the risk of malignancy. Testicular prostheses are placed after puberty.

An *ectopic testis* may lie anywhere in the inguinal, supra-pubic and femoral regions. Management is identical with that of the undescended testis, but orchidopexy is easier because the cord is usually long enough for the testis to reach the scrotum.

HIGHLIGHTS

- The processus vaginalis communicates with the peritoneal cavity in a congenital hydrocele
- It is obliterated at the deep inguinal ring in infantile hydrocele
- In a vaginal hydrocele the normality of the testis should be established
- A scrotal haematocele should be explored if it fails to resolve in 2 weeks
- A suspected testicular torsion must be explored within 6 hours
- A testicular tumour is diagnosed by ultrasound but if in doubt the testis is explored
- Orchidopexy should be done by the age of 2 years in unilateral, and by 5 years in bilateral, undescended testes

12

Voiding disturbance; urine retention; anuria

JULIAN SHAH AND ANTHONY R MUNDY

AIMS

1 Recognize the significance of urinary symptoms
2 Distinguish between irritative and obstructive symptoms
3 Appreciate the role of investigative methods in management

INTRODUCTION

Symptoms of voiding dysfunction are known as lower urinary tract symptoms (LUTS) and have a number of causes. LUTS may be sub-classified as *irritative* and *obstructive* symptoms. *Irritative symptoms* may be due to infection or bladder instability. *Obstructive symptoms* result from bladder neck or prostatic obstruction or may be neuropathic in origin and are associated with obstruction by the external sphincter mechanism (*detrusor sphincter dyssynergia*) (DSD). These symptoms may develop into retention of urine and/or incontinence.

Although haematuria may be a part of LUTS, detailed investigation is necessary in case it is a separate phenomenon.

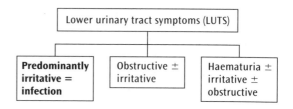

LUTS

Clinical assessment

A detailed history of symptoms of urinary tract dysfunction should be taken (Table 12.1), with a general medical history to elucidate any systemic causes.

Daytime urinary frequency is quantified by the period of time in minutes or hours between each act

Table 12.1 *Voiding disturbance*

Obstructive	Irritative
Hesitancy	Frequency
Poor stream	Nocturia
Terminal dribbling	Dysuria
Feeling of incomplete emptying	Strangury
Straining	Urgency/urge incontinence

of micturition. *Nocturia* is measured by the number of times the patient is woken from sleep to pass urine. The main causes of the frequency/nocturia syndrome are: excess fluid intake, particularly prior to sleep; bladder irritation due to urinary tract infection or stone in the bladder – this gives rise to a constant desire to pass urine; incomplete bladder emptying caused by outflow obstruction – residual urine reduces the functional capacity of the bladder and thus gives rise to frequency; detrusor instability (unstable or overactive bladder) which is commonly associated with prostatic outflow obstruction; and a small-capacity bladder due to inflammatory fibrosis which occurs with tuberculosis, schistosomiasis or idiopathic interstitial cystitis. Urinary *frequency* should be differentiated from *polyuria* in which urinary frequency and the volume of urine voided are excessive. This is accompanied by polydipsia commonly due to diabetes mellitus, diuretics, renal failure and less commonly diabetes insipidus.

Hesitancy is delay in starting to pass urine due partly to inhibition of the start of the voiding contraction and partly to the time it takes for the voiding pressure to rise sufficiently to overcome the outflow resistance. *Poor stream* is diminution in the force or calibre of the urinary stream. Interruptions in urinary flow may occur because the detrusor muscle cannot sustain the increased pressure required to overcome the outflow obstruction. *Dysuria* is pain or discomfort on micturition; the pain is often described as burning or scalding. Dysuria is commonly due to urinary tract infection and can follow urethral instrumentation and catheterization because of urethral irritation or trauma. *Strangury* is severe pain, referred to the base of the penis and down the urethra, that usually occurs at the end of micturition and is not relieved by voiding. It is associated with an abnormality in the region of the trigone of the bladder or bladder neck, such as a bladder or prostatic stone, bladder tumour or bladder infection.

Terminal dribbling at the completion of voiding must be distinguished from *post-micturition dribbling* (PMD). PMD is the leakage of a few drops of urine from the penis after voiding has been completed. It is almost universal in men though it may be associated with urethral strictures and urethral diverticula.

Urgency is the sudden desire to void with a feeling of impending incontinence. Bladder infection causes a sensory urgency. Uninitiated detrusor contractions due to detrusor instability are the most common cause of urgency. Urgency with pain is also seen in small-capacity painful bladders. *Urge incontinence* is less common in men than in women because of a stronger external sphincter that can hold urine against the high bladder pressures that may occur in bladder instability. *Stress incontinence* is urine leakage that occurs during coughing, sneezing, laughing or lifting and is most commonly seen in women due to pelvic floor and sphincter weakness complicating childbirth. Stress incontinence in men usually follows prostatic surgery. Incontinence can be continuous.

Straining is the forceful attempt to pass urine that is characteristic of urethral strictures and poor bladder contractility; it may also be seen in neuropathic bladders. Patients with prostatic outflow obstruction do not strain to void.

Haematuria is either noticed by the patient (*macroscopic*) or is discovered by dipstick testing (*microscopic*).

A number of systemic symptoms may be associated with urological disease and therefore system review is an important component of the assessment. Non-specific symptoms include: headaches and visual disturbances (hypertension); sweating and rigors (infection); peripheral oedema and dyspnoea or orthopnoea (cardiac and renal disease); general malaise (infection or renal disease); anorexia, nausea, vomiting and weight loss (malignancy).

Other relevant points to be considered are smoking and occupational exposure to dye, rubber, cable or sewage industries as these have been implicated in urothelial cancer; a history of hypertension, diabetes mellitus or neurological disease; and in women an obstetric history which should include information about difficult deliveries and previous gynaecological procedures.

Physical examination

A full general examination looks for a sallow complexion or anaemia and signs of weight loss which may indicate uraemia or malignancy. Blood pressure must always be measured, as hypertension may be a feature of renal disease. The abdomen is palpated for tenderness or masses. Loin tenderness is uncommon in non-acute renal disorders. Except in very thin patients, the kidneys are impalpable unless they are enlarged. A distended bladder is palpable in the lower abdomen. It is domed in shape, fixed to the anterior abdominal wall, dull to percussion and pressure on it may induce an urge to void. In the male the prepuce is retracted and the external urinary meatus inspected; the scrotum is inspected and palpated for masses or tenderness in the epididymis or testicle; and rectal examination allows palpation of the prostate for its size and configuration. In females, inspection of the genitalia includes the position and appearance of the urethra, the presence of urinary leakage or prolapse of the anterior vaginal wall (*cystocele*) or the posterior vaginal wall (*rectocele*), which may be particularly evident when the patient is asked to cough. Vaginal examination of the uterus and adnexae should also be carried out.

Finally, perineal sensation should be tested and also the leg reflexes which reflect the innervation of the bladder.

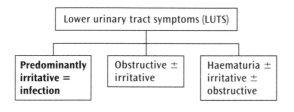

INFECTIONS OF THE LOWER URINARY TRACT

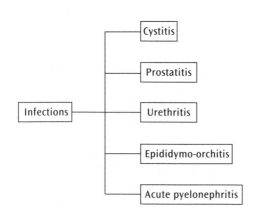

Clinical findings

Patients generally present with irritative voiding symptoms. Pyrexia is infrequent unless the kidneys are also inflamed (*pyelonephritis*). Supra-pubic pain and low back pain occur commonly with acute cystitis. Urinary frequency, nocturia, urgency and dysuria are the most common symptoms of cystitis. Strangury may occur in cystitis and is a painful sensation that occurs at the end of voiding. It is also a characteristic of bladder stone and tumours near the bladder neck.

Females are particularly susceptible to cystitis as ascending infection may reach the bladder because of the short female urethra. Rectal flora colonize the perineum and vaginal vestibule and reach the urethra and bladder. The onset of sexual activity in the female may cause cystitis (*honeymoon cystitis*). The presence of pruritus and vaginal discharge suggests vaginitis.

In males, purulent or mucoid urethral discharge and pruritus at the meatus are indicative of gonococcal or non-gonococcal urethritis. Acute prostatitis is a painful, febrile condition (though relatively rare) that often results in perineal discomfort and acute urinary retention.

Abdominal examination may elicit supra-pubic tenderness in cystitis. In females, pelvic examination may be normal, although the presence of vaginal discharge is suggestive of vulvo-vaginitis. In males, the urethral meatus is examined for discharge, erythema and oedema. On rectal examination, an exquisitely tender, swollen, warm and firm prostate is indicative of acute bacterial prostatitis. The scrotum is examined for epididymo-orchitis secondary to retrograde infection from the bladder, prostate or urethra.

A full blood count is often normal but occasionally leucocytosis may be present. Urine analysis usually shows pyuria, microhaematuria and bacteriuria. *Escherichia coli*, coagulase-negative staphylococci and enterococcus are the common bacteria isolated; proteus and pseudomonas are less commonly seen. In women, urine cultures may show no growth or low bacterial counts or cultures may reveal sexually transmitted organisms, *Chlamydia trachomatis* or *Neisseria gonorrhoeae*. Patients with vulvo-vaginitis may have sterile urine cultures, whereas vaginal cultures will show *Trichomonas vaginalis* and *Candida albicans* or *Gardnerella vaginalis*.

Prostatic massage should not be performed in *acute prostatitis* as the prostate is very tender and there is a risk of causing bacteraemia. Massage of the prostate is performed to collect prostatic fluid for microscopy, culture and sensitivities when *chronic prostatitis* is suspected, or *prostatodynia* when inflammatory cells are absent.

When there is urethral discharge, a calcium alginate swab is inserted into the urethra and rotated, and rolled onto a glass slide for Gram staining. The presence of intra-cellular Gram-negative diplococci on Gram stain is diagnostic of gonococcal urethritis but if only extra-cellular Gram-negative diplococci are seen, diagnosis will rely on culture results. When *N. gonorrhoeae* is not isolated non-gonococcal urethritis (NGU) is the likely diagnosis. Gram stain of a urethral swab reveals numerous polymorphonuclear leukocytes. The most common organisms are *C. trachomatis* and occasionally *T. vaginalis*. *C. trachomatis* is detected by fluorescein-conjugated monoclonal antibody or nucleic acid amplification, for example PCR or LCR.

Management

The principles of management are to treat the infection with an appropriate antibiotic, initially empirically until the urine culture and sensitivity results are available. High fluid intake and potassium citrate may relieve dysuria. Women with acute symptoms of cystitis but a low bacterial count should be treated with the antibiotic to which the organism is sensitive, whereas those with no identifiable organism paradoxically may respond to antimicrobial treatment. Agents commonly used are trimethoprin or an oral cephalosporin. Vaginal infections are treated with the appropriate antibiotic according to the organism isolated. Gonococcal urethritis is treated with a penicillin, although because of the emergence of β-lactamase-producing and other resistant strains, a third-generation cephalosporin (e.g., ceftriaxone, 250 mg intramuscularly) and in addition a 7-day course of oral doxycycline or erythromycin to cover concurrent chlamydial infections, are recommended. Non-gonococcal urethritis is treated with a 7-day course of doxycycline to which *C. trachomatis* is sensitive, but non-responders are treated with

erythromycin and those with *T. vaginalis* should be treated with metronidazole. The patient's partner should also be treated and they should refrain from sexual intercourse until cured.

In acute bacterial prostatitis, hospitalization is usually necessary, particularly if retention develops, as catheterization will be necessary. Intravenous antibiotics should be commenced for an acute pyrexial episode before changing to oral therapy. Prostatitis tends to respond to trimethoprim, doxycycline and norfloxacin. Anti-inflammatory agents may be necessary for pain. Alpha-blockers alleviate the outlet spasm that occurs in these patients. Regular prostatic massage may help patients with chronic prostatitis.

An abdominal X-ray excludes associated urinary stones, and radiological investigation of the urinary tract is required in those who do not respond to antibiotic treatment. Cystoscopy is mandatory when haematuria occurs. It should be recognized that cystitis secondary to radiation therapy, chemotherapy, bladder cancer and carcinoma *in situ*, eosinophilic cystitis and interstitial cystitis produce acute and recurrent symptoms without infection, when cystoscopy is necessary to establish the diagnosis.

Management of complications

Prostatic abscess is a rare complication of acute bacterial prostatitis and should be suspected when a patient with acute prostatitis is not responding to treatment. The prostate feels swollen, and is tender and fluctuant. Urine culture reveals the causative organism, commonly *E. coli* and, if the diagnosis is uncertain, a trans-rectal ultrasound scan of the prostate assists in diagnosis. Drainage is achieved by trans-urethral incision of the prostate and appropriate antibiotic therapy.

Chronic bacterial prostatitis presents with irritative voiding symptoms, perineal discomfort and low back pain. It may or may not be associated with urinary tract infection and the causative organisms are not always easily identified. Examination may reveal a normal, a boggy or indurated prostate gland, and prostatic massage produces secretion with numerous inflammatory cells, pus cells and bacteria. A urine specimen obtained after prostatic massage grows the same causative organism as the prostatic fluid.

Table 12.2 *Diagnosis of prostatitis*

	Expressed prostatic secretion (EPS)	
	White cells	Organisms
Chronic bacterial prostatitis	+	+
Chronic abacterial prostatitis	+	–
Prostatodynia	–	–

Trimethoprim, doxycycline or norfloxacin are effective agents but may need to be given for prolonged periods (1–3 months depending upon response).

When prostatic secretions contain excessive inflammatory cells but bacteriological investigations fail to isolate any organism including unusual organisms such as chlamydia or ureaplasma in the prostatic fluid or the urine, a diagnosis of abacterial prostatitis is made; if inflammatory cells are also absent then the diagnosis is prostatodynia (Table 12.2). These patients are often difficult to treat.

Acute epididymo-orchitis is associated with retrograde infection of the epididymis from the urethra or prostate. It starts in the tail of the epididymis and progresses to involve the entire epididymis and may also affect the testis (*orchitis*). It complicates sexually transmitted diseases in young men and is due to urinary tract infection and prostatitis in older patients. Patients with indwelling catheters are particularly susceptible to develop acute epididymo-orchitis. The presenting symptoms are the sudden onset of scrotal pain and swelling with redness of the overlying skin. The epididymis is thickened and tender. The patient is usually pyrexial. Associated symptoms of prostatitis or cystitis are usually present. Antibiotic treatment according to culture and sensitivities is commenced and in severe cases hospitalization and intravenous antibiotics are required.

Acute pyelonephritis manifests with pyrexia, rigors, loin pain and tenderness. Laboratory findings include marked leucocytosis, pyuria, bacteruria and microscopic haematuria with positive cultures. An ultrasound study of the kidney to rule out dilatation of the collecting system due to distal obstruction is a useful examination and may demonstrate oedema of the kidney. Antibiotic therapy should be initiated immediately and urine sent for urine culture and

sensitivity. If obstruction is present the kidney is drained, usually percutaneously and under ultrasound control. The underlying cause will need to be determined by further investigations and treated at a later date after the acute episode has settled.

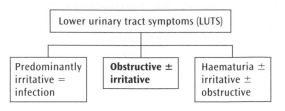

LOWER URINARY TRACT OBSTRUCTION

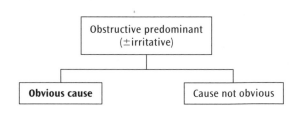

Clinical findings

Obstructive as well as irritative symptoms are the features of bladder outlet obstruction. Chronic retention most commonly presents with constant dribbling (*overflow incontinence*) and nocturnal enuresis. A number of patients will present with chronic retention as an incidental finding when the bladder is found to be palpable with no associated symptoms.

In adult males, a history of inflammation of the glans penis (*balanitis*) resulting in meatal stenosis or, in uncircumcised males, chronic inflammation and scarring of the prepuce resulting in narrowing of the preputial orifice (*phimosis*) may cause difficulty in urination. A urethral stricture is suspected if there is a history of previous catheterization, instrumentation, pelvic fracture or urethritis and if the patient admits to straining when voiding.

In males above 50 years of age, the most common obstructive lesion is benign prostatic hypertrophy (BPH) due to benign prostatic hyperplasia – hyperplasia of the para-urethral glands.

Sexual function should be documented with special attention to the presence or absence of erection and ejaculation. In both sexes, any disturbance of bowel function should be noted. Patients may already be known to have a neurological disorder, such as spinal cord injury, multiple sclerosis or peripheral neuropathy, or they present with generalized neurological symptoms, such as disturbed cerebral function, weakness, sensory loss or altered co-ordination. Enquiry should be made about associated medical conditions, such as diabetes mellitus. Certain drugs cause a change in bladder function, notably those with anticholinergic effects, such as antidepressants and drugs with atropine-like properties. Drugs that may affect relaxation of the bladder neck and prostatic urethra include pseudoephedrine, ephedrine and phenylpropranolol.

Physical examination looks for the general features of illness seen with uraemia due to renal failure which is associated to some degree with half of all patients with chronic retention and includes anaemia, hypertension, tachycardia and tachypnoea from metabolic acidosis. In chronic retention the bladder is painlessly distended and palpable.

In males, the external meatus and prepuce are examined for stenosis and the epididymis for signs of inflammation. Rectal examination is carried out and by palpation enlargement of the right and left lateral lobes is determined. The benign gland is smooth. Nodularity or a hard consistency is more likely with carcinoma. A prostate that feels normal can still be associated with obstruction. Urodynamic testing is necessary to diagnose obstruction in these circumstances and particularly in the younger male (i.e., aged less than 50 years).

In females, the urethral meatus is examined for stenosis or the presence of a urethral caruncle, which is a polypoid lesion at the meatus. A total uterine prolapse (*procidentia*), uterine fibroids or an ovarian or pelvic mass detected by vaginal examination, may predispose to voiding difficulty.

Neurological examination is essential and involves assessment of cerebral function, sensory level, muscular tone, power and reflex activity.

Management

Urinalysis using proprietary dipsticks will assist in the diagnosis of infection and haematuria and is an important initial investigation. Although haematuria may be associated with infection, other causes must be considered. A mid-stream specimen of urine (MSU) should be examined by microscopy and culture as urinary infection may be responsible for the presenting symptoms. Urine cytology for cancer cells is necessary in patients with haematuria and patients aged over 50 years with irritative symptoms.

If surgery is planned, infection should be eradicated to minimize the risk of peri-operative septicaemia and secondary haemorrhage. Serum electrolytes, creatinine and urea will give an indication of any disturbance in renal function due to obstruction. All men with outflow obstruction should be investigated by a free urine flow rate followed by bladder ultrasonography which estimates the volume of residual urine. Upper tract ultrasound demonstrates distension of the pelvicalyceal system by backpressure if present and provides as much useful information as an intravenous urogram (IVU) in these circumstances.

Subsequent investigations depend on the clinical findings and may not be required if the cause is obvious. In males, meatal dilatation will resolve the majority of meatal stenoses. A meatoplasty, which is a fairly demanding procedure that involves reconstructive surgery, is rarely necessary. Phimosis is treated by circumcision.

A suspected urethral stricture is diagnosed with an ascending urethrogram. Strictures are treated either by endoscopic incision with an optical urethrotome or by open surgical urethroplasty.

The patient with prostatic symptoms should be investigated by measurement of prostate specific antigen (PSA). If the PSA is raised a trans-rectal ultrasound scan of the prostate is performed. Sextant biopsies are obtained by the use of ultrasound guidance. The histological features will demonstrate the differentiation of the cancer according to the Gleason grading (Table 12.3). The carcinoma is clinically staged according to the physical examination and ultrasound: T_0 the prostate feels normal; T_1 a hard nodule in one of the lobes; T_2 a hard area which has spread into the opposite lobe but confined to the gland; T_3 a hard mass spreading outside the boundaries of the prostate and involving the seminal vesicles or T_4 the side wall of the pelvis.

A CT scan of the pelvis further outlines the extent of local disease and lymphatic spread. A chest X-ray

Table 12.3 *The Gleason grading system*

Gleason score*	Histological characteristics	Ten-year likelihood of local progression (%)
<4	Well-differentiated	25
5–7	Moderately differentiated	50
>7	Poorly differentiated	75

*The Gleason score is the sum of the two most prominent grades.

and an isotope bone scan will define distant metastases. On X-ray, prostatic bony metastases are typically sclerotic rather than lytic as in other bony secondaries.

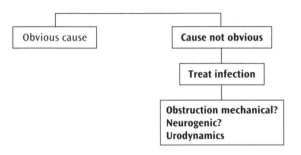

Cystourethroscopy is a prerequisite to the treatment of prostatic obstruction or any other intravesical lesion. However, cystoscopy is not particularly useful for the diagnosis of obstruction which should be made using urodynamic investigations prior to surgery.

When there is uncertainty whether the cause of obstruction is mechanical, as in BPH, or dysfunctional, *urodynamics* is required. By providing a dynamic assessment of the storage and voiding functions of the urinary tract, objective signs of benign prostatic hypertrophy can be measured and differentiated from functional abnormalities of the bladder muscle (detrusor) or of the urethral sphincters due to neurogenic lesions. As the bladder distends with urine, the detrusor muscle is stretched. There is an awareness of filling at a volume of 150–250 ml and a desire to void when normal bladder capacity (400–500 ml) is reached. The trigone contracts, opening the bladder neck and closing the ureteric orifices. The pelvic floor musculature, including the voluntary urethral sphincter, relaxes, the detrusor contracts and micturition is achieved. These functions are under neurological control. The

pelvic nerves supplying the bladder and urethra with afferent and efferent fibres synapse in the micturition centre located in the S2–S4 segments of the spinal cord, which corresponds with T12–L1 vertebral level. This centre is under voluntary control from higher centres in the pons and cerebrum.

Lesions above the micturition centre are characterized by detrusor overactivity and uncoordinated increased urethral sphincter activity. Lesions at the level of the micturition centre or lower are characterized by decreased activity of the detrusor and sphincter. Therefore, the patient may suffer from obstructive symptoms or incontinence. However, clinically, the pattern of symptoms is mixed and assessment of the dysfunctional elements as determined by urodynamics allows rational treatment. Via special catheters, the bladder is filled with saline or contrast medium, and a continuous recording of intra-vesical pressure is obtained via a transducer. A fine rectal catheter provides a simultaneous measure of abdominal pressure in order to separate the effect of straining from the intrinsic vesical pressure.

Cystometry measures the bladder capacity (400 ml), intra-vesical pressure during filling ($<15\,cmH_2O$), bladder pressure during voiding ($<60\,cmH_2O$ in males and $<40\,cmH_2O$ in females) and premature unstable contractions. The patient's ability to perceive filling is tested. The first sensation of filling occurs at between 150 and 250 ml.

Urethral pressure profilometry measures the urethral pressure with the bladder at rest and during voiding and is employed when the above measurements fail to determine neuropathic abnormality.

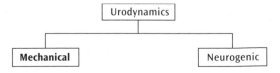

Management of BPH

Non-surgical treatment of prostatic obstruction includes α-adrenergic blockers, for example alfuzosin, doxazosin or tamsulocin, that improve the flow rate by acting on α-adrenergic receptors present in the bladder neck and prostatic smooth muscle, and finasteride that acts by reducing the size of the gland by inhibiting the conversion of testosterone to dihydrotestosterone.

Surgical treatment. The indications for surgical treatment are symptoms that are troublesome to the patient and complications which include recurrent urinary infection, bladder calculi, acute or chronic urinary retention, hydronephrosis and uraemia.

Pre-operatively, infection is actively treated with antibiotics. If the patient is in chronic retention, the bladder is drained by an indwelling catheter to allow the detrusor muscle and renal function to recover. Fluid and electrolyte balance is monitored and corrected, especially as on decompressing the bladder massive diuresis may occur.

Cystourethroscopy precedes prostatic surgery to exclude the presence of a urethral stricture, a bladder carcinoma or a calculus and to inspect the bladder wall for trabeculation and diverticula secondary to obstruction.

Trans-urethral resection of the prostate (TURP) is the most common procedure and involves excising strips of prostate tissue with a resectoscope using a cutting diathermy wire loop via a cystourethroscope. This removes the adenomatous portion of the prostate leaving the peripheral compressed portion of the gland that forms an outer capsule. Care is taken to avoid damage to the external sphincter mechanism.

Retro-pubic prostatectomy (RPP) is limited to patients with large prostate glands (>70 g) that are not suitable for TURP because of gland size and time required for resection. It is also considered when it is necessary to deal with bladder diverticula or large stones complicating BPH when prostatectomy is combined at the same time. RPP is rarely performed nowadays as most prostates may be removed by TURP. An indwelling catheter is left in the bladder after surgery and the bladder is irrigated with saline via the catheter to prevent clots forming within the bladder that may prevent adequate drainage resulting in clot retention. The catheter is removed once the urine is clear. Open prostatectomy is associated with a longer hospital stay and slightly higher morbidity and mortality.

Complications of TURP and open prostatectomy

During TURP the bladder is irrigated with 1.5% glycine to maintain a clear visual field and allow the use of the cutting current. Absorption of a substantial volume of glycine irrigant may occur into the extra- and intra-vascular space through the raw surface in the prostatic bed. This fluid is electrolyte free and, although it is generally tolerated by patients, occasionally a hyponatraemic, hypochloraemic metabolic acidosis develops with serious complications, including hypertension, tachycardia and confusion. This condition is known as *TUR syndrome*. Other immediate complications include intra- and post-operative haemorrhage, clot retention, urinary tract infection and failure to void when the catheter is removed. A late complication is retrograde ejaculation as the mechanism at the bladder neck that prevents semen entering the bladder during ejaculation is disrupted, hence patients fail to ejaculate through the penis, although the sensation of orgasm is unaffected. Other complications are incontinence as a result of sphincter damage and bladder neck stenosis from post-operative fibrosis and urethral stricture from the effects of intra-operative trauma and post-operative catheterization.

Other interventional therapeutic modalities that are particularly suitable for unfit patients include intra-prostatic urethral stents, microwave hyperthermia, trans-urethral needle ablation and high-intensity focused ultrasound.

Management of prostatic cancer

The management of prostatic cancer depends on a number of factors: stage, grade, PSA and patient performance status. A clinically *inapparent carcinoma* of the prostate is diagnosed either in prostatic tissue after TURP or on a needle biopsy (T_1), performed for an elevated PSA or a palpable nodule within the prostate (T_2). This can be treated either by radical prostatectomy, radical radiotherapy, brachytherapy or observation. Radical prostatectomy is associated with urinary incontinence in 10% of patients. Erectile dysfunction occurs in up to 60% of patients and can be reduced by a pelvic nerve-sparing technique. Radical radiotherapy is associated with a 50% risk of impotence and a smaller than 10% risk of bowel or bladder dysfunction. There are no randomized data comparing the outcomes of radical prostatectomy and radical radiotherapy.

Locally advanced disease (T_3 and T_4) can be managed by endocrine therapy alone, or in combination with radiotherapy. In patients presenting with bladder outlet symptoms TURP may be required.

Metastatic disease (M_1) is treated by hormone manipulation. Since the prostate gland is androgen-sensitive, androgen deprivation is effected by subcapsular orchidectomy or chemical orchidectomy with luteinizing hormone releasing hormone (LHRH) agonists or anti-androgens, such as cyproterone acetate or bicalutamide.

Hormonal therapy will often relieve the symptoms of urinary outflow obstruction, but if it does not TURP may be necessary. Local radiotherapy can be administered for painful bony metastases.

The histopathological features based on the Gleason system which recognizes five levels of increasing aggressiveness determine the long-term outcome:

- Grade 1 tumours consist of small, uniform glands with minimal nuclear changes.
- Grade 2 tumours show medium-sized acini, still separated by stromal tissue, but more closely arranged.
- Grade 3 tumours are the most common finding, and show marked variation in glandular size and organization, and generally infiltration of stromal and neighbouring tissues.
- Grade 4 tumours show marked cytological atypia with extensive infiltration.
- Grade 5 tumours are characterized by sheets of undifferentiated cancer cells.

Because prostatic cancers are often heterogeneous, the numbers of the two most prominent grades are added together to produce the Gleason score. This score provides useful prognostic information; Gleason scores above 4 are associated with a risk of more rapid disease progression, increased metastatic potential, and decreased survival (*see* Table 12.3).

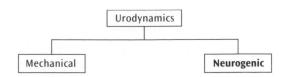

Management of neuropathic bladder

Two principal types of neuropathic bladder dysfunction occur: the *acontractile* or *arreflexic* bladder and the *hyperreflexic* bladder (with detrusor sphincter dyssynergia), distinguished by urodynamics.

Acontractile or arreflexic bladder

Patients with detrusor hypocontractility or an acontractile bladder may empty the bladder by abdominal straining or by suprapubically applied manual pressure (*Crede manoeuvre*). This approach is not to be recommended. Medication such as bethanecol or distigmine should not be given. The mainstay of treatment is clean intermittent self-catheterization (CISC) using a 12Ch catheter every few hours with the bladder volume kept below 500 ml.

Hyperreflexic bladder

In hyperreflexia there is detrusor overactivity. The urethral sphincter is usually uncoordinated (*detrusor sphincter dyssynergia*). Strategies for management depend upon the physical ability of the patient, gender and preference. The simplest and preferred management is with anticholinergic suppression of bladder hyperactivity and CISC. External sphincterotomy converts the patient from retention to incontinence, and in males, an applied condom to collect the urine is an alternative option for the patient who is too disabled to perform CISC. Some patients opt for a long-term indwelling supra-pubic catheter. Although an effective method of draining the bladder, it is prone to complications and there is a long-term risk of bladder cancer at 20 years. An implanted nerve stimulator (SARSI) is suitable for the patient with a complete transection of the spinal cord. Bladder augmentation with small intestine (*clam cystoplasty*) or urinary diversion that involves an ileal conduit is reserved for selected patients.

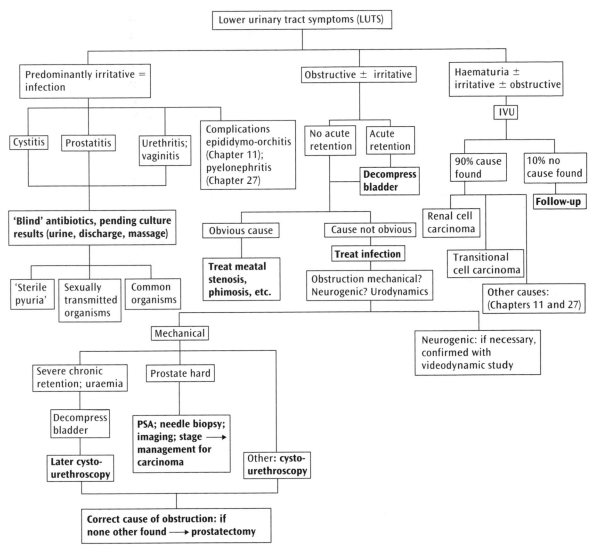

Algorithm 12.1

RETENTION OF URINE

In a patient who is not passing urine, *acute retention* must be distinguished from *anuria*. The patient in retention, except when in chronic urinary retention, is acutely distressed with abdominal or perineal pain and the bladder is palpable. Once the pain is relieved by catheterization, clinical assessment is conducted as described already. This may arise post-operatively (Chapter 16) and may follow spinal cord injury (Chapter 21).

Management

Catheterization

Acute retention is treated by urethral or supra-pubic catheterization. In either case, strict aseptic precautions must be taken to avoid introducing infection. For urethral catheterization, the external genitalia should be carefully washed with soap-based antiseptic. A 1% lignocaine hydrochloride with 0.25% chlorhexidine in a jelly base should be gently inserted into the urethra. A Foley catheter size 12 or 14 F is advanced along the urethra. In a male this is carried out with the penis being held taut and upright. Once the catheter is in the bladder, the self-retaining balloon is inflated to 10 ml. The catheter is then connected to a closed system drainage bag.

When there is history of previous difficult catheterization, prostatectomy or urethral stricture or the finding of a non-retractile foreskin, inserting a supra-pubic catheter is quick and safe provided the bladder is palpably distended. This avoids bleeding and the creation of a false passage from forceful instrumentation.

Reviewing the patient

A catheter is left in place while the patient is being fully assessed and a decision is made either to test whether the patient can void urine satisfactorily when the catheter is removed or proceed with definitive treatment. In either case, any urinary infection must be treated aggressively before a trial without catheter or an operation.

Trial without catheter

The catheter is removed usually either at midnight or early in the morning so that if the trial fails a catheter can be replaced at a convenient time. Success is judged if the patient can pass reasonable volumes of urine with each voiding, that is, >100 ml, and examination at intervals shows the bladder is not distended with retained urine which would indicate chronic retention with overflow. When in doubt an ultrasound examination of the bladder should provide a more accurate measure. Unsuccessful trial without catheter is an indication for cystourethroscopy and definitive surgical treatment. The bladder should never be allowed to overdistend and any patient who has not passed urine for 4 hours should be assessed.

OLIGO-ANURIA

Anuria is defined as absence of urine excretion for 12 hours, whereas *oliguria* is a urine output of less

than 0.5 ml/kg bodyweight per hour. It is classified as pre-renal, renal or post-renal. *Pre-renal oligo-anuria* is due to inadequate perfusion of the kidneys and can complicate acute fluid loss. Mean blood pressure in the glomeruli is usually above 60 mmHg; when it falls much below 60 mmHg filtration ceases. This level may be much higher in previously hypertensive patients. *Renal oligo-anuria* is often due to *acute tubular necrosis*. This is the result of primary damage or ischaemia of the renal tubular epithelium, or damage by nephrotoxic agents such as intravenous contrast media used in radiology or drugs (e.g., aminoglycosides and cephalosporins). It may complicate pre-renal oligo-anuria if not treated promptly, especially in septic or jaundiced patients and those with pre-existing renal disease or if there is distal obstruction. Other causes of renal failure may involve the glomeruli, for example glomerulonephritis. *Post-renal* (syn. *obstructive*) *anuria* arises if a calculus or clot becomes impacted in the ureter of the only functioning kidney, the other kidney being congenitally absent, previously removed or damaged by disease. Alternatively, both ureters are obstructed by calculi, or rarely by retro-peritoneal fibrosis or malignancy. An 'abdominal compartment syndrome' is also well-recognized where any cause of raised intra-abdominal pressure is thought both to occlude the ureters and to impair renal venous drainage.

Management

Causes of fluid loss, renal or hepatic disease, sepsis and intake of drugs should be considered. Although a history of urinary lithiasis is helpful, calculous anuria may arise without previous symptoms. A past history of prostatic or cervical cancer suggests retroperitoneal ureteric involvement with malignant infiltration or retro-peritoneal fibrosis if the patient has taken drugs such as methysergide.

Anorexia, hiccoughs, vomiting and drowsiness are earlier features of uraemia before the patient develops delirium and coma. The patient is examined for signs of hypovolaemia or cardiac failure. The loins are examined for tenderness, and rectal and vaginal examinations are carried out to rule out pelvic malignancy.

A urinary catheter is inserted to monitor urine output. If one is already *in situ*, its patency must be confirmed. In the case of hypovolaemia, blood transfusion, electrolyte solution or plasma expanders are administered. A central venous pressure line would be appropriate in a patient with cardiac insufficiency. A specific gravity of the urine exceeding 1020 is indicative of a concentrated urine and probably intact renal function. Pre-renal causes should be sought. However, if the specific gravity is 1010, and the blood urea mounting by 3.0–5.0 mmol or more daily, this suggests that the patient may be developing acute tubular necrosis and should be treated accordingly. An ultrasound examination to detect renal obstruction is essential as renal recovery is enhanced once the kidneys are decompressed. The obstructed kidney can be drained by percutaneous nephrostomy, allowing drainage of urine and pus. Obstructing ureteric stones are removed by ureteroscopy.

Management of acute renal oligo-anuria

In the absence of vomiting, the loss of water in an anuric patient is limited to extra-renal routes, that is, lung, skin and faeces. A daily intake of 500 ml should be sufficient plus the volume vomited or lost by gastric aspiration, diarrhoea or fistulae. An extra 200 ml is allowed for each 0.5° increase in temperature above 37°C. Care should be taken to avoid salt- and water-overload. Nitrogen intake should not be heavily restricted as this would encourage increased catabolism and breakdown of body protein. The aim is to provide 2000 calories per day and this can usually be achieved with the use of products taken orally or via a feeding tube. It is important to maintain meticulous fluid balance records and have regular estimations of urea and electrolytes.

Should the potassium rise to dangerous levels, a calcium resonium enema and/or intravenous glucose with insulin are simple corrective measures, plus restriction of potassium intake. Metabolic acidosis is likely to develop and may require administration of sodium bicarbonate provided that non-renal causes of metabolic acidosis, such as tissue ischaemia, have been excluded first.

Renal replacement therapy (RRT) should be considered in the case of rising urea and creatinine, acidosis, hyperkalaemia and/or fluid overload. The method of RRT depends on the facilities available and can either be continuous or intermittent dialysis and/or filtration. Peritoneal dialysis, whereby a catheter is placed into the peritoneal cavity to enable the infusion and drainage of dialysis fluid from the peritoneal cavity, is now rarely performed acutely. It relies for its effect on an osmotic gradient, allowing fluid and ions to be exchanged across the peritoneal membrane. The solutions used are either isotonic or hypertonic. In haemodialysis or haemofiltration, a double-lumen venous catheter is connected to a pump-driven apparatus in which exchange of fluid, electrolytes and small molecules is effected across a biocompatible membrane. The pressure gradient provides filtration and/or a counter-current of fluid is used to provide dialysis. The membrane is distributed over a large surface area by means of hollow fibres or flat plates to achieve adequate filtration. Acute tubular necrosis may last for 6–8 weeks. In the recovery phase, diuresis then commences and the patient passes a large volume of dilute urine with large losses of sodium and potassium. Therefore, amounts of water and ions equal to those passed the previous day are added to the daily allowance. Should oliguria persist for a longer period, renal investigations are indicated such as a renal biopsy.

Incontinence

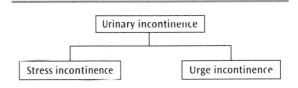

Incontinence is the involuntary loss of urine. Urine loss may occur through the urethra or less commonly from an abnormal extra-urethral route such as an ectopic ureter or a vesico-vaginal fistula. This section will mainly cover urethral incontinence due to urethral or bladder abnormalities.

Clinical findings

Incontinence presents either as *stress* or *urge incontinence*. *Stress incontinence* is loss of urine when intra-abdominal pressure rises during coughing, straining or lifting in the absence of detrusor activity. It is usually due to urethral incompetence but may also occur with an over-distended bladder with normal sphincters. *Urge incontinence* is due to idiopathic unstable detrusor contractions or detrusor hyperreflexia due to a neuropathic bladder. Increased sensory stimulation by stones, tumours or infection may also precipitate similar symptoms.

The assessment of a patient with incontinence is not different from that with retention. The diagnosis of the abnormality is either anatomical or functional.

Uroflowmetry shows decreased flow rates in patients with bladder outflow obstruction and eliminates the patient with overflow incontinence. Cystometry demonstrates unstable detrusor contractions in patients with urge incontinence but not in patients with stress incontinence. In addition, on video-urodynamics, descent of the bladder neck with leakage during coughing is demonstrated in patients with stress incontinence.

Cystoscopy is necessary where tumour, stone or fistula is suspected. Vaginal speculum examination and a cystogram will aid in diagnosis of vesico-vaginal fistula when suspected.

Management of stress incontinence

Minor degrees of incontinence may be treated with pelvic floor exercises and oestrogen therapy for associated atrophic vaginitis. In females, surgical treatment will produce continence in 60–80% of patients. The procedures employed include: *colposuspension* (still considered the 'gold standard') which is an open operation in which the vagina is sutured to the pectineal ligament; the *sling procedure*, which employs either the patient's own tissue – an autograft made of a strip of rectus sheath or allografts from donors or a prolene mesh (such as tension-free vaginal tape) (TVT); *peri-urethral injection of a bulking agent* such as silicon macroparticles, collagen or Teflon paste; an *artificial urinary sphincter*, although this method is rarely used in females; and *ileal conduit urinary diversion*, which is the final option.

In males, stress incontinence is rare but may complicate pelvic fractures, spinal cord injury or prostatectomy. Post-prostatectomy incontinence is treated with sub-mucosal injection of bulking agents or the artificial urinary sphincter. Incontinence due to sphincter injury is treated by surgical repair or reconstruction or by the implantation of an artificial urinary sphincter.

Management of urge incontinence

Urge incontinence due to bladder instability is treated by bladder exercises, the patient gradually increasing the intervals between voiding, or by biofeedback or acupuncture. However, the main-stay of treatment rests with medication. Anticholinergic agents, such as oxybutynin, tolterodine, propiverine and imipramine, suppress the overactive contractions.

Bladder distension under anaesthesia will rarely produce sustained benefits in treating unstable bladder contractions. Severe cases and failure to respond to these simple measures may demand augmentation cystoplasty (a segment of ileum is anastomosed to the bi-valved bladder – *clam cystoplasty*).

Haematuria

Clinical findings

Haematuria due to tumours of the urinary tract is typically painless, although flank pain may be present with renal tumours, and ureteric colic (*clot colic*) may occur from clots causing ureteric obstruction. When due to stone or infection, haematuria is usually accompanied by pain or dysuria but bladder tumours may predispose to unexplained recurrent urinary tract infection, and when near the bladder neck may cause strangury or urine retention. Enquiry is always made about renal or stone disease, trauma and voiding disturbances. Oral anticoagulants and a history of atrial fibrillation or rheumatic heart disease can be relevant since renal infarcts from an embolus can cause haematuria. The stage of micturition at which blood appears is sometimes diagnostically helpful. Blood from the kidneys, ureters or bladder wall will mix with the urine and be present throughout the urinary stream. Urethral bleeding may leak out independently of micturition or be seen only at the beginning or end of the urinary stream.

Blood arising from the bladder neck or posterior urethra may sometimes be present as terminal haematuria. In males more often than females above the age of 50, a history of smoking and exposure to industrial carcinogens used in the rubber, cable, dye and printing industries should raise suspicion of malignancy.

Examination involves looking for signs of anaemia, hypertension which may be due to renal disease but can be associated with polycythaemia caused by excessive erythropoietin secreted by renal cell carcinoma, tenderness or a mass in the loin or the upper abdomen, a palpable bladder or a mass in the supra-pubic region or blood in the urethral meatus. The testicles are examined for a right-sided varicocele that may be present due to right renal vein obstruction which may block the drainage of the gonadal vein. Rectal examination of the prostate and vaginal examination for a pelvic mass are carried out.

Management

A mid-stream specimen of urine (MSU) is sent for bacteriological examination; microscopy is performed in all patients as well as cytology for malignant cells. When haematuria is confirmed, and whether the cultures reveal infection or not, and even in the presence of irritative or obstructive symptoms, an ultrasound investigation of the urinary tract is performed. IVU is particularly useful for the diagnosis of urothelial tumours. Cystourethroscopy is required in all patients. In 10% no cause is identified and in the remaining patients an abnormality will dictate further investigations. Except for tumours, most conditions that may cause haematuria have been discussed already in this chapter and are considered further in Chapters 21 and 27.

Management of tumours of the kidney and urinary tract

Two types of cancer arise from the renal parenchyma, *renal cell carcinoma* confined to adults and also known as *renal adenocarcinoma* (syn. *hypernephroma, Grawitz tumour*) and *nephroblastoma* present in infancy or early childhood. *Transitional cell carcinoma* is at least four times as common as renal cell carcinoma and arises mainly in the bladder but also in the pelvicalyceal system of the kidney, the ureters or anywhere in the tract. Bladder tumours histologically are nearly all transitional cell carcinomas, the remainder are *squamous cell* (7%) or *adenocarcinomas* (1%) that develop from glandular epithelial remnants of the embryological urachus.

Renal cell carcinoma

A renal carcinoma may show obliteration or distortion of the calyceal system, whereas a transitional cell carcinoma may show a filling defect in the collecting system. Better definition is obtained by ultrasonography as it reliably distinguishes simple benign cysts from solid masses. CT scanning can be valuable for assessing invasion of the renal vein and inferior vena cava, peri-nephric invasion, regional lymph nodes and liver metastases. Arteriography is no longer used to diagnose renal cell carcinoma but to outline the arterial anatomy if partial nephrectomy is being considered if one kidney is missing or bilateral renal tumours are present. Other investigations are a full blood count for anaemia or polycythemia and a chest X-ray for pulmonary metastases. Liver function tests may on occasion be abnormal even in the absence of metastatic disease but this can be suggestive of poor prognosis. The staging of renal cell carcinomas is described in Table 12.4.

Table 12.4 *Staging of renal cell carcinomas*

T_1	Tumour 7 cm or less in greatest dimension, limited to the kidney
T_2	Tumour more than 7 cm in greatest dimension, limited to the kidney
T_3	Tumour extends into major veins or invades adrenal gland or peri-nephric tissue, but not beyond Gerota's fascia
T_{3a}	Tumour invades adrenal gland or peri-nephric tissues, but not beyond Gerota's fascia
T_{3b}	Tumour grossly extends into renal vein(s) or vena cava below diaphragm
T_4	Tumour invades beyond Gerota's fascia

Surgical treatment

The mainstay of treatment for renal tumours in adults is surgery. *Radical nephrectomy* through a trans-peritoneal, loin or trans-thoracic approach involves removal of the affected kidney and upper ureter in addition to the adrenal gland and Gerota's fascia. Isolated pulmonary metastases can be resected at the same time. Renal artery embolization is rarely employed nowadays. Immunotherapy using interferon and interleukins, with or without chemotherapy, are being evaluated in specialized centres for metastatic disease and in the adjuvant setting. The overall survival is 40% at five years.

Transitional cell carcinoma (TCC)

TCC accounts for only 7% of all renal tumours and tumours of the ureter and renal pelvis account for only 2–4% of all transitional cell tumours. Patients who develop a transitional cell carcinoma of the pelvis or ureter have a 30–50% chance of developing a transitional cell tumour of the bladder in the future. The presence of a transitional cell carcinoma of the bladder is associated with only a 2–3% chance of a tumour in the upper urinary tract. This is relevant in the follow-up of these patients.

The diagnosis of tumours of the renal pelvis or ureter is based on ultrasound and IVU, ureteroscopy and urine cytology. These tumours are managed by nephroureterectomy and partial cystectomy. Patients require annual cystoscopic follow-up.

A bladder tumour may show on an IVU or ultrasound scan as a filling defect or can be found at cystoscopy. Staging of bladder tumours is achieved by a combination of cystoscopic examination and palpation under anaesthesia and histological examination of resected specimens (Table 12.5). Bi-manual palpation of the bladder between a finger in the rectum or in the vagina and a hand on the anterior abdominal wall is performed before and after resection of the tumour. This gives an idea of the extent of bladder wall penetration and spread into the pelvis. The lesion is completely excised down to muscle using a resectoscope and multiple random mucosal biopsies are taken. If an invasive tumour is found, a chest X-ray and CT scan of the abdomen

Table 12.5 *Staging of bladder tumours*

T_a	Non-invasive papillary tumour
T_{is}	Carcinoma *in situ*, 'flat tumour'
T_1	Tumour invades sub-epithelial connective tissue
T_2	Tumour invades muscle
T_{2a}	Superficial muscle
T_{2b}	Deep muscle
T_3	Tumour invades peri-vesical tissues
T_{3a}	Microscopically
T_{3b}	Macroscopically

and pelvis will further outline the extent of the disease.

Superficial tumours (T_a, T_1)

Initial treatment is by trans-urethral resection of the tumour and is followed by regular flexible cystoscopy under local anaesthesia every 3 months for the first year, 6 months for the second year and every year thereafter. If recurrence develops an intensive follow-up schedule is recommended. The risk of recurrence and invasion is high in smokers, those with large tumours, multiple tumours, severe dysplasia or carcinoma *in situ* in random biopsies and high-grade superficial tumours. Intra-vesical chemotherapy instillation should be considered in these patients. The agents used are BCG, Thiotepa, Epodyl, Adriamycin, and Mitomycin C given once-weekly for 6 weeks. Five-year survival is 75%.

Invasive tumours (T_2, T_3)

When muscle has been invaded, local treatment by trans-urethral resection must be supplemented by a more radical form of treatment, either radical radiotherapy or radical surgery. Both offer a 35–40% five-year survival. Radical radiotherapy preserves the bladder but troublesome symptoms of radiation cystitis and proctitis may complicate the treatment. If the patient fails to respond, salvage cystectomy may be difficult and associated with significant morbidity. Radical cystectomy is followed either by the formation of a surface urinary diversion (*ileal conduit*) or by a bladder reconstruction (*orthotopic neobladder*) or by a continent catheterizable urinary diversion. Pre-operative radiotherapy or chemotherapy does not seem to offer added survival benefit, but is still under investigation with randomized clinical trials.

Metastatic tumours

The treatment options are palliative chemotherapy, which includes MVAC (methotrexate, vinblastine, adriamycin, cisplatin) and CMV (cisplatin, methotrexate, vinblastine); palliative radiotherapy; or both. Median survival in these patients is 1 year.

Unusual tumours of the urinary tract

Squamous cell carcinoma is rare, although it commonly complicates bladder schistosomiasis and may result from the presence of a long-term catheter. This tumour is treated along similar lines to transitional cell carcinomas except if the lesion is in the distal

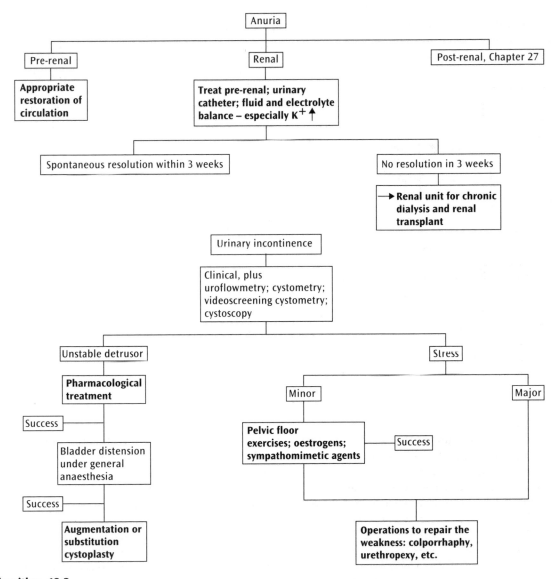

Algorithm 12.2

urethra when it is treated as penile carcinoma by partial amputation of the penis and block dissection of the inguinal lymph nodes if involved. *Adenocarcinoma* is resected as it arises solely in the urachal remnant.

Nephroblastoma arises in the kidney from embryonal renal tissue and presents in early childhood, usually before the age of 3 years, as a large abdominal mass. Surgical resection, radiotherapy and chemotherapy give an excellent prospect of complete cure even when distant metastases are present.

HIGHLIGHTS

- Women with cystitis with no identifiable organisms may respond to antimicrobial treatment
- Prostatic message to obtain prostatic fluid should be avoided for bacteriological examination if acute prostatitis is suspected
- A prostate that feels normal can still be associated with obstruction
- Urodynamic studies are of value in differentiating between mechanical and dysfunctional bladder outlet obstruction due to neurological disorders, and in urinary incontinence
- A patient with acute retention who has not passed urine for 4 hours after trial without a catheter should be reassessed for definitive treatment by flowmetry and bladder ultrasonography
- Cystourethroscopy should always precede open prostatic surgery
- Microscopy, bacteriological examination and cytology for malignancy cells should be performed in all patients with haematuria, and patients aged over 50 years with irritative symptoms
- In a patient with oligo-anuria the urine specific gravity and ultrasound scan of the kidneys are essential diagnostic investigations
- Renal replacement therapy should be considered in the case of rising urea and creatinine, acidosis, hyperkalaemia and/or fluid overload

13

Chronic lower limb ischaemia

M ADISESHIAH

AIMS

1 Demonstrate the method of diagnosis and assessment of severity of chronic limb ischaemia by clinical means alone
2 Demonstrate the significance of intermittent claudication
3 Understand the significance of the combination of rest pain/ischaemic ulceration/gangrene (critical ischaemia)

INTRODUCTION

The most common cause of death in Europe is from the various forms of atherosclerosis. This is a generalized disease and the clinician has to define priorities in treatment according to the principal organ that is affected. In this respect vital structures such as the heart, brain, kidneys and bowel take precedence over the limbs.

The clinical picture in chronic limb ischaemia is typical. The salient symptoms are *intermittent claudication* and *rest pain*, and the physical signs are coldness of the limb, ischaemic ulceration and gangrene. The presence or absence of pulses affords valuable information about the patency of the large arteries, but gives little information about the presence or degree of ischaemia. The pulse may be absent but an effective collateral circulation can maintain perfusion, whereas tissue ischaemia may develop in the presence of full limb pulses because of arterial occlusion as in Raynaud's syndrome and Buerger's disease. Other signs which are more likely in severe disease are trophic changes, coldness of the skin, pallor of the limb when elevated and guttering because of empty veins, with a change in colour into a blueish-red when the leg is hung down.

Intermittent claudication runs a relatively benign clinical course. Rest pain, on the other hand, with or without the physical signs of gangrene and/or ischaemic ulceration, is commonly referred to as *critical ischaemia*. It is more sinister and constitutes an absolute indication for intervention.

INTERMITTENT CLAUDICATION

The word *claudication* means limping. The symptom is described as pain, usually in the calf, which comes on after a variable amount of running or walking, and is relieved by stopping exercise, usually within 15 minutes. When the time required to obtain relief on resting is longer, the pain is most likely due to arthritis or some other musculoskeletal cause. The pain is distal to the level of arterial obstruction, is usually sited in the calf (*femoro-popliteal*) and may extend into the thigh or even the buttocks (*common iliac*) with loss of erection in the male (*aortic/internal iliac artery*). The pain is typically variable in onset and sometimes hardly obtrudes on the patient's consciousness. Characteristically, the pain is more severe when walking uphill or upstairs. At other times the pain is crippling and prevents the performance of simple chores, such as shopping, or leisure activities.

Intermittent claudication is due to arterial stenosis or occlusion with sufficient blood flow via collateral channels at rest, but on exercise the collaterals do not accommodate the increase in blood flow that is called for with increased activity.

It is important to distinguish between true intermittent claudication and spinal (*cauda equina*) claudication caused by compression of the cauda equina within the spinal canal by disc prolapse or spinal stenosis. In the latter, the complaint is of effort pain in a similar anatomical distribution, that is, calves, back of thighs and buttocks. Some important differences from true vascular claudication include a paraesthetic quality sometimes described as 'pins and needles'; the pain takes a longer time to disappear with rest, up to 30 minutes; there is usually a history of backache; and most typically, complete relief is obtained only on sitting down, whereas vasculogenic claudication subsides shortly after standing still. The diagnosis becomes clearer when the physical signs are elicited. Invariably, there are no signs to suggest ischaemia, and signs of a lower motor neurone lesion, such as diminished or absent tendon reflexes, may be present. The diagnosis may be established by measuring the ankle blood pressure at rest and after exercise. In spinal stenosis these are usually within normal limits, whereas in vascular insufficiency they are reduced.

Investigations

Arteriography is only required if the clinical picture suggests that intervention is necessary. A standard non-invasive investigation to determine the severity of the ischaemia is measurement of the blood pressure at the ankle.

The ankle/brachial blood pressure index (ABPI)

In the supine position, the blood pressure (systolic, diastolic and mean) is approximately the same in all four limbs at any level from the proximal to the distal parts of the limb. For unclear reasons, the blood pressure in the normal human at the ankle is slightly higher than the brachial. The normal ankle blood pressure, whether it be systolic, diastolic or mean, divided by the corresponding brachial pressure comes out as an average of 1.1 with a standard deviation of 0.1. This fraction is known as the ankle/brachial blood pressure index (ABPI).

An index of less than 0.8 is diagnostic of lower limb ischaemia. In intermittent claudication uncomplicated by rest pain, resting ABPI may be normal and indicates adequate perfusion at rest. However, when the patient is exercised by treadmill walking, the index drops to significantly low levels, providing proof of chronic limb ischaemia. In cases of rest pain the index falls to 0.3 or less.

It is possible to obtain falsely high estimates of ABPI in instances where the brachial blood pressure is low due to upper limb arterial disease. In diabetes mellitus, the ankle arteries are stiff and uncompliant due to medial calcification, again giving rise to falsely elevated ABPI levels.

Sphygmomanometry, which is most commonly used for brachial blood pressure measurement, is unsuitable for ankle pressure measurement. Therefore, the usual method of obtaining ABPI is to use a hand-held continuous wave doppler probe which emits the characteristic sound of an arterial flow signal when placed over an artery. A pneumatic cuff connected to a sphygmomanometer is applied above the malleoli and the pressure noted at which the flow signal disappears and reappears on inflation and deflation of the cuff. The mean of the two pressures is the ankle pressure. The artery that is insonated in the arm is the brachial in the antecubital fossa. At the ankle, both the dorsalis pedis and the posterior tibial arteries are insonated and the higher reading is taken as the ankle pressure.

By use of automatic oscillotonometric machines it is possible to obtain the systolic, diastolic and mean ABPI in all four limbs. However, this technique does not accurately measure blood pressures below 40–50 mmHg.

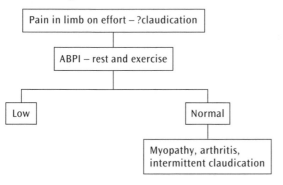

Risk factors

More than 90% of patients presenting with chronic limb ischaemia suffer from arteriosclerotic disease. It is essential to recognize contributing risk factors in the clinical evaluation and take steps to eliminate or minimize them in the hope of improving the overall prognosis. These are smoking, hypertension, diabetes mellitus and hyperlipidaemia.

Smoking is by far the most common and the most important risk factor. *Hypertension* is easily diagnosed during the physical examination and should be investigated and treated. The possibility of renal artery stenosis should be borne in mind. *Diabetes mellitus* may be diagnosed by a positive family history, the symptoms of polydypsia and polyuria, a raised fasting blood sugar and the classical abnormal glucose tolerance curve. Diabetes produces limb ischaemia in two main ways: premature arteriosclerosis in the classical distribution in large arteries, or arterial occlusive disease in the infra-geniculate arteries with relative sparing of the aorto-iliac-femoral segment. Another manifestation is the infected foot with ulceration or abscesses in the plantar spaces in the presence of normal foot pulses. A family history of circulatory disorder – myocardial infarction, stroke or limb ischaemia in men under 55 years, women under 65 years, is characteristic of *hyperlipidaemia*. The presence of xanthelasma and/or corneal arcus with raised fasting serum lipids

is diagnostic of a monogeneic familial disorder of lipid metabolism, *familial hyperlipidaemia*.

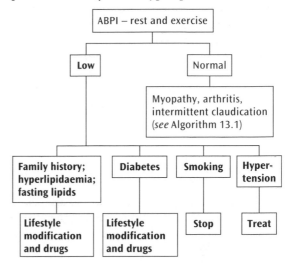

Associated ischaemic disorders (co-morbidities)

The two systems that are commonly affected are the cardiovascular and the cerebrovascular. In addition, there may be involvement of the visceral blood supply, mesenteric and renal, and these require attention prior to managing limb ischaemia.

Cardiovascular ischaemia is detected in the history by the presence of angina pectoris and/or a history of myocardial infarction. The severity of the disease is measured by cardiac scintigraphy and angiography.

Cerebrovascular ischaemia is elicited by enquiry about a previous stroke, transient ischaemic attack (TIA), amaurosis fugax, total or partial monocular loss of vision. *TIA* is a stroke with complete recovery within 24 hours. *Amaurosis fugax* is transient blindness, described by the patient as the descent of a black curtain in one eye that clears within a few minutes. These symptoms are usually due to particulate emboli which travel up through the cerebral arteries from the heart or an arteriosclerotic plaque at the origin of the internal carotid artery and lodge in the brain or the retinal arteries to cause ischaemia. Duplex colour ultrasonography is the method of choice in measuring the type and degree of carotid stenosis.

Mesenteric ischaemia is uncommon, but when it occurs, it presents as post-prandial abdominal pain with weight loss. This clinical picture is more often due to a visceral disorder, which should be thoroughly investigated before selective mesenteric angiography is considered.

Renovascular hypertension due to renal artery stenosis is encountered in less than 10% of all hypertensive patients and should be considered in those with severe hypertension. The diagnosis is established by isotope renography, angiography and renal vein assay.

Management

It is essential to appreciate that the management of the patient with claudication is different from that of the patient with the rest pain/ischaemic ulceration/ gangrene (*critical ischaemia*) complex. Intermittent claudication on its own is a common presentation. When the diagnosis is confirmed, it is essential to take into account and actively treat any risk factor or associated ischaemic disease as already discussed. The natural history of intermittent claudication is that a majority of patients will either improve with the formation of collaterals, or they will remain the same indefinitely. Less than 10% will deteriorate to develop critical or acute ischaemia. On the other hand, approximately 50% of patients presenting with intermittent claudication will die of myocardial ischaemia or stroke within five years. It is for these reasons that intermittent claudication on its own is not treated by angioplasty or bypass surgery which bears a morbidity and mortality. Every effort should be made to assist the patient to give up smoking. Patients are also encouraged to walk daily for one hour as this improves tissue oxygenation. Drugs are of doubtful value in the effort to improve walking distance. Aspirin 75 mg/day offers survival benefit in patients with atherosclerosis from the point of view of prevention of stroke and myocardial infarction. It is reasonable to offer the claudicant who is symptomatically disabled the option of balloon angioplasty in order to open up the occluded or stenosed artery, thereby extending the claudication distance. Although less successful than bypass surgery, balloon angioplasty carries a much lower morbidity and mortality. When the patient's livelihood or leisure activity is significantly restricted and when

the patient is young, there is a relative indication for angioplasty in the first instance, and if this fails, bypass surgery.

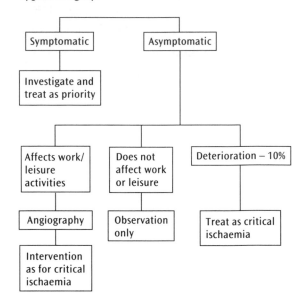

CRITICAL ISCHAEMIA

The clinical combination of rest pain, gangrene and ischaemic ulceration, accompanied by a resting ankle blood pressure index of <0.3, is known as *critical ischaemia*.

Rest pain

This is probably one of the most excruciating types of pain. It is a harbinger of impending gangrene. Typically felt in the digits and the dorsum of the foot, it is associated with coldness and numbness. When severe, it extends up the shin and higher. It is thought to be due to ischaemia of the pain nerve endings. The pain is felt all the time, but is particularly severe at night. It often wakens the patient or prevents him sleeping. This is because the mechanical advantage of gravity on the poor arterial circulation in the foot in the erect position is lost when the patient is recumbent. Indeed, the pain is typically relieved by dependency of the limb. In a severe case, the patient gets out of bed at night and walks around the room for relief, or will abandon the bed altogether and take to sleeping

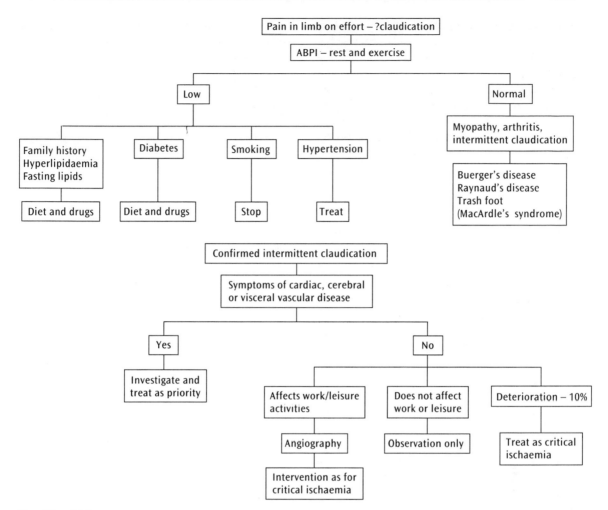

Algorithm 13.1

in a chair. This causes the limb to swell owing to the effect of this posture on the venous return. The limb swelling mimics that seen in venous insufficiency with the important difference that the ischaemic limb will feel icy-cold to touch.

ISCHAEMIC ULCERATION

This is a sign of severe ischaemia. The ulcer does not show any specific signs and an ischaemic aetiology is based on other features in the history and the physical examination. The ulcer is usually painful and occurs at pressure points such as the heel, malleoli or the head of the first and fifth metatarsals (Fig. 13.1). A characteristic but uncommon site for ischaemic ulceration is the outer side of the gaiter area, although it can also occur above the medial malleolus at the classic site for venous ulcers. Occasionally, a number of small scabs affecting the superficial layers of the skin will form and these are a variety of ischaemic ulcers.

Gangrene

Gangrene results from saprophytic digestion of dead tissue produced by ischaemia. This physical sign, whilst perhaps the most visually dramatic, should be interpreted with caution in the assessment of the

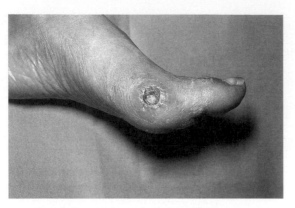

Fig. 13.1 *Painful ischaemic ulcer on the medial aspect of the head of the first metatarsal due to popliteal artery occlusion.*

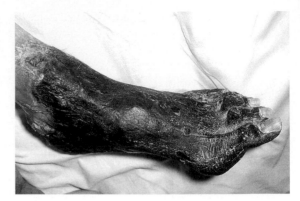

Fig. 13.2 *Painless, sharply demarcated gangrenous foot due to proximal large arterial ocdusion, indicating good proximal perfusion due to collaterals.*

severity of ischaemia. The gangrenous part will have suffered complete loss of blood supply, but paradoxically, when the demarcation line is sharp and distinct, it can be safely assumed that the blood supply proximal to the gangrenous area is adequate and therefore this part of the limb is viable (Fig. 13.2). Demarcation can only occur if the proximal blood supply is adequate. In more extensive ischaemia, the gangrenous area is confluent with a grey zone where the tissues appear viable but are severely ischaemic. This zone is of variable size and merges with obviously viable tissue. In the event of successful revascularization of the limb, the grey area recovers while necrosis in the ischaemic part progresses, resulting in a contracted, sharply demarcated area. It is, therefore, unwise to perform amputation for ischaemic gangrene until revascularization has been attempted and demarcation is obvious, unless the gangrenous area becomes infected proximally or there is evidence of septicaemia.

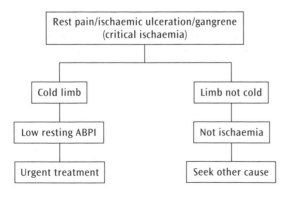

Management

Critical ischaemia is a relatively stable but extremely distressing condition and constitutes an absolute indication for intervention. The patient is admitted as an emergency. Often, the patient is disorientated because of insomnia and pain. The best analgesia is the administration of a long-term opiate and/or local anaesthetic epidural using a tunnelled line to minimize infection of the meninges. The patient should be rested in bed flat to reduce any oedema in the legs. Urgent angiography should be carried out at the next elective session to ascertain the site and degree of the arterial occlusion and the length of the segment affected. Once a plan for intervention is made, this is discussed with the patient.

In a patient with a short history, an attempt should be made to thrombolyse the occlusion using stretokinase, urokinase or tissue plasminogen activator (TPA) in low dose delivered by a special intra-arterial catheter directly into the clot. In approximately 60% of cases, complete clot lysis will be achieved.

In short, less than 5 cm, stenoses and occlusions a balloon angioplasty carries an immediate success rate of 70% with relief of critical ischaemia. However, when the occlusion is long and after failed angioplasty, bypass surgery must be considered. Upstream disease in the aorto-iliac segment is treated by angioplasty with or without stenting in short length stenoses/occlusions and aorto-femoral bypass by use of a Dacron trousers prosthesis in more diffuse disease.

A single long iliac artery occlusion is treated by ipsilateral ilio-femoral or cross femoral bypass. When the disease is infra-inguinal or infra-genicular or both, femoro-popliteal or femoro-crural bypass to the tibial arteries is indicated. The donor artery is usually the common femoral and the recipient artery is the first artery below the block showing the best run-off. The best material for bypass is the saphenous vein, but if it has been stripped because of varicose disease or if the vein is itself varicose, prosthetic materials such as Dacron, knitted polyester or Teflon tubes are used. In mixed upstream and downstream (i.e., multi-level) disease, a useful 'rule of thumb' is to treat the upstream disease first, which, if successful, is usually all that needs to be done for relief of critical ischaemia.

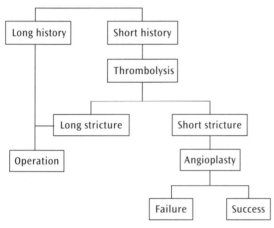

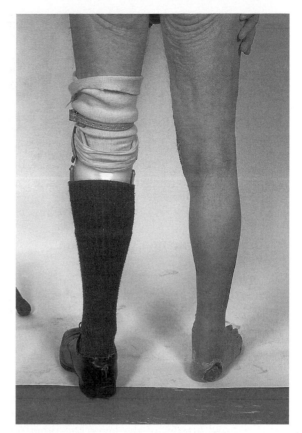

Fig. 13.3 *Bilateral critical ischaemia, right limb salvaged by bypass surgery, but left limb lost below knee due to failure of revascularization.*

In the event of successful thrombolysis/angioplasty/bypass surgery, relief of critical ischaemia is achieved and a pain-free salvaged limb obtained. If revascularization is unsuccessful, a major amputation will be required (Fig. 13.3). However, it is important to note that it is possible to precipitate acute limb ischaemia during the mangement of chronic limb ischaemia. This is tragic when the primary problem was uncomplicated claudication. In the event of failure of critical limb ischaemia, the definitive treatment is major amputation to achieve permanent relief from pain and give the patient a chance to walk again with the aid of a prosthetic limb.

Complications of arterial surgery

The main complications of revascularization are myocardial infarction and stroke because of generalized atherosclerosis. Infection of the bypass, particularly when prosthetic materials are used, carries significant morbidity and occasional mortality with a high incidence of limb loss. This complication should be suspected if there is recurrent pyrexia or a persistently discharging wound sinus.

Occlusion of the bypass can occur at any time in the post-operative period, for technical reasons and/or myointimal hyperplasia within or adjacent to the graft. Early occlusion requires re-exploration to unblock the graft and correct any predisposing factor such as inflow or outflow narrowing or a fault in the graft itself. Infra-inguinal grafts have a 75% one-year patency rate. Some 10–15% occlude within the first 10 days and the remainder within the first 6 months. A lower late occlusion rate continues through the years.

Early occlusions are usually due to poor 'run-off', and those occurring 3–6 months after operation are due to myointimal hyperplasia. This latter phenomenon is due to hyperplastic activity in smooth muscle cells either within the graft or at the recipient arterial end of the artery. Neither problem is amenable to treatment at the present time, although myointimal hyperplasia is the subject of much research. Limb loss is a frequent consequence of early graft failure. Although late graft failure also renders the limb ischaemic, it often remains viable due to the development of collateral circulation.

Peripheral ischaemia with normal proximal pulses

The three common conditions are thromboangiitis obliterans, Raynaud's disease and 'trash foot' (see Algorithm 13.1).

Buerger's disease

Thromboangiitis obliterans or *Buerger's disease* is characterized by thrombotic occlusions of small and medium-sized arteries in the lower and often the upper limb, and is strongly associated with smoking. It occurs mostly in men. Its onset at a younger age, the absence of embolic source, trauma or autoimmune disease, diabetes or hyperlipidaemia, with normal proximal pulses are diagnostic clinical features.

Management here presents the most difficult challenge of all, the task of persuading the patient to give up smoking! The common condition requiring surgery is painful digital gangrene. Apart from adequate analgesia, it is important to wait for demarcation of the digit before amputation. There is no surgical or drug therapy that offers a prospect of cure. In the long term the disease may remit, especially if the subject stops smoking.

Raynaud's disease

Raynaud's disease is due to episodic digital vasospasm in response to cold, usually affecting the digits of the hands, and is characterized by blanching of the fingers and cyanosis due to ischaemia, then redness due to hyperaemia on rewarming of the hands. There may also be associated pain and paraesthesia.

It is relevant to distinguish between the two clinical manifestations of the disease as it bears relevance to prognosis. *Primary (vaso-spastic)* disease occurs in young females with a long history of cold sensitivity and is rarely complicated by trophic changes or tissue loss. In *secondary (vaso-obstructive)* Raynaud's disease the digital circulation is already compromised by occlusive disease due to arteritides commonly associated with autoimmune connective tissue disease, malignancy or myeloproliferative disorders. It may also occur with the prolonged use of vibrating tools in susceptible individuals, so-called 'vibration white finger'. Patients with vaso-obstructive disease are older and do not have a history of cold sensitivity. The digital involvement is asymmetrical and trophic changes with ulceration or gangrene may be present. Blood count, ESR, serum rheumatoid factor and antinuclear antibody titre identify those patients with systemic disease requiring specific therapy. Arteriography is necessary only when Raynaud's syndrome is unilateral as it then might be due to subclavian embolic disease.

Treatment consist of avoiding stimuli that provoke the symptoms and the positive steps of stopping smoking and wearing mittens rather than gloves. Nifedipine provides symptomatic relief by producing vasodilatation. A course of intravenous iloprost, a prostacyclin analogue, is effective in severe and prolonged attacks. Surgery plays a role only when the disease is complicated with painful digital gangrene.

'Trash foot'

'Trash foot' or 'hand' is an iatrogenic or self-inflicted phenomenon. Particulate emboli are either introduced, as in intra-vascular drug abuse when colloid and semi-particulate debris is injected into the arterial lumen, or disturbed and released as microparticles of thrombus or plaque during angiographic or surgical manipulations of the arterial wall, especially from aneurysmal sacs and friable arteriosclerotic plaque. The particulate emboli lodge in the small arteries and arterioles giving rise to severe ischaemia of the digits as well as the superficial and deep tissue layers of the limbs. Prostacycline analogues given intravenously or into the artery of supply to the limb may be of some benefit. Muscle involvement is complicated by the compartment syndrome for which fasciotomy is indicated. Over a period of time, demarcation and separation of the necrotic areas will take place requiring surgical extirpation. In severe cases, reperfusion syndrome with the risk of renal failure and muscle necrosis, as described in Chapter 28, may complicate the picture.

McArdle's syndrome

McArdle's syndrome is a rare condition in which pain is associated with full peripheral pulses. The pain is true ischaemic pain, resulting not from reduction in arterial perfusion but from accumulation of pain factors due to the congenital lack of an enzyme (phosphorylase) vital to the efficient aerobic metabolism of the Krebs cycle. The diagnosis is suggested by the youth of the patient, and confirmed by special histochemical staining techniques of material obtained by muscle biopsy.

Acrocyanosis

Acrocyanosis is an ill-understood but benign condition. It presents in middle-aged females as a spectacular symmetrical mauve discoloration, usually in the skin over the shins. It is characterized by an absence of symptoms, a normal skin temperature and good pulses from femoral to pedal level. The patient is often alarmed by the appearance of the legs, but may be safely reassured after clinical assessment.

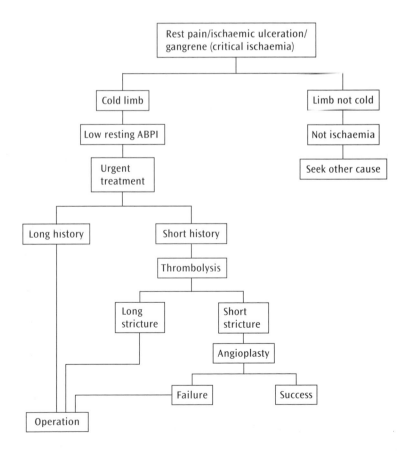

Algorithm 13.2

HIGHLIGHTS

- Intermittent claudication is not usually an indication to attempt revascularization
- In true intermittent claudication the ankle blood pressure index is less than 0.8
- In intermittent claudication, look for risk factors and arterial disease elsewhere, especially in the coronary and cerebral circuits
- If the pulses are full despite peripheral ischaemia, consider Buerger's disease, Raynaud's disease, 'trash foot' (and McArdle's syndrome)
- Rest pain/ischaemic ulceration/gangrene (critical ischaemia) is an urgent indication to attempt revascularization
- If vascularization fails, major amputation is necessary and worthwhile

14

Varicose veins and leg ulcers

PHILIP COLERIDGE SMITH

AIMS

1 Relate the physical signs and treatment of varicose veins to their pathophysiology
2 Distinguish the symptoms and signs of varicose veins from other complaints
3 Understand the management of varicose veins
4 Differentiate between the various types of leg ulcer

VARICOSE VEINS

Varicose veins are a common problem occurring in about 20% of the adult population in Western countries and increasing with age, but only 15% of those affected have symptoms or develop complications.

Pathophysiology

The aetiology of varicose veins remains unclear. Primary varicose veins are probably familial and their frequency in women implicates pregnancy as a contributing factor. Secondary varicose veins are a consequence of the post-phlebitic limb where the deep valves are incompetent or the deep system is occluded as a sequel to deep vein thrombosis.

Normally, blood flows from the superficial to the deep venous system via the mid-thigh, the mid-knee and other smaller *perforating* veins. The deep veins of the calf are surrounded by muscle which contracts and compresses the veins during walking. Blood is ejected from the calf against gravity towards the heart via the calf muscle pump and is prevented from flowing towards the feet by valves in the deep veins.

The physiological definition of a varicose vein is a superficial vein in which reverse flow can be demonstrated, often by special investigation when clinically it is not apparent. A vein in which reverse flow has been demonstrated is known as an *incompetent vein*. This may not yet have become dilated or tortuous, especially in the main trunk of the saphenous vein. Valves in the long saphenous vein probably fail first, allowing reverse flow in this vein. The vein distends in response to this abnormal flow. At a later stage, the valve at the sapheno-femoral junction fails, leading to worsening of the varicose veins. The long saphenous system is involved in 80% of cases and the short saphenous system in 20%.

```
┌─────────────────────────────────────┐
│    Complaint of varicose veins       │
└─────────────────────────────────────┘
                  │
┌─────────────────────────────────────────┐
│ Examine for superficial venous incompetence │
└─────────────────────────────────────────┘
```

Clinical features

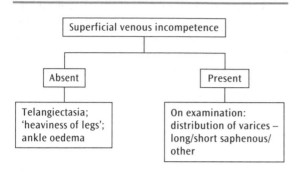

Many patients attribute their complaints to varicose veins which, although common in the population, are frequently asymptomatic, therefore careful assessment is essential. Thread veins or telangiectases are often confused with varicose veins.

Although aching of the legs is a symptom commonly associated with varicose veins, worse on prolonged standing and relieved by lying down, it is important to consider the possibility of referred pain from the back, the hip or the knee joint, and from claudication, even when there are obvious varices.

Heaviness of the legs and ankle oedema are more likely to be post-thrombotic sequelae, particularly if long-standing and there is a history of pregnancy or bed confinement because of illness or surgical operation. Lymphatic obstruction is a rare cause unless there is a history of chronic infection or radiotherapy in the region of the groin or pelvis. Lymphoedema is differentiated from venous oedema by the absence of skin pigmentation and pitting oedema. Cardiac, hepatic or renal failure causes bilateral leg oedema and other associated features easily distinguish these conditions. Large pelvic tumours causing obstruction in the large veins should be considered in a patient who presents with progressive or bilateral limb swelling.

Examination

This is best performed with the patient standing and is aimed at confirming the presence of varicosities and identifying their source and level of communication with the deep veins. The varices are filled in this position and on digital compression they can be emptied which distinguishes them from thread veins. Their location in relation to the saphenous vein is usually obvious. Varices in the medial aspect of the calf and above the knee usually arise from the long saphenous vein and those on the postero-lateral aspect of the calf are from the short saphenous vein. A prominently distended long saphenous vein at the sapheno-femoral junction (saphena varix) and a palable thrill over the sapheno-femoral junction on coughing are signs of sapheno-femoral incompetence. The skin around the ankle is also examined for discoloration, eczema or ulceration (described later).

In skilled hands, the tourniquet test gives useful information about the level of communication with the deep veins, especially in patients with primary varices. With the patient lying down, the examiner elevates the patient's leg and empties the veins by massaging the leg, then occludes the proximal end of the long saphenous vein by applying a tourniquet around the thigh a few centimetres from the groin. The patient stands and filling of the veins is observed. If the veins remain empty but refill rapidly on removing the tourniquet then the communication is at the sapheno-femoral junction. Digital pressure over the sapheno-femoral junction preventing retrograde filling of the saphenous vein is called the *Trendelenburg test*. If the veins fill rapidly despite the tourniquet this indicates a communication distally and the test is repeated with the tourniquet above the knee. If this controls filling, the main communication is an incompetent mid-thigh perforating vein but if the tourniquet fails to control filling, the tourniquet is applied below the knee as the communication is likely to be at the short sapheno-popliteal or medial knee perforator. By gentle palpation along the medial side of the leg, the sites of perforating veins are recognized as defects in the deep fascia. A tourniquet above the suspected perforating vein, and emptying and refilling on digital pressure, will identify any communication within the calf perforating veins.

Investigation

Clinical tests are now recognized as being of limited accuracy in the diagnosis of venous disease, especially in patients with recurrent varices and leg ulceration. More sophisticated investigations are usually used to obtain a reliable diagnosis and a Doppler ultrasound is particularly helpful (Algorithm 14.1). A simple hand-held probe is positioned over the vein under investigation with the patient in the standing position. Examination begins at the sapheno-femoral junction. The femoral vein is located 1 cm medial to the femoral artery. With the patient standing still, the blood flow in the femoral vein may be difficult to hear because it moves at only a few centimetres per second at rest with occasional accelerations due to respiration. By grasping the calf of the leg with the free hand and squeezing firmly, the examiner can eject blood from the calf muscle pump resulting in an audible signal from the Doppler machine. Reverse flow is heard in an incompetent vein as the examiner releases the grip on the calf. With practice, the examiner can locate each superficial vein and test its competence. It is advisable to test the main trunk of the long saphenous vein in the thigh and at the knee since there may be an incompetent saphenous trunk in the presence of a competent sapheno-femoral junction.

Further improvements can be made by the use of ultrasound imaging combined with Doppler ultrasound, referred to as *duplex ultrasound*, which demonstrates blood flow by superimposing a colour flow map on the B-mode ultrasound image. This investigation has been shown to be at least as accurate as venography and avoids intravenous contrast media and ionizing radiation.

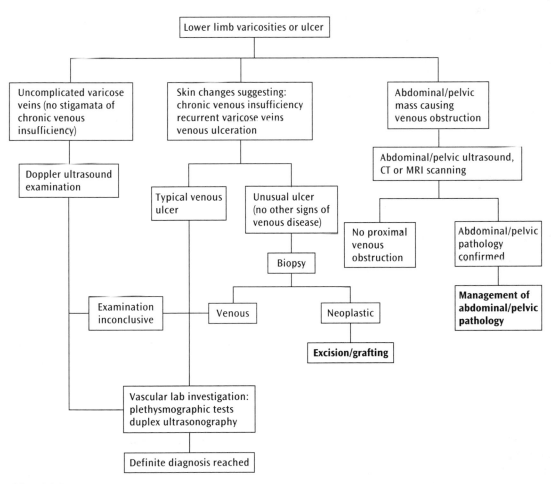

Algorithm 14.1

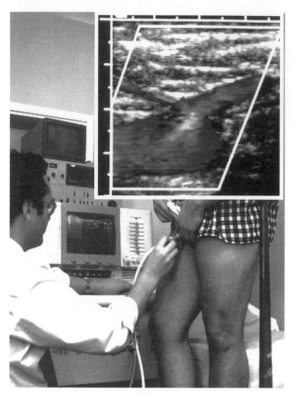

Fig. 14.1 *Duplex ultrasonography used to diagnose venous disease. The procedure is described in the text.*

A duplex ultrasound examination for varicose veins is carried out in a very similar manner to the hand-held Doppler study (Fig. 14.1). The vein is located using the ultrasound image, compression to the calf is applied, and the effect on blood flow is observed by use of the colour Doppler mode. The forward and reverse blood flow is recognized with accuracy by an experienced investigator and in this manner the state of competence of the long saphenous, short saphenous and deep veins is defined. This examination can also detect evidence of previous venous thrombosis which may have caused damage to the deep veins of the limb. It is the method of choice in investigating suspected deep vein thrombosis (DVT). In patients with recurrent varices following treatment, a duplex ultrasound examination determines the type of surgery previously performed and the source of the new varicose veins, which may recur following sapheno-femoral

or sapheno-popliteal ligation or may arise in a previously normal vein due to progression of the disease.

Management

Symptomless varicose veins require no treatment. However, patients presenting with aching legs after standing, unsightly veins or with complications, namely superficial thrombophlebitis, haemorrhage, venous eczema or ulceration deserve appropriate treatment (Algorithm 14.2).

Ligation and stripping

The widely applied procedure for patients with long or short saphenous vein incompetence involves saphenous ligation at the sapheno-femoral or sapheno-popliteal junction and stripping the saphenous vein, which offers the best chance of permanently removing the varices. If the long or short saphenous vein is left in place it often re-establishes a communication with other veins and venous reflux continues resulting in early recurrence of varices. The long saphenous vein in the calf is accompanied by the saphenous nerve which is at risk of damage during removal of the vein. It is standard practice to strip the saphenous vein from the groin to the upper calf to avoid damaging this nerve. The short saphenous vein is accompanied by the sural nerve and great care must be taken to identify and protect the nerve when removing this vein.

The saphenous vein is usually removed after identifying it in the groin at its junction with the femoral vein where it is divided and ligated, and all its tributaries are also divided and ligated. A wire is passed down the saphenous vein to a small incision in the upper calf. The *Babcock method* of removing the vein involves attaching a 10–15 mm diameter olive to the wire in the groin and pulling it down the calf. An inverting technique causes less damage to the tissues surrounding the vein. In this method after the wire has been passed through the vein a ligature is used to tie the proximal saphenous vein to the wire (Fig. 14.2 (a)). Traction to the distal end of the wire inverts the vein at its proximal end. When

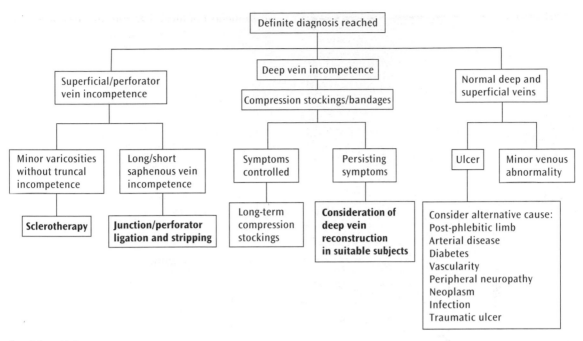

Algorithm 14.2

successful, this technique removes the saphenous vein through a small incision in the calf (Fig. 14.2 (b)). Should the vein break, the Babcock technique can be used as a rescue method (Fig. 14.2 (c)).

The varicosities are marked before the operation with an indelible marker and can often be removed through small incisions not longer than 2 mm in length that do not require suturing and may simply be covered by an adhesive dressing. A fine artery for ceps or a vein hook is used to bring the varicosity to the surface. It is then grasped by a larger forceps, divided and traction applied to one end until it breaks. This procedure is repeated until all viscosities have been removed. Only the main communications between the superficial viscosities and the deep veins are ligated. The leg is firmly bandaged with crepe and elastic bandages or graded compression stockings at the end of the operation to prevent bleeding from unligated vessels. Operative treatment used to require a hospital stay of two or three days, but now the majority of patients are treated in day surgery units. Patients are encouraged to walk about a mile every day and to keep the leg elevated when sitting. The bandages are removed at a week, but the stockings should be worn for longer. Patients

should be warned that their legs are likely to be bruised when the bandages are removed.

Injection treatment (sclerotherapy)

Injection therapy or sclerotherapy is used in the treatment of superficial varicosities below the knee but is not suitable for large varicosities, in particular above the thigh. It is effective in patients in whom the saphenous veins are competent or have been removed at an earlier operation, but should not be considered for the treatment of incompetence of the main saphenous veins. The principle of the treatment is to produce a fibrous destruction of the varicose veins by injecting an irritant solution and then applying strong compression to the limb. The patient is examined while standing and the varicosities to be injected are marked on the skin. Syringes containing 1 ml of sodium tetradecyl are prepared. The patient then lies recumbent and a fine needle is inserted into the most distal varices. The leg is then elevated to empty the varicosities and the sclerosant injected to destroy the endothelial lining of the vein. A firm bandage is then applied which sticks together the interior surfaces of the vein.

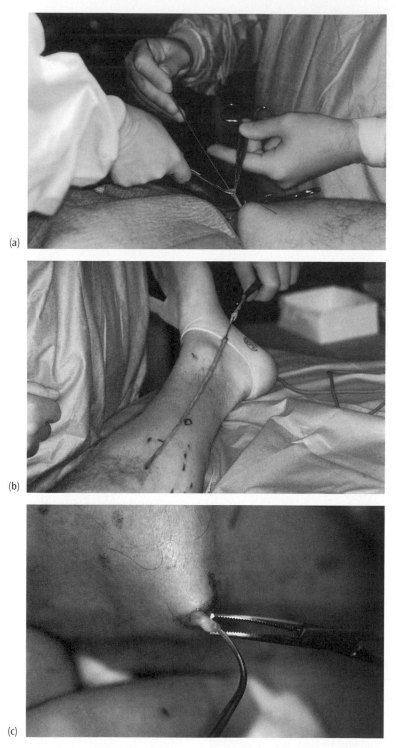

Fig. 14.2 *A long saphenous vein removed by the inverting stripping technique. (a) Tying the proximal saphenous vein to the wire; (b) Removing the saphenous vein through a small incision in the calf; (c) Using the Babcock technique to rescue a broken vein.*

The process is repeated in the rest of the varices, working proximally along the limb. The patient is encouraged to walk for about a mile a day. Compression bandaging should be continued for about two to three weeks following this treatment. Further sessions of sclerotherapy are continued at weekly intervals until all varicosities have been treated.

Care is required during sclerotherapy to avoid injection of sclerosant outside the vein. This solution is extremely damaging to the tissues and if more than 0.5 cc leaks there is a serious risk of skin ulceration. Before each injection, the position of the needle within the vein should be confirmed by withdrawing blood through the needle. No more than 0.5 cc of sclerosant should be injected at the one site, which with the vein empty is sufficient to achieve the desired result. Superficial thrombophlebitis may occur if compression bandaging is not carefully applied and breakdown of the haemoglobin in this area may result in brown pigmentation of the skin due to deposition of haemosiderin.

Sclerotherapy is also used for the cosmetic treatment of thread veins. A practitioner of this technique is able to canulate these veins with a 30-gauge needle. A very dilute sclerosant is injected which is sufficient to eradicate these vessels. Again, great care is necessary to ensure that the injection is given within the vein since skin ulceration may occur otherwise.

Laser therapy

Lasers are effective in treating telangiectases and other cutaneous vascular lesions where these arise above the level of the umbilicus. Lasers and machines producing flashes of light are largely ineffective in the management of thread veins in the lower limbs. Cosmetic veins of the lower limbs are best managed by sclerotherapy.

LEG ULCERS

An ulcer is a macroscopic breach in the skin or the mucous membrane. Varied factors (*see* Algorithm 14.2) are responsible for chronic ulceration in the lower limb. The history and clinical features of the ulcer can be diagnostic.

Aetiological factors

Although trauma, even trivial, is a common precipitating incident, this may not always be vivid in the patient's memory and perpetuating causes that should be considered are venous insufficiency, arterial ischaemia and diabetic neuropathy. A malignant ulcer is suspected when a proliferative growth develops in a long-standing ulcer (*Marjolin's ulcer*) or a history of a skin lump precedes the ulcer. A uniform feature, irrespective of the underlying cause, is failure to heal.

Pain

Ischaemic ulcers are usually painful and associated with a history of claudication or rest pain. *Venous ulcers* are also often painful, but can be recognized because they are associated with the skin changes at the ankle of haemosiderosis (brown pigmentation) and lipodermatosclerosis (woody induration). *Diabetic ulcers* are usually painless because of sensory neuropathy.

Site

The site of an ulcer may offer some indication as to its cause. Post-thrombotic and varicose ulcers are typically above the medial malleolus and may extend circumferentially. Diabetic neuropathic ('perforating') ulcers occur on the feet overlying the metatarsal heads or other bony prominences, commonly the toes, the ball of the great toe and the malleoli. Ischaemic ulcers may occur anywhere in the leg below the mid-calf on the anterior aspect of the shin and dorsum of the foot. The back of the heel is a particularly common site because of pressure necrosis.

Characteristics of the ulcer

The characteristics of the ulcer must be precisely defined. The *floor* of a healing ulcer is covered with healthy pink granulation tissue, but is pale and covered with slough when it is healing poorly or is infected, as in venous or neuropathic ulcers. Neuropathic ulcers are distinctly deep and penetrating. In ischaemic ulcers, the underlying structures are exposed in the floor of the ulcer as diminished blood supply delays healing and the formation of granulation tissue.

The *base* of an ulcer, the tissue around and underneath the ulcer, is usually indurated because of surrounding cellulitis or neoplastic infiltration from the floor of the ulcer. A distinguishing feature is absence of tenderness in a malignant ulcer. The *edge* of a healing ulcer is sloping or terraced as new epithelium grows in towards the centre, it is sharp and the ulcer is punched out in neuropathic ulcer, is undermined in decubitus ulcers due to pressure necrosis, is rolled in basal cell carcinoma, and everted in squamous cell carcinoma.

Other features

Firmness of the regional lymph nodes is not necessarily indicative of malignancy, whereas tenderness is more suggestive of secondary inflammation.

Examination for the presence of varicose veins, the peripheral pulses and sensation are helpful differentiating features. The peripheral neuropathy of diabetes is identified by the impairment of superficial sensation, in particular pain, the diminution of tendon reflexes and muscle wasting.

Management

Duplex scanning and Doppler ultrasound measurement of the ankle blood pressure, with blood glucose levels, are relevant investigations in most cases. Biopsy of the edge of the ulcer and its floor may be required if there is a suspicion of malignancy. Necrotic tissue and slough should not be removed unless ischaemia has been excluded, as removal could aggravate ischaemia and delay healing. Treatment of the primary disease and regular dressings with a mild antiseptic solution after gentle debridement of the ulcer are essential. Bedrest may be necessary. Antibiotics are not prescribed unless there is evidence of cellulitis. Skin grafting should be considered for large, slow-healing ulcers provided that swabs from the ulcer are

clear of organisms such as pseudomonas that may threaten the viability of the graft.

Venous ulcers

One the characteristic features of a venous ulcer is its location to the regions above the medial or lateral malleolus. In severe cases, medial and lateral ulcers may merge to form a circumferential ulcer surrounding the leg above the ankle, and with scarring there is reduction in the diameter of the leg. The appearance of a narrowed ankle and a wide calf is described as the *inverted champagne bottle abnormality*. Venous ulcers are always associated with other features of venous disease and varicosities are sometimes visible in the limb. The earliest change is brown pigmentation of the skin (*haemosiderosis*), which progresses to thickening and induration of the skin and subcutaneous tissues (*lipodermatosclerosis*) and eventually the skin breaks down and ulcerates.

The floor of the ulcer is covered with a yellow layer of slough and is colonized by bacteria. However, infection is infrequent but may present as cellulitis surrounding the ulcer. When the ulcer is healing the floor will show pink granulation tissue with new epithelium growing in as a thin, transparent layer covering a typically terraced edge.

Pathophysiology

The mechanism that produces venous ulceration is not fully understood but the physical abnormality of the venous system has been elucidated. During walking, calf muscle contraction actively pumps blood from the legs which reduces the venous pressure in the deep veins and allows the flow of blood from the superficial into the deep veins of the leg. Whilst sedentary, the pressure in the superficial veins is 80–90 mmHg and diminishes to 20 mmHg during walking, but it does not drop below 40–50 mmHg if the valves in the deep or superficial veins are damaged (Fig. 14.3). The physiological disturbance in leg ulceration is failure to reduce the pressure in the superficial veins during walking due to valve incompetence, in the superficial and

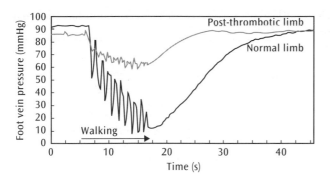

Fig. 14.3 *Reduction in superficial venous pressure on walking in a normal limb and in a limb with venous valvular incompetence.*

the deep veins in the majority of patients, or in the perforating veins in a few patients. The venous hypertension damages the capillaries in the skin, leading to varicose 'eczema' due to red cell escape and breakdown with deposition of haemosiderin in the tissues (haemosiderosis), replacement of the subcutaneous tissue with fat (lipodermatosclerosis) and eventually ulceration.

Histological examination of the liposclerotic skin of patients with chronic venous disease of the leg shows capillary proliferation and infiltration of the peri-vascular tissues with T-lymphocytes and macrophages. The capillary endothelium is damaged and abnormal. It is believed that the leucocyte activation due to venous hypertension results in free-radical injury to the endothelium and a chronic inflammatory process, referred to as *lipodermatosclerosis*. It is unclear how this leads to leg ulceration. It has been suggested that venous hypertension results in transudation of plasma and peri-capillary fibrin cuffs which interfere with oxygen transfer, causing tissue hypoxia. An alternative explanation is that massive activation of the peri-vascular macrophages releasing cytokines results in destruction of the microcirculation of the skin and tissue damage.

Management

The treatment of venous ulcers depends on the venous abnormality which should be determined by duplex scanning. When this is not available, an alternative reliable but invasive investigation is venography. This demonstrates the anatomy of the venous system, the site of obstruction and the competence of the valves. If there is superficial venous incompetence, which is the case in half of the patients presenting with venous ulcers, the standard surgical treatment for the varicosities is indicated. The remaining patients show deep venous or a combination of deep and superficial venous incompetence. In these patients no simple surgical procedure is available. Ligation of the perforating veins used to be recommended in this situation, but is not a long-term effective treatment. These ulcers are better treated by compression bandaging. A method known as four-layer bandaging which safely applies 45 mmHg compression at the ankle is now widely used. In clinical trials this has produced healing rates of 70% in 12 weeks. The ulcer itself requires regular cleaning and excision of dead tissue. Several specially designed wound dressings have been introduced but none seems to accelerate ulcer healing. Although some drugs have been shown to improve healing, they have failed to demonstrate a consistent benefit for wider clinical application. Stanazolol, an anabolic steroid with minimal androgenic effect, enhances fibrinolysis and is worth trying in resistant cases. Defibrotide, an anti-thrombotic and fibrinolytic agent, prostaglandin E1 and Pentoxfiline do not seem to be effective without compression therapy. Systemic antibiotics should only be administered if there is spreading cellulitis. Topical application of drugs, particularly antibiotics, is unwise since these may cause sensitization and a severe skin reaction that will complicate healing. In large or slow-healing ulcers, split- or pinch-skin grafts enhance healing.

Once an ulcer has healed, the high risk of recurrence can be reduced by advising the patient to put on a compression below-knee stocking during the day and to elevate the leg when sitting. In the UK stockings are graded 1, 2 or 3, according to the degree of compression applied; grade 3 stockings provide 30 mmHg compression at the ankle. Although very effective, elderly patients often find them particularly difficult or uncomfortable to apply.

Patients with venous leg ulcers often have associated arterial disease, and in these patients, ischaemia of the leg may develop if high levels of compression are used on the leg. It is therefore essential to assess the peripheral circulation in any patient in whom compression bandaging or stockings are to be applied, clinically and by measuring ABPI. In patients with an ABPI of less than 0.85, a lower level of compression should be applied.

HIGHLIGHTS

- Treatment of varicose veins is dependent on the site of venous incompetence determined clinically and by duplex scanning
- Injection sclerotherapy is not suitable if there is incompetence of major veins
- Duplex scanning is an essential investigation for varicose veins that recur after treatment or in patients with leg ulceration
- In leg ulcers, examination of the peripheral arterial pulses, the veins and the nervous system (for evidence of peripheral neuropathy) is essential

15

Before operation

PAUL B BOULOS AND CELIA L INGHAM CLARK

> **AIMS**
>
> ---
>
> 1 Understand the requisites in pre-operative management
> 2 Appreciate the relevance of recognizing and treating co-morbid conditions

INTRODUCTION

The surgical team is responsible for ensuring that a patient's admission for a surgical procedure is made safe and that recovery is speedy. This task, usually delegated to trainees, requires careful assessment to determine the appropriateness of the planned procedure and to identify morbid conditions that require treatment in order that the operation may be undertaken safely and with minimal threat to the patient's full recovery. Morbidity is related to the physiological state of the patient before surgery (Table 15.1).

PRE-OPERATIVE ASSESSMENT

Patients are admitted with a provisional or a definitive diagnosis, based on a history and examination carried out in a crowded clinic, where some information that could totally alter the planned treatment

Table 15.1 *Physiological status scale: American Society of Anesthesiologists (ASA)*

ASA class	Physical status
1	A normal healthy individual: no organic, physiological, biochemical or psychiatric disturbance
2	A patient with mild to moderate systemic disturbance; this may or may not be related to the disorder requiring surgical treatment
3	A patient with severe systemic disease which is not incapacitating
4	A patient with incapacitating systemic disease that is a constant threat to life with or without surgery
5	A moribund patient who is not expected to live and where surgery has been performed as a last resort
6	A patient who requires an emergency operation

might have been overlooked; or else the patient's condition might have improved or deteriorated, or the patient might have developed an inter-current disease. A detailed history and clinical examination are undertaken with these possibilities in mind.

To secure the patient's safety, it must be ensured that the proposed operation provides the best treatment for the patient and that the risk to the patient's life imposed by the operation and general anaesthesia is minimal.

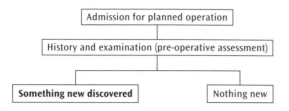

After the clinical evaluation, which includes history and physical examination, further investigations to re-affirm the primary diagnosis or to evaluate an existing or suspected inter-current illness may need to be arranged (Table 15.2). Patients at high risk of complications are identified and special therapeutic measures instituted as explained later. When necessary, a second opinion should be sought for any condition that requires specialist input. Information thus

Table 15.2 *Routine pre-operative assessment*

History
Respiratory disease, smoking
Cardiovascular disease
Other medical disorders: bleeding diathesis, hypertension, diabetes
Previous general anaesthesia
Drugs and alcohol intake

Physical examination
Mental state
Nutrition and hydration
Oral hygiene and dentures
Abnormalities of jaw and neck
Respiratory system
Cardiovascular system

Investigations
Full blood count, blood group
Blood urea and electrolytes: in patients undergoing major surgery, patients on diuretics, on intravenous fluids, patients with renal disease
Liver function tests: in patients undergoing major surgery, patients with history of excessive alcohol intake, patients with history of liver disease
Urinalysis
Chest X-ray: in patients with cardiovascular or respiratory disease, >60 years and smokers
ECG: in patients >50 years, cardiac disease and hypertension

obtained determines if circumstances have changed with respect to the planned treatment, and in consultation with the anaesthetist, a decision is made on the patient's fitness for the operation to be undertaken and on the appropriateness of the planned procedure.

PRE-OPERATIVE PREPARATION

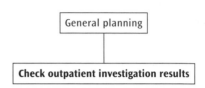

General planning

All laboratory and imaging results should be available and the reports filed in the patient's hospital notes. It is inadvisable to rely on verbal reports not substantiated by written documentation.

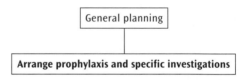

Routine pre-operative prerequisites include antibiotic (Table 15.3) and deep vein thrombosis (DVT) prophylaxis (Table 15.4), bowel preparation when necessary, ordering blood if significant blood loss is anticipated, arranging for specific investigations, for example laryngoscopy for vocal cord movements prior to a thyroidectomy, and for per-operative requirements such as imaging for cholangiography, central vein cannulation or internal fixation of bone.

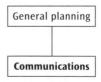

Special supportive measures should be arranged. The stoma therapist is informed in advance about a patient who requires a stoma, to allow ample time to explain the implications of living with a stoma and its management, and to position the site of the stoma

Table 15.3 *Guidelines for antibiotic prophylaxis*

- Indicated if risk of infection exceeds 5%, i.e., all operations except clean operations with no pre-operative infection and no opening of gastrointestinal, respiratory or urinary tracts
- Operations involving prosthetic implants or where ischaemic or necrotic muscle is retained
- Operations likely to induce bacteraemia in patients with haemodialysis shunts, trans-venous pacemakers and ventriculo-atrial and ventriculo-peritoneal shunts for hydrocephalus, established prosthetic arterial grafts or joint prostheses
- A single pre-operative dose is given either 1 hour before the operation or intravenously at induction; a second per-operative dose is given in long operations; a maximum of two further doses should be sufficient; longer courses are only indicated in operations for peritonitis
- In biliary and bowel surgery, the risk is from Gram-negative bacilli (Enterobacteriaceae), faecal anaerobes (*Bacteroides fragilis*), *Staphylococcus aureus* and enterococci, notably *Enterococcus faecalis*. The most commonly used prophylactic regimen is a combination of cephalosporin and metronidazole; for appendicectomy, rectal metronidazole is given 2 hours before operation
- In vascular grafts and joint replacements, the organisms implicated are *S. aureus*, coagulase-negative staphylococci (e.g., *S. epidermidis*) and, rarely, coliforms. Flucloxacillin is the agent of choice but gentamicin is added for extra protection
- Ischaemic or injured muscle is susceptible to gas gangrene and tetanus. Clostridia are sensitive to benzylpenicillin and metronidazole, one of which should be given in a high dosage early after major trauma and before amputations for ischaemia

Table 15.4 *Options for thromboembolism prophylaxis*

- Low-dose subcutaneous heparin given as standard unfractionated heparin 2–3 times a day or as low molecular weight heparin in a single daily dose
- Calf compression devices for intra-operative use; their efficacy is less than that of low-dose heparin
- Graded-compression stockings must be worn during operation and in the post-operative period
- Intravenous dextran – intravenous dextran 70 is almost as effective as low-dose heparin; 500 ml is given daily from the time of operation until the third post-operative day; its disadvantages are the need for an intravenous line, the large volume of fluid infused and the occasional hypersensitivity

prior to the procedure. The physiotherapist is alerted about a patient with chronic respiratory disease or one undergoing an amputation or a joint replacement and is actively involved in preparing the patient and in following the post-operative course and rehabilitation.

A bed should be reserved if a patient is likely to require admission to a high dependency or intensive care unit. It is prudent to forewarn the patient and arrange a visit to the unit beforehand, to minimize his or her anxiety on waking up from the anaesthetic in an unfamiliar environment.

Plans for rehabilitation and convalescence should be discussed with the patient and relatives in order to arrange in advance domestic or home nursing help.

The anaesthetist is informed about any high-risk patient, to allow time for any investigations or treatment that the anaesthetist may feel necessary before the operation.

The operation list should include the patient's details and the proposed operation, and theatre staff are informed of any special requirements for instruments, intra-operative imaging or patient positioning, and alerted about patients with a high risk of cross-infection.

Patient information and informed consent

The medical condition and the reasons for the proposed treatment are clearly explained to the patient in simple terms, if necessary aided with diagrams, in a sympathetic and unhurried approach. The justification for a surgical approach, or for a specific procedure against other options, reassures the patient about the decision taken. The patient is informed of potential complications with a greater than a 5% risk, either as a result of surgery in general, or specifically related to the intended operative procedure. Any complication that may be life-threatening or result in a permanent disability, no matter how rare it may be, should be explained.

A signed consent for the operation is not sufficient without written details of the main risks and complications that have been discussed with the patient and are either stated in the consent form or in the patient's notes. At the time of consent, the operation site is marked on the patient's skin with indelible ink, and in the case of bilateral structures the side is highlighted on the consent form.

MANAGEMENT OF MEDICAL CONDITIONS

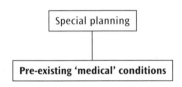

The physiological disturbances of general anaesthesia and surgery may exacerbate a pre-existing medical condition, posing a threat to the patient's recovery and survival. Such patients require special therapeutic and supportive measures, including elective transference to a high-dependency or intensive care unit.

The elderly

These patients are particularly vulnerable, because of limited mobility, generalized atherosclerosis, intercurrent disease and compromised cardiac, respiratory and renal function. They are slow to recover and this prolongs their hospital stay and increases the risk of acquired hospital infections. They are prone to postoperative confusion, DVT, respiratory and cardiac complications. Therefore, analgesics and sedatives are prescribed sparingly and care is taken in fluid replacement in order to avoid extremes of hypotension and hypertension, which disturb the cerebral circulation and cause circulatory overload, cardiac decompensation and renal failure. Physiotherapy to the chest and the encouragement of mobility are essential components of management.

Obesity

Obese patients have a high morbidity because of their predisposition to hypertension, ischaemic heart disease and diabetes mellitus. They are prone to cardiorespiratory complications, because of the strain on the cardiovascular system and decreased chest wall compliance. With impaired mobility, they are also prone to DVT and pulmonary embolism. Clinical signs can be difficult to elicit, which hampers pre-operative assessment.

These patients should be considered as at high risk. Pre-operative investigations, even in the asymptomatic, should include a chest X-ray, ECG and blood glucose estimation. In some instances, peak flowmeter measurement or spirometry might be necessary.

Cardiovascular disorders

Cardiovascular disorders account for most postoperative medical complications. Atherosclerosis is the most common cause of cardiovascular disease complicating surgery. The risk of death in these patients is significantly higher when emergency surgery is undertaken than when performed electively after the cardiac condition has been stabilized.

Hypertension

Anxiety about the operation may give a high blood pressure measurement that should fall with bedrest; therefore, measurements should be repeated to ensure a reliable reading. Patients with a systolic pressure less than 180 mmHg and a diastolic pressure less than 110 mmHg, unless associated with other cardiovascular disease, are not particularly at risk of cardiac complications. Hypertensive patients are usually on β-adrenergic blockers, calcium antagonists, angiotensin-converting enzyme (ACE) inhibitors, vasodilators or methyldopa; these medications should not be stopped even if oral intake is restricted – the normal dose of the drug can be given with a small amount of water. Patients with severe or poorly controlled hypertension are at risk of cardiac failure or stroke and should not undergo general anaesthesia or surgery until adequately controlled.

Ischaemic heart disease

Stable angina carries a small risk, compared to unstable angina; 15% of patients with unstable angina develop a myocardial infarction following a surgical operation and therefore cardiac surgery to revascularize the myocardium is desirable, if deferring the planned procedure is not crucial. Otherwise, nitrates to dilate the coronary arteries and reduce pre-load and, unless the patient is in heart failure, β-adrenergic blockers which reduce cardiac strain and oxygen demand, should also be continued during the peri-operative period. The risk of post-operative myocardial infarction is low in patients with no previous history, but increases to 30% if an operation is performed within 3 months of a myocardial infarction, and is 10–15% at 6 months, before it stabilizes at 5%. Therefore, surgery should be deferred as long as feasible after a heart attack.

Cardiac failure

This is commonly caused by ischaemic heart disease and hypertension, and if present should be recognized and treated with diuretic therapy whilst carefully monitoring the serum sodium and potassium levels. If untreated there is the risk of severe pulmonary oedema that develops soon after reversal of general anaesthesia, and of myocardial infarction or cerebrovascular accident because of poor myocardial function that is further compromised by low blood pressure as a result of vasodilatation caused by general anaesthesia.

Arrhythmias

Atrial fibrillation is usually secondary to ischaemic heart disease, mitral valve disease or thyrotoxicosis. Uncontrolled fibrillation may precipitate cardiac failure and increases the risk of arterial embolism. It is treated prior to surgery with digoxin, verapamil or a β-adrenergic blocker and treatment should be continued in the peri-operative period. These patients are usually on warfarin, and it will be necessary to modify the anticoagulation therapy.

Bradycardia, that is, an apex rate below 60 per minute, if not due to digoxin toxicity or beta-blockade, is caused by complete heart block and diagnosed on ECG. This condition requires urgent trans-venous pacing. A temporary or permanent cardiac pacemaker is not a particular problem for general anaesthesia, but a monopolar surgical diathermy should not be used close to the control box as it may interfere with a permanent pacing system. A bipolar diathermy machine can be safely used instead.

Valvular heart disease

A patient with a previous history of rheumatic heart disease may or may not have a cardiac murmur; if the history has not previously been recognized, a cardiological opinion is essential to assess any functional deficit. Careful monitoring is required during and after the operation, which otherwise may pose a considerable risk. Antibiotic prophylaxis is essential, to minimize the risk of endocarditis. A detectable murmur, in the absence of history or clinical features of rheumatic heart disease, may indicate a hyperdynamic circulation associated with anxiety, anaemia or thyrotoxicosis, or may be an innocent flow murmur, as in aortic sclerosis in the elderly; however, the latter must be distinguished from aortic stenosis which is a serious valvular disorder. The operation is better deferred until a specialist opinion is obtained.

Patients with replacement valves carry the risk of infective endocarditis and therefore require antibiotic prophylaxis. Patients with mechanical valves, but not with bioprosthetic (pig) valves are usually maintained on oral warfarin anticoagulation to prevent valve thrombosis. Anticoagulation with warfarin therapy in the lower range of prothrombin ratios (1.5–2.0) can safely be continued prior to operation. For major surgery in patients with a high risk of thrombosis, especially those with mitral valve prostheses, intravenous heparin is substituted for warfarin at least 48 hours before the operation and continued during the operative period.

Infective endocarditis

Disruption of laminar flow through a narrow orifice in damaged valves predisposes to local thrombus formation and deposition of circulating bacteria.

Streptococcus viridans is the most common organism. Many surgical procedures and invasive investigations cause bacteraemia. Patients with prosthetic valves, valvular heart disease, hypertrophic obstructive cardiomyopathy or a previous history of bacterial endocarditis require antibiotic prophylaxis. The indication for and choice of antibiotics need to be discussed with the clinical microbiologist in cases of uncertainty.

Cerebrovascular disease

Cerebrovascular disease should be suspected if there is a history suggestive of stroke or transient ischaemic attacks (TIAs), and in patients with ischaemic heart disease or peripheral vascular disease. In the presence of bruits on auscultation, the carotid arteries should be assessed by duplex scanning. Patients with a stenosis greater than 70% should be considered for carotid endarterectomy, especially if symptomatic. Other factors that may precipitate stroke include hypoxia, hypotension or increased blood viscosity secondary to dehydration and must be avoided during anaesthesia and the peri-operative period. These patients are usually on aspirin (75–300 mg daily) to inhibit platelet aggregation, and this causes excessive bleeding. After a stroke, general anaesthesia should be avoided for at least 3 months.

Investigations

The relevant investigations in a patient with suspected or confirmed cardiac disease include:

- Chest X-ray for cardiomegaly, pulmonary oedema and pleural effusion.
- ECG on all patients over 50 years of age and on any patient with cardiac symptoms or signs.
- Echocardiography with Doppler assessment of the gradient across the valve is an important measurement of the extent of valvular disease and demonstrates the presence or absence of vegetations.
- Duplex Doppler scanning is required in patients with suspected carotid stenosis.
- Plasma urea, electrolytes and creatinine should be measured because patients taking diuretics and ACE inhibitors may have abnormalities of fluid and electrolytes, such as chronic dehydration or hypokalaemia, and may have renal insufficiency.
- A clotting screen is required in all patients on warfarin or aspirin.

Respiratory disease

Respiratory complications and cardiovascular disorders account for the majority of post-operative complications. Physiotherapy, hydration and bronchodilators are the mainstay of peri- and post-operative management and some patients may require assisted ventilation.

Chronic obstructive airways disease

Chronic bronchitis, emphysema and asthma are associated with broncho-constriction, bronchial wall oedema, excessive secretion of mucus and plugging of the airways. Physiotherapy is started before the operation, teaching the patient breathing exercises and the correct posture for draining various segments of the lungs. Adequate hydration reduces the risk of retained secretions. In asthmatic patients, appropriate medications are given; alternatively, inhaled preparations with selective β-2 adrenoceptor stimulants (e.g., salbutamol or terbutaline) are administered via a nebulizer. Whenever possible, β-blockers and non-steroidal anti-inflammatory drugs (NSAIDs) that cause bronchospasm, and morphine which has a central respiratory inhibitory effect, should be avoided. Operation should be deferred during an acute exacerbation.

Smoking

The risk of complications affecting the cardiovascular and respiratory systems is five times greater in smokers than in non-smokers and is caused by carbon monoxide and nicotine. Carboxyhaemoglobin reduces the availability of haemoglobin for combination with oxygen, and it alters the oxygen dissociation curve so that the affinity for oxygen is increased, and hence less oxygen is released for tissue oxygenation. Nicotine through catecholamines increases the demand on the myocardium by increasing the heart rate and blood pressure. Smoking also impairs the immune function.

Smoking should be stopped at least 4 weeks before operation to improve pulmonary function and reduce post-operative pulmonary morbidity. However, cessation of smoking even for only 24 hours has measurable benefits on cardiovascular function. Other measures, which include physiotherapy and adequate hydration, apply in those with chronic bronchitis.

Other pulmonary disorders

Upper respiratory tract infection, viral or bacterial, accompanied by pyrexial illness reduces resistance to trauma and infection, and in children, airways obstruction because of mucosal oedema and excessive secretion may result in lobar collapse or bronchopneumonia. Therefore the presence of productive cough, wheeze, moist sounds in the lungs and fever is an indication for deferring the operation until full recovery. Antibiotic treatment is recommended if sputum culture is positive.

Chronic pulmonary disease, such as chronic bronchiectasis and cystic fibrosis, require intensive physiotherapy and prophylactic antibiotics pre-operatively. A history of *spontaneous pneumothorax* is important because it may recur during anaesthesia or in the post-operative period. *Pulmonary surgery* or *radiotherapy* and *post-operative pulmonary complications* in the past may have compromised pulmonary function, which must be assessed and physiotherapy instituted before and after the operation. A history of *pulmonary embolism* requires prophylactic anticoagulation.

Patients are usually aware of their respiratory disease, but the degree of disability must be assessed by asking about exercise tolerance, cough, sputum and chest infections, and the need for specific medications and antibiotics.

Investigations

A chest X-ray is required in any patient with symptoms or signs of chest disease or cardiac disease, and this should include patients who previously had chest surgery or radiotherapy, and those with a history of post-operative pulmonary complications at previous surgery. A routine chest X-ray in asymptomatic patients has a low yield of abnormalities to influence management. Patients with significant chronic pulmonary disease require evaluation by blood gas analysis, spirometry and exercise tolerance testing. Peak flow measurements before and after bronchodilators determine the reversible benefit of bronchodilators in those with obstructive airways disease. Bacteriological examination of the sputum is necessary in those producing purulent sputum.

Renal disease

Chronic renal failure or renal dysfunction is common in the elderly owing to atherosclerosis and hypertension. The kidneys are particularly vulnerable to fluid and electrolyte disturbances. Fluid overload due to impaired glomerular filtration should be avoided by cautious fluid replacement and correction with diuretics may be required, whereas dehydration and hypovolaemia reduce renal perfusion and precipitate acute renal failure. Therefore, fluid replacement, especially in patients with excessive fluid losses due to vomiting or diarrhoea, is best monitored with central venous pressure.

Regulation of serum osmolality is disturbed, and hypo- or hypernatraemia are easily precipitated if sodium replacement is inappropriate and this should be avoided. Hyperkalaemia may develop if potassium load is increased by blood transfusion or tissue damage, or by reduction in glomerular filtration as a result of diminished renal perfusion caused by cardiac failure or hypotension. Drugs such as digoxin are given carefully because their excretion is impaired and raised blood levels can exacerbate renal damage, particularly if the drug is nephrotoxic, such as gentamicin. Chronically uraemic patients usually have a normochromic normocytic anaemia as a result of decreased renal erythropoietin, but pre-operative treatment by blood transfusion is unnecessary as tissue oxygenation is maintained by compensatory physiological mechanisms and indeed contraindicated because it may cause fluid and electrolyte disturbance.

Endocrine disorders

Diabetes mellitus

No special pre-operative treatment is required for operations performed under local anaesthesia. Patients having an operation under general or regional anaesthesia require special care according to the type of diabetes.

Type II (non-insulin dependent) diabetes. Diabetic patients controlled on diet alone require no special measures provided their glucose levels are monitored. Patients on oral hypoglycaemic drugs, if on long-acting agents such as chlorpropamide or metformin, should be changed several days before the operation to a short-acting sulphonylurea (tolbutamide). On the day of the operation, the patient is starved. The morning dose of oral hypoglycaemic is omitted and is not re-introduced until the patient is allowed oral intake. During this period, the blood glucose is monitored and if the level rises above 13 mmol/l, it is controlled with small doses of soluble insulin given subcutaneously. After a major operation or if the period of starvation is prolonged, the patient is treated with insulin and glucose infusion as for insulin-dependent diabetes.

Type I (insulin-dependent) diabetes. The patient is admitted to hospital a few days before the operation and good control established; usually a twice-daily mixture of short- and intermediate-acting insulin is adequate. The patient is starved from midnight and the operation should be planned for early the next day. If the glucose level is higher than 13 mmol/l or the electrolytes are disturbed, the operation is postponed. On the day of the operation, the first dose of insulin is omitted and 5% dextrose and insulin infusion (125 ml/hr) is commenced before the operation, and continued during the operation. The rate of insulin infusion is titrated against hourly blood glucose estimations using the standard sliding scale, with the aim of maintaining the blood glucose level at 8 mmol/l. Post-operatively, the electrolytes are checked regularly and blood glucose is estimated 2–4 hourly, 5% dextrose or dextrose saline with potassium (20 mmol/l) infusion is continued at 125 ml/hr until oral diet is established when subcutaneous insulin is re-introduced using the pre-operative regime.

Thyroid disease

Thyrotoxicosis if untreated before surgery carries a risk of thyrotoxic crisis which has a high mortality. The effectiveness of anti-thyroid therapy is reflected in a falling pulse rate, particularly the sleeping pulse, and a reduction in the hyperkinetic state. β-adrenergic blockers, such as propranolol, can achieve the same effect and can be used for rapid pre-operative preparation. Potassium iodide is given for 10 days before the operation to reduce the vascularity of the gland. Before surgery, laryngoscopy is performed to check that both vocal cords are moving normally in case of subsequent damage to the recurrent laryngeal nerves.

Hypothyroidism predisposes patients to fatal coma, due to hypothermia, sensitivity to depressant drugs, decreased cardiovascular reserve and susceptibility to electrolyte disturbance. If suspected, the operation is postponed, thyroid function checked by measuring the free thyroxine (T_4) and thyroid stimulating hormone (TSH) levels and oral replacement therapy is commenced. If surgery is urgent, a thermal blanket during the operation and heavy covers after the operation are employed to avoid hypothermia, fluid and electrolyte replacement is carefully maintained and sedatives are given cautiously. Treatment with oral thyroxine is started as early as possible.

Disorders of the adrenal glands

Adrenal insufficiency is commonly due to hypothalamo-pituitary-adrenal suppression by long-term corticosteroid therapy. *Addison's disease* due to primary adrenal failure or pituitary ablation by tumour or surgery, or following adrenalectomy is infrequent.

These patients are usually on steroids, and under the stress of surgery, the adrenal response to stimulation to secrete glucocorticoids is diminished which may lead to acute cardiovascular failure with hypotension and shock (*Addisonian crisis*). This should be suspected following unexplained collapse in a surgical patient, and treated rapidly with intravenous hydrocortisone, saline and glucose infusion. All patients on steroid therapy are usually given steroid cover during the peri-operative period (e.g., 100–200 mg hydrocortisone prior to the operation and 100 mg daily until restarted on their oral regime).

Phaeochromocytoma

This condition is usually suggested by paroxysmal hypertension, palpitations, tremor and flushing, or revealed by a grossly fluctuating blood pressure during an operation. The diagnosis is confirmed by 24-hour urinary estimations of dopamine, adrenaline, noradrenaline and vanillyl mandelic acid (VMA). CT scanning, ultrasonography and 131 MIBG-isotope scanning localize the tumour. The tumour is composed of chromaffin cells derived from sympathetic nervous tissue. The majority occur in the adrenal medulla and are benign, the remainder arise in the sympathetic chain from neck to pelvis. Pre-operatively, α-adrenergic blocking drugs (e.g., phenoxybenzamine) and β-adrenergic blockade with propranolol are used to control the blood pressure and prevent arrhythmias. Anaesthetic agents are carefully selected: nitrous oxide, isoflurane and enflurane are suitable; halothane is not. Phentolamine (a short-acting α-blocker) and propranolol are used during the operation. The tumour is handled gently to limit the release of catecholamine, and when it is removed, large volumes of plasma and plasma substitutes are required to prevent a catastrophic fall in blood pressure.

Liver disease

Patients can be classified as those with known liver disease and those who are likely or suspected to have liver dysfunction.

Chronic hepatitis, whether viral or alcoholic, increases morbidity. Detoxification of endogenous metabolites and drugs and synthesis of plasma proteins, including clotting factors, are defective. In liver cirrhosis, portal hypertension and hypersplenism causing thrombocytopenia add to the risk of bleeding.

Water and salt retention due to impaired aldosterone metabolism in the liver is often accompanied by hypokalaemia and alkalosis. In obstructive jaundice, biliary back-pressure disturbs drug metabolism and the synthesis of clotting factors, besides diminishing absorption of fats, including vitamin K, the substrate for prothrombin synthesis. Endotoxins reaching the liver via the portal circulation are not detoxified, spill over into the systemic circulation and predispose to organ failure. Renal function is particularly vulnerable if renal perfusion is impaired by dehydration (*hepato-renal syndrome*).

In patients with liver dysfunction drugs and anaesthetic agents should be prescribed cautiously. Encephalopathy is prevented by correction of hypokalaemic alkalosis, use of enemas and oral lactulose to empty the colon of nitrogenous residue, and by metronidazole or neomycin to sterilize the gut of ammonia-producing bacterial flora. Clotting is corrected by administering vitamin K parenterally as its oral absorption is diminished in biliary obstruction, and is ineffective when liver function is impaired. Infusion of fresh frozen plasma or clotting factors is the preferable treatment and platelet infusion may be necessary in cirrhotic patients. In jaundiced patients, renal function is protected in the pre-operative period of restricted oral intake, by liberally administering intravenous fluids overnight and during the procedure. The patient should be catheterized and the urine output monitored carefully. Systemic antibiotics, usually cephalosporin with or without metronidazole, are given to prevent endotoxaemia.

A history of liver disease is easy to elicit as jaundice with prolonged illness are usual antecedent features. Liver dysfunction should be considered in male homosexuals and intravenous drug abusers, as well as alcoholics.

Investigations include full blood count (MCV is raised in alcoholics), liver function tests (an elevated serum gamma glutaryl transferase level is an indicator of excessive alcohol intake), clotting screen and platelet count, plasma urea and electrolytes. Screening for hepatitis B and hepatitis C should be performed.

Gastrointestinal disease

Gastro-oesophageal reflux increases the risk of gastric contents spilling into the oesophagus and overflowing into the trachea and lungs. This is a hazard during anaesthesia, particularly in obese and pregnant patients. *Peptic ulcer disease* may be exacerbated by the stress of surgery. Patients not already on anti-ulcer therapy are started on an H_2-antagonist or proton pump inhibitor. NSAIDs and other similar oral analgesics should be avoided. Patients with *inflammatory bowel disease* can be anaemic and malnourished;

a period of nutritional supplementation until the haemoglobin and plasma proteins are within acceptable levels is beneficial if surgery can be deferred. These patients may be steroid-dependent and will require steroid cover during the peri-operative period, as previously explained. Other drugs, such as azathioprine, increase the predisposition to septicaemia when colonic dissection translocates bacteria into the portal and ultimately the systemic circulation. Prophylactic antibiotic treatment needs to be prolonged during the post-operative period in patients with inflammatory bowel disease.

Haematological disorders

Anaemias

Chronic anaemia does not pose any special risk because physiological compensatory mechanisms develop. However, in order to minimize morbidity and mortality, the haemoglobin should not be less than 10 g/dl. The decision whether to transfuse pre-operatively depends on the level of anaemia, the anticipated blood loss during the operation and the age and fitness of the patient. When anaemia is acute, if the patient is elderly with poor cardiac and respiratory reserve, and is undergoing major surgery with the likelihood of excessive bleeding, blood transfusion a few days before the operation will better stabilize the patient. Otherwise, blood is transfused during the operation.

Haemoglobinopathies

Sickle cell disease is a hereditary haemolytic anaemia, occurring mainly among those of African origin, in which the normal haemoglobin A is replaced by haemoglobin S (HbS). The HbS molecule crystallizes when the blood oxygen tension is reduced and this distorts and elongates the red cell (*sickling*). This increases blood viscosity and obstructs the blood flow, causing vascular occlusion and ischaemic infarcts. Patients with *sickle cell trait* are at less risk and are usually asymptomatic. A sickle cell test by haemoglobin electrophoresis must be performed before operation on any black patient so that the anaesthetist can be prepared. In the peri-operative

management, hypoxia, dehydration, hypothermia, acidosis and infection are particularly avoided.

Polycythaemia

This is either *primary* due to a myeloproliferative disorder (*polycythaemia rubra vera*) or *secondary* to chronic cardiac or pulmonary disease. The increased red cell mass raises blood viscosity. A high haematocrit in the absence of hypovolaemia therefore deserves attention. The increased blood viscosity may lead to thromboembolic complications. In polycythaemia rubra vera the platelet count may be high, which adds to the risk of arterial or venous thrombosis, but paradoxically, haemostasis is defective and may lead to haemorrhage.

These patients require treatment by venesection or myelosuppression prior to elective operations. In an emergency, the haematocrit is reduced by pre-operative venesection and the volume is restored by colloid infusion.

Leukaemia and leucopenia

Patients with myeloproliferative disease, or bone marrow suppression commonly drug-induced or secondary to radiotherapy or chemotherapy, should only be considered for surgery if absolutely indicated, because of high mortality from sepsis and haemorrhage. Fresh blood, platelet and leucocyte transfusion is essential until the blood count indices and the clotting screen are optimized. Prophylactic antibiotics are required in neutropenia.

Bleeding disorders

Inherited clotting diseases are *haemophilia* and *von Willebrand's disease*. Haemophilia occurs in males and is an X chromosome-linked deficiency of factor VIII or IX. The anti-haemophilic factor is administered before operation and for 2 weeks after operation. von Willebrand's disease is an autosomal condition with abnormal platelet function and factor VIII deficiency. It is managed peri-operatively with fresh frozen plasma or cryoprecipitate.

Idiopathic thrombocytopenic purpura (ITP) is due to the development of antibodies which damage the patient's own platelets, resulting in a tendency to spontaneous bleeding. The platelet count is reduced, the bleeding time is increased but the clotting and pro-thrombin times are normal. In preparation for an operation, steroids and fresh blood transfusion or transfusion with platelet concentrates are necessary. In resistant cases, the antiplatelet immune response is blocked by IgG transfusion to saturate the splenic Fc binding sites and reduce platelet destruction in order to allow the platelet count to rise at the time of surgery.

Liver disease is associated with a bleeding tendency because of deficient synthesis of clotting factors and, in patients with cirrhosis, hypersplenism results in thrombocytopenia. The clotting abnormality can only be corrected by fresh frozen plasma and platelet trans-fusion prior to the operation. There is no place for vitamin K therapy when liver function is poor.

Intestinal malabsorption as a result of pancre-atic dysfunction in chronic pancreatitis or previous pancreatectomy, small intestinal disease or resection, or biliary obstruction, impairs fat, and consequently vitamin K absorption. Pre-operative vitamin K injec-tions correct the clotting deficiency but in emergency fresh frozen plasma is required.

Anticoagulation therapy, usually with warfarin, is commonly prescribed to patients after venous thromboembolism, or with a mechanical heart valve prosthesis or atrial fibrillation. In these patients war-farin is continued while reducing the prothrombin ratio (INR 1.5–2.0) during the peri-operative period. Alternatively, especially in major surgery, the more common practice is to discontinue warfarin 4 days before the operation and convert to intravenous heparin infusion or subcutaneous low-dose heparin in those on anticoagulation for venous thrombo-embolism. Heparin is continued until the patient is ready to be discharged, when warfarin is recommended.

Aspirin is frequently prescribed for patients with atheroma affecting the coronary (*ischaemic heart disease*), carotid (*cerebrovascular*) or limb arteries (*peripheral vascular disease*). Aspirin and many NSAIDs reduce platelet adhesiveness and aggrega-tion by inhibiting thromboxane and prostaglandin. Aspirin intake causes excessive oozing during and after operation, although this is rarely serious. How-ever, for major arterial surgery, aspirin should be stopped at least 2 weeks before the operation.

In all patients undergoing surgery a history of abnormal bleeding from simple cuts or previous surgery, dental extraction or childbirth should be obtained. Patients are asked about any intake of anti-coagulant drugs or aspirin, a history of haemato-logical, liver disease, malabsorption or previous intestinal resection and a family history of bleeding disorders.

If a bleeding disorder is suspected, a platelet count and clotting screen must be performed. A clotting screen includes prothrombin time or ratio and acti-vated partial thromboplastin time. No operation should be performed until any clotting disorder is corrected.

Musculoskeletal and neurological disorders

Impaired mobility exposes these patients to chest complications, thromboembolism and pressure sores, particularly if there is a sensory deficit due to neuro-logical disease. These patients are frequently on aspirin, steroids or other anti-inflammatory agents, and therefore all relevant measures should be under-taken to prevent the complications associated with these medications as already described.

Gold and penicillamine cause renal parenchymal damage and bone marrow depression and NSAIDs may exacerbate chronic renal failure. Special care should be taken during positioning on the operat-ing table, particularly in those with stiff or replaced joints. In rheumatoid arthritis, hyperextension of the neck during intubation may cause subluxation of the odontoid joint resulting in serious injury to the spinal cord. Therefore, these patients should have a lateral X-ray view of the cervical spine pre-operatively.

DRUG THERAPY

Many drugs prescribed interact with anaesthetic or analgesic agents or through side-effects that can be serious during the post-operative period. The rele-vant drugs in common use are:

- *Antihypertensives* – abrupt discontinuance may result in rebound hypertension.

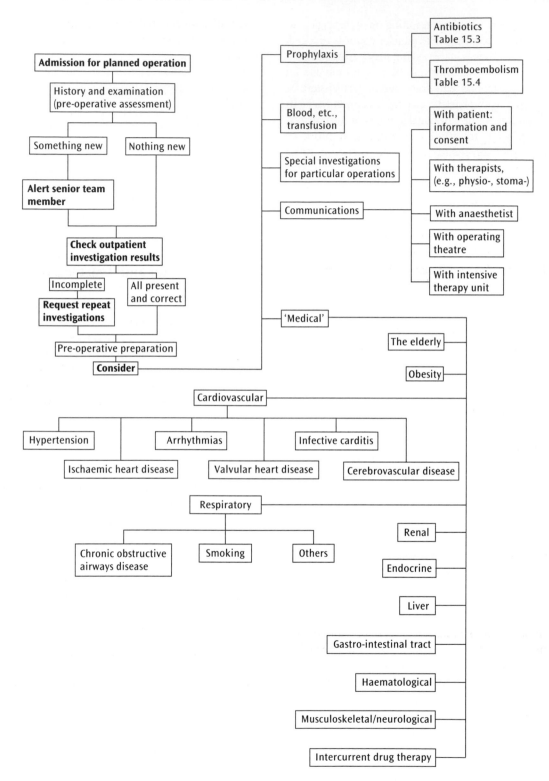

Admission for planned operation

History and examination
(pre-operative assessment)

Something new | Nothing new

Alert senior team member

Check outpatient investigation results

Incomplete | All present and correct

Request repeat investigations

Pre-operative preparation

Consider

Prophylaxis
— Antibiotics Table 15.3
— Thromboembolism Table 15.4

Blood, etc., transfusion

Special investigations for particular operations

Communications
— With patient: information and consent
— With therapists, (e.g., physio-, stoma-)
— With anaesthetist
— With operating theatre
— With intensive therapy unit

'Medical'

The elderly

Obesity

Cardiovascular
— Hypertension
— Ischaemic heart disease
— Arrhythmias
— Valvular heart disease
— Infective carditis
— Cerebrovascular disease

Respiratory
— Chronic obstructive airways disease
— Smoking
— Others

Renal

Endocrine

Liver

Gastro-intestinal tract

Haematological

Musculoskeletal/neurological

Intercurrent drug therapy

Algorithm 15.1

- *Diuretics* – may cause electrolyte abnormality and dehydration. The relevant clinical measurements are vital and should not be overlooked in these patients.
- *Anticoagulants* – warfarin predisposes to haemorrhage and reversing its effect cannot be achieved as rapidly as with heparin. Preparation of patients on warfarin for surgery has been described. Aspirin also interferes with clotting. The platelet count and clotting screen are essential in these patients.
- *Glucocorticoids* – may lead to acute adrenal insufficiency causing cardiovascular collapse. This is avoided by increasing the therapeutic dose during the perioperative period. Anti-ulcer therapy is also recommended because of the associated risk of peptic ulceration with glucocorticoids.
- *Oral contraceptives* – increase the risk of DVT and pulmonary embolism, although the risk is less with the progesterone than with the combined pill. Prophylactic low-dose heparin is recommended and for major surgery, especially if on the combined pill, the patient is advised to discontinue the pill 4 weeks prior to surgery.
- *Antidepressants* – monoamine oxidase inhibitors (MAOIs) interact with sympathomimetic amines and narcotic analgesics, which may cause a hypertensive crisis and potentiate narcotic effects.

SAFETY OF ANAESTHESIA

The anaesthetist is responsible for ensuring that the patient is fit for operation and for deciding on the best mode of anaesthesia. A history of previous operations or any difficulties that the patient may be aware of are worth noting, and past anaesthetic records that may be available in the hospital notes are reviewed. The anaesthetist pays particular attention to problems related to the conduct of the anaesthesia and these include:

- *Direct trauma to mouth or pharynx* (e.g., teeth, artificial crowns and bridges). This exposes the patient to the risk of aspirating infected material from carious teeth causing pharyngeal obstruction or aspiration pneumonia. Pre-operative dental care may be necessary.
- *Difficult intubation* in patients with rheumatoid arthritis or ankylosing spondylitis, and patients who previously had tracheostomy that may have caused some stenosis.
- *Inherited disorders* may be difficult to elicit unless the patient had a previous operation and is aware of it. These are malignant hyperpyrexia which may follow any inhalational anaesthetic, or pseudocholinesterase deficiency, causing prolonged apnoea after succinylcholine.
- *Idiosyncratic or allergic reaction* to anaesthetic agents which may be minor in the form of nausea and vomiting or major cardiovascular collapse or respiratory depression or halothane jaundice. The anaesthetist is fore-warned if there is a past history.

HIGHLIGHTS

- Patient selection for surgery determines outcome and depends on careful assessment of fitness
- Cardiovascular and respiratory diseases are the most common causes of morbidity
- Optimizing patients with medical conditions prior to surgery diminishes morbidity
- Inter-current drug therapy can be potentially dangerous if the necessary precautions are not taken
- The anaesthetist should be involved in the pre-operative assessment

Pulmonary embolism may also be acute or insidious in onset and is commonly due to small pulmonary emboli, causing breathlessness, pleuritic chest pain, haemoptysis and low-grade fever. The presence of a pleural rub, or bronchial breathing (*consolidation*) on auscultation is non-specific, and clinical signs of DVT may not be apparent. Chest X-ray appearances of pleural effusion, pleural thickening and segmental consolidation are suggestive but not diagnostic. In radio-isotope ventilation/perfusion (V/Q) scanning, the patient inhales radioactive gas and the distribution of radioactivity within the air spaces of the lung is compared with distribution of injected radionuclide-labelled albumin microspheres in the pulmonary bed, detected by gamma camera. In pulmonary embolism, distribution of isotope in the ventilation scan is normal, but areas of pulmonary under-perfusion because of emboli show as defects in the perfusion scan. The same information can be obtained by helical or spiral CT scanning of the lungs, which is faster and more reliable.

When these diagnostic tests cannot be performed promptly, because of the difficulty in distinguishing between chest infection and pulmonary embolism, it is safer to combine anticoagulation therapy with intravenous heparin (bolus dose of 10,000 units, followed by a continuous infusion of 24,000–48,000 units daily) with antibiotics until a definitive diagnosis can be made.

When embolism is massive, sudden dyspnoea is accompanied by chest pain and cardiovascular collapse. ECG may show evidence of right heart strain (S wave in lead I, Q wave and inverted T wave in lead III). When non-fatal, pulmonary angiography is performed, placing a catheter into the embolus in the pulmonary artery for instillation of thrombolytic drugs, or alternatively, surgical embolectomy is carried out under cardiopulmonary bypass.

Adult respiratory distress syndrome (ARDS) should be suspected after aspiration into the lungs, a major blood transfusion reaction or massive blood transfusion, disseminated intravascular coagulation and sepsis. The patient usually has rapid shallow breathing, but no cough, chest pain or haemoptysis and on auscultation there are scattered crepitations. PaO_2 is low and $PaCO_2$ remains normal except in severe cases. Chest X-ray may be normal in the early stages,

progressing rapidly until diffuse alveolar infiltrate ('white out') becomes evident. Until this progression, ARDS may be difficult to distinguish from congestive cardiac failure except that the cardiac diameter is normal in ARDS and cardiac failure usually responds to diuretic therapy.

Patients require urgent transfer to the intensive care unit. Management consists of ventilation with positive end expiratory pressure (PEEP), and careful monitoring of fluid balance and cardiac output by measurement of the right atrial pressure via a central venous line and of the left atrial pressure by a Swann–Ganz catheter.

Inotropic agents (e.g., dopamine) may be required to maintain cardiac output. Antibiotics are used for suspected or established infection as described above.

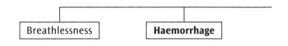

HAEMORRHAGE

Bleeding in the immediate post-operative period is known as *reactionary haemorrhage*. It is due to inadequate haemostasis. Causes include a large raw surface, a slipped ligature and coagulopathy as a result of aspirin medication, anticoagulation or massive blood transfusion of stored blood deficient in coagulation factors. When haemorrhage is slow, the blood loss is compensated by increased cardiac output without a significant fall in blood pressure. If the bleeding does not cease or the fluid loss is not restored, the circulation is compromised, the blood pressure falls and the patient develops shock: tachycardia, dryness of the mouth, poor peripheral venous filling and diminished urine output. Abdominal distension or frank blood or blood-stained fluid with high haemoglobin concentration in the drainage bags are suggestive evidence of significant blood loss.

Management entails securing venous access, inserting a central venous and a bladder catheter, infusion of plasma substitutes such as gelatin solutions until whole blood is available, and checking the clotting screen. Abnormal clotting is corrected with protamine sulphate if the patient had prophylactic heparin, or fresh frozen plasma, platelet concentrate or fresh blood transfusion. If these measures fail and the clotting is corrected or was normal, re-exploration should not be delayed.

Late post-operative haemorrhage occurring several days after the operation is known as *secondary haemorrhage*. It is infrequent and usually due to infection that causes erosion of vessels and may require re-exploration to secure haemostasis if treating the infection is unsuccessful in stopping the bleeding.

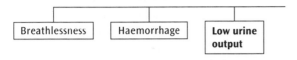

LOW URINE OUTPUT

Low urine output is a frequent post-operative problem. The decision to make is whether the patient is in *retention*, that is, the kidneys are secreting urine normally but the bladder is failing to empty; or is *oliguric*, that is, secreting urine at a less than normal rate. Instant assessment that would help to identify the underlying problem is whether the patient senses a full bladder and whether it is palpable. The pulse volume and rate, blood pressure, peripheral venous filling and presence of a raised jugular and basal crepitations are useful indices of cardiac function and tissue perfusion.

The patient in *urinary retention* is usually distressed and uncomfortable, although this may be masked by the effect of sedatives. It is more common in males, particularly when there is a degree of prostatic hypertrophy. Predisposing factors include immobility, the difficulty of passing urine in the supine position, lack of privacy, neurological bladder dysfunction caused by general or spinal anaesthesia or pelvic operations and inability to use the abdominal wall or perineal muscles in voiding because of wound pain. The diagnosis of retention is made by finding a palpable supra-pubic mass which is dull on percussion, and if in doubt, by an ultrasound examination or passing a urinary catheter.

Management involves adequate post-operative analgesia, the use of a commode or urine bottle at the bedside (although the privacy of a bathroom may be more conducive) and the sound of running tap water encourages micturition. Catheterization is the last resort if all these measures fail; the catheter is left in not more than 24 hours, unless the patient is known to have prostatic hypertrophy when a urological opinion is sought for definitive treatment.

Having excluded urinary retention, *oliguria* (less than 300 ml in 12 hours) is considered. In the absence of signs of haemorrhage or sepsis, this is invariably due to reduction in the volume of the extra-cellular fluid. At the end of a long surgical procedure the patient is cold and peripherally vasoconstricted, but once back on the ward in a warmer atmosphere vasodilation occurs and, if the fluid losses have not been adequately replaced, this results in diminished renal perfusion and urine output. If the patient has an indwelling catheter, an abrupt fall in urine output suggests a blocked catheter. This would be confirmed by observing a free flow when the catheter has been flushed with saline and improved output in the ensuing period, whereas a steady fall in urine output over several hours, in the absence of sepsis or blood loss, is likely to be due to a fluid deficit. If the patient is hypotensive, fluid is administered rapidly and a urinary catheter inserted (unless one is already present) in order to monitor the urine output which should be not less than 30 ml/hour. However, even in the absence of signs of circulatory decompensation (tachycardia and hypotension) hypovolaemia should be suspected and managed by a 'fluid challenge', the rapid infusion of 250 ml of crystalloid or colloid over half an hour. If this restores the urinary output, fluid replacement is continued.

If these measures fail, *bilateral ureteric injury* must be considered if the surgical procedure might have endangered the ureters, as in pelvic operations. An ultrasound examination demonstrates bilateral hydronephrosis if the ureters have been ligated, or free fluid in the pelvic cavity if the ureters have been divided. When these conditions have been excluded, the only possible diagnosis is acute renal failure.

Anuria due to acute renal failure is defined clinically as cessation of urine output (less than 300 ml in 24 hours) with a rise in blood urea concentration. It is due to renal tubular necrosis as a consequence of poor renal perfusion associated with *hypotension* due to hypovolaemia, cardiac failure or sepsis, *antibiotic nephrotoxicity* due mainly to the aminoglycosides, the *hepatorenal syndrome* following operative procedures in jaundiced patients, and *occlusion of the renal arteries* complicating aortic surgery.

Management consists of restricting fluid replacement to obligatory losses only during the oliguric phase. When the tubules recover, a diuretic phase occurs, recognized by spontaneous diuresis of a large volume of dilute urine of low osmolality, which should be compensated with intravenous fluids until the kidneys recover and regain their function to concentrate the urine. Haemofiltration or renal dialysis is required if serum urea, creatinine and potassium levels continue to rise and the patient remains anuric.

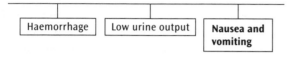

NAUSEA AND VOMITING

Nausea, with or without vomiting, in the early post-operative period is usually a side-effect from anaesthetic agents and analgesics, especially opiates. It is treated with anti-emetics, such as metoclopromide or cyclizine, which are usually prescribed with post-operative analgesics. Antibiotics, in particular metronidazole, can also cause nausea. However, *intestinal obstruction*, either *paralytic* or *mechanical*, can occur after operations.

Paralytic ileus complicates abdominal, spinal, pelvic and retro-peritoneal surgery and causes vomiting. Although it usually presents with abdominal distension and an absence of bowel sounds, vomiting that persists after the resolution of these clinical signs is suggestive of a persistent failure of gastric emptying (*gastric ileus*). Naso-gastric intubation and correction of electrolyte imbalance promote intestinal recovery provided that intra-abdominal sepsis, which can be an underlying factor, is eliminated by the absence of pyrexia and leucocytosis and by appropriate imaging.

Mechanical small bowel obstruction, although rare, can occur after abdominal operations due to fibrinous adhesions or defects in the mesentery or the peritoneum which allow entrapment. It is differentiated from paralytic ileus by the high-pitched bowel sounds. If conservative treatment fails, re-exploration is unavoidable.

Having reviewed the patient's medications and examined the abdomen for signs of paralytic or mechanical obstruction, electrolyte disturbances, particularly *hypokalaemia* and *uraemia*, are other likely causes.

Vomitus that looks like coffee grounds and tests positive for blood is likely to be the result of a *Mallory–Weiss tear* if it follows forceful vomiting; or else to *reflux oesophagitis* associated with recumbency, particularly in those patients with pre-existing symptoms, although *gastritis* or *peptic ulcer* disease should be considered especially if the patient had been on aspirin or NSAIDs. Treatment is with an H_2-antagonist or a proton pump inhibitor, reserving endoscopy only if symptoms persist. Major bleeding is a rare post-operative complication but may occur in patients with peptic ulcer or oesophageal varices when therapeutic endoscopy is the first line of treatment.

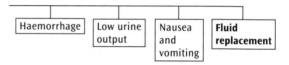

FLUID REPLACEMENT

Unless the patient is allowed oral intake, intravenous fluid replacement is essential because the patient is likely to be fluid-depleted as a result of starvation, bowel preparation and insensible losses during prolonged operations. After major surgery patients may not be able to commence oral intake because they are under sedation, or are feeling nauseated or are vomiting because of the effect of the anaesthetic agents and analgesics. After abdominal surgery, oral intake may be delayed because of paralytic ileus.

An average adult requires 2.5–3.0 l of water to compensate for obligatory fluid losses via skin and lungs, stool and urine, as well as 70 mmol of sodium ions and 60 mmol of potassium ions daily. In the immediate post-operative period there is sodium retention caused by aldosterone secretion in response to the metabolic insult of surgery, and also excessive potassium release from the damaged tissues. Hence, fluid replacement in the same volume of 5% dextrose, and without added sodium or potassium, is adequate. However, if a patient requires intravenous fluids for more than 48 hours, 500 ml isotonic ('normal') saline (0.9 g/dl sodium chloride = 154 mmol sodium/l) satisfies the body's need for sodium, and the remaining water requirement is made up of 5% glucose. A potassium supplement of 60 mmol is also required and is provided in pre-mixed intravenous solutions which contain 20 mmol of potassium chloride in 500 ml or 1000 ml, or 40 mmol in 1000 ml of 5% dextrose or normal saline. Potassium chloride should never be given in a concentration greater than 40 mmol per 500 ml of solution or administered as a bolus injection as this may cause a cardiac arrest.

Whilst a patient is on intravenous fluid therapy, an accurate record of fluid input and output is kept. The *basic daily ration* of water and electrolytes as described above compensates for insensible losses and urine output. The patient is monitored carefully for *abnormal* losses (vomiting or gastric aspirate, diarrhoea, ileostomy output, fistula discharge, abdominal distension due to accumulated liquid in the gastrointestinal tract) and signs of fluid or electrolyte imbalance. Abnormal losses during the previous 12 hours are replaced with an approximately equal volume of normal saline. The common problems encountered are as follows.

Dehydration (this commonly used term is a misnomer because the loss is not of pure water but of salt and water) as a result of inadequate replacement of excessive fluid losses mentioned above. The clinical signs are dryness of the mouth, loss of skin turgor, tachycardia, poor urine output, high urine osmolality, an elevated serum urea but not creatinine, and a high haematocrit and plasma protein concentration. This condition should not occur if abnormal losses are adequately replaced. If it does, extra normal saline is given and attention concentrated on the accurate recording of the fluid balance chart.

Overhydration or fluid overload results from excessive intravenous fluid administration or cardiac failure and, less commonly, liver or renal disease. It is recognized by shortness of breath, a raised jugular venous pressure, tachycardia, crepitations in the lung bases and peripheral or sacral oedema. Urine osmolality is low and the serum sodium is low because of dilution. Overhydration is managed by restriction of water intake.

Hyponatraemia, that is, serum sodium concentration below 130 mmol/l, is associated with overhydration, and also with dehydration when the blood urea has risen. Less commonly, it is due to excessive anti-diuretic hormone (ADH) secretion, which is suspected in a patient who appears to be normally hydrated but in whom urine osmolality is high while the plasma osmolality is low. When the serum sodium falls below 120 mmol/l, the patient is confused and below 110 mmol/l convulsions and coma may develop. Treatment is directed at the underlying cause. Sodium losses can be replaced by increasing sodium intake, whereas water retention is treated by fluid restriction; in other words, hypertonic saline solution is used.

Hypernatraemia is uncommon and is usually due to excessive sodium administration or water loss, and very rarely is caused by Conn's syndrome (*primary hyperaldosteronism*). Clinically, there is thirst, drowsiness, and if the serum sodium rises above 160 mmol/l, hypernatraemic encephalopathy and coma. Treatment is by slow intravenous replacement with hypotonic saline solution. Rapid infusion with 5% dextrose is contraindicated as it will cause water intoxication with coma and convulsions.

Hypokalaemia is usually due to diuretic therapy with inadequate potassium supplementation. Hypokalaemia causes lethargy, muscle weakness, paralytic ileus and ventricular dysrhythmias which may progress to cardiac arrest. ECG shows a prolonged P–R interval, T-wave inversion and classical U-waves. Hypokalaemia can be corrected by oral potassium supplements as effervescent or slow release tablets. For patients on intravenous fluids, potassium chloride in a concentration of not more than 40 mmol/l may be administered, at an infusion rate not exceeding 15–20 mmol/hour and the therapy should be monitored by ECG as cardiac dysrhythmias may develop and require the infusion to be interrupted.

Hyperkalaemia is commonly due to renal failure, although it can be caused by excessive potassium administration or a large transfusion of old stored blood. It is also encountered in acidotic, hypoxic and ischaemic states. A potassium concentration above 6.0 mmol/l is a medical emergency, especially if peaked T-waves are seen on ECG. Treatment involves treating the underlying cause while measures to reduce the level of plasma potassium are instituted, including intravenous infusion of calcium gluconate or sodium bicarbonate or insulin and glucose, a combination that promotes the movement of potassium ions into the intra-cellular compartment. The cation exchange resin calcium resonium, orally or rectally, removes excess potassium. Renal dialysis is required for severe hyperkalaemia associated with renal failure.

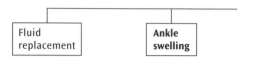

ANKLE SWELLING

The diagnosis depends on whether the swelling is bilateral or unilateral.

Bilateral swelling with pitting oedema is usually due to hypo-albuminaemia following major surgery and prolonged starvation in patients with compromised nutritional status because of malignancy or sepsis. Congestive cardiac failure due to intravenous fluid overload in a patient with hypertension or heart disease is another cause of bilateral ankle swelling, and can be distinguished by looking for other signs of heart failure. The diagnosis is easy to reach from the presenting clinical features, and is confirmed by the serum albumin, ECG and chest X-ray.

A diagnostic catch is that bilateral thrombosis of the leg veins extending to the inferior vena cava can produce swelling of the whole of *both* lower limbs.

Unilateral ankle oedema should always raise the suspicion of DVT. The classical features besides swelling of the leg, are increased warmth of the leg and tenderness of the calf muscles. Increased pain on passive dorsiflexion of the foot (*Homans' sign*) is still often described, although Homans himself ultimately decided that it was worthless. Half the cases of DVT are asymptomatic.

Ilio-femoral thrombosis produces diffuse painful and pale swelling of the whole limb as a result of fluid transudate causing oedema; this is known as *phlegmasia alba dolens* ('white leg') which may progress to *phlegmasia caerulea dolens* when the limb is blue because of venous ischaemia that ultimately develops into gangrene.

Diagnosis of DVT is best made by duplex Doppler ultrasonography which has outmoded venography and radionuclide-labelled fibrinogen.

Treatment is started with intravenous heparin, which has an immediate anticoagulant effect (bolus of 10,000 units, followed by continuous infusion of 24,000–48,000 units over 24 hours, adjusting the dose to maintain the partial thromboplastin time at two to three times normal). In the meantime, warfarin, which has a delayed therapeutic effect, is commenced and continued for 3–6 months. In patients who develop several episodes of thromboembolism or in whom anticoagulation is contraindicated, a filter is placed percutaneously in the inferior vena cava under radiological control to prevent any emboli from reaching the pulmonary circulation.

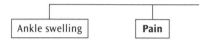

POST-OPERATIVE PAIN

Prevention of pain is better than starting treatment after it has developed. Satisfactory pain control by eliminating the discomfort caused by the wound improves breathing and coughing reducing respiratory complications, relieves anxiety, ensures sleep, early mobilization and recovery.

Pre-emptive analgesia administered during the operation is being employed more frequently. It includes intravenous long-acting analgesic drugs, infiltration of the wound edges with long-acting bupivacaine, regional nerve block (e.g., intercostal nerve block), epidural analgesia using morphine and local anaesthetic, and NSAIDs given by suppository or intramuscularly.

In minor and intermediate surgery, in addition to pre-emptive analgesia, oral analgesics are sufficient. Preparations commonly prescribed are paracetamol or paracetamol compound agents (plus codeine-co-dydramol; plus dextropropoxyphene, co-proxamol) and NSAIDs (ibuprofen, indomethacin, diclofenac) as tablets or suppositories. NSAIDs are prescribed with caution in patients with peptic ulcer, asthma or renal disease.

In many hospitals, the management of pain following major surgery is the responsibility of the 'acute pain service' run by specialist nurses and anaesthetists. The conventional method of intramuscular opioid analgesia at regular intervals as required is inadequate and has been abandoned but, if necessary, morphine is probably the most effective. Better pain control is achieved by *continuous infusion of opiates* using a programmed pump, but because the drug concentration may reach levels which cause respiratory depression and hypoxia, careful respiratory monitoring or pulse oximetry is required. *Continuous subcutaneous infusion* of more soluble opioids, such as diamorphine, achieves similar results with less risk of respiratory depression. *Pain-controlled analgesia* (PCA) allows the patient an incremental dose to the pre-set infusion dose through a delivery system with lock-out to prevent overdosing. The nursing staff should be familiar with PCA and with the effects of opiate overdose (drowsiness, slow respiratory rate) whilst ensuring that effective analgesia is being provided. *Epidural analgesia*, delivered via a cannula placed in the epidural space using drugs such as lignocaine and morphine is very effective, but requires careful monitoring because it may cause hypotension, urine retention and respiratory depression.

Site of pain:

- Chest: myocardial infarction, pulmonary embolism, pneumothorax, pneumonia, oesophagitis
- Wound: haematoma, infection, deep abscess, haematoma
- Abdomen: anastomotic leakage, abscess, ileus or mechanical obstruction, ischaemic bowel, constipation
- Limb: DVT, arterial ischaemia, compartment syndrome

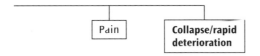

COLLAPSE OR DETERIORATION

Instant management is to ensure that the airway is clear, administer oxygen by mask and secure intravenous access. The patient's level of consciousness is assessed, the temperature, respiratory rate, pulse and blood pressure are measured. Information is obtained about associated medical conditions, the nature and extent of operation, the course of recovery since the operation and any symptoms preceding the current event. The operation and anaesthetic

Table 16.1 *Causes of post-operative collapse or deterioration*

Inadequate reversal of anaesthesia
Hypovolaemic shock
Severe infection and sepsis
Hypoxia due to respiratory disorder or depressant drugs
Pulmonary embolism
Myocardial infarction or cardiac dysrhythmias
Cerebrovascular accident
Hypoglycaemia
Adrenal insufficiency by steroid therapy
Electrolyte disturbances
Drug reactions

notes, the drug and fluid balance charts are also reviewed. Physical examination focuses on signs of respiratory, cardiovascular, circulatory or neurological complications, peritonitis and signs of sepsis or anaphylaxis. The likely causes are listed in Table 16.1. Special tests are determined by the clinical findings and the results of ECG, blood gases, serum enzymes, serum electrolytes and full blood count and blood cultures.

HIGHLIGHTS

- Pulse, blood pressure, temperature and urine output are crucial post-operative measurements
- Antibiotics should be carefully selected for respiratory infection
- Wound infection is more likely with contaminated or dirty operations
- Prolonged catheterization should be avoided to prevent urinary infection
- When intra-abdominal sepsis is suspected CT scan is the investigation of choice
- A central venous line is the likely cause of pyrexia until proven otherwise
- Acute breathlessness is more likely to be due to pulmonary embolism or acute cardiac ischaemia
- Blood clotting profile should be checked before re-exploring a patient for haemorrhage
- When the urine output is low, frusemide should not be given if the patient is hypovolaemic
- Medications are a common cause of post-operative nausea and vomiting
- Ankle oedema in the post-operative patient is commonly due to hypoproteinaemia

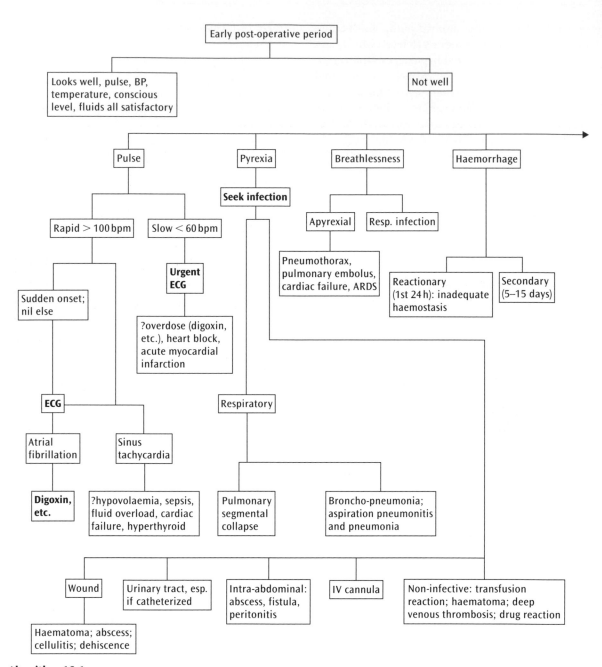

Algorithm 16.1

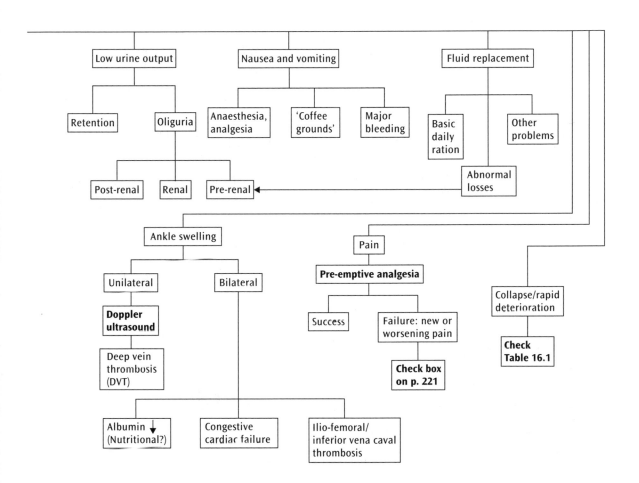

17

Ear, nose and throat

MARTIN J BURTON

INTRODUCTION

Otorhinolaryngology – head and neck surgery – encompasses a broad spectrum of disorders of the ear, nose, throat and neck. At its boundaries it interacts closely with neurosurgery and neurology (skull base problems), oncology (head and neck cancer), medical audiology (hearing and balance dysfunction), ophthalmology (intra-orbital disease) and plastic surgery (reconstruction and cosmesis).

Ear, nose and throat disorders present many problems which are addressed in the ensuing sections. A knowledge of head and neck anatomy and pathophysiology of the special senses is required to understand the nature and effect of the disease processes encountered. Examination and treatment require special equipment, mirrors, endoscopes and magnification to view the areas of concern. Skills in microsurgery and endoscopy in addition to the general surgical skills ranging from the handling of individual tissues to the overall care of the critically ill patient are the basics of overall management. Patients range in age from the premature infant to the extremely elderly, potentially taxing communication skills.

The ensuing sections address the most important and common ear, nose and throat problems.

RECURRENT 'TONSILLITIS'

> **AIMS**
>
> 1 Be familiar with the clinical features of tonsillar disease
> 2 Recognize potentially malignant disease of the tonsils

Soreness of the throat is common. A diagnosis of acute, infective pharyngitis or tonsillitis is often made on the basis of the history and clinical examination. Recurrence of this symptom requires further assessment. Examination of the tonsils by use of a tongue depressor and suitably bright light-source allows the patient to be categorized into one of two broad groups.

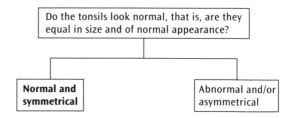

Normal symmetrical tonsils

Sinister disease is unlikely in tonsils which appear normal and are of equal size, even if both tonsils are relatively large. However, between bouts of acute tonsillitis the tonsils often appear normal. Some tonsils contain more crypts than others and the presence of multiple crypts need not cause concern. The presence of white, cheesy material within the crypts may produce an unpleasant taste in the patient's mouth but is of no more serious significance.

The findings of normal tonsils should prompt a careful review of the history. A history of recurrent episodes of acute tonsillitis, responsive to antibiotics or of almost continual soreness of the throat with acute exacerbations, suggests recurrent acute or chronic tonsillitis, respectively.

Does the history support a diagnosis of recurrent acute/chronic tonsillitis?

Recurrent acute or chronic tonsillitis

Several treatment options are available – medical and surgical. Antibiotics may be prescribed as single courses, repeated as necessary to eliminate infections. Alternatively, a low, prophylactic dose of antibiotic may be prescribed for an extended period of, for example, 3 months. In an adult, more than a single episode of tonsillitis per year necessitating time off work is a relative indication for tonsillectomy. Two quinsies, or a single quinsy following recurrent tonsillitis, also provide such an indication.

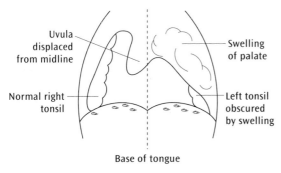

Fig. 17.1 *Diagram of clinical appearances in quinsy. Note the uvula displaced by the bulging left peri-tonsillar swelling.*

A *quinsy* is a peri-tonsillar abscess and usually presents as a severe sore throat with trismus and consequent difficulty in speaking and swallowing. On examination, the uvula is displaced from the midline by a marked swelling usually arising between the superior pole of the tonsil and the anterior faucial pillar (Fig. 17.1).

Whilst tonsillectomy prevents future tonsillitis, patients may still experience episodes of viral pharyngitis in common with the rest of the population.

Diagnosis of recurrent acute or chronic tonsillitis not possible

The history and examination should aim at establishing other causes for throat pain. These may include pharyngitis, laryngitis, etc., and, more importantly, malignant disease of the upper aerodigestive tract. Examination should therefore include indirect laryngoscopy.

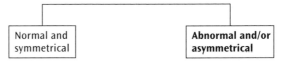

Abnormal and/or asymmetrical

Tonsils which are either asymmetrical or abnormal in appearance may contain tumours derived from either their lymphoid component (*lymphoma*), squamous epithelial covering (*squamous cell carcinoma*) or, much less commonly, from the minor salivary glands and connective tissue contained therein. Comparison of the size of the tonsils may suggest one or other of these diagnoses.

Unilaterally large tonsil

A tonsil which is larger than the other, but is otherwise of normal appearance, may contain a *lymphoma*. The history and clinical examination should focus on a search for symptoms and signs of lymphoma elsewhere in the head and neck and more distantly. The tonsil should be removed by unilateral tonsillectomy and submitted to histological examination to allow accurate typing of the tumour using immunocytochemical techniques. Further treatment will depend upon the stage of the disease as established by bone marrow aspiration and computer tomographic (CT) scanning of the head and neck, chest and abdomen.

One tonsil may *appear* larger than the other if it is pushed medially by an underlying structure. Tumours of the deep lobe of the parotid may do this as may lesions of other structures in the parapharyngeal space. If there is any doubt about apparent unilateral enlargement a CT scan of the neck is undertaken before the tonsil is approached surgically.

Ulcerated/bleeding tonsil

Squamous cell carcinoma of the tonsil usually presents with an ulcer or friable, bleeding mass of one tonsil. Clinical examination should focus on determining the size and extent of the primary tumour, the presence of any local metastases in the cervical lymph nodes, the presence of another synchronous primary tumour in the upper aerodigestive tract and a search for distant metastases. Examination is complemented by special investigations, including chest radiography

and CT scanning of the neck. Diagnostic endoscopy with biopsy of the lesion should precede any therapeutic intervention. Treatment may be either medical (radiotherapy ± chemotherapy) or surgical (tonsillectomy ± resection of adjacent tissues ± neck dissection) or a combination of the two.

Both tonsils abnormal

When acutely or chronically infected, both tonsils may appear abnormal. This may be accompanied by erythema and swelling of the surrounding tissues. These relatively non-specific signs of infection and inflammation are usually indicative of a simple *bacterial* or *viral* infection. The presence of a white, creamy slough over both tonsils is characteristic of *infectious mononucleosis (glandular fever)*; the diagnosis may be confirmed by a positive Monospot test and the presence of atypical lymphocytes in the peripheral blood smear. Although uncommon in the developed world, diphtheria may be seen in immunocompromised patients. A fibrinous exudate forms a

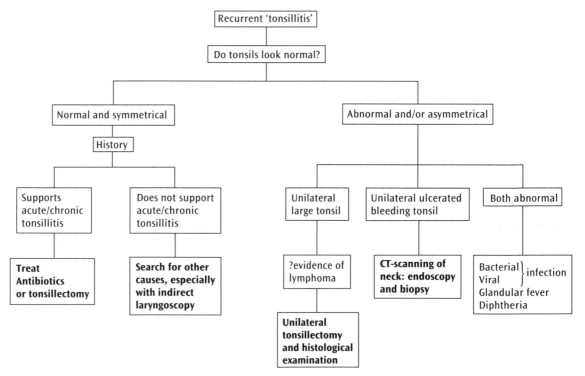

Algorithm 17.1

membrane over the tonsils. The diagnosis will only be made if the index of suspicion is high and the appropriate cultures undertaken.

HIGHLIGHTS

- Normal and symmetrical tonsils do not exclude recurrent acute or chronic tonsillitis
- A unilateral large or ulcerated tonsil may be due to an underlying malignancy
- Bilateral abnormal tonsils may be due to infectious mononucleosis or diphtheria

---

DISCHARGING EAR

AIMS

1 Be familiar with the examination of a discharging ear
2 Distinguish 'safe' from 'unsafe' tympanic membrane perforations
3 Understand the rationale underlying this distinction
4 Know when to suspect cholesteatoma

Discharge from the ear, or *otorrhoea*, is one of the six cardinal symptoms of ear disease. In establishing and treating its cause one needs to consider the source of the discharge and how it relates to the other five symptoms of: deafness, dizziness, otalgia (pain in the ear), tinnitus (noises in the ear) and facial weakness.

The nature of the discharge may provide a clue as to its origin. There are no mucus secreting glands in the skin of the external auditory canal but there are plenty in the middle ear cleft. Therefore, a mucoid discharge suggests communication between the middle ear and external auditory canal.

The ear is examined carefully as the pinna may be tender to touch. Otoscopic examination allows determination of the first important sign.

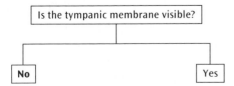

Tympanic membrane not visible

If the tympanic membrane is not visible this is usually because the ear canal is swollen, or full of debris.

Ear canal swollen

With a discharging ear and a swollen ear canal the diagnosis is *otitis externa*. Unless the tympanic membrane is seen it is not possible to decide whether or not this is secondary to *otitis media*. Treatment should proceed expectantly until the membrane is visible.

Furunculosis is a specific type of otitis externa in which a hair follicle in the external meatal skin becomes infected, often with a staphylococcus. This is associated with severe pain and discharge is often scanty unless and until the abcess points and bursts. Treatment consists of analgesia, oral anti-staphylococcal antibiotics and a hygroscopic wick.

Swelling due to diffuse non-specific, or *acute infective otitis externa* (*see later*) should be treated with gentle suction clearance if possible and topical steroid/antibiotic ointment which, as the swelling subsides, is substituted with drops. In time, the eardrum becomes visible and management proceeds as described below.

Canal full of debris

Gentle cleaning of the canal with a wisp of cotton wool, avoiding rigid objects, is sometimes possible, or else aural toilet by suction clearance under the operating microscope is recommended. Antibiotic/steroid drops should then be prescribed and the patient reviewed regularly for further cleaning and inspection until the eardrum is visualized.

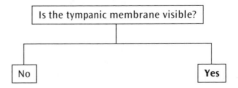

Tympanic membrane visible

An *intact tympanic membrane* indicates that the source of the discharge is the external canal itself. The most common cause is *otitis externa*. This acute or chronic inflammatory condition of the skin of the ear canal can arise in several ways. Some patients have underlying *eczema* of the canal skin, others traumatize their ears with cotton-buds, towels, fingers, etc. Whatever the cause, the canal skin becomes swollen and oedematous and watery discharge is produced. *Acute infective otitis externa* may supervene, usually with pseudomonas, staphylococcal or streptococcal species, and occasionally fungi or yeasts, particularly if prolonged courses of topical steroid/antibiotic combinations have been used – *otomycosis*. Associated symptoms include pain and deafness with swelling of the pinna and inflammation of the peri-auricular lymph nodes.

The principles of treatment are:

- Careful cleaning of the ear canal (ideally using suction under the operating microscope).
- Prevention of water or objects (fingers, hair-grips, etc.) entering the ear.
- If the canal is swollen, insertion in the canal of a dressing such as small foam wicks ('Otowicks').

In many *acute* cases there is infection and it is reasonable to prescribe a steroid/antibiotic combination as ointment or drops. In *chronic* cases, and following initial treatment of infected cases, allergy may develop to the antibiotic content of the drops; drops or ointment containing steroid alone is often more appropriate.

If the *tympanic membrane is not intact* the primary problem is likely to be in the middle ear. Any degree of otitis externa which is present may be a secondary phenomenon caused by infected material from the middle ear.

An important consideration is whether the problem is acute, chronic or recurrent.

Acute

In *acute otitis media* the tympanic membrane often ruptures allowing mucopus from the middle ear to enter the external canal. Acute otitis media is

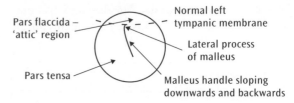

Fig. 17.2 *Diagram of the normal left tympanic membrane.*

particularly common in children. It usually follows an upper respiratory tract infection and common organisms include *Streptococcus pneumoniae, Haemophilus influenzae* and *Branhamella catarrhalis*. As pus accumulates in the middle ear cleft, pressure increases and the most striking symptom – otalgia – develops in association with deafness. Further increase in pressure leads to rupture of the eardrum with sudden production of aural discharge and immediate improvement in the otalgia. At this stage a perforation is present in the pars tensa of the membrane (Fig. 17.2). It is usually not marginal, that is, the perforation does not extend to the very margin of the drum and a rim of drum surrounds the perforation. Treatment consists of antibiotics, analgesia and decongestant nasal drops. The perforation usually closes spontaneously within 6 weeks.

Chronic or recurrent

In *chronic suppurative otitis media* a *chronic* perforation exists and the patient usually complains of *chronic* deafness with *recurrent, intermittent* discharge. The patient falls into one of two categories depending on the type and position of the perforation.

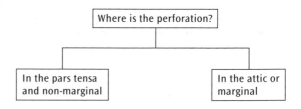

A non-marginal perforation in the pars tensa is defined as the 'safe' type of *chronic suppurative otitis media* (CSOM) or 'tubotympanic' CSOM. A perforation which extends to the margin of the drum,

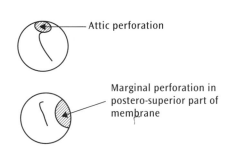

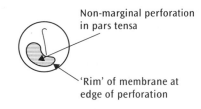

Fig. 17.3 *Three types of perforated eardrum.*

or one in the pars flaccida or 'attic' region defines *'unsafe' CSOM* or *'attico-antral' CSOM* (Fig. 17.3).

The terms 'safe' and 'unsafe' arise because serious, life-threatening disorder in the middle ear or mastoid of patients with 'safe' perforations rarely arise, whereas there *may* be (but by no means certainly is) the more serious disorder of *cholesteatoma* in patients with the 'unsafe' perforation.

Pars tensa and non-marginal perforation

The disease is usually confined to the middle ear cleft (*mesotympanum*) and *Eustachian tube* – hence, the other term for this condition is *tubo-tympanic CSOM*. In these patients organisms enter the middle ear cleft via the Eustachian tube or through the perforation. Patients complain of *intermittent discharge* associated with upper respiratory tract infections or after swimming, hair washing, etc., where water entered the ear. They also complain of *deafness*. The condition is not painful. An acute infection may resolve spontaneously but usually oral and/or topical antibiotics are necessary. There is a general reluctance to prescribe antibiotic-containing ear drops because of their theoretical ototoxic effect. In practice this does not occur and steroid/antibiotic ear drops are regularly prescribed if a middle ear infection fails to settle.

Commonly, there is *no* active infection in the middle ear cleft and the patient has deafness only with no discharge. Examination reveals a clean, dry perforation. To avoid infection the patient should keep the ear dry. It is reasonable not to interfere, especially in those who have no, or few, episodes of discharge. It is possible to repair the membrane with a *myringoplasty* procedure. A piece of fascia is taken from over the temporalis muscle and used as a 'patch' on the tympanic membrane. The primary aim is to close the perforation, *not* improve the hearing. If the patient wishes to avoid recurrent discharge and/or wants to be able to get the ear wet with impunity, surgery may be considered. However, any operation on the ear carries a small risk of total deafness.

Pars flaccida ('attic') and marginal perforation

Perforation in the attic region or a marginal perforation in the postero-superior part of the drum means there is an underlying disease in the *attic* and in the passage between the middle ear cleft and mastoid air cells – the *antrum*. Hence the term *attico-antral CSOM*. The word 'perforation' is often a misnomer, as it implies a *hole* in the membrane. In most of these cases, chronic Eustachian tube dysfunction produces persistent negative middle ear pressure. As a consequence the 'weakest' parts of the tympanic membrane – the pars flaccida and the postero-superior quadrant – are sucked into the middle ear creating a small *retraction pocket*. The lining of the pocket is the normal external layer of the tympanic membrane – keratinizing, squamous epithelium. The 'perforation' is simply the 'mouth' of such a pocket (Fig. 17.4).

Provided that the keratin shed by the lining of the pocket is extruded into the ear canal the situation is safe and stable. When the pocket is large, keratin debris accumulates forming a *cholesteatoma* (*see* Fig. 17.4) which enlarges, usually into the attic and antrum and thence back into the mastoid. The 'pocket' becomes a keratin-containing 'sack' which destroys bone and can erode parts of the ossicular chain (producing *conductive deafness*), over the facial

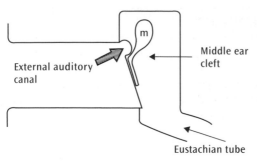

Diagrammatic representation of coronal section of:
(i) external auditory canal;
(ii) middle ear cleft;
(iii) Eustachian tube.

The malleus (m) is the only ossicle shown

Large arrow = pocket of skin beginning to develop in pars flaccida

Fig. 17.4 *Development of a cholesteatoma.*

Middle ear cleft

External auditory canal

Eustachian tube

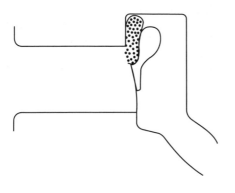

Pocket has enlarged and now contains retained keratin = cholesteatoma

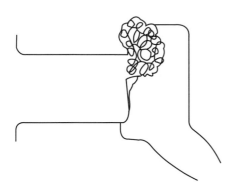

Larger cholesteatoma has eroded malleus head and bony boundaries of middle ear

nerve (producing *facial weakness*) and the inner ear (producing *vertigo and sensorineural deafness*). Further bone erosion may expose the dura or intracranial sinuses and complications of cholesteatoma include meningitis, brain abcess and lateral sinus thrombosis. These complications of cholesteatoma are not common but are of such importance that this disorder must be treated promptly, and are the reasons an ear with a cholesteatoma is regarded as unsafe.

In patients with cholesteatoma, discharge is due to intermittent infection of the cholesteatoma debris, commonly with anaerobic organism producing a foul-smelling discharge.

The practical difficulty is that examination of the ear and the mouth of the cholesteatoma does not give an indication of the size of the underlying cholesteatoma sack. The clinical features described above may help. A CT scan may demonstrate anatomical variations in the mastoid or other features such as erosion into the lateral semi-circular canal.

Principles of treatment include cleaning of the ear canal under the microscope followed by a short period of topical steroid/antibiotic therapy. Occasionally, the full limits of a retraction pocket can be seen and inspected and a cholesteatoma excluded. More commonly, following aural toilet and a course of drops, the mouth of a cholesteatoma becomes evident. These ears need formal surgical exploration designed to eradicate disease, prevent recurrence and complications, and restore hearing, but this must not compromise the other aims of surgery, designed to render the ear 'safe'.

Usually some form of *mastoidectomy* is performed; the classical procedure is a modified radical mastoidectomy. This exteriorizes the cholesteatoma pocket, preventing further retention of cholesteatoma debris within the ear.

HIGHLIGHTS

- Ear discharge can be from the middle or the external ear
- A clear external ear is essential in order to visualize the tympanic membrane and to allow topical medication
- A tympanic membrane which is not intact suggests middle ear disease
- Topical antibiotic/steroid combinations are useful in many discharging ears
- Chronic discharge and deafness may be due to cholesteatoma, especially if the discharge is foul-smelling or there is an attic or marginal perforation

---

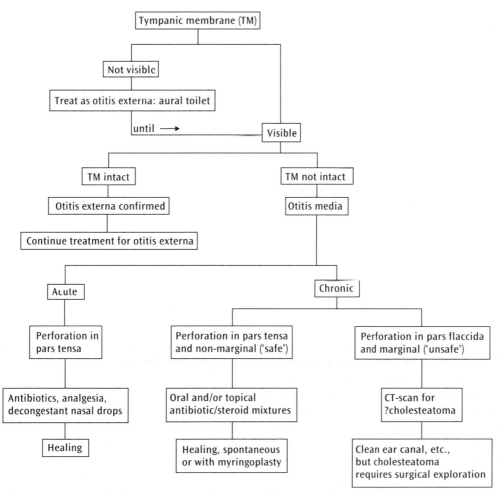

Algorithm 17.2

EPISTAXIS

AIMS

1 Appreciate the seriousness of nose-bleeds
2 Recognize the causes of nasal bleeding
3 Become familiar with the overall
   management

Bleeding from the nose – *epistaxis* – is common and usually self-limiting. Yet a patient may die from a nosebleed, as a consequence of mismanagement. Elderly patients in particular may ooze over a long period before seeking medical attention and the problem may appear trivial until they collapse from hypovolaemia. The patient with an epistaxis should be managed in a systematic way. This involves controlling the bleeding by simple measures, maintaining the circulation, ruling out predisposing factors and identifying the few patients who require hospital care or more active treatment.

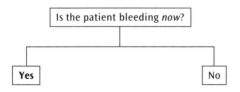

Patient actively bleeding

In the patient who is actively bleeding, first aid measures should be instituted while the vital signs are monitored. The measures include *pinching the soft, anterior, cartilaginous part of the nose firmly against the anterior septum*. The patient sits up, and leans forwards with the mouth open to allow blood dripping down the back of the nose into the pharynx to be spat out and collected in a receiver. The patient is discouraged from swallowing blood – it is an emetic. A pack of 2 ml of 4% cocaine on 1 cm ribbon gauze or lignocaine and topical adrenaline solutions may be used, and should stop the bleeding within 15 minutes. The patient should not be sitting up if there are signs of hypovolaemia.

Patient not bleeding

The patient's pulse and blood pressure and other signs of circulatory decompensation must be measured, as well as the haemoglobin and haematocrit estimations as the patient may still require fluid or blood replacement.

The second question should be considered at the *same time as the first.*

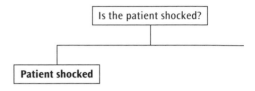

If the patient is shocked *full resuscitation measures* should be instituted immediately. These are discussed elsewhere (Chapter 23).

Patient not shocked

The patient may not be shocked at presentation but may become so later. It is vital to continue to monitor the patient's pulse and blood pressure at regular intervals whilst bleeding continues *and* when bleeding has stopped, particularly if this involved a major intervention. A steady trickle down the back of the throat in a patient whose bleeding has 'stopped' may be easily overlooked.

Most nosebleeds occur from *Little's area* just inside the nose on the antero-inferior part of the nasal septum. The patient is asked to blow the nose to remove any clots from this area, which is inspected after spraying the nose with topical anaesthesia (lignocaine or cocaine) whilst any new bleeding is sucked away with a sucker. A good light is essential, preferably a head-light to leave both hands free.

Is there an obvious bleeding point?

Obvious bleeding point

An obvious bleeding point can be *cauterized* with *silver nitrate* or electrocautery in a circle 2–3 mm around the bleeding point before applying cautery directly to it. If this fails, the anterior nasal cavity can be packed with layers of ribbon gauze soaked in bisthmuth iodoform paraffin paste (BIPP). Artificial sponge tampons as well as a range of balloons are now available and easier to use.

No obvious bleeding point

This may arise if the bleeding point is posterior or when an anterior bleed has stopped leaving no trace. A thorough search is made if possible by examining the nasal cavity with an endoscope.

When bleeding is clearly coming from the posterior part of the nose it may be controlled by a long intra-nasal tampon or nasal balloon. Should the bleeding point remain unidentified while bleeding continues, then the anterior part of the nose is packed initially, adding a post-nasal balloon if bleeding is still not controlled.

Are there any predisposing factors which need treatment?

Predisposing factors

Whilst measures are in hand to stop bleeding, a thorough history should be taken to elicit any predisposing factors (Table 17.1). Blood for full blood count, biochemistry profile, clotting factors, grouping (and cross-matching if necessary) are essential investigations which can be of diagnostic value and would allow specific treatment to be instituted.

Patient's admission to hospital

Patients with packs *in situ*, the elderly and infirm, those who live alone at home or have poor local support should all be admitted, for bedrest and regular observation, monitoring the blood pressure to rule out unsuspected hypertension. Packs are usually left *in situ* for at least 24 hours but if they are to be left longer than 48 hours prophylactic antibiotics should be given – the packs obstruct the sinus ostia and *sinusitis* and *intra-nasal infection* can develop. If the patient is anxious, a light sedative is prescribed. Patients with pre-existing chest or heart disease,

Table 17.1 *Causes of epistaxis*

Idiopathic
Vascular disease – arteriosclerosis
Coagulation defects – leukaemia
Drugs – anticoagulants, aspirin
Tumours – malignant, benign
Infection
Iatrogenic – post-nasal surgery
Hereditary haemorrhagic telangiectasia
  (Osler–Weber–Rendu disease)
Trauma

especially the elderly, can become hypoxic with nasal packs *in situ* and it is wise to consider giving 24% O_2. After removal of the packs there should be a period of observation before the patient is discharged home. It is mandatory that at this stage, or at follow-up in the clinic, the nasal cavity is examined to ensure that there is no lesion responsible for the bleeding.

Patients discharged home

Patients who can be discharged home should be given written instructions on the management of nose-bleeds. Some will need follow-up to ensure that no intra-nasal pathology has been overlooked.

Bleeding not controlled

If bleeding has not been controlled up to this point there are several alternative courses of action.

First, alternative anterior and/or posterior packs can be inserted. This may fail to control bleeding because anatomical variations such as a grossly deviated nasal septum may make it impossible to insert a pack and apply pressure to the bleeding point. If and when the patient is adequately resuscitated it may be necessary to examine the nose under general anaesthesia, correct a septal deformity with a *submucous resection* (SMR) or *septoplasty* (*see* 'Blocked and runny nose', p. 249) and pack the anterior and posterior nose tightly.

If at this stage bleeding has still not been controlled, the next possible treatment is ligation of the anterior ethmoid artery, the external carotid artery or the maxillary artery. These procedures aim to reduce the pressure in the vessels supplying the nose. The upper anterior part of the nose derives its blood supply from the internal carotid circulation via the anterior ethmoid arteries which can be approached through a canthal incision. The remainder of the nose receives its supply from the external carotid artery which can be ligated in the neck, under local anaesthetic if necessary. Alternatively, the maxillary artery can be identified behind the posterior wall of the antrum and ligated.

Another approach is by *embolization* of branches of external carotid artery. This is effective when the bleeding point can be clearly identified, usually when the patient is actively bleeding.

HIGHLIGHTS

- Epistaxis can be controlled by simple measures
- Cardiovascular resuscitation may be required
- Local or systemic causes should be ruled out by thorough examination
- Submucous resection, septoplasty and ligation or embolization of the arterial branches may be necessary with persistent bleeding

---

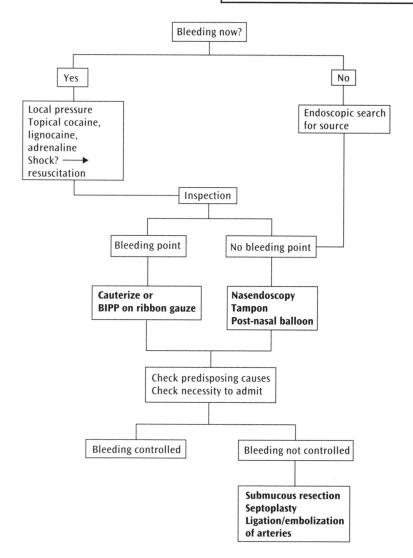

Algorithm 17.3

UNILATERAL FACIAL WEAKNESS

AIMS

1 Be able to distinguish Bell's palsy from facial weakness due to other causes
2 Understand the indications for medical treatment
3 Be able to minimize the morbidity associated with the condition

---

There is a tendency to call all facial weakness 'Bell's' palsy. This is inaccurate: the name should be reserved for *idiopathic* facial palsy. It is worthwhile at the outset to assume that a facial weakness is *not* a Bell's palsy *until* all other possibilities have been excluded.

Bell's palsy accounts for 60–75% of acute facial palsies. The onset is usually rapid (over less than a 48-hour period) and may be accompanied by pain and numbness in the ear, mid-face and tongue. Taste is disturbed if the chorda tympani is involved and other cranial nerves may also be affected.

History and examination seek evidence of disease along the full course of the nerve from the cerebellopontine angle to the facial musculature. A systematic approach following this route in reverse is described here.

Is there evidence of parotid disease, for example tumour or trauma?

Evidence of parotid disease

Parotid disease is covered in Chapter 2. If there is no evidence of parotid disease, the intimate relationship of the nerve with the *middle ear* and *skull base* explains the need for careful examination of this region. The facial nerve enters the middle ear from the internal auditory canal and immediately turns posteriorly to run horizontally along the medial wall of the middle ear cleft. Not infrequently, the bony canal covering the nerve is dehiscent. The nerve turns through 90° at the back of the middle ear cleft to run downwards towards the skull base, exiting through the stylomastoid foramen.

Is there evidence of external or middle ear disease?

Evidence of external ear disease

Vesicles on the pinna or tympanic membrane are classic signs of *Ramsay Hunt syndrome – herpes zoster oticus*. This accounts for 2–7% of acute facial palsies. The VIIth nerve is infected with the herpes zoster virus producing facial weakness and a varicelliform eruption over some or all of the external ear, the deep ear canal skin and the soft palate. The patient may have other cranial nerves affected (V, IX and X) and complain of hearing loss and vertigo (VIIIth nerve involvement). Patients are treated with a course of an appropriate anti-viral agent. Only a minority recover completely and are free of sequelae.

Evidence of middle ear/skull base disease

Significant middle ear or skull base disease is evidenced by conductive hearing loss and/or abnormal findings on examination of the tympanic membrane, and/or an abnormal appearance of the skin and bone of the floor of the external auditory canal.

The facial nerve may be involved in *acute otitis media* if the nerve is dehiscent. In addition to the standard treatment (*see* 'Discharging ear', p. 227), a myringotomy is performed if the drum has not burst spontaneously. This small incision in the tympanic membrane will relieve middle ear pressure. Weakness arising from *chronic suppurative otitis media* with *cholesteatoma* has been discussed (*see* 'Discharging ear', p. 229). Rarer middle ear causes of facial weakness include uncommon tumours arising in or extending into the middle ear; these may be visible behind an intact tympanic membrane or may have eroded through it. In all these cases one would expect to find evidence of a conductive hearing loss.

Malignant otitis externa is a severe form of otitis externa due to *Pseudomonas aeruginosa* infection in diabetic or otherwise immunocompromised patients. Infection erodes the bone of the floor of the external auditory canal leading to osteomyelitis of the skull base. Nerves emerging through this region can be 'picked off' by the spreading infection. A history of discharge is accompanied by signs of exposed bone, even sequestrum, in the floor of the canal. Intensive antibiotic treatment is required. Although not 'malignant' in the oncological sense, the high morbidity and mortality associated with this condition give rise to the epithet.

No evidence of middle ear disease

With normal hearing and normal examination findings middle ear disease is unlikely.

The facial nerve arrives at the middle ear having exited from the brain stem at the junction of the pons and medulla, crosses the cerebellopontine angle and traverses the internal auditory canal within the temporal bone.

Is there clinical evidence of inner ear or temporal bone disease?

Clinical evidence of inner ear or temporal bone disease

Sensorineural hearing loss or 'dizziness' may be evidence of dysfunction of the cochlea or vestibular system, or to either of the respective branches of the VIIIth nerve arising from the inner ear. An uncommon but important cause of such symptoms is an *acoustic neuroma* – more correctly termed a *vestibular schwannoma* – a benign tumour arising from the vestibular nerve. Facial nerve involvement is unusual as the nerve seems remarkably resistant to physical pressure. When this lesion expands it grows into the cerebellopontine angle (CPA). This or any other CPA tumour may affect adjacent cranial nerves, especially the Vth, and all cranial nerves should be examined paying particular attention to the Vth.

When the physical examination is complete all patients should have an audiogram and tympanometry to look for hearing loss and to assess middle ear function. Various tests have been described to examine the function of the branches of the facial nerve in order to determine the site of a facial nerve lesion. These tests include:

- *Schirmer's test* for tear production (greater superficial petrosal nerve).

- *Stapedial reflex testing* (branch to stapedius muscle).
- *Taste and salivary flow testing* (chorda tympani).

So-called 'topodiagnostic' testing has limited practical usefulness.

No clinical evidence of inner ear or temporal bone disease

In the absence of any abnormality, at this point it is reasonable to treat the palsy *pro tem* as *Bell's palsy*. The next practical question is the following.

Is the palsy complete?

Complete facial palsy

When the palsy is complete, a short, reducing course of oral steroid may improve outcome. A formal systematic review of the use of steroids in Bell's palsy has not been undertaken but it is widely accepted management if there are no contraindications. Steroids work best when given early in the course of the palsy and should be started if the patient is seen in the first week. A suitable regimen would be prednisolone EC 60 mg/day, reduced by 15 mg every 3 days and discontinued at the end of 15 mg for 3 days. The 'cut-off' point in time after onset of palsy after which steroid therapy is *inappropriate* is a matter of conjecture.

Patients with facial weakness are at risk of *eye problems* as they are unable to blink normally. The eyes must be kept moist (artificial tears and taping at night) and any hint of a more serious problem (e.g., pain and/or grittiness and redness of the eye) should initiate urgent referral to an ophthalmologist.

It has been suggested that Bell's palsy is due to a viral infection of the herpes group. However, the evidence for the efficacy of anti-viral therapy is inconclusive.

Incomplete facial palsy

Although steroids are not indicated in incomplete palsies, eye care as described above is pertinent. Patients are asked to return if the palsy becomes complete and thence managed as above.

A period of observation should now ensue. One-third of Bell's palsy patients have partial weakness only and have an excellent prognosis. The majority of patients with a complete palsy will have signs of recovery 4–6 weeks after onset and complete recovery is likely in these patients. The remainder will recover more slowly but *if there are no signs of recovery at 2–3 months*, further investigation is necessary

Has *all* other pathology, including a *retro-cochlear or posterior fossa lesion*, been excluded?

The aim is to identify rare causes of facial weakness. Many of these patients have other symptoms and signs which may be evident from the general history and examination. Appropriate investigations include chest X-ray (sarcoid), full blood count and ESR (autoimmune disease) and MRI scanning (facial neuroma and CPA tumours).

> **HIGHLIGHTS**
>
> - Facial palsy can be due to parotid, ear or temporal bone disease
> - Physical examination and investigations are required to determine the level and extent of facial palsy
> - Eye care is crucial in a patient with a facial weakness

NASAL TRAUMA AND NASAL DEFORMITY

> **AIMS**
>
> 1 Be able to recognize nasal injury
> 2 Be familiar with the management of nasal trauma
> 3 Understand the indications for surgery for nasal deformity

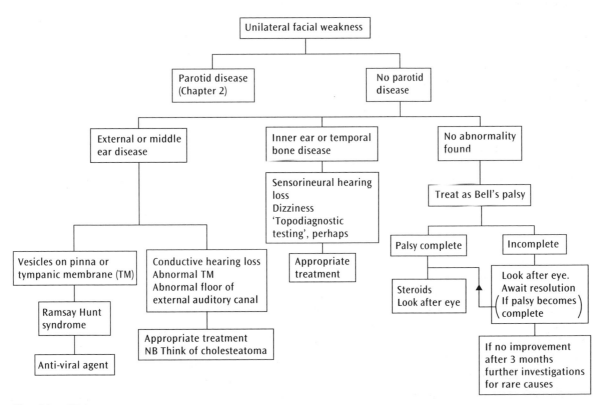

Algorithm 17.4

Nasal trauma

Nasal injuries are common and usually result from a blow to the nose. In the *multiply injured patient* a nasal injury is usually of low priority, but if bleeding from the nose is significant the procedure outlined in the section on epistaxis should be followed. Usually, bleeding settles and the more common situation is the patient who appears to have an isolated nasal injury.

Assessment of such a patient focuses on three areas – *nasal skeleton*, *nasal septum* and *associated injuries.*

Nasal skeleton

Assessment of the nasal skeleton is often difficult immediately following an injury because of swelling of the overlying and surrounding tissues which may also cause a deformity without underlying structural damage.

Is the nose deformed? When the nose was normal previously, the observed deformity in the shape of the nose must be assessed. Two parts of the external nose should be considered: the *nasal bones* (comprising the bony nasal bridge) and the *cartilaginous dorsum* (running from the tip of the nasal bones to the tip of the nose). Palpation of the nasal bones is often unnecessary and painful but may be appropriate if the bony bridge appears straight and the deviation is in the cartilaginous dorsum. If it is felt that the nose may be deformed the patient is reviewed 7 days post-injury, to allow the swelling to subside and a more accurate assessment to be made.

When a patient is convinced that the nose is deformed, a fracture can be obvious on gentle palpation, although firm palpation is sometimes required to feel a fracture and to elicit pain or discomfort. If deformity is minimal, a history of previous trauma should be queried since often a patient may be unaware of a slightly deviated nose from an old fracture. Photographic records may be helpful. In general radiography of the nasal bones at this stage (or indeed at the time of injury) is of no benefit. With reasonable evidence of a fracture, *manipulation* of the nose under anaesthetic is carried out. Lateral deviations are corrected by digital pressure laterally and if the reduced bones are unstable a Plaster of Paris (POP) splint is applied in order to prevent re-fracture when the patient rolls over in bed. Treatment of fractures in which the nasal bones have been pushed posteriorly and been depressed relative to the surrounding bony structures is more complex and may involve intra- and extra-nasal splinting or packing.

If the deformity is entirely due to a deviated cartilaginous dorsum, with intact nasal bones, manipulation is unlikely to be effective.

Nasal septum

The nasal septum should be assessed at the time of initial presentation. An important complication of nasal trauma is a *septal haematoma*: the blood collects between the mucoperichondrium of the septum and the septal cartilage. This leads to bilateral nasal obstruction but more importantly it deprives the septal cartilage of the blood supply it receives from the mucoperichondrium and can result in necrosis of the cartilage. A haematoma may become infected producing a *septal abscess*, and spread of infection to the cavernous sinus with serious intra-cranial sequelae. A nasal septal haematoma should be drained immediately. Aspiration is rarely as successful as formal drainage. Drainage should be followed by nasal packing to keep the mucoperichondrium against the septal cartilage.

Bilateral nasal obstruction due to a septal haematoma is rare. *Unilateral* obstruction due to a *fracture of the nasal septal cartilage* is much more common. It manifests as deviation of the cartilaginous dorsum. Repositioning displaced nasal bones may improve the position of the dorsum but it is rarely possible to reposition an internally displaced septum successfully. Manipulation of a deviated cartilage under anaesthetic is not warranted.

Associated injuries

It is easy to overlook associated injuries unless these are specifically sought. Examination should aim at assessing tenderness or deformity of the zygomatic arches and maxilla, sensation in the distribution of the three divisions of the trigeminal nerve, external ocular movements and jaw opening and closure.

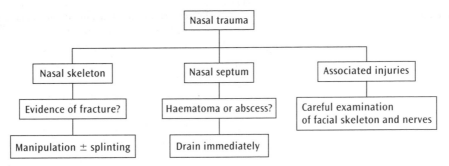

Algorithm 17.5

In this way fractures of other bones of the facial skeleton are not overlooked.

NASAL DEFORMITY

Nasal deformities may be congenital or acquired. The distinction can be difficult but is rarely of practical concern. The subject of congenital deformities, including cosmetic surgery to noses deemed to be of imperfect size or shape, is beyond the scope of this chapter. Acquired deformities of the nose are however relatively common. They are often accompanied by deformities of the nasal septum which may produce nasal obstruction (*see* 'Blocked and runny nose', p. 249).

The patient with an abnormal nasal appearance is usually seeking some form of surgical correction of a perceived deformity: that is, a *rhinoplasty*, and if a nasal septal deformity also needs correction, a *septo-rhinoplasty*. In assessing these patients the primary care physician and general otolaryngologist or plastic surgeon might require the assistance of a psychologist or psychiatrist. Advanced surgical techniques have been developed for correcting some of the more complex nasal deformities that require the expertise of a specialist rhinoplasty surgeon.

It is important to establish the nature of the deformity.

Deviated nose

A deviated nose may result from deviation of the nasal bones, the cartilaginous septum or both. A hump along the dorsum of the nose may also be primarily bony or cartilaginous or may be a combination of these two.

Other nasal deformities include: *'saddle' deformity*, where there is a hollow depression about a centimetre above the tip of the nose, due to loss of the internal support of this part of the cartilaginous dorsum; *abnormalities of the nasal tip* – too wide or narrow, protruding from the face too much or too little, or pointing upwards or downwards; and *deformities of the alar rim of the nose or the columella*.

When no deformity is evident, explanation, reassurance and counselling are clearly required.

The patient with an obvious deformity should be introduced to the concept of the rhinoplasty 'ladder', which grades noses as *Beautiful*, *Normal*, *Deformed*, *Horrible*. Whatever the starting point, it is generally possible only to move one step up to the next 'rung' of the ladder. For example, to go from a *horrible* nose to a *beautiful* nose is impossible, whereas a *deformed* nose can be rendered *normal* but not *beautiful*. The patient who understands this is less likely to be disappointed with the result of his surgery. The management pathway adopted should be:

- *Deformity amenable to surgery and patient expectations appropriate*: proceed to rhinoplasty surgery.
- *Deformity amenable to surgery but expectations inappropriate*: further counselling and discussion required before proceeding to surgery.
- *Deformity not amenable to surgery*: as always, if a specific surgeon does not have the specialist skills required to correct a specific type or degree of deformity the patient should be referred to a specialist colleague. Whilst this opportunity must

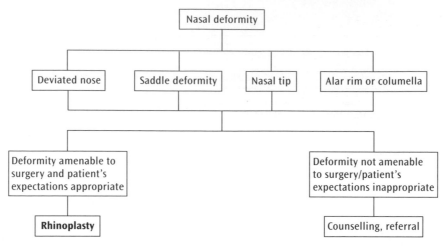

Algorithm 17.6

never be denied to patients when appropriate advice or treatment is available elsewhere, the patient with unrealistic expectations and subtle or difficult deformities should be warned against seeking treatment without proper consultation with the general practitioner.

Rhinoplasty surgery

Many techniques are available for correcting nasal deformities. Most procedures are undertaken intra-nasally, avoiding scars on the outside of the nose, although external rhinoplasty is preferred in some cases. The incisions for such surgery usually only produce small scars across the columella. Cartilage and bone can be removed from the nasal dorsum after the skin and soft tissues have been elevated from the nasal skeleton. The nasal bones can be re-positioned after they have been mobilized.

After surgery, the skin over the nose is taped to prevent haematoma and soft tissue swelling in the planes created when the tissues were elevated, and a plastic or POP splint is applied externally to prevent displacement of the nasal bones in the immediate post-operative period.

The 'final' result of rhinoplasty surgery will not be evident for 12–18 months following surgery and the patient should be warned of this. Maturation and remodelling of soft tissues is a dynamic process which lasts for at least this period.

HIGHLIGHTS

- Examination of the nasal skeleton can be difficult immediately following an injury because of tissue oedema
- A septal haematoma or abscess requires immediate drainage
- An associated maxillo-facial injury should be excluded
- Patients should be carefully selected for cosmetic rhinoplasty

OTALGIA

AIM

1 Be aware of the causes of otalgia

Pain in the ear – earache or *otalgia* – is common. Sometimes it is caused by disease of the ear and it is important always to consider the other cardinal symptoms of ear disease (*see* 'Discharging ear', p. 227). But more importantly it must always be borne in mind that pain in the ear does not necessarily reflect disease in this region. 'Referred' otalgia – pain referred to the ear from disease at another site – is common.

The first practical question to be addressed is the following. Is there evidence of *local ear* disease?

Local ear disease present

The initial history and examination should focus on the pinna, external auditory canal and middle ear. One should look particularly for signs of inflammation and infection in these regions as these are the main causes of pain at this site.

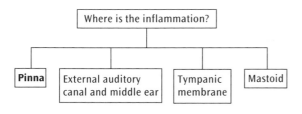

Pinna

Inflammation of the pinna is usually secondary to *otitis externa* and reflects spread of infection from the tissues of the cartilaginous external canal. Infection of the cartilage of the pinna results in *peri-chondritis*. This is an exquisitely tender condition that may also complicate injury or any operation involving the cartilage (e.g., mastoid surgery for the treatment of cholesteatoma, drainage of a haematoma of the pinna). Prompt treatment, with systemic antibiotics and if necessary incision and drainage of any resulting abscess, is mandatory if destruction of the cartilage is to be avoided.

Herpetic lesions may be seen on the pinna in *herpes zoster oticus* (*Ramsay Hunt syndrome*).

Tumours of the pinna are rare and not usually painful unless infected or involving nerve or cartilage. An unusual condition – *chondrodermatitis nodularis helicis* – presents with small painful lesions on the rim of the helix, most often in elderly men. Inflammation of the cartilage and skin (*chondrodermatitis*) occurs in nodules (*nodularis*) on the helix (*helicis*).

External auditory canal

Otitis externa is the most common cause of otalgia due to disease of the external auditory canal (EAC). *Furunculosis* can be particularly painful. Severe pain may be a sign of so-called *malignant otitis externa*.

The herpetic lesions of herpes zoster oticus may only be visible within the EAC.

Tympanic membrane and middle ear

An abnormality of the tympanic membrane in the patient with otalgia may reflect disease of the membrane itself or the middle ear. *Bullous myringitis* is thought to be due to a viral infection of the tympanic membrane, often associated with an upper respiratory tract infection. Red vesicles appear on the surface of the drum, and occasionally a secretory middle ear effusion is seen. It is a painful but self-limiting condition. Treatment is with analgesics.

Acute otitis media is one of the most common causes of otalgia, especially in children. In this group *otitis media with effusion* (*glue ear*) is also common and children complain of intermittent otalgia without necessarily suffering from superimposed acute infections. Otitis media with effusion may also occur in adults with acute onset. It may follow an upper respiratory tract infection or an episode of *barotrauma*. The pressure changes associated with changes in altitude and depth whilst in planes or when diving can result in the rapid accumulation of middle ear effusion. Treatment is with analgesics, decongestants and drainage via a myringotomy.

Mastoid

Swelling and pain behind the ear over the mastoid may be a feature of *mastoiditis*. However, this condition is much rarer than it used to be and more often the symptoms and signs are due to infection in the post-auricular lymph nodes, secondary to otitis externa or otitis media. When mastoiditis *does* occur it is due to spread of infection to the mastoid air cells from the middle ear cleft and so one expects to see an abnormal tympanic membrane with signs of middle ear infection. In the current age of antibiotics usage, '*masked*' *mastoiditis* is sometimes seen. Mastoid infection follows partially treated acute otitis media and the symptoms of mastoid infection are in part 'masked' by the effect of the antibiotics in reducing the degree of infection. Although rare, it is important not to miss the diagnosis of mastoiditis.

Normal appearance of vocal cords

Assessment of the normality or otherwise of the vocal cords requires considerable expertise. The range of 'normality' is broad. Subtle oedematous changes or small areas of *leukoplakia* (white patches) may be missed as may small polyps suspended below the free edge of otherwise normally appearing cords. It is imperative to examine the *full* length of the cords. The anterior commissure may be difficult to visualize with the mirror and nasendoscopy might be more effective.

If one is satisfied that the cords are indeed normal in appearance, a second question is posed.

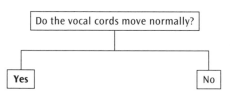

Normal vocal cord movement

It is unusual to find perfectly normal vocal cord movement and normal vocal cord appearance in a hoarse patient. This should raise the possibility that the cause of the hoarseness might lie elsewhere (in the sub-glottis or poorly visualized supra-glottis). Normal voice requires a steady column of exhaled air which may be compromised by pulmonary pathology resulting in dysphonia; a full respiratory assessment may be required.

Abnormal vocal cord movement

There are several well-recognized patterns of abnormal vocal cord movement. The simplest of these is a *unilateral vocal cord palsy*.

Unilateral vocal cord palsy

The palsied cord may be in an abducted or adducted (in the latter case in either the median or paramedian) position. The non-paralysed cord may meet the palsied cord satisfactorily on phonation or may fail to do so, resulting in a persistant glottic 'chink'. Left vocal

Table 17.2 *Causes of recurrent laryngeal nerve palsies*

Malignant disease (lung carcinoma, thyroid tumours, etc.)	25%
Surgical trauma (thyroid surgery)	20%
Inflammatory (pulmonary TB)	13%
Idiopathic	13%
Non-surgical trauma (aneurysm, neck trauma, left atrial hypertrophy)	11%
Other	11%
Neurological (CVA, etc.)	7%

cord palsies are more common than right due to the longer course of the left recurrent laryngeal nerve.

Although many unilateral cord palsies are idiopathic, the patient requires comprehensive investigation to exclude underlying disease (Table 17.2).

Investigations include a plain chest radiograph and a CT scan of the neck from (and including) the skull base to the aortic arch, in order to encompass the full extra-cranial course of the recurrent laryngeal nerves. In some patients, pan-endoscopy (laryngoscopy, pharyngoscopy, oesophagoscopy, bronchoscopy and formal examination of the post-nasal space) will be required if these investigations are negative. A positive investigation result may dictate more specific invasive investigations.

In many cases, treatment of the underlying condition will not be followed by recovery of the palsy. However, a process of compensation often occurs in which the non-palsied cord is able to cross the midline to meet its neighbour resulting in complete closure of the glottic aperture and an improvement in the voice. In some cases this does not occur. In this instance surgical procedures are available to medialize a palsied cord lying in an abducted position. These include *medialization thyroplasty* with a silastic strut and *vocal cord injection* with Teflon or collagen, and are only to be performed when it is clear that a palsy will not recover. Idiopathic vocal cord paresis may recover spontaneously up to 6 months after onset, and hence these procedures should not be considered in such patients within this time period.

Bilateral vocal cord palsies

These are uncommon and are most often seen as a consequence of thyroid surgery. If the cords are both adducted the patient often has a good voice, but at the expense of breathing difficulties which are more likely to present immediately post-operatively (when airway obstruction follows extubation) or later with stridor. If both cords are abducted the patient is *aphonic*. A normal voice can usually only be restored if the patient is provided with a tracheostomy for breathing.

Reduced vocal cord movement

Patients with so-called functional dysphonia secondary to inappropriate voice use may have bowing of the vocal cords so that the glottic aperture is not completely closed on phonation. Other abnormalities characterized by reduced vocal cord movement are rare.

Abnormal appearance of vocal cords

Both benign and malignant pathology may result in an abnormal appearance of the vocal cords. In some cases it is possible to distinguish these on clinical examination. Symmetry of clinical findings is more often found in benign conditions, but when in doubt as to the nature of laryngeal pathology the appropriate biopsy should be undertaken.

As a guide to which patients need such an intervention, the following question should be asked.

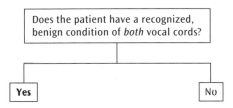

Pathognomonic benign appearance of vocal cords

In patients who have abused their voices by shouting, singing, talking excessively, etc., certain conditions are often encountered. *Singer's nodules* (a misnomer as they frequently occur in non-singers) are small, white nodules arising on the free edge of both vocal cords at the junction of the anterior and middle third. *Reinke's oedema* refers to a condition in which both vocal cords are oedematous and swollen, with a dull, gray appearance. This oedema may progress to *polyp*

formation of one or both cords. Small nodules and limited oedema can often be corrected by a course of speech therapy and vocal hygiene advice. Further management is highly specialized and somewhat controversial; expert advice should be sought.

Abnormal appearance or diagnostic uncertainty

Malignant or benign disease may produce a larynx of abnormal appearance. The appearances of malignant disease (almost invariably *squamous cell carcinoma*) vary. At one extreme, *carcinoma in situ* may appear as an area of leukoplakia. This is a descriptive term referring simply to a 'white patch' and should not be taken to be synonymous with any particular diagnosis. Although malignancy is a possibility it may also be caused by *epithelial hyperplasia* and *hyperkeratosis*. Carcinomas may also appear as small plaques or polyps, or as ulcerating or exophytic lesions. Infiltration of surrounding tissues may be manifested as limitation of vocal cord movement or complete fixation.

In all these situations, and in any case of diagnostic uncertainty, the patient should undergo *direct laryngoscopy* or *microlaryngoscopy* (direct laryngoscopy using a microscope) to obtain tissue for histological examination. Chest radiography rules out metastatic disease as may CT of the neck. This will also help determine local spread of malignancy. A contrast swallowing study may be indicated for similar reasons.

A full description of the treatment of benign and malignant laryngeal disease is beyond the scope of this chapter. Suffice to say that treatment may involve local excision, extended local excision (laryngectomy – complete or partial, or laryngo-pharyngectomy), radiotherapy with or without chemotherapy and

---

HIGHLIGHTS

- Hoarseness for more than 4 weeks should be investigated
- Abnormality in vocal cord appearance is indicative of local pathology
- Abnormal vocal cord movement is the result of recurrent laryngeal nerve palsy, and when unilateral is usually due to malignancy

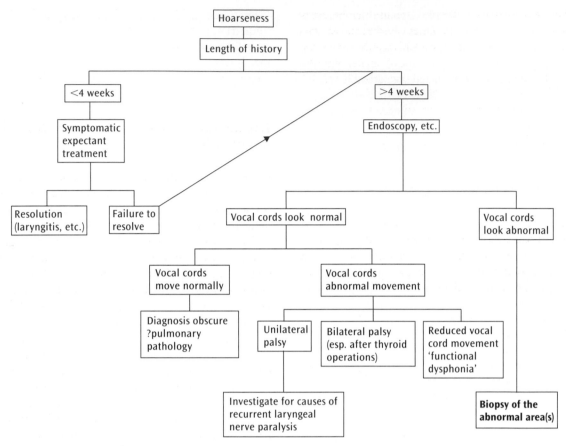

Algorithm 17.8

radical or selective neck dissection. One or more of these treatments may be used simultaneously or sequentially.

STRIDOR IN ADULTS

AIMS

1 Develop a clear and rational approach to the management of the stridulous patient
2 Be aware of the options available in management

Stridor is the noise made when breathing is obstructed in the upper airways. It is an important and serious

sign which requires specialist ENT assistance for further treatment unless the patient is *in extremis* when immediate action may be life-saving.

The type of stridor acts as a *guide* to the site of obstruction:

- *Inspiratory stridor*: larynx or above.
- *Biphasic stridor*: trachea.
- *Expiratory stridor*: bronchi.

On encountering a stridulous patient the patient's respiratory condition should be assessed as rapidly as possible. Intervention is required well before the point at which respiratory failure develops into respiratory arrest. Assessment includes looking for cyanosis and pallor, signs of use of the accessory muscles of respiration, tachycardia and tachypnoea. Stridor which is becoming quieter *may* be an ominous sign reflecting *reduced* air entry and a tiring patient.

If pulse oximetry is available it is a useful measure of oxygenation. These measurements determine whether the patient's airway must be secured instantly or not.

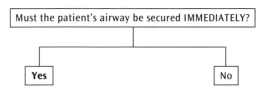

Airway needs securing immediately

Immediate securing of the airway demands intubation or some form of tracheostomy. The help of the resuscitation team should be sought, and in the interim, *Heliox* administered by mask. Heliox is a mixture of oxygen and helium. It has a lower viscosity than pure oxygen and so can more easily pass narrowed airways to the lungs. Dependent on the clinical response, a decision as to whether intubation is necessary can be made.

If an anaesthetist or other experienced personnel are present it is reasonable to attempt per oral intubation which, if successful, leads to further management as described below (*see* 'Airway secure', p. 248). However, if the facilities for intubation are unavailable, or the attempt unsuccessful, the airway can be secured by puncturing the cricothyroid membrane, which is found by running a finger down the front of the neck from the laryngeal prominence and feeling for the gap between the lower border of the thyroid cartilage and the cricoid ring. Various devices are available for performing a cricothyroidotomy but any sharp blade or a wide bore needle (such as a large intravenous cannula) can be used. Once the airway is entered a tube of some form is placed. A large gauge needle is suitable for the entire procedure.

If this is ineffective and a more formal emergency tracheostomy is required a mid-line incision is made over the upper trachea (so as to avoid other vital structures) and through soft tissue (which may include the highly vascular thyroid isthmus) until the trachea is reached. The second, third and fourth tracheal rings are divided longitudinally and a tube is inserted. Once the airway is secure, 100% oxygen is administered, and assisted artificial ventilation can be instituted if required (*see* 'Airway secure').

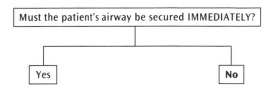

The airway does not need to be secured immediately

If there is time to assess the patient's clinical situation more fully and to institute supportive treatment, it is still advisable to seek anaesthetic and ENT involvement at this stage.

Supportive treatment includes Heliox or oxygen by mask, establishing intravenous access, and since in many causes of stridor there is an element of oedema, an intravenous bolus injection of corticosteroid is often appropriate. Nebulized adrenaline should also be considered to dilate the lower airways.

The patient's clinical response is reconsidered. Should the condition be deteriorating then the airway needs to be secured immediately as already described. Should the patient remain stable, a full history and examination are carried out. It may be evident that the patient's condition has remained stable over a period of some days or weeks even though the stridor may be loud and the breathing laboured. Alternatively, the stridor may progress and deteriorate over 12–24 hours, when the question of concern is:

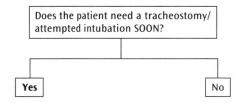

Patient needs airway securing soon

In these circumstances immediate arrangements are made to transfer the patient to the operating theatre for urgent tracheostomy. The anaesthetic team should be advised of the situation and should assess the patient. Senior anaesthetic personnel are required. In general, *intubation*, if this can be done safely, is preferable to *tracheostomy*.

Once the surgical team has prepared the patient's neck with antiseptic and injected local anaesthetic into the tracheostomy site in readiness for a formal tracheostomy, the anaesthetic staff should attempt intubation. This is a difficult procedure. It may be preferable to attempt intubation with the fibre-optic bronchoscope and the patient sitting up. Failed intubation may result in two situations. If an airway can be maintained using a mask, the tracheostomy can proceed under local anaesthetic, the patient lying or sitting, speedily but without undue haste; otherwise, urgent tracheostomy should be performed.

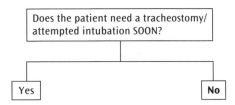

Patient does *not* need airway securing soon

A patient whose airway is not critically embarrassed gives an opportunity for further examination and investigation. The most important part of the examination is that of the larynx, indirectly with a mirror, but in many patients the fibre-optic nasendoscope is necessary. If the supra-glottis and glottis are completely normal the problem must lie in the sub-glottis or trachea. It is important to know this in the event that the patient's condition deteriorates. Obstruction below the sub-glottis will not be alleviated by a cricothyroidotomy which by definition enters the sub-glottis. Obstruction of the middle or lower trachea may make entering the trachea at the level of rings two to four difficult or impossible.

A soft-tissue radiograph of the neck will demonstrate the upper trachea, larynx, epiglottis, tongue base and retro-pharyngeal tissues, all of which may be abnormal. A chest radiograph will demonstrate any soft tissue swelling impinging on the trachea or narrowing it. Further information may be obtained from a CT scan of this region. However, radiology departments are not safe places for people with significant airway obstruction and it may be appropriate to delay investigations to a later stage.

Table 17.3 *Causes of stridor in adults*

Congenital	Usually present in childhood
Acquired	Traumatic
	Direct injuries: blunt trauma; penetrating injuries; burns and scalds; radiotherapy; foreign bodies; intubation injuries or sequelae
	Infection: acute laryngitis; acute supra-glottitis; diphtheria; peri-chondritis
	Inflammatory: Wegener's granulomatosis; peri-chondritis; rheumatoid arthritis
	Neoplastic: benign: laryngeal papillomata; laryngeal polyp(s); malignant: squamous cell carcinoma of the supra-glottis, glottis, and sub-glottis
	Neurological: bilateral vocal cord palsies with cords adducted

Airway secure

Once the airway is secure there is often the opportunity for further investigation. Successful *intubation* should be followed by laryngoscopy to determine the cause of the stridor. If this is likely to be temporary, for example an infective supra-glottitis, tracheostomy should be avoided and the patient is left intubated in an appropriate high dependency unit until the problem has resolved and extubation is safe. If a long-term problem is identified, such as a large laryngeal tumour, appropriate biopsies should be taken and then a formal tracheostomy performed. If a *tracheostomy* has been necessary it should also be followed by direct laryngoscopy to establish a diagnosis. Table 17.3 outlines the causes of stridor in adults. The most common causes in hospital practice are malignant disease and supra-glottitis.

HIGHLIGHTS

- Securing the airway is the initial primary objective
- Intubation can be a difficult procedure
- Laryngoscopy should be a standard investigation

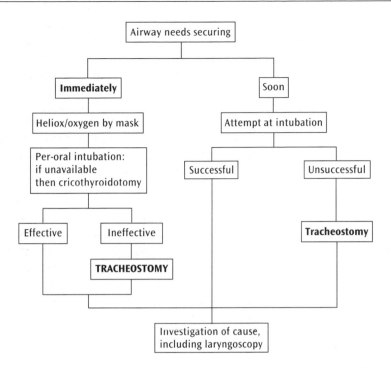

Algorithm 17.9

BLOCKED AND RUNNY NOSE

AIMS

1 Understand the difference between nasal problems due to localized structural abnormalities and those due to systemic disturbances
2 Recognize the symptoms and signs of sinister sino-nasal disease

Nasal blockage and nasal discharge – *rhinorrhea* – are common nasal symptoms. The nostrils are separated by the nasal septum. If a patient has *unilateral* symptoms it is reasonable to expect a localized disease process. Conversely, *bilateral* symptoms are more likely to be due to a systemic disorder. For example, allergy affects the nasal lining bilaterally, producing bilateral blockage or discharge, whereas nasal blockage due to a tumour is likely to affect one side of the nose only, unless and until it is huge.

The majority of cases of nasal blockage and rhinorrhea can be considered under two broad headings: *rhinitis* and *mechanical obstruction*. Rhinitis implies inflammation of the nasal lining. Inflammation is associated with swelling and, in the nose, often with the production of excess mucus. As the nasal lining is continuous with the lining of the paranasal sinuses, the latter may also become inflamed, resulting in rhino-sinusitis.

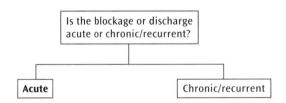

Acute nasal blockage and/or rhinorrhea

The blockage or discharge may be bilateral or unilateral.

Acute bilateral nasal blockage and/or rhinorrhea

Acute rhinitis. Infection, usually the *common cold*, is the most common cause of acute rhinitis. Several organisms have been identified; most are viral, commonly of the rhinovirus group. Bacterial infection can supervene and bacterial sinusitis follows a 'cold' in up to 10% of patients. In most cases of 'cold', antibiotics are not indicated. Simple measure such as rest, increased fluid intake and a short course (not more than 10 days) of a nasal decongestant, such as ephedrine or xylometazoline, are usually sufficient.

Acute sinusitis is characterized by purulent nasal discharge, pain in the regions of the sinuses (cheeks, inter- and supra-orbital regions) and systemic disturbance with fever, malaise, etc. Oedema of the mucosa of the nose and sinuses produces obstruction of the relatively narrow sinus ostia. This process is more likely to occur in those with pre-existing mucosal oedema and with narrow sinus ostia. This patient group includes a large proportion who have so-called 'ostio-meatal complex disease' as a result of allergic or non-allergic rhinitis (*see below*).

Initial treatment is with oral antibiotics, decongestants and topical nasal steroids. If this regime fails it may be necessary to use more potent intravenous antibiotics and to drain surgically the sinus or sinuses involved. The maxillary antrum alone may be affected or infection may involve the frontal or ethmoid sinuses. Infection of these sinuses can spread to adjacent regions, including the orbit, and intra-cranially. Hence sinusitis should be taken seriously if simple therapeutic measures are unsuccessful. This is particularly true of children with ethmoidal sinusitis where the orbital contents may be at risk.

Septal haematoma; *septal abcess*. See 'Nasal trauma and nasal deformity', p. 237.

Acute unilateral nasal blockage and/or rhinorrhea

Foreign body in the nose. Nasal foreign bodies are common in children and may produce a discharge which in turn may lead to *vestibulitis*. Inorganic materials are less irritant and may remain undetected for long periods. Foreign bodies should be removed, which can be difficult in children, particularly if attempted with inappropriate instruments and inadequate illumination. Often, a short general anaesthetic is required. Sometimes the object is best retrieved via the nasopharynx. Both nasal cavities should be inspected after removal and suction of the nose as there may be more than one foreign body.

Acute nasal septal deviation. See 'Nasal trauma and nasal deformity', p. 237.

CSF rhinorrhea. If the dura and bone separating the CSF space and nasal cavity is breached CSF escapes into the nose or the ear. This may occur as a result of *trauma* causing a basal skull fracture or, more rarely, *spontaneously* as a result of hydrocephalus or a brain tumour eroding bone and dura. It may be *iatrogenic*, following intra-nasal surgery. A clear watery nasal discharge of CSF is distinguished from nasal mucus by its high glucose content, but now it is more usual to look for the presence of beta-2-transferrin. Management depends on the precise cause. Most leaks settle spontaneously, although prophylactic broad spectrum antibiotics (e.g., ampicillin and flucloxacillin) are advisable. Surgical repair of the dural tear is necessary if the discharge persists.

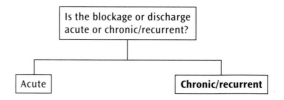

Chronic or recurrent nasal blockage and/or rhinorrhea

Chronic bilateral nasal blockage and/or rhinorrhea

This is an extremely common combination of symptoms and one which consumes huge resources. A clue to the possible cause of the obstruction can be obtained by asking: Is the blockage or discharge intermittent or constant?

Intermittent. Intermittent symptoms, obstruction which fluctuates in severity or from side to side, implies a fluctuating pathological process. The most common cause is *chronic rhinitis*. Although some patients with these symptoms also experience frequent pain in the sinuses and are labelled as suffering from chronic 'sinusitis' it is more correct, and clinically more appropriate, to consider these patients as having *chronic rhinosinusitis* – almost invariably the symptoms are related to nasal problems.

Blocked and runny nose 251

Patients fall into two broad groups, the allergic and non-allergic, which may be identified by the symptoms and signs. There are few *nasal* signs which allow allergic patients to be distinguished from the non-allergic. Nor is the nasal history always helpful; nasal obstruction, rhinorrhea and sneezing are common to both.

Allergic rhinitis. The history may reveal an allergic tendency with asthma, eczema, etc., or a strong family history thereof. The patients may say that they have 'hay fever', are allergic to cats, dust, etc. Allergy of this type is very common and two sub-groups of patients can often be identified. Those with *seasonal allergic rhinitis*, the allergens being pollens, etc., of different types present only at certain times of the year, and those with *perennial allergic rhinitis*, allergic to material present year-round such as feathers, cats, or dust, who suffer all the time. House dust mite is ubiquitous in even the cleanest home and is a common allergen. Allergens may be ingested; these include eggs, milk, nuts, etc. The practical difficulty is to determine to what exactly the patient is allergic. Skin testing is possible but usually only against a specific set of allergens. Radio-allergosorbent testing (RAST) aims to determine the presence of circulating IgE specifically produced in response to a battery of tested substances. There has been much argument about the value of these tests. Skin testing has an established place in British practice, RAST less so.

Management of allergic rhinitis involves: *allergen avoidance* if possible, this may include changing bedding containing feathers, removing carpets and curtains, vacuuming matresses, etc.; *regular topical nasal steroids* in the form of beclomethasone diproprionate or related compounds; *occasional courses of more potent topical steroids,* such as betamethasone sodium phosphate, or in severe cases, a *short course of oral steroids*. In addition, *oral anti-histamines* may be useful; the newer non-sedating varieties are preferred. Nasal sodium cromoglycate may be of some value. The only role for surgery is in reducing the bulk of tissue obstructing the nose. Often, the *inferior turbinates (conchae)* are swollen and these can be trimmed or debulked in a variety of ways. Surgery on this highly vascular region may be associated with significant post-operative bleeding. A deviated septum may be contributing to nasal obstruction. Correction of this deformity with a septoplasty or SMR

procedure, although it will not alter the underlying allergic tendency, may improve the airways.

Non-allergic rhinitis. This is a heterogeneous group, including rare chronic infective problems, uncommon inflammatory conditions but most importantly a disorder referred to as *vasomotor rhinitis*. In this condition the normal fine balance between the sympathetic nerve supply to the nasal vasculature (producing shrinkage of the nasal lining and decreasing mucus production) and the parasympathetic supply (producing swelling of the lining and increasing mucus production) is disturbed. A relative predominance of parasympathetic tone produces symptoms similar to those in allergic rhinitis. A variety of causes have been identified, including medication, hormonal, emotional and environmental factors such as dust, irritants and temperature changes.

Management is similar to that described above. *Non-invasive measures* include humidification of the ambient environment, maintaining a cool moist rather than a warm, dry environment, elimination of smoke and irritants, etc. *Topical nasal steroids* can be used; nasal *ipratropium bromide* has been shown to be effective in patients in whom rhinorrhea is the predominant symptom. Anti-histamines are of value only if there is an allergic *element*. Surgical treatment in the form of turbinate surgery as described above is also possible. Similarly, septoplasty or SMR may be of value.

Constant symptoms. If a patient's symptoms are constant, this may be because the degree of allergy or intra-nasal swelling is such that the nose is constantly blocked. Alternatively, the patient may have *nasal polyps*.

Nasal polyps. Classical nasal polyps are a result of prolonged mucosal oedema in the nose and sinuses. The consequence of this process is that the lining of the ethmoid sinuses prolapses out through the ostia into the nasal cavity. The 'polyp' looks like a peeled grape and consists of a mucosal sac full of fluid. Allergy and infection are believed to be responsible. As the polyps grow they produce nasal obstruction which is usually bilateral. They can be treated medically or surgically. Smaller polyps will shrink when *topical nasal steroids* are applied, and this effect may be enhanced by the use of a short course of *oral steroids*, although the risks and benefit of this course of action must be assessed carefully. Alternatively, the polyps may be removed surgically. *Intra-nasal polypectomy* was traditionally performed by use of a nasal 'snare', but increasingly this is being done under endoscopic control. If polyps recur, as many do, the 'roots' can be removed by performing an *ethmoidectomy*. Again, the classic *external ethmoidectomy* approach is being replaced by *endoscopic ethmoidectomy*, one of the procedures which constitutes '*functional endoscopic sinus surgery*' (FESS).

Unilateral nasal polyps require separate consideration.

Chronic unilateral nasal blockage and/or rhinorrhea

Chronic and predominantly unilateral symptoms, in particular nasal blockage, may be seen in some patients with the conditions outlined above: foreign bodies in the nose; nasal septal deviation; nasal and para-nasal polyps. The unilaterality sometimes reflects the fact that there is a minor degree of asymmetry within the nose and only one side appears to be compromised by mucosal swelling.

Several of the conditions mentioned above under 'acute' problems may become chronic. These are: *foreign body in the nose*; *nasal septal deviation*; and nasal and para-nasal polyps or tumours.

Nasal polyp. A unilateral nasal polyp is a cause for concern as it may indicate more sinister, localized pathology. A truly unilateral nasal polyp should always be removed for histological examination to exclude a *sino-nasal malignancy*. However, endoscopic examination of the nose will often reveal that an apparent unilateral polyp is not so, smaller and symptomless polyps being present on the opposite side.

Antrochoanal polyp. This type of polyp is not malignant but is closely related to ordinary nasal polyps. The maxillary sinus lining becomes swollen and prolapses into the nasal cavity, it is drawn backwards towards the posterior choana as it enlarges,

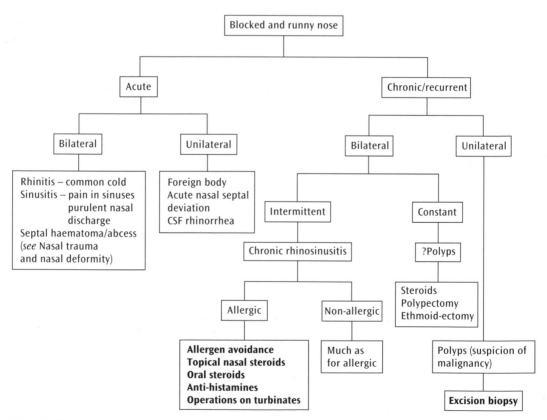

Algorithm 17.10

resulting in a large polyp, dumb-bell in shape; one bulbous end occupying the antrum, the isthmus passing through the maxillary ostium and the other bulbous end in the posterior choana. The polyp can usually be snared.

Malignant and other polyps. Malignant polyps are rare. *Tumours of the para-nasal sinuses* can erode into any adjacent structure, including the facial skin, orbit, roof of the mouth, pterygoid fossa, etc. Swelling and inflammation of the facial skin is 'never' due to simple sinusitis. Usually this is related to dental disease but if the teeth are normal one must always suspect malignancy in the antrum. CT scan is a helpful investigation when in doubt. Nasal polyps are extremely rare in children except those with *cystic fibrosis* and hence a child with polyps should have a sweat test and a paediatric referral.

HIGHLIGHTS

- A unilateral nasal discharge in a child is due to a foreign body until proven otherwise
- Allergic and non-allergic rhinitis can be difficult to differentiate
- Unilateral sino-nasal symptoms may herald the presence of an underlying malignancy
- Swelling of the cheek is 'never' due to maxillary sinusitis

---

HEARING LOSS

AIMS

1 Understand the difference between conductive and sensorineural deafness and be able to distinguish them
2 Appreciate which patients with hearing loss require further investigation

---

The assessment and management of patients with hearing problems is an important field. The specialties of audiology and audiological medicine are devoted to it. For the generalist faced with a patient who believes that his or her hearing is sub-optimal, or indeed whose relatives are convinced of this even if the patient is not, what follows is a simple initial approach.

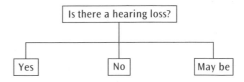

Most adults will present with the certainty that they have a hearing problem. In a few cases formal audiological testing with a *pure-tone audiogram* (PTA) will be the only way of assessing this. The management of young children is beyond the scope of this chapter but in this group the presence or otherwise of a hearing loss may be extremely difficult to determine.

In the clinic or surgery, simple voice tests may allow a rough assessment of the presence or otherwise of a hearing loss and the side which is involved if it is unilateral.

Hearing loss present

Hearing loss may be due to: disease of the mechanical part of the hearing mechanism in the external or middle ear (the external canal, tympanic membrane or ossicular chain) or to damage to the sensory cells in the inner ear (cochlea) or its neural connections (the VIIIth cranial nerve). Disease confined to the more central neural connections is extremely rare. In the first instance the hearing loss (HL) is said to be *conductive* (CHL), in the second, *sensorineural* (SNHL). The two types may occur independently or together. It may be possible to distinguish between them with simple tests but this distinction may require a PTA or other audiological tests.

When hearing problems are unilateral and uncomplicated *tuning fork tests* can be helpful. However, complex losses make interpretation of the results very difficult.

Weber's test (Fig. 17.5) involves placing a tuning fork (usually a 512 Hz fork, not a low-frequency fork) in the centre of the forehead and asking the patient whether it is heard louder in the middle or at one side. If it *lateralizes to the deaf ear* then there is a conductive loss in that ear, if it *lateralizes to the non-deaf ear*, that is, to the 'good' ear, the patient has a sensorineural loss in the deaf ear. Only a small hearing loss (5 dB or more) is required for Weber's test to lateralize.

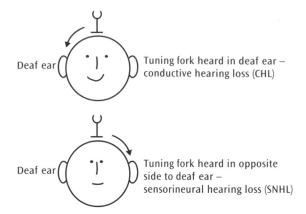

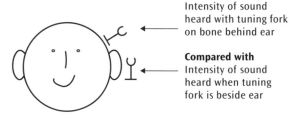

Deaf ear — Tuning fork heard in deaf ear – conductive hearing loss (CHL)

Deaf ear — Tuning fork heard in opposite side to deaf ear – sensorineural hearing loss (SNHL)

Fig. 17.5 *Weber's test.*

Intensity of sound heard with tuning fork on bone behind ear

Compared with
Intensity of sound heard when tuning fork is beside ear

Fig. 17.6 *Rinné's test.*

In *Rinné's test* (Fig. 17.6) the fork is placed beside the ear (tines 2.5 cm from the EAC, parallel to the side of the head) and pressed firmly on the mastoid process – the head supported with the other hand. This compares hearing by air conduction (AC) with hearing by bone conduction (BC). The *normal* patient will hear through air conduction better than bone (AC > BC) as will the patient with a *sensorineural hearing loss* in that ear. This is a 'Rinné positive' result. The patient with a *conductive hearing loss* of 15–20 dB or more will hear bone conduction better than air conduction (BC > AC). This is a 'Rinné negative' result. Thus, there remains a group of patients with a small conductive loss (5–15 dB) who, although their Weber test lateralizes to the deaf ear, will still be Rinné positive – air conduction > bone conduction.

It is important to perform both tests and confirm with voice testing, preferably with a 'masking' device on the ear not being tested, using a 'Baranay box', which is a mechanical clockwork device that produces a loud masking noise. The importance of this lies in the 'false negative Rinné' test. A patient who has no hearing *whatsoever* in one ear may still find

that the tuning fork behind is heard louder than the fork beside that ear. In this situation the vibrations are passing from the mastoid to the *opposite* cochlea. It would obviously be a mistake to assume 'Rinné negative, BC > AC therefore conductive hearing loss in this ear' – only by checking with voice testing will the true situation 'Dead ear' be recognized.

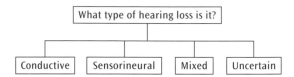

Conductive hearing loss (CHL)

If the patient appears to have a conductive hearing loss one is searching for an abnormality which is disrupting the normal passage of vibrations through the EAC, tympanic membrane and middle ear.

Abnormalities of the EAC and tympanic membrane and their treatment have been described elsewhere in this chapter. Many will be associated with at least some degree of conductive hearing loss. These include otitis externa, furunculosis and tympanic membrane perforations of the 'safe' and 'unsafe' types, as well as patients with fluid in the middle ear cleft behind an intact eardrum, that is, secretory otitis, or *otitis media with effusion* (OME), known in children as *'glue ear'*.

When the EAC and tympanic membrane are normal the problem must lie within the middle ear cleft. The most common disorder is *otosclerosis*, a familial disease of the bone surrounding the stapes footplate which fixes the stapes and hence reduces its ability to vibrate within the oval window. Other causes include fixation or disruption of the ossicular chain.

Patients with purely conductive hearing losses do well with hearing aids. Surgical intervention is also possible, often with good results, but there are no 'absolute' indications for such procedures and risks of surgery (including sensorineural hearing loss) must be weighed against the benefits.

Sensorineural hearing loss (SNHL)

Sensorineural hearing loss (SNHL) is often the manifestation of a systemic process and both ears

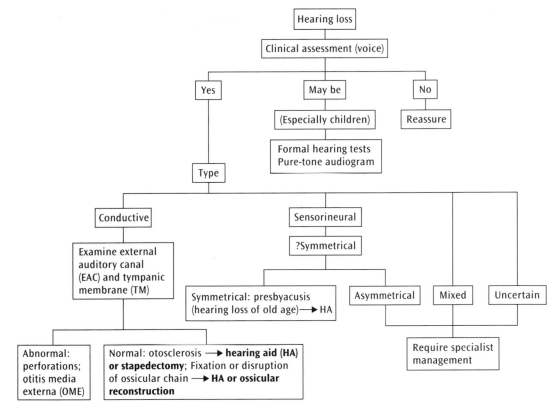

Algorithm 17.11

are affected. It is important, however, to identify that small group of patients in whom a localized disorder is present.

Symmetrical SNHL

SNHL as a consequence of ageing (*presbyacusis*) is extremely common and the diagnosis is easy to make in the elderly patient. Usually both ears are equally affected. Other congenital and acquired causes of sensorineural deafness are less common.

Asymmetrical SNHL

Patients with asymmetrical hearing, or indeed unilateral tinnitus or evidence of unilateral vestibular hypofunction, should be investigated further for a remediable lesion affecting the inner ear or VIIIth

cranial nerve. This involves an MRI scan to image the full course of the nerve from the cochlea to the brainstem. The most common lesion is an *acoustic neuroma*, better termed a *vestibular schwannoma*, which is a benign growth from the neurilemmal covering of the vestibular portion of the VIIIth nerve that produces symptoms by pressure on adjacent structures.

Hearing loss absent

Some patients are found to have normal hearing despite being convinced that their hearing is reduced. In some of these patients a disorder of auditory function probably is present but the PTA is not sufficiently sensitive to detect it. Recently, a phenomenon termed 'obscure auditory dysfunction syndrome' (OADS) has been described in some of these patients.

Possible hearing loss

In children in particular it may not be possible to determine accurately a hearing loss. In these circumstances repeated testing may be necessary but under no circumstances must a deaf child be 'missed'. When in doubt, a specialist referral is mandatory as objective tests of hearing may be required.

HIGHLIGHTS

- Never assume a child can hear; if there is any suggestion of deafness – refer
- Unilateral audio-vestibular symptoms require investigation
- Never forget the 'false negative' Rinné test in the patient with a 'dead' ear

18

Eyes

LYDIA CHANG, MARK WILKINS AND D JOHN BRAZIER

AIMS

1 Differentiate those ocular problems that threaten sight from those that do not
2 Describe the clinical features associated with common ocular problems
3 Understand the treatment principles of these ocular problems

INTRODUCTION

A basic understanding of the anatomy of the eye and visual pathways (Fig. 18.1) allows a non-specialist to recognize the important ocular conditions of relevance in clinical practice. Sometimes there is overlap between systemic and ophthalmic disorders, emphasizing the importance of a comprehensive evaluation of patients with eye symptoms. An essential objective is to recognize those potentially sight-threatening conditions.

CLINICAL EVALUATION

A careful ocular history and clinical examination should be obtained with particular reference to the following.

Ocular history

Visual disturbance can present as a gradual or sudden, painful or painless, uni-ocular or binocular, partial or complete loss of vision. Associated symptoms can include redness, photophobia, discharge, headache, and nausea and vomiting. It is important to elicit a history of trauma, previous intra-ocular surgery and a history of short- or long-sightedness.

- *Medical history*: systemic conditions such as hypertension, diabetes mellitus, inflammatory bowel disease, allergies and other serious illnesses can present with ocular problems.
- *Drug history*: some drugs affect the eye, including steroids, antidepressants, (hydroxy)chloroquine, ethambutol, anticholinergics and tamoxifen.
- *Family history*: squint, some types of glaucoma and early onset cataract may be familial.

Physical examination

This includes all the components of the eye: the orbit, eyelids, conjunctiva, cornea, sclera, anterior chamber and the fundi. Visual function, including visual acuity, visual fields, pupillary reflexes and eye movements, should also be examined (*see* Fig. 18.1 below).

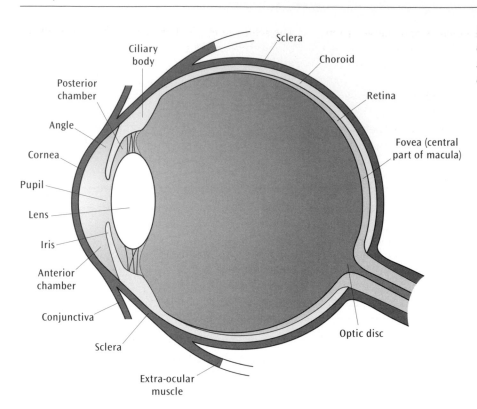

Fig. 18.1 *The anatomy of the eye; horizontal section through the eyeball.*

Eye components

A pen torch is used to examine the external eye. It is possible to identify the following abnormal features: eyelid problems such as oedema, xanthelasma, ptosis, ectropion, exophthalmos, chalazion and basal cell carcinoma. Conjunctival injection or pallor, and swelling due to accumulation of serous fluid leaking from capillaries causing chemosis. Corneal oedema giving it an opaque, ground-glass appearance, corneal ulcers and arcus senilis. The scleral colour may be yellow due to jaundice and blue due to osteogenesis imperfecta.

Digital palpation with the eyelids shut is used to estimate the intra-ocular pressure of the eyeball – a stony hard sensation suggests raised intra-ocular pressure. The orbital margins are examined for tenderness and anaesthesia.

Eye function

The resting position of the eye should be established – with a squint it is abnormally deviated. Eye movements in all directions should be checked, noting the presence of double vision observed by the patient, to determine the function of the IIIrd, IVth and VIth cranial nerves. The corneal reflex is a measure of the function of the Vth cranial nerve – the patient should blink when the cornea is touched.

Visual acuity can be measured with the patient's distance spectacle correction and a Snellen's Chart. If patients have forgotten their glasses or have an uncorrected refractive error the acuity can be improved by asking them to look through a pinhole. Visual fields are tested using confrontation: the patient sits in front of the examiner with a distance of about 40 cm between them, and both cover the eye that is not being tested, that is, when the patient covers the left eye, the examiner covers the right eye. Whilst the patient looks at the examiner's open eye, the examiner moves a pin into the visual field from the non-seeing periphery until the patient sees the white head of the pin.

Pupillary reflexes to light and accommodation measure the anterior visual pathways. An important sign to elicit is the relative afferent pupil defect (or *'Marcus Gunn pupil'*) which develops when there is optic nerve or retinal disease. It is tested for by briskly swinging a bright pen torch between the pupils and noting their reactions – the abnormal pupil will dilate. It is present when there is optic nerve or retinal disease, but absent with disorders of the ocular media, such as cataract or vitreous haemorrhage.

Direct ophthalmoscopy is used to examine the ocular media and the fundus. When the eye is viewed at an arm's length with the ophthalmoscope's lens setting on zero, the reflection from the fundus gives the pupil a red appearance and this is called the 'red reflex'. This is diminished in the presence of opacities between the cornea and the fundus, such as cataract or vitreous haemorrhage.

With the ophthalmoscope close to the eye, the lens setting is adjusted until a clear view of the retina is obtained. The optic disc is identified and the retina examined for exudates, haemorrhages or new vessel formation. The central posterior part of the retina is called the macula – it can be discoloured white and/or black with haemorrhages in age-related macular degeneration.

The pupil can be dilated to allow better inspection of the fundus – a drop of tropicamide 1% dilates the pupil within 20–30 minutes and the effect lasts for between four and 10 hours. Pupillary dilation is safe to use in the general population. However, it may precipitate angle closure glaucoma in susceptible people, inducing iridotrabecular contact and obstructing aqueous flow out of the eye, resulting in an increase in the intra-ocular pressure. Therefore such patients must be advised of the symptoms of angle closure glaucoma and told to seek immediate medical attention if the symptoms occur.

Investigations

Fluorescein testing identifies abrasions or ulcers of the cornea as green areas when the cornea is examined with a blue light after instillation of fluorescein drops. Angiography, ultrasound scanning of the eyeball, CT or carotid duplex ultrasound scans are additional tests when required.

THE RED EYE

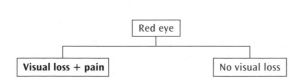

The acute red eye is characterized by redness of the conjunctiva or sclera. Vision may be unaffected or be gradually or suddenly reduced. Patients may complain of pain, varying from a mild discomfort to a severe pain that may keep the patient awake at night. There are numerous causes depending on whether there is an associated deterioration in vision or not, which determines the need for an ophthalmic referral (Plate 1).

Red eyes with visual loss and pain

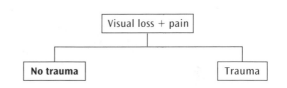

Deterioration or loss of vision demands a specialist opinion. The examiner enquires about a history of trauma. The following conditions may present with a red eye with reduced vision.

No history of trauma

Acute angle closure glaucoma. This results from acute obstruction to the circulation of aqueous humour, resulting in a large increase in intra-ocular pressure. Vision can be permanently reduced because of damage to the optic nerve due to a high intra-ocular pressure. The aqueous humour, fluid produced in the ciliary body, passes from the posterior chamber through the pupil into the anterior chamber, where it is drained out of the eye via the Canal of Schlemm located in the angle of the eye between the iris and the cornea. Primary acute angle closure glaucoma has a prevalence of less than 1% and is less common than primary open angle glaucoma (to be discussed later).

The most common mechanism causing angle closure is pupillary block. This usually results from an increase in lens size with age, which presses against the posterior surface of the iris, obstructing the flow of aqueous and narrowing the drainage angle. Groups at risk are women, long-sighted (*hypermetropic*) individuals, patients of Oriental ethnicity, patients with a family history for angle closure and patients

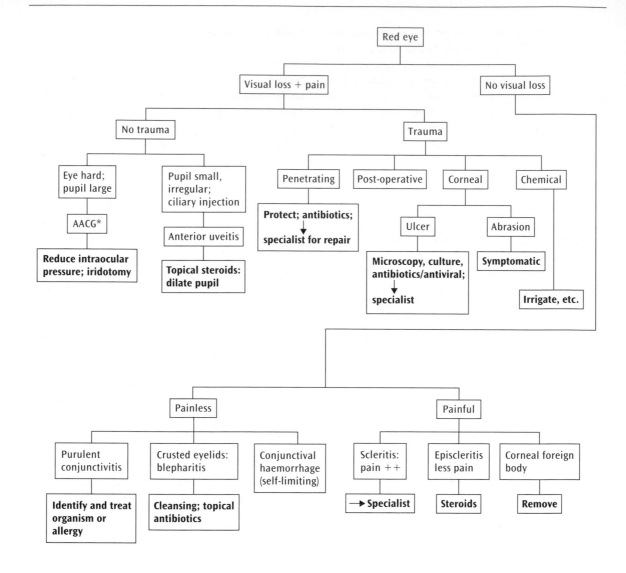

*AACG = acute angle closure glaucoma.

Algorithm 18.1

taking anticholinergic drugs, including tricyclic anti-depressants, anti-emetics and antispasmodics. In predisposed patients, angle closure glaucoma may be induced by the pupillary dilating effects of topical mydriatics.

The patient develops an acutely painful, red eye with a severe reduction in vision. The pain can be very intense, and the patient may also complain of nausea and vomiting, and of seeing haloes around lights. Sight is reduced because of corneal oedema, which can give the cornea a ground-glass appearance and may obscure examination of the rest of the eye. The pupil is irregularly or oval-shaped, moderately dilated and reacting sluggishly to light. The eyeball will feel stony hard on digital examination.

Urgent treatment to reduce the intra-ocular pressure includes the use of intravenous acetazolamide, a topical beta-blocker (e.g., timolol or levobunolol) and an α-adrenoceptor stimulant (e.g., brimonidine or apraclonidine) to reduce aqueous production.

Topical steroids are needed to reduce the intra-ocular inflammation. Topical pilocarpine pulls the iris away from the occluded angle. However, in angle closure glaucoma, the iris becomes ischaemic and does not absorb pilocarpine – therefore it should not be used until later. Oral or intravenous osmotic agents may be required if the initial measures do not reduce the intra-ocular pressure.

Definitive treatment consists of a laser peripheral iridotomy to both eyes: a hole is made in the iris to overcome the pupillary block and to provide an alternative route for aqueous flow from the posterior to the anterior chamber. Sometimes further medical or surgical treatment is required following laser treatment.

Anterior uveitis. Anterior uveitis, iritis or *iridocyclitis* are terms that describe inflammation of the uveal tract which consists of the iris, ciliary body and choroid. The cause in most patients is idiopathic, but it can be associated with systemic disease, such as ankylosing spondylitis, Reiter's syndrome, juvenile chronic arthritis, sarcoidosis, inflammatory bowel disease and infective diseases. Hence, patients with symptoms of other organ dysfunction or general malaise should be investigated appropriately. Other than a red eye, the patient complains of pain and photophobia. Early on in the disease, vision is usually unaffected but may later be reduced. On examination, the redness is more marked around the corneal margin, a pattern termed *ciliary injection*. Inflammation and adhesions (*posterior synechiae*) between the iris and the anterior surface of the lens result in the pupil being irregularly shaped, small and poorly reactive to light (*see* Plate 1 above). If the posterior synechiae are circumferential, aqueous drainage may be blocked resulting in a secondary rise in intra-ocular pressure.

It is important to differentiate between anterior uveitis with a small pupil requiring dilation and acute angle closure glaucoma with a large pupil requiring constriction. Treatment consists of topical steroids to reduce the inflammation, pupillary dilatation to relieve the pain and prevent posterior synechiae formation.

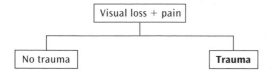

History of trauma

Traumatic red eye. Penetrating injuries can result from high-speed projectile objects. The details of the injury are important, for example, a patient hammering metal or being in close proximity to machinery that could have produced a projectile foreign body.

Suggestive signs are the presence of pigmented uveal tissue in a conjunctival laceration, a deep or flat anterior chamber compared to the other eye and a positive Seidel test. This test consists of administering a drop of topical anaesthetic and wiping a moistened 2% fluorescein strip over the site of injury, which is then examined with the blue light of the slit lamp. If a bright green stream of aqueous appears through a pool of dark fluorescein this is a positive test and indicates a leak from the anterior chamber.

In cases of obvious penetrating trauma, the eye should not be examined any further but protected with an eye shield since it will require an examination under anaesthesia. Orbital X-rays or CT scans with the eyes looking straight ahead, and in the upgaze position may be needed to rule out an intra-ocular foreign body. Magnetic resonance imaging (MRI) is contraindicated because the magnets can move a metallic intra-ocular foreign body and cause further damage.

A penetrating injury needs to be urgently repaired and the posterior segment should also be examined for a second perforation site. Systemic antibiotics must be administered to prevent intra-ocular infection, and the patient's tetanus toxoid vaccination status updated.

Post-operative uveitis is an inflammatory sequela of intra-ocular surgery. It often develops after post-operative steroids have been discontinued prematurely. Patients present with a painful, red eye and vision may be disturbed. It usually resolves once topical steroids are restarted.

Post-operative endophthalmitis results from an infective inflammation of the vitreous cavity and the anterior chamber following intra-ocular surgery. It is usually caused by organisms which live on the patient's eyelids and conjunctiva. Although rare, it is an ophthalmic emergency usually presenting within 2 weeks after surgery. The patient presents acutely with a severely painful, red eye, eyelid oedema, conjunctival chemosis and a cloudy cornea, and marked visual loss. On slit lamp examination, there may be a level of pus in the anterior chamber called a *hypopyon*, which often makes it difficult to see any details of the iris. In addition, the inflammation of the vitreous cavity, termed *vitritis*, often obscures the fundal view resulting in absence of the red reflex. A relative afferent pupil defect is a poor prognostic sign for recovery of vision. Distinguishing clinically between a sterile uveitis and an infective endophthalmitis can be difficult.

Prompt specialist treatment is necessary to save the patient's vision, which involves the injection of broad-spectrum antibiotics into the vitreous cavity. At the same time, a sample of vitreous and aqueous humor is obtained for microscopy and culture. Topical antibiotics and cycloplegics are also used. Topical steroids are administered later to reduce the accompanying inflammation. Despite treatment, the final visual acuity in most patients is poor. The risk factors for final reduced vision are visual acuity at presentation of light perception only, absence of the red reflex and an afferent pupil defect.

Corneal ulcer. A corneal ulcer can be due to a viral or bacterial infection. The extended wear of contact lenses is a risk factor. Characteristically, besides redness, the eye is painful, watering and photophobic with reduced vision if the lesion is located centrally. There can also be a purulent discharge and the cornea immediately around the infective lesion may be opaque. The ulcer is coloured green when a drop of minims 2% fluorescein is put in the eye and viewed with the blue light of the slit lamp. A corneal ulcer caused by Herpes simplex can look branch-like, stains with fluorescein and is called a *dendritic ulcer*.

These patients should be referred to an ophthalmologist for further evaluation and management. Scraping the ulcer for a sample and sending it for microscopy and culture can identify the infecting organism. Treatment consists of administering the appropriate antibiotic drops and acyclovir ointment for a Herpes simplex infection.

Corneal abrasions are breaks in the corneal epithelium, usually caused by trauma. The patient presents with an acutely painful, red, watering and photophobic eye. Vision may be reduced if the abrasion is located centrally. After the instillation of one drop of minims 2% fluorescein, corneal abrasions appear as green areas when viewed with the blue light of the slit lamp. Abrasions usually resolve within 24–48 hours, therefore symptomatic treatment consists of a combination of a topical cycloplegic, antibiotic ointment and/or firm pressure patching.

Chemical burns are caused by acids, alkalis and any irritant substances coming into contact with the eye. Alkalis potentially cause more severe injuries than other chemicals because they saponify the corneal proteins allowing greater penetration.

Chemical burns are usually immediately painful and visual acuity is reduced if the injury is severe. Clinical signs include eyelid oedema, conjunctival injection and chemosis. However, severe alkali burns blanch the conjunctiva because of ischaemia. Corneal signs range in severity from minimal punctate staining with fluorescein to larger defects with areas of thinning and cloudiness in severe injuries. There may be an iritis, which may be difficult to detect through a cloudy cornea. In severe injuries, the eye feels hard if the intra-ocular pressure is raised.

The most important step before a detailed examination is to irrigate the eye using at least one litre of normal saline or even water for at least half an hour. During this, pain can be controlled with a topical anaesthetic. Before and after irrigation, the pH of the tear film should be checked using litmus paper or a urine dip stick in order to be able to confirm that it has returned to 7. Specialist advice should be sought after completing the initial treatment.

Mild cases of chemical burns heal spontaneously and in the meantime, firm pressure patching, cycloplegic eyedrops and a topical antibiotic will provide symptomatic relief. Severe burns require more intensive treatment to promote epithelial healing, to prevent the cornea from perforating and to reduce the risk of conjunctival scarring and secondary infections.

A note on topical steroids

Although effective in the treatment of conditions such as iritis, they should be prescribed sparingly and only when the diagnosis is established. Importantly, Herpes simplex corneal ulcerations may be worsened by steroids and prolonged use can increase the intra-ocular pressure, resulting in steroid-induced glaucoma. An ophthalmologist should be involved if prolonged use of topical steroids is envisaged.

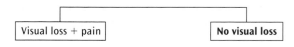

Visual loss + pain	No visual loss

Red eyes without visual loss

Red eyes without visual loss are caused by a wide variety of conditions. Sometimes this presentation can initially be managed without specialist involvement. However, on review if there is no improvement then the patient should be referred to an ophthalmologist – and this should be prompt if any visual disturbance develops.

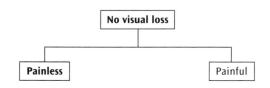

Painless

Conjunctivitis. Conjunctivitis is bacterial, viral, allergic or chlamydial in aetiology. Bacterial conjunctivitis is caused by organisms such as *Staphylococcus aureus*, *Haemophilus influenzae* and *Streptococcus pneumoniae*. Patients present acutely with a sticky, red eye and a purulent discharge. They usually complain of a gritty sensation rather than pain, and vision is generally unaffected unless the cornea is involved. Other signs may include swollen eyelids and chemosis. This type of conjunctivitis usually resolves after a week's treatment with a topical antibiotic such as chloramphenicol.

Viral conjunctivitis may accompany a flu-like illness, particularly when due to adenovirus. The eye may be photophobic and painful and vision may be reduced if there is corneal involvement. The patient may have a sore throat and/or pre-auricular lymphadenopathy. *Adenoviral keratoconjunctivitis* can sometimes present with small, roundish, whitish lesions in the cornea which stain green with fluorescein. Mostly, a viral conjunctivitis is self-resolving and therefore treatment is for symptomatic relief. Topical steroids if there is corneal involvement and reduced vision should be managed by an ophthalmologist.

A *non-infectious conjunctivitis* may occur seasonally, particularly during the pollen season, or may develop in patients with atopic dermatitis. The use of topical medications can sometimes induce a toxic conjunctivitis. Such eyes are usually red, itchy, watering and there may be a whitish discharge unlike the yellowish discharge associated with a bacterial conjunctivitis. Treatment includes topical antihistamines and/or steroids and stopping the topical medication where necessary.

A *chlamydial infection* should be considered if a conjunctivitis does not resolve spontaneously after 2 weeks or after using topical antibiotics. *Chlamydia trachomatis* causes a chronic conjunctivitis called *adult inclusion conjunctivitis*. It can be transmitted venereally or by hand-to-eye contact. Typical features are a mucopurulent discharge, pre-auricular lymphadenopathy and accompanying genitourinary symptoms. A conjunctival scrape should be taken for microscopy and culture. Treatment is with oral erythromycin or tetracycline and topical tetracycline. Importantly, all sexual partners need to be examined and treated to prevent recurrence of the condition.

Blepharitis is a common, inflammatory, non-sight-threatening disorder of the eyelids. Vision is usually unaffected; most patients complain of intermittent, recurrent discomfort and redness of the eyes and eyelids. Scaly crusts around the eyelashes, injected eyelid margins and a conjunctivitis may be seen in staphylococcal blepharitis. Sometimes the crusts are more greasy-looking, as in seborrhoeic blepharitis. The meibomian glands can secrete oily droplets on the lid margin, which may also produce a foamy tear film. This condition may also cause a painless, localized swelling of the eyelid called a *meibomian cyst* or an infection of a lash follicle called a *stye*. Some patients have dry eyes, which may result in punctate staining of the cornea. Management consists of treatment of the staphylococcal infection with a topical antibiotic, eyelid cleaning to remove the crusts and the oily secretions and artificial tear drops for the dryness.

Conjunctival haemorrhages are usually idiopathic or may be associated with minor trauma. Rarely, they may be associated with hypertension, bleeding disorders, the use of anticoagulants and anterior cranial fossa fractures. They are usually painless, do not affect vision and are self-resolving so no specific treatment is required.

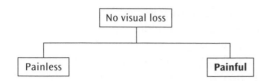

Painful

Scleritis is a rare inflammatory disorder of the sclera and is usually idiopathic. It can be associated with systemic diseases, in particular, rheumatoid arthritis, systemic lupus erythematosus, Wegener's granulomatosis and infective conditions such as herpes zoster and tuberculosis. Scleritis is a severely painful condition and may keep a patient awake at night. It may involve the anterior or the posterior segment of the eye and therefore reduced vision is a potential risk. On examination, the eye is tender to touch, there may be diffuse, sectoral or nodular redness and eyelid oedema. The severity of the pain associated with this condition usually indicates a specialist referral. Treatment consists of systemic steroids and sometimes, cytotoxic agents.

Episcleritis refers to a relatively common, idiopathic inflammatory disorder involving the connective tissue between the sclera and the conjunctiva. It can be easily distinguished from scleritis because it is much less painful and vision is generally unaffected. The eye can be diffusely or sectorally reddened. Episcleritis is usually self-resolving, and treatment includes non-steroidal anti-inflammatory eyedrops and/or topical steroids.

Foreign bodies on the conjunctiva or the cornea may cause a painful red eye but vision is rarely affected. They can be easily removed with the use of the slit lamp – a drop of topical anaesthetic allows proper examination of the eye and the foreign body may be washed out or removed with a cotton bud or a 25 gauge needle. Then chloramphenicol ointment and an eyepad should be applied for at least 24 hours. Foreign bodies can leave imprints on the cornea called *rust rings*. Unless they are removed such eyes will remain persistently uncomfortable, red and watering. A rust ring or an incompletely removed foreign body should be referred to an ophthalmologist for removal.

Corneal wound sutures may present many years postoperatively and, unless removed, can predispose to corneal infections and endophthalmitis. Patients will describe a foreign body-like sensation associated with a red eye whilst vision will usually be unaffected. If the cornea is infected this may be recognized by a white area around the suture, called an *infiltrate,* associated with conjunctival congestion, a yellow discharge and sometimes signs of an anterior uveitis. A more severe infection can result in a corneal abscess with a hypopyon. Residual sutures should therefore be referred to an ophthalmologist for removal.

VISUAL LOSS

Visual loss may present unilaterally or bilaterally.

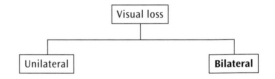

Bilateral loss of vision

Bilateral loss of vision is rare and may be due to diabetic retinopathy or lesions involving the visual pathways posterior to the optic chiasm or the visual cortex. On examination, these patients present with visual field defects – a lesion of the optic chiasm results in a bitemporal hemianopia, and a lesion behind the optic chiasm produces a homonymous hemianopia. These patients need a full neurological examination and should be referred to a neurologist or an ophthalmologist.

Unilateral loss of vision is the more common complaint, and may present suddenly or gradually and with or without pain.

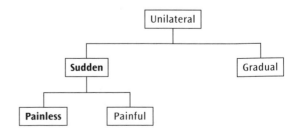

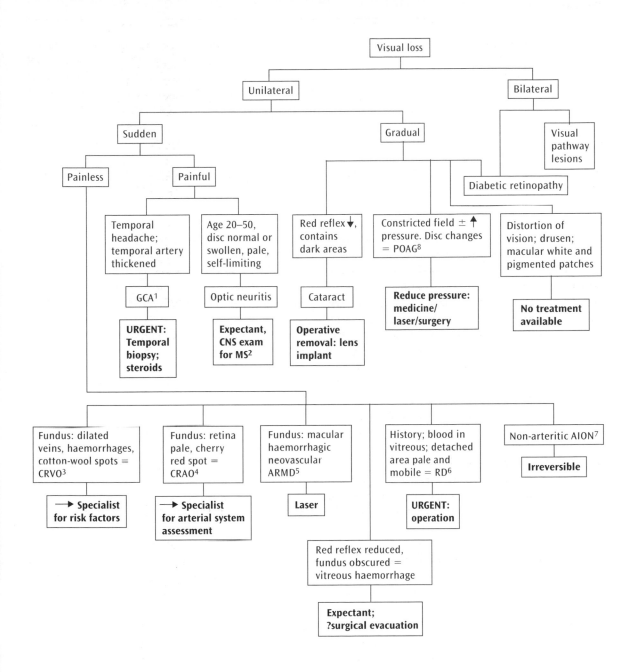

Visual loss

Unilateral — Bilateral

Unilateral branch:

Sudden — Gradual

Bilateral branch: Visual pathway lesions; Diabetic retinopathy

Sudden: Painless — Painful

Painful:
- Temporal headache; temporal artery thickened → GCA[1] → **URGENT: Temporal biopsy; steroids**
- Age 20–50, disc normal or swollen, pale, self-limiting → Optic neuritis → **Expectant, CNS exam for MS[2]**

Gradual:
- Red reflex↓, contains dark areas → Cataract → **Operative removal: lens implant**
- Constricted field ± ↑ pressure. Disc changes = POAG[8] → **Reduce pressure: medicine/laser/surgery**
- Distortion of vision; drusen; macular white and pigmented patches → **No treatment available**

Lower row:
- Fundus: dilated veins, haemorrhages, cotton-wool spots = CRVO[3] → **→ Specialist for risk factors**
- Fundus: retina pale, cherry red spot = CRAO[4] → **→ Specialist for arterial system assessment**
- Fundus: macular haemorrhagic neovascular ARMD[5] → **Laser**
- History; blood in vitreous; detached area pale and mobile = RD[6] → **URGENT: operation**
- Non-arteritic AION[7] → **Irreversible**

Red reflex reduced, fundus obscured = vitreous haemorrhage → **Expectant; ?surgical evacuation**

[1]GCA   = giant-cell (temporal) arteritis.
[2]MS   = multiple sclerosis.
[3]CRVO   = central retinal vein obstruction.
[4]CRAO   = central retinal artery obstruction.
[5]ARMD   = age-related macular degeneration.
[6]RD   = retinal detachment.
[7]AION   = anterior ischaemic optic neuropathy.
[8]POAG   = primary open angle glaucoma.

Algorithm 18.2

Unilateral, sudden visual loss

Central retinal vein occlusion (CRVO)

This is a blockage of the central retinal vein by a thrombus, and commonly develops in patients over 50 years of age. Hypertension, diabetes and atherosclerotic cardiovascular disease are the most frequently associated underlying systemic conditions. Other less common factors to consider are blood dyscrasias, dysproteinaemias (e.g., myeloma) and vasculitides (e.g., sarcoidosis). A branch retinal vein occlusion involves a part of the retinal vasculature, and if the blockage involves the macula, vision may be reduced.

A CRVO occurs *painlessly* in a white eye with sudden loss of vision. On examination, there may be a relative afferent pupil defect, and funduscopy shows dilated, tortuous retinal veins with numerous retinal haemorrhages, white lesions called cotton-wool spots, which are localized areas of retinal ischaemia (Plate 2).

The patient should be referred promptly to a specialist. Although there is no effective treatment at present, these patients need to be investigated for underlying risk factors. Patients with severe ischaemic changes and with a vision acuity less than 6/60 have the greatest risk of developing abnormal new blood vessels in the anterior segment of the eye, for example the iris. Therefore, these patients need regular review, since retinal laser photocoagulation can prevent neovascular glaucoma from developing.

Central retinal artery occlusion (CRAO)

CRAO is a sudden decrease in blood flow through the central retinal artery resulting in retinal ischaemia. A CRAO is a less common occurrence than a CRVO. The most common pathogenesis is atherosclerotic disease of the ophthalmic or carotid artery resulting in thrombus formation, which breaks off and blocks the central retina artery. Associated systemic conditions may be cardiac diseases (e.g., valvular problems, arrhythmias), vasculitides (e.g., systemic lupus erythematosus, temporal arteritis), coagulopathies (e.g., antiphospholipid antibodies, Protein C or S deficiency) and oncologic diseases.

A patient with a CRAO should be referred promptly to an ophthalmologist. There is sudden, *painless* and usually permanent loss of vision. Sometimes this is preceded by transient episodes of visual loss lasting only minutes at a time called *amaurosis fugax*. Within the first few minutes to hours after the blockage the retina may appear normal. Subsequently, the retina turns pale and whitish due to the decreased blood flow and the retinal arterioles look thin and attenuated. An embolus may be visible in the central retinal artery or one of its branches. The centre of the macula is devoid of the layers forming the neurosensory retina (the nerve fibre and ganglion cell layers) and shows up as a red area due to the underlying choroidal vessels. This area stands out red against the rest of the white retina and is called a *cherry red spot*. There may also be a relative afferent pupil defect.

A thorough cardiovascular examination should be performed, for example carotid bruit may indicate ipsilateral carotid artery disease. Investigations, including echocardiography and carotid artery duplex scanning, may be necessary. There is no proven treatment for CRAO; however, some treatment approaches aim to increase retinal arterial blood flow by reducing the intra-ocular pressure via paracentesis, ocular massage and the inhalation of carbogen (a mixture of 95% oxygen and 5% carbon dioxide). These measures are often not successful and many ophthalmic units have stopped using carbogen.

Age-related macular degeneration (ARMD)

Age-related macular degeneration is a common, *painless*, chronic degenerative disorder of the retina affecting individuals over the age of 50 years. It involves the central part of the retina called the *macula*, which is the part of the retina responsible for visual acuity and colour vision. There are two types of ARMD: non-neovascular (dry) and neovascular (wet), with the former occurring most commonly.

Neovascular ARMD is associated with the formation of new blood vessels from the choriocapillaris under the retina (*choroidal neovascularization*, CNV). Only a small proportion of all patients with ARMD develop CNV. This type of ARMD can present with an acute deterioration in vision due to bleeding from the blood vessels. On examination, there is no relative afferent pupil defect and funduscopy shows an elevated and haemorrhagic area at the macula.

Laser photocoagulation is the only proven treatment for neovascular ARMD. Unfortunately, only about 15–20% of patients with this type of ARMD are suitable for laser treatment.

Vitreous haemorrhage

A vitreous haemorrhage is *painless* and develops when the vitreous gel detaches from its peripheral retinal attachments (a *posterior vitreous detachment*, PVD). This can occur spontaneously or be caused by trauma. It may also be associated with a retinal detachment or the rupture of abnormal new blood vessels in diabetic subjects who have developed a proliferative retinopathy due to severe retinal ischaemia.

The visual loss ranges from a moderate to a severe reduction, sometimes preceded by symptoms of flashing lights and floaters. On examination, there is no relative afferent pupil defect and the red reflex may be diminished due to the intra-ocular haemorrhage. In addition, the blood may obscure fundal details. Investigations include an ultrasound scan to assess the integrity of the retina. Treatment consists of bedrest and stopping any unnecessary anticoagulants. An uncomplicated vitreous haemorrhage usually resolves within 6 months but, if persistent, intra-ocular surgery to evacuate the haemorrhage may be required. The treatment for proliferative diabetic retinopathy is laser photocoagulation (*see later*).

Retinal detachment (RD)

A retinal detachment is *painless* and arises from a break in the retina allowing fluid from the vitreous to separate the neurosensory retina from the retinal pigment epithelium. A retinal break is usually caused by a posterior vitreous detachment (PVD). The vitreous gel liquefies with age which may then detach from the retina, exerting traction on it and tearing it at its strong points of attachment.

High myopia, cataract surgery, proliferative diabetic eye disease, blunt and penetrating trauma all increase the risk of a retinal detachment. Trauma results in compression of the anterior–posterior diameter of the globe and expansion along the equatorial plane, which exerts traction on the vitreous

tearing the retina. Systemic diseases, such as Marfan's syndrome and Ehlers–Danlos syndrome may also be associated with this condition.

Visual loss may be preceded by symptoms of flashing lights and floaters. When the retina detaches a field defect develops, which patients may describe as a black veil or curtain being drawn across the field of vision. Visual acuity is reduced when the detachment involves the macula. On examination, there can be a relative afferent pupil if a large area of the retina is involved and the red reflex may be diminished. Funduscopy reveals blood in the vitreous and the detached retina looks white and is mobile.

The patient should be referred to an ophthalmologist urgently. Treatment is usually surgical and consists of the use of laser, cryotherapy, gas and/or liquids to flatten the retina, seal the retinal break and treat prophylactically any other suspicious areas.

Anterior ischaemic optic neuropathy (AION)

AION predominantly develops in people over the age of 50 years. It is categorized into *arteritic* and *non-arteritic* AION. Non-arteritic AION is more common and generally occurs in hypertensive patients, with a mean age of 60 years. An AION presents with sudden, painless, severe and usually irreversible loss of vision. On examination, there may be a relative afferent pupil defect and an altitudinal field defect is common.

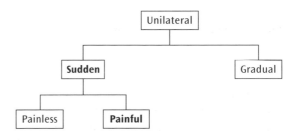

Arteritic AION generally occurs in older patients (mean age 70 years). Another name for arteritic AION is *giant cell* (or) *temporal arteritis* (GCA). It is caused by a vasculitis affecting the superficial temporal, ophthalmic and posterior ciliary arteries.

Patients with GCA most commonly complain of a severe, generalized or temporal headache sometimes associated with jaw claudication. Systemic symptoms include malaise, weight loss, fever and proximal muscle stiffness and pain due to polymyalgia rheumatica. In GCA, the temporal artery is tender, thickened and non-pulsatile. In the acute stage, the optic disc looks swollen and is surrounded by haemorrhages.

The differentiation between a giant cell arteritis and a non-arteritic AION is important because the treatments differ. In GCA, the erythrocyte sedimentation rate (ESR) and C-reactive protein (CRP) are markedly raised and the diagnosis should be confirmed with a temporal artery biopsy. GCA is an ocular emergency as visual loss may develop in the other eye in 55–95% of patients if left untreated. The treatment for GCA is to administer high-dose systemic steroids. There is no proven treatment for non-arteritic AION.

Optic neuritis

Optic neuritis is an inflammatory disorder of the optic nerve, sometimes located behind the optic disc (*retrobulbar*) or including the disc (*papillitis*). It generally occurs in people aged between 20 and 50 years and is more common in women. Patients present with an acute reduction in vision, which continues to deteriorate over several days before stabilizing and gradually recovering. Pain in or around the eye occurs in most patients and may be exacerbated by eye movements.

On examination, as well as reduced visual acuity there may also be reduced colour vision and a visual field defect (e.g., a central scotoma). A relative afferent pupil defect is common. The optic disc often looks entirely normal when the site of involvement is retro-bulbar. Otherwise, it may look swollen and disc pallor develops later.

There is a close association between optic neuritis and multiple sclerosis. Therefore, a thorough neurological examination is essential, looking for limb weakness, sensory disturbances and brain stem problems such as nystagmus and ataxia. The risk of developing multiple sclerosis within 2 years of the optic neuritis is 20%. The treatment for optic neuritis is usually conservative because it usually resolves spontaneously. Intravenous methylprednisolone may accelerate visual recovery but will not improve its final outcome.

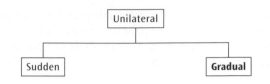

Gradual visual loss

The two most common causes of gradual visual loss in older patients are cataract and glaucoma. However, specific enquiry may suggest other causes – glare is often associated with cataract, distortion may be associated with age-related macular degeneration and a history of diabetes mellitus may indicate a diabetic retinopathy.

Cataract

Cataract is the process of opacification of the lens and is the most common cause of reversible blindness worldwide. Age is the most important risk factor. Other risk factors include radiation exposure (e.g., infra-red causes cataract in glassblowers and furnace workers), systemic disorders such as diabetes and galactosaemia, atopy and the prolonged use of steroids (both systemic and topical). Diabetic cataracts present at an earlier age and progress faster. Severe dehydration, poor nutrition and smoking are associated with a higher risk of cataract. It is also likely that as yet unidentified recessive genes are responsible for a predisposition to cataract. Local ocular problems, for example, uveitis and trauma, are also risk factors.

Some patients complain of monocular diplopia and glare. On funduscopy, the red reflex is usually diminished and the lens opacities look like dark areas in the red reflex. The view of the retina may be obscured if the cataract is significant. This condition is not an ocular emergency and can be assessed in an ophthalmic outpatient clinic. Management is surgical, consisting of removing the cataract and replacing it with an artificial lens called an *implant*.

Cataracts may be congenital, due to a maternal infection (e.g., rubella), a systemic disease or an hereditary disorder. On examination, there may be a dull red reflex or a white pupil. A child with a suspected cataract must be referred promptly to an ophthalmologist to assess for the risk of development of *amblyopia*, a developmental defect of the visual processing in the brain which can result in permanently reduced visual acuity.

Non-neovascular age-related macular degeneration (ARMD)

ARMD is a degenerative condition of the central retina and may occur bilaterally. It presents with a gradual loss of central vision with accompanying distortion. The distortion is tested for with an Amsler chart – the patient looks at the centre of the chart, which consists of a grid of horizontal and vertical lines with a spot in the centre, and is asked if any of the lines are distorted.

Funduscopy typically reveals small, circular, yellow-white spots in the retina called *drusen*. At the macula the retinal pigment epithelium and photoreceptors atrophy, exposing the underlying choriocapillaris and sometimes the white sclera. This appears as a well-circumscribed area consisting of white and hyperpigmented patches. There is at present no treatment for non-neovascular ARMD.

Diabetic retinopathy (DR)

Diabetic retinopathy is the progressive development of dysfunction of the retinal vasculature due to chronic hyperglycaemia. The longer a patient has diabetes the greater the risk of developing diabetic retinopathy; 71–90% of individuals with insulin-dependent diabetes mellitus for more than 10 years have the condition. Not all patients with DR complain of visual loss. However, any diabetic patient presenting with visual loss should promptly be referred to an ophthalmologist. Diabetic retinopathy can be classified into two types: non-proliferative (early and advanced) and proliferative.

In *early non-proliferative DR*, the earliest change is the development of microaneurysms, which look like small, red dot- or blot-shaped haemorrhages. Other types of haemorrhages can be splinter- or flame-shaped. Fluid may leak from the retinal blood vessels resulting in either the formation of lipid-containing *exudates* or *macular oedema*. Exudates are well-defined, yellow, glistening lesions in the retina forming a circular pattern around leaking microaneurysms (Plate 3). Macular oedema is very difficult to see with a direct ophthalmoscope and results from fluid leakage without exudate formation: it represents a leading cause of blindness in diabetic subjects.

Advanced non-proliferative DR results from increasing retinal ischaemia. The clinical signs include *multiple haemorrhages*, white lesions called *cotton-wool spots* which are areas of retinal infarction, and *dilated* and *looped venules*.

Severe retinal ischaemia can progress to *proliferative diabetic retinopathy*, which is characterized by the growth of new blood vessels from the optic disc or from one of the retinal vessels. These abnormally friable vessels are prone to bleed resulting in a vitreous haemorrhage. Another possible complication is a retinal detachment due to the vitreous detaching and exerting traction on the retina via these vessels.

Fluorescein angiography involves the intravenous injection of the dye sodium fluorescein and then photographing the fundus as it circulates through the retinal vasculature. It is a useful imaging test to assess the severity of the diabetic retinopathy, demonstrate the sites of blood vessel leakage, evaluate the extent of areas of retinal ischaemia and confirm the development of proliferative retinopathy. It can help the ophthalmologist decide whether or not laser treatment would be appropriate.

Clinical trials have shown that patients who controlled their blood glucose tightly (four measurements per day) did far better than those who did not (one measurement per day). Argon laser photocoagulation is used to treat the leaking microaneurysms causing macular oedema, or to stop the progression of neovascularization in proliferative retinopathy.

Glaucoma

Glaucoma is a term used to describe a group of diseases characterized by the progressive development of an optic neuropathy and visual field defects. Intraocular pressure is the most important risk factor for the development of glaucoma. Primary open angle glaucoma (POAG) is the most common type of glaucoma, and major population studies indicate that in Caucasians over 40 years of age its prevalence is about 2% and about four times this in African-Caribbeans. The risk of POAG increases with age and most patients are aged over 80 years. Susceptibility to POAG can be inherited; recent research into the genetics of glaucoma indicates that multiple, as yet unidentified genes may be responsible for the development of POAG.

POAG is a chronic, bilateral, asymmetrical disease, and usually presents asymptomatically. A patient may only complain of visual loss when the disease is quite advanced, when there may also be a relative afferent pupil defect and marked constriction of the visual field. Intra-ocular pressure can be raised but not necessarily. Suspicious signs on funduscopy include deepening or enlargement of the cup of the optic disc ('cupping' of the disc, Plates 4 and 5) or loss of or pallor of the neuroretinal tissue around the rim of the optic disc.

POAG should be managed by an ophthalmologist and most treatments are aimed at reducing intra-ocular pressure. The treatment options include medical therapy consisting of eyedrops or oral medication, and the use of laser and surgery. In the differential diagnosis, trauma, compressive lesions, toxic agents or nutritional deficiencies may result in optic neuropathies which exhibit similar optic nerve changes.

DOUBLE VISION (DIPLOPIA)

Double vision or *diplopia* is defined as the perception of a double image. *Monocular diplopia* is present when one eye is covered and a double image is seen, and *binocular diplopia* occurs when both eyes are open.

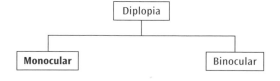

Monocular diplopia

This may be due to some irregularity in the ocular media, such as cataract and keratoconus. A cataract due to an opacity in the inner layers of the lens produces a different refractive area compared to the rest of the lens and can result in this symptom.

Keratoconus is a rare, progressively worsening conical irregularity of the cornea. Patients may also present with increasing myopia and astigmatism. The diplopia may be corrected with prisms incorporated into glasses or contact lenses, but sometimes a penetrating keratoplasty may be indicated.

Binocular diplopia

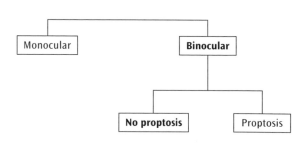

Distinguishing features include whether the diplopia is constant or variable and whether there is forward displacement of the eyeball called *proptosis*. Diplopia caused by neuromuscular disorders of the extra-ocular muscles such as cranial nerve palsies, myasthenia gravis or head injuries occurs without proptosis, whereas diplopia due to thyroid eye disease and orbital cellulitis is usually accompanied by proptosis.

Diplopia without proptosis

Cranial nerve palsies. The nerves that move the extra-ocular muscles of the eye are the oculomotor (III), the trochlear (IV) and the abducent (VI) cranial nerves. Palsies of these nerves can produce diplopia. The diplopia is sometimes intermittent because the patient adopts a compensatory head position to overcome the abnormal eye movements. A *squint*, which is an abnormal resting position of the eye, is often present. The eye movements of the affected eye may be restored by occluding the vision of the fellow eye, because this results in increased nerve stimulation to the affected cranial nerve and therefore increased muscle action. It is important to remember that an isolated nerve palsy may present with distinctive

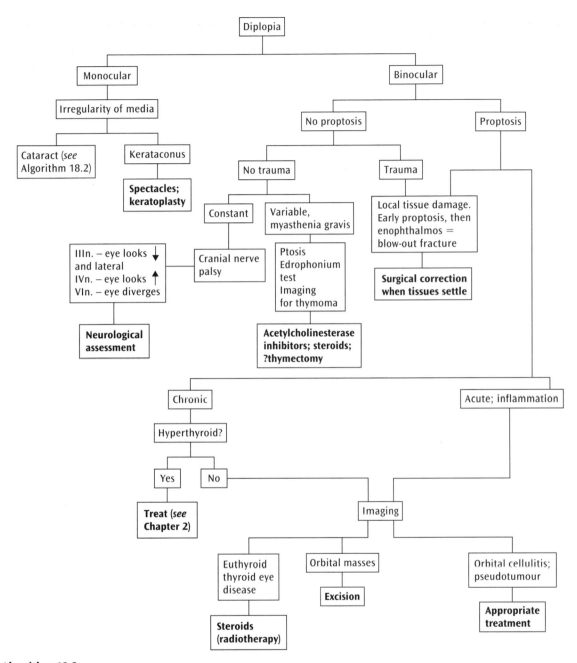

Algorithm 18.3

signs, but the clinical picture may be confused if several nerves are involved.

In adults, most nerve palsies are idiopathic. Another common cause is atherosclerotic disease of the blood vessels supplying the cranial nerves. These palsies generally occur without pupillary involvement and mostly resolve spontaneously. A cerebral aneurysm is a less common cause and usually involves the IIIrd nerve. Head injuries commonly affect the fourth nerve. Herpes zoster infection can involve any of the cranial nerves – patients may also present with a painful, vesicular rash on the forehead associated with a painful red eye and reduced vision. Demyelination is another possible cause. Tumours only rarely cause cranial nerve palsies: in children, they generally affect the VIth nerve.

A IIIrd nerve palsy affects all the extra-ocular muscles except the lateral rectus and superior oblique. The eye is deviated laterally and down, and the eyelid may droop, a condition called *ptosis*.

Adduction, elevation and depression of the eye are reduced. Complete paralysis of the IIIrd nerve prevents constriction of the pupil so that it is dilated and fails to react to light; the patient may also complain of blurred vision because of loss of accommodation. If the pupil is involved, the diagnosis may be a cerebral aneurysm compressing the parasympathetic component of the IIIrd nerve. Such compressions are often, but not always, painful.

A IVth nerve palsy results in an elevated eye due to weakness of the superior oblique muscle. The patient may complain of vertical diplopia, maximal when the patient looks downwards with the affected eye turned inwards, as there is limited depression on adduction. The head may be held in an abnormal position, tilted towards the opposite shoulder.

A VIth nerve palsy results in a convergent squint due to weakness of the lateral rectus muscle and an inability of the eye to abduct.

Management of a patient presenting with a cranial nerve palsy includes a full neurological examination and investigations including a CT or MRI scan of the cranium. The treatment depends on the cause.

Myasthenia gravis is an autoimmune disorder characterized by an antibody blocking acetylcholine receptors at the neuromuscular junctions of skeletal muscles, resulting in an incapacity to sustain muscular activity. Early ocular symptoms are intermittent; diplopia and/or ptosis are variable, periodic and usually worse in the evening. Muscle fatiguability confirms the diagnosis, for example eye movements become increasingly diminished after repetitive attempts and the eyelid droops increasingly after prolonged upgaze. Other muscular groups can be affected, resulting in weakness of chewing, swallowing, speaking and of limb movements.

The diagnosis is confirmed by the *edrophonium test*: an intravenous injection of the anticholinesterase inhibitor, edrophonium, increases muscle action.

Electromyography demonstrates the fatiguability of the muscles on repetitive stimulation. A blood test measuring antibodies to acetylcholine receptors is positive in 90% of cases. Patients should also be investigated radiologically for a thymoma, although this is present in only 10% of patients. Treatment includes the use of acetylcholinesterase inhibitors to enhance acetylcholine muscle stimulation, with steroids and other immunosuppressants. A thymectomy is of benefit in the majority of patients, irrespective of the presence of a thymic tumour.

Diplopia with proptosis

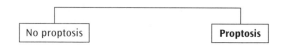

The presence or absence of pain and inflammatory signs distinguishes between underlying causes.

Blow-out fracture. A blow-out fracture of the orbital floor is a fracture of the thin bone overlying the intra-orbital canal, caused by a sudden increase in orbital pressure. Patients present with a *painful* diplopia caused by entrapment of the supporting septa and/or the inferior rectus or inferior oblique muscles within the fracture. An initial proptosis develops because of orbital tissue oedema and haemorrhage. This is usually temporary and once the inflammation subsides the eye may become sunken (*enophthalmos*). Other features include numbness overlying the cheek and upper lip due to infra-orbital nerve damage and emphysema in the orbit and the eyelids due to the escape of air from an adjacent sinus into the subcutaneous tissues.

This condition should be referred to an ophthalmologist to assess the extent of injury. Plain X-ray films and CT imaging are necessary to confirm the diagnosis. Treatment is delayed until the soft tissue oedema has resolved, and for residual diplopia, the fracture is reduced to release the entrapped tissue.

Orbital cellulitis is a *painful* infective condition of the soft tissues behind the orbital septum. It is less common than pre-septal cellulitis when the infection is localized to the eyelid tissues anterior to the septum. This condition is an ophthalmic emergency because the infected, oedematous orbital tissues can compress the optic nerve and permanently damage vision. Sometimes when untreated this can be a fatal condition because of spreading intra-cranial sepsis.

Orbital cellulitis can follow a sinus infection in children and young adults (especially of the ethmoid sinus, which may spread to the orbit), penetrating trauma, or after ocular operations such as orbital, retinal detachment and squint surgery.

The patient presents acutely with diplopia associated with painful and restricted eye movements. A unilateral proptosis develops rapidly. Other features include eyelid oedema and erythema, chemosis, decreased visual acuity and colour vision, and a relative afferent pupil defect. *Management* of orbital cellulitis requires joint ophthalmic and ENT care consisting of CT scanning of the sinuses, the prompt administration of intravenous antibiotics and sometimes surgical drainage of the sinuses.

Orbital pseudo-tumour is a rare, idiopathic, non-infective, non-neoplastic inflammation of the orbital tissues. It can mimic orbital cellulitis so that a trial of antibiotics may sometimes be necessary. It causes a *painful* diplopia associated with restricted eye movements and a red, proptosed eye. Ultrasonic and radiological imaging may show characteristic changes consisting of extra-ocular muscle thickening. An histological diagnosis may sometimes be necessary to confirm the diagnosis. The treatment usually consists of the systemic administration of steroids.

Thyroid eye disease is an autoimmune disease, which commonly develops in middle-aged women with hyperthyroidism. The extra-ocular muscles are involved in a restrictive myopathy; in the acute stage of the disease, the extra-ocular muscles become hypertrophied and the surrounding orbital soft tissues become oedematous due to an inflammatory infiltration, which restricts the patient's eye movements.

It is the most common cause of bilateral proptosis. Other complaints include diplopia, a foreign body sensation due to dry eyes, and sometimes, reduced visual acuity, colour vision and a relative afferent pupil defect due to compression of the optic nerve by the hypertrophied recti muscles. Other signs are eyelid retraction, lid lag, eyelid oedema and conjunctival injection with chemosis. Such a patient should also be examined systematically for clinical evidence of hyperthyroidism, although the eye disease can occur in the absence of systemic problems.

Investigations include establishing the patient's thyroid status by measuring serum TSH, T3 and T4 levels. A CT scan may show fusiform extra-ocular muscle enlargement.

Management of thyroid eye disease includes the use of artificial teardrops for dry eyes, incorporating prisms into glasses or squint surgery to treat the diplopia, and using oral systemic steroids and occasionally radiotherapy to reduce the orbital inflammation and to treat an optic neuropathy. An endocrinologist should manage the treatment of the patient's hyperthyroidism.

Other conditions

Finally, the differential diagnosis of a unilateral, *painless* proptosis in the absence of thyrotoxicosis includes orbital lesions such as lacrimal gland tumours, mucoceles, gliomas, meningiomas, cavernous haemangiomas and varices. Orbital imaging, for example ultrasound, CT and MRI scanning will help identify these conditions.

HIGHLIGHTS

- An urgent ophthalmic opinion is required in a patient with a painful red eye, deterioration of vision or diplopia

19

Orthopaedics

GEORGE BENTLEY, CHRISTOPHER BD LAVY AND DISHAN SINGH

AIMS

1 Learn the methods of clinical assessment in orthopaedics
2 Define the clinical and pathological features of common bone and joint disease

INTRODUCTION

Musculoskeletal disorders present with pain because of a rich nerve supply, structural deformity and disturbance or loss of function. These symptoms can be acute after trauma and infection, or chronic, due to conditions arising in childhood or later in life as a result of degeneration from wear and tear or precipitated by a prior injury, or due to inflammatory and neoplastic disease. These salient aspects must be borne in mind when history and examination, the crucial components of clinical assessment, are carried out, especially if surgical treatment is being considered as the risk involved may outweigh the outcome which may not attain the patient's expectation.

HISTORY

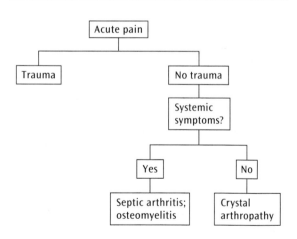

Acute pain commonly follows injury causing *fractures* and *dislocations*. The pattern of an injury indicates the tissue damage that may have occurred. The cardinal signs are swelling, discoloration, bruising, loss of function and the presence of crepitus when there is a fracture. When there is no history of trauma but systemic signs, namely pyrexia and malaise, are present and accompany local signs of inflammation, septic arthritis or osteomyelitis should be considered. In the absence of systemic signs crystal arthropathy is likely.

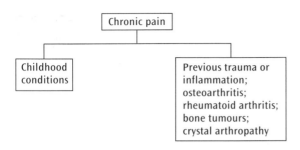

Chronic pain can be due to conditions that arise in childhood and are related to the age of the child, or to residual damage from previous trauma or inflammatory arthritides and osteoarthritis and bone malignancies. The local signs are similar apart from absence of signs of acute inflammation, and a consistent feature is restricted movement of the involved part.

The precise site of the pain, its origin, its radiation and its association with other sites of pain should be established. The relationship of pain to the degree of activity at work, during exercise outdoors or indoors, at rest and at night, as well as the type and quantity of analgesia required to relieve the pain, are measures of its severity.

EXAMINATION

The scope of examination is limited following injury, but should include the bones, the adjacent joints, the soft tissues and the skin as well as the peripheral neurological and circulatory function. The joints are examined in three stages: look, feel and move. 'Looking' involves comparing the diseased joint with the opposite side for discrepancy in shape or size, signs of skin inflammation or discoloration, swelling, scars or sinuses, deformity and wasting of the adjacent musculature, taking into account that when a joint is inflamed the patient puts it into the position of greatest ease. 'Feeling' assesses the overlying skin temperature, the bony or joint contours, lumps, thickening of or fluid in the joint, and tenderness. 'Moving' the limb by asking the patient to put the joint through as much movement as possible without causing pain, gives the range of passive movement. Limitation of all movements indicates arthritis, whereas restriction of certain movements suggests an extra-articular lesion or

mechanical block within the joint. Instability in a joint indicates ligament laxity related to pathological disease of the joint or secondary to an injury.

Methods of assessing individual areas will be considered in the relevant sections.

Acute pyogenic arthritis can be difficult to distinguish from acute osteomyelitis; indeed, acute suppurative arthritis is not an uncommon complication of acute osteomyelitis of adjacent bone. It should be considered in children, immunocompromised patients and the elderly with degenerative joint disease. Infection is usually blood-borne from a distant site of trivial infection due to *Staphylococcus aureus*, streptococcus and pneumococcus, although a gonococcus should be suspected in the sexually active. Local extension from a neighbouring focus such as osteomyelitis, and direct infection by a penetrating wound or a compound fracture are other causes.

Tuberculous arthritis or *osteomyelitis* still prevails in developing countries. Although it usually starts in childhood, it should be suspected in all age groups in otherwise unexplained monoarticular arthritis, particularly in patients with a history of tuberculosis. It is haematogenous in origin, from a primary pulmonary focus caused by the inhalation of the human strain or from the gastrointestinal tract if the disease was acquired by the ingestion of bovine tubercle. It starts either in the synovial membrane, especially where extensive, as in the hip and knee, and progresses to destroy the articular cartilage and adjacent bone; or primarily in intra-articular bone and spreads to the synovium. The spine is also commonly involved, and the disease process results in collapse of the vertebral bodies and an abscess which tracks along the tissue planes, for example pus from the thoraco-lumbar region tracks along the psoas muscle and presents in the groin (*psoas abscess*). The 'pus' is necrotic rather than purulent material and therefore does not show local signs of inflammation: hence the term a 'cold abscess'.

Osteomyelitis complicates open fractures and bone surgery, but in the intact bone is due to haematogenous infection, commonly by *Staphylococcus aureus*, streptococcus, pneumococcus, *Haemophilus influenzae* and salmonella, and begins in the metaphysis. There may therefore be a history of pyrexial illness associated with septicaemia. In *acute osteomyelitis*, the inflammatory exudate collects under the periosteum and along the length of the medulla producing toxic symptoms. Pus forms, tracks around the bone and bursts through the periosteum, then tracks through the muscles to present subcutaneously. If not, or inadequately treated, chronic osteomyelitis develops. In *chronic osteomyelitis*, as the periosteum is stripped off the bone thrombosis of the vessels results in bone infarction and necrosis (*sequestrum*), around which the elevated periosteum lays down new bone that surrounds the dead bone (*involucrum*), and where pus breaks through the periosteum there are defects in the involucrum (*cloacae*). Another form of chronic osteomyelitis is a *Brodie's abscess* which consists of pus and granulation tissue encased by dense sclerotic bone.

Crystal arthropathy comprises gout in the middle-aged and pseudogout in the elderly and can be mistaken for acute bacterial arthritis in its presentation. In *gout*, urate is deposited in the joint. The urate is a product of nucleic acid metabolism, and excess results either from a metabolic disorder, or chemotherapy with anti-metabolites, dehydration or intake of diuretics. High uric acid blood levels and the presence of birefringent crystals in the fluid aspirated from the joint are diagnostic. *Pseudogout* mimics gout but has a less acute presentation, is caused by the deposition of pyrophosphate, results in calcification of the joint surfaces, commonly in the knee, and its source is obscure. Crystal arthopathies cause chronic degenerative changes and osteoarthritis.

Rheumatoid arthritis is a chronic inflammatory autoimmune multisystem disease which is more common in females and below the age of 40. The synovial membrane, infiltrated with chronic inflammatory cells, enlarges and encroaches (*pannus*) upon the articular cartilage, destroying it. The intra-articular ligaments are also destroyed, the underlying bone is eroded and becomes porotic from hyperaemia, and instability and deformity result. The small joints of the hands and feet are most frequently and symmetrically affected with characteristic signs: metacarpo-phalangeal joint swelling and subluxation of the metacarpo-phalangeal joints, spindling of the proximal interphalangeal joint, muscle wasting and finger deformity and ulnar deviation of the fingers and hand. Other joints that may be affected are the cervical spine, temporo-mandibular joints, the wrists and the knees. The clinical features are usually clear. A raised erythrocyte sedimentation rate (ESR) and the presence of rheumatoid factor in the blood as well as radiological changes aid in the diagnosis. The joint space is narrowed as in osteoarthritis, but osteophytes are small or absent and the bone adjacent to the joint is porotic, and collapsed.

Osteoarthritis is the most common cause of joint pain, and is either primary, possibly related to mechanical stress, poor cartilage nutrition and cartilage fragmentation leading to inflammation, or secondary, due to predisposing factors. It is particularly noticeable in the weight-bearing joints such as the hip and knee. The surface of the articular cartilage is roughened, a change known as *fibrillation*, and progresses until bone is exposed, where it gradually becomes thickened (*sclerosis*) and *cysts* form in the cancellous bone. Detached fragments of cartilage become attached to the synovial membrane and cause inflammation which results in fibrosis that limits joint movement. New bone formation around the periphery of the joint leads to typical excrescences, known as *osteophytes*. These changes are seen radiologically as narrowing of the joint space, sclerosis in the sub-chondral bone and cysts and new bone formation.

Bone tumours. Most of the benign tumours of bone occur in children and, except for giant cell tumours which are regarded as locally malignant and osteoid osteoma, often stop growing with the cessation of skeletal growth.

Osteochondroma can be solitary or multiple and originates in the epiphysis of bones. The complaint of severe or persistent pain should raise the suspicion of malignant change. *Osteoid osteoma* is seen in patients aged between 5 and 25 years, more commonly in males, and usually involves the femur and tibia. Severe pain is not relieved by rest, and the only abnormal physical sign is bone tenderness. *Chondroma* is a lobulated mass of cartilage that may arise in any bone but most frequently in the metacarpals, phalanges or metatarsals. When it arises in the medulla (*enchondroma*), the bone is thinned and expanded by the tumour, causing pain and deformity. *Aneurysmal bone cysts* arise mainly in the ends of growing long bones and consist of expanding osteolytic lesions containing bloody fluid that may cause pathological fracture.

The main malignant tumours are *osteosarcoma* and *chondrosarcoma*. *Osteosarcoma* has a maximum age incidence between 15 and 20 years of age and occurs in the metaphyseal region of long bones, especially those of the leg. In the elderly, osteosarcoma can complicate Paget's disease of bone. The tumour is composed of pleomorphic cells which destroy normal bone but also produce abnormal bone that is deposited sub-periosteally as the tumour elevates the periosteum (*Codman's triangle*) and along the tissue strands as irregular spicules of bone radiating from the shaft to give a 'sunray' appearance. Metastases occur via the bloodstream. *Chondrosarcoma* occurs between 15 and 60 years, can start in an osteochondroma and can arise in any bone; it is graded as low-grade (well-differentiated), average-grade (moderately differentiated) and high-grade (poorly differentiated). The tumour is cartilaginous with patchy calcification, is locally invasive and gives rise to blood-borne pulmonary metastases. *Fibrosarcoma* is composed of spindle-shaped fibroblasts which produce a cartilaginous matrix, and in bone may arise centrally or periosteally. *Synovial sarcoma* consists of elements of synovium mixed with malignant fibroblasts and arises close to major joints, often the knee, ankle or wrist. Like other fibrosarcomas it can arise in soft tissue and metastasizes by the lymphatics and the bloodstream. *Osteoclastoma* or *giant cell tumour* occurs most often in the third and fourth decades of life and is more common in women. It is composed of undifferentiated spindle cells and multinucleate giant cells in a vascular stroma and arises in the epiphyseal regions of the long bones, especially around the knee and occasionally in the humerus, radius and ulna. Recurrence after local excision is common, is more malignant than the initial tumour and spreads via the bloodstream. *Ewing's tumour* is believed to arise from the endothelial cells in the bone marrow or immature reticulum cells or the myeloid cell, and occurs in the middle of a long bone in childhood or adolescence. Radiography shows a number of sub-periosteal new bone formations expanding the shaft and giving the characteristic appearance of a cut onion. *Secondary bone tumours*, are more common than primary and arise from carcinomas of the breast or prostate, bronchus, kidney and thyroid; they are mostly osteolytic but a few arising from the prostate are osteosclerotic.

The diagnosis of a bone tumour is based on important clinical features: the age of the patient; the attachment to bone; the location of the tumour; and whether there is a primary neoplasm elsewhere. The more malignant the tumour, the more likely is it to present with severe pain or pathological fracture rather than as a mass.

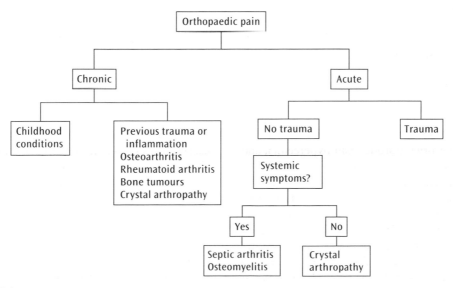

Algorithm 19.1

PAIN IN THE ARM

AIMS

1 Differentiate between conditions that present with acute pain and those that cause chronic pain
2 Distinguish between causes of localized pain and tenderness and of diffuse pain in the arm
3 Recognize extrinsic causes of pain in the arm

Introduction

The arm includes the shoulder girdle which consists of the scapula that articulates with the chest wall, the humerus (*glenohumeral joint*) and the clavicle (*acromioclavicular joint*); the elbow, where the humerus articulates with the radius and ulna; the wrist where these articulate with the carpal bones; and the phalanges which articulate with the carpus.

Pain can arise from any of the anatomical compartments of the arm and may be localized or diffuse. Pain in the arm can also originate from the cervical spine. Visceral pain from pulmonary or myocardial disease and from pathological conditions arising under the diaphragm can also be referred to the shoulder or arm. It is important, therefore, to bear in mind all these possibilities when taking a history and to examine the neck, arm, forearm and hand rather than focus on the painful area.

Examination

Look

An effusion in the shoulder joint may not be obvious because of the thick muscular covering of the capsule. Fluid in the subacromial bursa presents as a fluctuant swelling in front and to the lateral side of the humeral head and, with a large collection, posteriorly as well. The humeral head can be palpated separately and this differentiates it from an effusion into the shoulder joint.

The positions of ease taken when the joints are inflamed are: the shoulder in slight abduction; the elbow flexed at a right angle; the forearm pronated; and the wrist in slight flexion.

Feel

Feel the bony prominences of the cervical vertebrae, the para-vertebral muscles and the anterior aspect of the neck. Although structures on the front of the neck do not usually cause pain in the arm, a complaint of neck pain requires full examination of the neck. Three important bony points in the neighbourhood of the shoulder joint are the tip of coracoid, tip of acromion, prominence of greater tuberosity; around the elbow are the tip of the olecranon, the medial epicondyle and the lateral epicondyle. The wrist and hand, joint surfaces and soft tissues are palpated for tenderness and the overlying skin temperature. The arm and hand are examined for altered or absent sensation and the pulses at the wrist and elbow palpated.

Move

Observe the movements of the following joints:

- *Neck*: flexion, extension, rotation and lateral bending (this is the movement involved in trying to put the ear on the shoulder).
- *Shoulder*: flexion, abduction, external and internal rotation, noting pain especially on abduction (Fig. 19.1). Check for apprehension

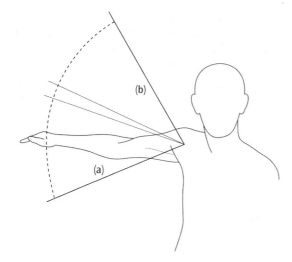

Fig. 19.1 *Low arc (a) and high arc (b) of shoulder pain on abduction of a shoulder. The low arc of pain is due to impingement of the rotator cuff muscles against the undersurface of the acromion, and indicates inflammation or a tear of the rotator cuff muscles. The high arc of pain is usually due to degenerative changes in the acromio-clavicular joint. Both arcs of pain may co-exist.*

when the shoulder is in the unstable position of abduction and external rotation.

- *Elbow*: flexion, extension, pronation and supination.
- *Wrist and hand*: wrist flexion and extension with the fist opened and closed. The power is examined by asking the patient to grip the examiner's fingers and pull, then push against the examiner's resistance. The triceps, biceps and supinator reflexes are examined.

Acute pain

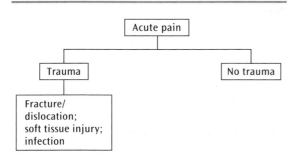

A history of trauma suggests a fracture or a dislocation, otherwise infection is the likely cause.

Following trauma, the pain is localized in the area of damage, although it may involve the whole arm. The clinical signs and radiography establish the diagnosis.

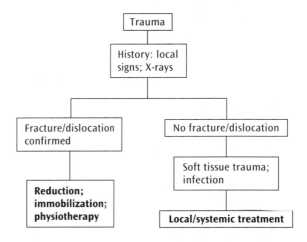

Fractures of the fingers are caused by direct trauma. Fractures are reduced and splinted to the adjacent finger, whereas fractures unstable after reduction are held in position by internal fixation with pins. Fracture at the base of the first metacarpal bone with proximal displacement of the thumb (*Bennet's fracture*) is treated by closed reduction and plaster of paris or by internal fixation. Hand injuries are treated by early mobilization to avoid stiffness and allow a good functional result.

Fractures at the wrist are caused by falls on the outstretched hand. *Scaphoid fracture* is identified by tenderness in the anatomical snuff box and the fracture is demonstrated on oblique X-ray views. Treatment is by scaphoid plaster, extending from below the elbow to the base of the proximal phalanges, for six weeks. The fracture may pass unnoticed until some time later when the patient presents with pain in the wrist and tenderness in the anatomical snuff box. This is usually due to avascular necrosis of the proximal fragment which is a recognized complication of this injury and is treated by excising the necrotic bone. A common fracture at the wrist joint is a *Colles' fracture* which produces the classical dinner-fork deformity in which the distal fractured end of the radius is shifted and tilted backwards and radially impacted, accompanied by a fracture of the ulnar styloid. When the radial fragment is displaced anteriorly, the fracture is a *Smith's fracture*. Treatment of both types of fracture is by reduction and immobilization in a plaster cast.

Fractures of the radius and ulna result usually from direct trauma and are treated by internal fixation. Fracture of the ulna with dislocation of the proximal radio-ulnar joint (*Monteggia fracture*) and a fracture of the radius with dislocation of the distal radio-ulnar joint (*Galeazzi fracture*) are best treated by reduction of the dislocation and internal fixation.

Fractures around the elbow include fractures of the olecranon and head of radius treated by immobilization in a plaster cylinder or internal fixation. A common and serious injury in children is a *supracondylar fracture of the humerus* with backward displacement as it carries a high risk of brachial artery injury which should be diagnosed if the arm is pulseless, pale and cold. The fracture is reduced carefully and if after the reduction the pulse, colour and temperature do not return to normal urgent arteriography or exploration is indicated. *Compartment syndrome* may develop, demonstrated by pain over the flexor compartment in the forearm with passive extension of the fingers. If not recognized and treated promptly, by splitting the plaster cast to relieve the pressure and performing fasciotomy, this condition will progress to *Volkmann's ischaemic contracture* of the flexor group of muscles with clawing of the fingers. Fractures around the elbow may result in median and/or ulnar nerve injury.

Fractures of the mid-shaft and neck of the humerus are treated by collar and cuff or a sling, with early mobilization to avoid shoulder stiffness. In mid-shaft fracture, radial nerve injury must be excluded. *Fractures of the clavicle* are managed similarly.

Dislocations

Finger dislocations are a common sports injury and are easily reduced under digital local anaesthesia with lignocaine. *Elbow dislocation* can result from a fall on the hand. The forearm is pulled backwards and the ulna dislocates posteriorly behind the

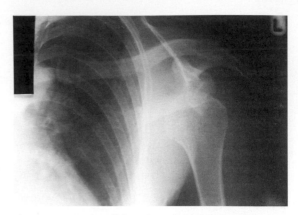

Fig. 19.2 *Anterior dislocation of the left shoulder (see also Fig. 21.6, p. 351, for posterior dislocation).*

humerus. The dislocation is reduced under general anaesthesia and immobilized for a few weeks. *Anterior dislocation of the shoulder* follows a similar injury; the humerus is pushed forwards tearing the capsule of the joint. The patient is unable to move the arm and supports the arm in slight abduction. On examination, there is loss of the rounded contour of the shoulder because of the flattening of the deltoid prominence and there is a depression below the acromion where the head of the humerus normally lies. It may be possible to feel the humeral head anteriorly. Injury to the circumflex nerve as it winds around the neck of the humerus can occur and is usually a neurapraxia that recovers spontaneously. It is, therefore, necessary to test for an area of anaesthesia over the deltoid region before reducing the dislocation. Radiography will show the head of the humerus in the sub-glenoid or sub-coracoid positions (Fig. 19.2). Reduction employing different manoeuvres under analgesia is usually successful but general anaesthesia may sometimes be required. Following reduction the arm is strapped to the chest wall with the arm flexed to prevent abduction. Early surgical repair of the avulsed capsule in shoulder dislocations appears to reduce the risk of recurrence.

When there is no history of trauma, and having eliminated the possibility of subcutaneous infection, acute septic arthritis or osteomyelitis is a likely cause.

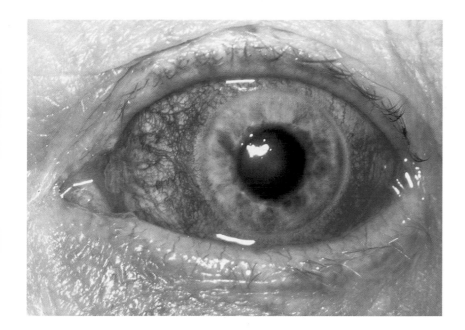

Plate 1 *An infected eye due to anterior uveitis. Typically, the inflammation of the conjunctiva is circumcorneal, but not in this case. The pupil dilates poorly because it is adherent to the anterior surface of the lens due to posterior synechiae.*

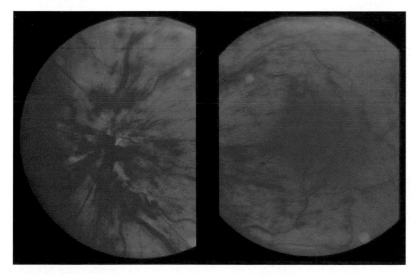

Plate 2 *The appearance of the fundus in central retinal vein occlusion. The optic disc (left) is swollen and numerous haemorrhages with cotton-wool spots surround it. There is also venous engorgement and tortuosity. The macular area (right) of the retina is involved and the haemorrhages and oedema shown may have reduced vision.*

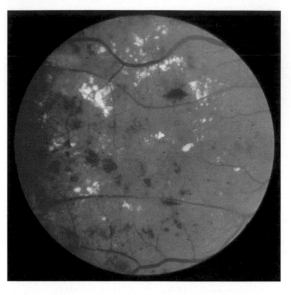

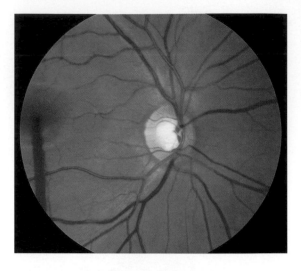

Plate 4 *Cupping of the optic disc; a normal optic disc.*

Plate 3 *The appearance of the fundus in diabetic retinopathy, showing numerous yellow exudates, blot haemorrhages and micro-aneurysms.*

Plate 5 *Cupping of the optic disc; loss of neural tissue at the rim of the optic disc results in excavation of the head of the optic disc, described as 'cupping' of the optic disc and seen typically in glaucoma patients.*

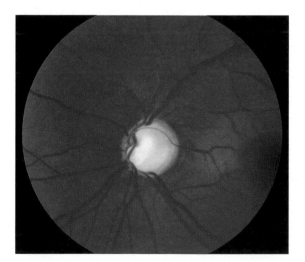

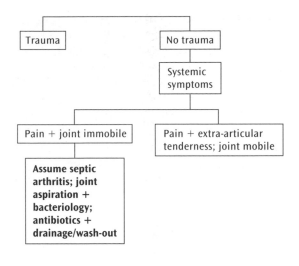

Acute septic arthritis

There is increasing pain, inability to move the joint and malaise. The patient is often toxic with a raised temperature and pulse rate. The arm is held in the position of ease, palpation reveals warmth and tenderness, an effusion can be difficult to demonstrate and movements are very painful and are therefore restricted. An X-ray of the joint will not show any change in the early stages of septic arthritis. When suspected, the joint is aspirated; the fluid is sent for bacteriology, and if purulent, the joint is drained or open wash-out by arthrotomy may be required. The appropriate antibiotics are administered intravenously. The joint is immobilized until the infection has resolved, in the position of optimal function.

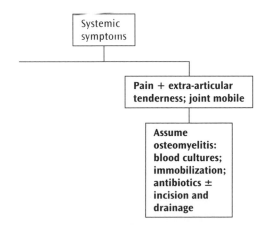

Acute osteomyelitis

The presentation is similar to septic arthritis, although the patient is more likely to be a child.

On palpation, an area of maximum tenderness over the metaphysis of a long bone should be regarded as diagnostic until proved otherwise. The adjacent joint may contain an effusion, raising the possibility of suppurative arthritis, but the ability to move the joint contrasts with acute suppurative arthritis. Days after onset, swelling, heat and tenderness are detected. Blood cultures are essential, but a raised ESR and white cell count is non-specific. An X-ray shows no abnormal features until at least 10 days, when it will demonstrate elevated periosteum and new bone formation, and rarefaction of the bone due to hyperaemia. MRI scan is more helpful in the early diagnosis of acute osteomyelitis; when MRI is not available, high uptake on an isotope scan is helpful.

Treatment consists of immobilization and systemic antibiotics; incision and drainage may also be required.

Chronic pain

This is more frequently local pain accompanied by tenderness than diffuse pain without a specific area of tenderness.

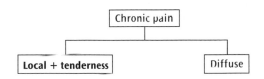

Local pain and tenderness

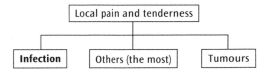

Local pain and tenderness in the arm can be due to infection or a bone tumour.

Chronic osteomyelitis may remain quiescent for considerable time but with acute or subacute exacerbations, with constitutional symptoms and local signs of inflammation. An X-ray may show a sequestrum. A *Brodie's abscess* causes intermittent pain and examination may reveal tenderness and thickening of the bone. A radiograph shows a band of sclerosis surrounding a lucent area. *Treatment* is by immobilization of the limb and administration of antibiotics; when ineffective, surgical intervention is required to remove dead bone and curette the abscess cavity which if large is packed with cancellous bone chips under antibiotic cover.

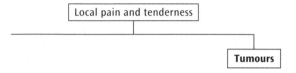

Bone tumours can also cause localized tenderness, particularly when malignant, the upper end of the humerus being a common site for osteosarcoma and chondrosarcoma. Ewing's tumour in the long bones of the arm may present with intermittent pyrexia and a painful, hot swelling that can be difficult to distinguish from acute haematogenous osteomyelitis. The radiographic appearances may be characteristic but if malignancy is suspected histological material should always be obtained by biopsy before treatment is undertaken. MRI is particularly useful in outlining the features of a bone tumour and its local extent. Benign tumours are not treated unless there is suspicion of a malignant change, for example osteochondroma, or if there is risk of pathological fracture as in chondromas and aneurysmal bone cysts, which are excised by curettage and the resulting cavity is packed with bone chips. Malignant bone tumours are treated by wide local excision with replacement of the defect by a custom-made prosthesis or allograft. Radiotherapy or chemotherapy or both are administered in combination with surgery depending on the sensitivity of the tumour.

However, malignant disease and infection are not common and most patients presenting with arm pain will usually have one of the following conditions best considered by anatomical areas.

Shoulder tenderness. Several conditions share a common clinical presentation of shoulder pain. There is tenderness during active movement within a painful arc (often the mid-part of the range of abduction, between 60° and 120°, whilst raising the arm above the head) sometimes associated with pain limited to a particular range of movement. It is common among those involved in heavy manual work and sports, and follows unusual activity among others. A useful aid to clinical examination is a syringe of local anaesthetic. Infiltration around the tender area may abolish pain and localize the site of pathology.

Although symptomatic treatment is effective in most cases, arthrography or arthroscopy is sometimes required to establish the diagnosis in those who are not responding. The following clinical entities are recognized:

- *Sub-acromial impingement* is a condition in which any of the structures below the acromion, such as the sub-acromial bursa or supraspinatus tendon, becomes inflamed. There is tenderness of the acromion and a painful arc when the arm is abducted. It is effectively treated by the injection of steroid under the acromion into the bursa or around it but not into the tendon.
- *Acute calcific tendinitis* has similar clinical features to sub-acromial impingement but is often acute in onset, the pain is very severe especially on abduction and there is exquisite tenderness just beneath the tip of the acromion. A radiograph shows an area of calcification in the supraspinatus tendon. This condition resolves spontaneously. Treatment is by local steroid injection in the sub-acromial region and, if calcification is detected early, aspiration or excision of the calcific deposit dramatically relieves pain.
- *Rotator cuff tears* complicate rupture of the supra-spinatus tendon which is part of the rotator cuff constituted by the muscles inserted around the shoulder joint and its capsule. This causes considerable pain and discomfort. The patient is able to abduct the arm to only about 40° to 50°, but the absence of injury and fullness of all passive movements exclude fracture or dislocation. Repeated injection for inflammation of the supraspinatus tendon or calcific tendinitis should be avoided as often further investigation will show degenerative change in the acromio-clavicular joint with osteophytic impingement on the supraspinatus tendon that

causes its rupture. Early diagnosis and excision of the impinging part of the acromion will result in pain relief and prevent rupture of the tendon that may extend to the rotator cuff, requiring its repair. Isolated tendon rupture leaves slight disability and repair is not essential, especially considering that the tendon holds the sutures poorly.

- *Frozen shoulder* is of unknown aetiology. Characteristically, it causes pain and stiffness of the shoulder with little or no glenohumeral movement. Usually it resolves within 2 years but physiotherapy, manipulation under anaesthesia and local steroid injection may help.

- *Biceps tendinitis* is inflammation of the synovial sheath of the intra-articular tendon of the long head of the biceps muscle. Like supraspinatus tendinitis, pain in the shoulder is felt especially on abduction and rotation. Local steroid injection can be effective, although it should be prescribed with caution to limit the risk of rupture of the tendon associated with this condition. Rupture is recognized by asking the patient to flex the elbow against resistance, when the affected biceps muscle bunches distally leaving a gap proximally.

- *Recurrent dislocation* follows damage to the glenoid labrum, the capsule or the bone of the humeral head following one or several shoulder dislocations. It is often not painful but is usually associated with a feeling of apprehension when the arm is in an unstable position of abduction and external rotation. A radiograph shows the characteristic Hill Sachs or 'Hatchet' lesion on the humeral head where the soft bone of the humeral head has been worn down by the anterior lip of the glenoid following several anterior dislocations. Treatment is usually by surgical reconstruction of the labrum and the capsule.

- *Acromioclavicular joint arthritis* is usually due to osteoarthritis and is commonly post-traumatic. It is frequently misdiagnosed as arthritis of the shoulder joint as the patient localizes the pain not on top of the shoulder but in the shoulder joint. The patient experiences sharp pain when the arm is raised above a right angle, which contrasts with tendinous cuff lesions. There is tenderness and an obvious swelling over the joint. An X-ray is likely to show a decreased joint space with osteophytes, cyst formation and sclerosis. Should this condition fail to respond to physiotherapy or local steroid injection, excision of the distal 1.5 cm of the clavicle is the simplest and safest treatment.

- *Glenohumeral pain* may be caused by an inflammatory condition such as rheumatoid arthritis or in the elderly by degenerative disease, although the shoulder is rarely affected by primary or secondary osteoarthritis. This is recognized by pain experienced when abduction is commenced and which continues throughout the movement. The treatment depends on the primary cause. In osteoarthritis, arthrodesis in the position of function (i.e., the position taken up by the shoulder when the hand is brought to the mouth) is easier to secure than in rheumatoid arthritis because the bones are hypertrophic rather than porotic and total joint arthroplasty is available in selected cases.

Elbow tenderness. Olecranon bursitis (*student's* or *miner's elbow*), the result of repeated pressure or slight injuries, appears as a swelling over the subcutaneous surface of the olecranon process. It is rarely due to an infection and usually responds to anti-inflammatory drugs and rest. When infected, it is hot, tender and painful. Spontaneous resolution may occur, although antibiotics, incision and drainage or excision may be required if the condition is persistently troublesome.

Other common causes of tenderness around the elbow are the *enthesopathies*, that is inflammation of the short fibrous origin of a muscle (*enthesis*) and these are of the common flexor muscle origin of the forearm at the lateral epicondyle or of the common extensor muscle origin at the medial epicondyle. The patient complains of throbbing pain especially on either flexion, with a point of considerable tenderness over the lateral epicondyle (*Tennis elbow*) or on extension, with a point of tenderness over the medial epicondyle (*Golfer's elbow*). In most cases, especially when over-use is the likely cause, rest results in spontaneous recovery but when severe or chronic, anti-inflammatory drugs, physiotherapy or local steroid injection into the point of tenderness can be effective. In a few, surgical release of the common extensor or flexor origin from the epicondyle to decompress the area allowing it to re-attach itself, is required. The new attachment of the muscle origin is often pain-free.

Arthritis of the elbow joint, either osteoarthritis or rheumatoid arthritis is also associated with tenderness with painful and restricted movement of the joint. In osteoarthritis, the joint is rarely painful enough to require surgery but when it is, arthrodesis of the humeroulnar joint is carried out.

In *rheumatoid arthritis* synovectomy is occasionally useful but arthrodesis is not always successful. Total replacement arthroplasty of the humeroulnar joint is promising treatment.

Forearm tenderness. Nerve entrapment syndrome usually involves the median or ulnar nerve and is a result of neurapraxia from continued pressure which if not relieved leads to irreversible nerve damage. The most common nerve lesion causing pain in the forearm is *carpal tunnel syndrome* in which the median nerve is compressed at the wrist where it passes through a fibrous canal bounded by the carpal bones and the flexor retinaculum. The compression results from wrist fractures and dislocations, fluid retention and oedema associated with pregnancy and myxoedema, or granulation tissue in rheumatoid arthritis. The classical symptoms are weakness of thumb abduction and numbness and tingling in the sensory distribution of the nerve (on the palmar surface of the medial three and a half fingers); they are worse at night and wake the patient who learns to shake the hand to relieve the discomfort. The examination can be normal, although flexing the wrist may reproduce the symptoms, and in advanced cases there is wasting of the thenar eminence. The sensation over the palm is preserved as it is supplied by a small branch from the median nerve which passes over the flexor retinaculum and this distinguishes a median nerve lesion at the wrist from a proximal lesion. It is self-limiting in pregnancy; otherwise, treatment is by decompressing the nerve by dividing the flexor retinaculum and, in rheumatoid arthritis, synovectomy at the wrist may be required.

Ulnar neuritis is due to entrapment of the nerve at the elbow. It results from overstretching by bony prominences following fractures at the elbow joint and entrapment by a fibrous band as it passes between the origins of the flexor carpi ulnaris muscle. The patient complains of tingling in the little finger and loss of intrinsic muscle function and fine finger movements. On examination, there is tenderness on tapping the nerve on the medial side of the elbow, dryness of the skin on the medial border of the hand and sensory changes. In advanced cases there is wasting of small muscles of the hand. Ulnar neuritis is distinguished from an enthesopathy by the history and examination, although nerve conduction studies might be required. Decompression by transposition of the nerve to the front of the elbow limits the neurological deficit but does not reverse it. Ulnar nerve entrapment at the wrist as it passes through its tunnel can occur with median nerve compression in rheumatoid arthritis and following trauma.

Tenosynovitis, commonly of the extensor tendons of the hand, is usually associated with rheumatoid arthritis, although it can follow excessive use. A splint to restrict movement of the hand, including the fingers, anti-inflammatory agents, physiotherapy and local steroid injection into the tendon sheaths offer pain relief. *Stenosing tenosynovitis* is of obscure aetiology; the tendon sheath thickens and entraps the tendon, resulting in pain and limitation of movement. It usually affects the common sheath of the abductor pollicis longus and extensor pollicis brevis tendons at the wrist (*de Quervain's disease*). This is treated by surgical release.

Diffuse pain

Having ruled out a referred pain from a visceral origin, and in the absence of local tenderness, there are a few extrinsic conditions that may account for the pain in the arm.

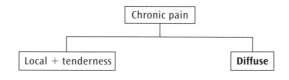

Cervical spondylosis (Fig. 19.3) in patients aged over 40 years and *cervical disc prolapse* in those under 40 years of age are common; rarely, *metastatic cervical deposits* are causes of pain. Those patients with cervical disc prolapse, unlike those with cervical spondylosis, do not usually have a long history

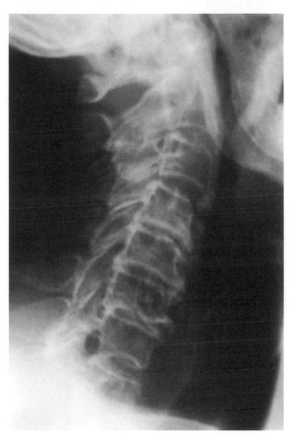

Fig. 19.3 *Cervical spondylosis. A lateral X-ray of the cervical spine shows narrowing of the disc spaces at multiple levels. There is sclerosis of the vertebrae and formation of osteophytes.*

of neck symptoms and characteristically show more marked neck muscle spasm and stiffness. The referred pain in the shoulder and arm and tingling in the arms is not necessarily due to nerve root entrapment which is usually accompanied with localizing neurological signs. A plain X-ray may not be contributory. In the presence of neurological signs a radiculogram combined with a CT or MRI scan better defines bony or disc compression. Nerve conduction studies or cervical myelography may be required when neurological signs from cervical bony entrapment are to be differentiated from local nerve entrapments. In the absence of neurological signs the patient is treated with non-steroidal anti-inflammatory drugs or a cervical collar and physiotherapy. With persistent symptoms, and especially if localizing neurological signs are marked, surgical anterior fusion should be considered.

Cervical rib occurs in 0.4% of people and in more than half is bilateral. The subclavian artery and the first dorsal nerve are angulated as they pass over it instead of the first thoracic rib. Especially if the shoulder sags, nerve pressure symptoms or less frequently vascular symptoms, or both are apparent and are precipitated by the patient's occupation, for example a decorator or a postman with his bag. A cervical rib as the cause of pain and tingling in the hand and forearm, whether wasting of the thenar and hypothenar muscles is present or not, should only be accepted after cervical spondylosis and nerve entrapment has been excluded. When vascular symptoms are present pain is the prevailing complaint; it is located in the forearm but may radiate to the upper arm and is precipitated by the use of the arm and relieved by rest. The hand on the affected side is colder than the opposite side, becomes pale when held aloft and blue when it is dependent, whereas the volume of the radial pulse is variable. In mild cases the use of a sling and exercises aimed at strengthening the muscles of the shoulder girdle may alleviate the symptoms; otherwise excision of the rib is required.

A *Pancoast tumour* is a peripheral lung carcinoma that arises at the apex of the lung, invades the brachial plexus, upper ribs and adjacent vertebrae and causes intractable pain. It is recognized by other associated features. The sympathetic chain is involved producing Horner's syndrome: the upper lid droops, the pupil is smaller and there is no sweating on the side of the lesion. The neck and chest wall veins are distended from pressure on the superior vena cava. The diagnosis is easily reached, and treatment is palliative.

Reflex sympathetic dystrophy is a rare condition characterized by persistent pain, swelling, hyperaesthesia, stiffness and disuse of the arm following an injury. The diffuse osteoporosis is usually accompanied with localizing neurological signs. *Treatment* is difficult and includes physiotherapy and pain control.

Repetitive strain injury (RSI)

This is a non-pathological diagnosis that describes a mix of arm and hand pains experienced by people who do heavy manual or repetitive work. Often, one of the pathological conditions described above is present. A normal physical examination of the arm and neck, a normal nerve conduction study, the absence of cardiac or systemic disease yet a patient with persistent symptoms, constitutes a management problem and deserves a specialized investigation. An isotope bone scan may demonstrate increased metabolic activity associated with endocrine or neoplastic disease. An MRI scan of the neck might demonstrate sub-clinical pathological changes producing referred pain in the arm. An X-ray and CT scan of the chest will exclude lesions at the apex of the lung. If all these investigations are normal then the patient should be kept under review with reassessment of symptoms and examination after a few weeks. Having excluded an underlying sinister pathology, if the pain persists and control is inadequate the diagnosis of RSI can be confidently made and the patient is referred to a pain clinic.

HIGHLIGHTS

- Fractures and dislocations are the most commonest cause of acute pain in the arm
- Early diagnosis and treatment of acute septic arthritis or osteomyelitis will prevent deformity or loss of function
- A painful shoulder should be managed carefully to prevent rotator cuff tears
- Elbow pain and tenderness is frequently not due to arthritis
- Nerve entrapment and tenosynovitis are the common causes of pain in the forearm and the wrist
- Cervical spondylosis, disc prolapse or rib and a Pancoast tumour are possible causes of diffuse pain in the arm

---

PAIN IN THE HIP

AIMS

1 Understand the principles of examination of the hip joint
2 Be familiar with common conditions that affect the hip joint
3 Recognize the relationship of hip disease to age

Introduction

The hip joint is a large weight-bearing joint, and therefore exposed to mechanical stress exhibited in its vulnerability to fractures and to disorders that affect the epiphysis and the articular surfaces. Because of its large synovial membrane it is particularly prone to inflammatory and infective processes. These constitute the common conditions encountered, and present with pain, usually in the groin but less frequently in the buttock, as tension in the hip joint causes pain and spasm in those muscles that share the nerve supply. The pain is sometimes felt solely in the knee, since both joints receive the same nerve supply.

Examination

It is fundamental that the spine, contralateral hip, and knees are also examined.

Look

Inspection is started in the standing posture. A patient with arthritis of the hip joint tends to bear weight on the sound leg to lessen weight-bearing, which results in slight flexion of the knee joint on the affected side. The adductors and glutei may appear wasted from disuse atrophy. The presence of scars and sinuses is relevant and can be due to chronic septic arthritis. In the position of ease the hip is partially flexed, abducted and externally rotated.

Feel

The bone and soft tissue landmarks around the hip are palpated for induration and swelling but the hip joint is mostly inaccessibly deep to thick muscles, although tenderness may be elicited around the greater trochanter, thigh or buttock. The capsule is prolonged down the neck of the femur and here is where it can be felt. A finger on the anterior superior iliac spine is rolled down the inguinal ligament until the femoral pulse is felt. A point below the inguinal ligament and lateral to the femoral artery overlies a small portion of the head which is not intra-acetabular; tenderness on pressure suggests arthritis,

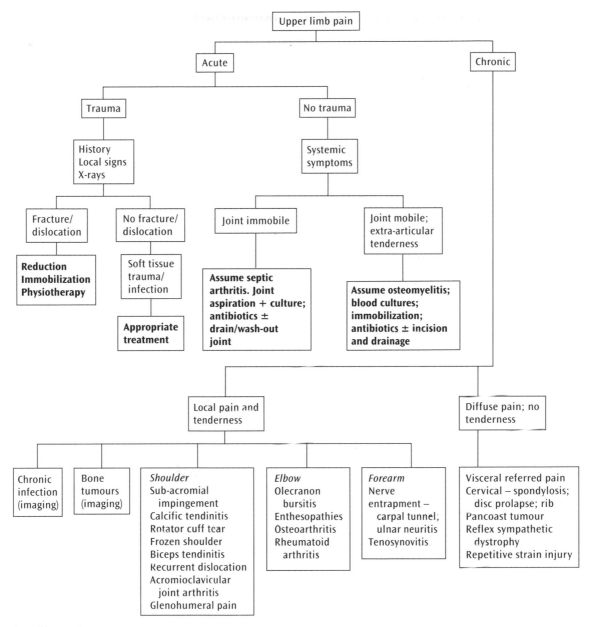

Algorthim 19.2

and crepitus can be felt when rotating the hip. Absence of the head of the femur signifies dislocation.

Move

A fixed flexion deformity is masked by increased lumbar lordosis which allows the affected leg to reach the ground when the patient is standing. This is demonstrated by the *Thomas test*; with the patient lying on the couch, one hand is placed under the lumbar spine and with the other hand the sound hip is flexed until the spine can be felt against the hand, thus straightening the lordosis. This puts the pelvis in a neutral position, and will reveal any flexion

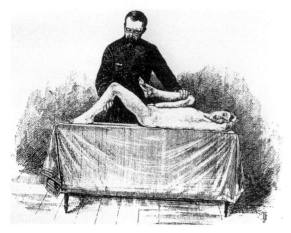

Fig. 19.4 *The Thomas test (see text).*

deformity in the affected limb (Fig. 19.4). When movements of the hip joint are tested, the anterior superior iliac spines must lie square with the couch and care must be taken that the pelvis does not move. Internal and external rotation, abduction, adduction, flexion and extension movements are compared with the other hip.

Measure

The true length of a lower limb is measured with the patient lying supine on a flat surface and the pelvis square. The normal limb must be placed in a similar position to the affected limb before measurement is taken, from the anterior superior iliac spine to the medial malleolus of the ankle. Any difference between the two sides is due to a real difference in length of the limb or of the small part of the pelvis between the anterior superior iliac spine and the acetabulum. When there is real leg shortening, viewing from the side while the patient is lying with the hips and knees flexed and the heels level, demonstrates the part of the limb involved. Apparent length is measured from any convenient mid-line point, such as the xiphisternum, to the medial malleolus of each ankle, and is not as important as real shortening.

Hip disease can affect true length by loss of height in the hip itself, and apparent leg length

because joint deformity such as fixed adduction of the hip can cause the pelvis to be held at an oblique angle to the upper body, and the adducted hip will appear short.

Assess function

The patient's *walking gait* is scrutinized. An *antalgic gait* occurs when there is pain on weight-bearing and the patient shortens the time spent on the painful hip. A *short leg gait* occurs when the shoulder on the affected side droops during the period of weight-bearing on the short leg; however, the head does not usually cross the mid-line. A *Trendelenburg gait* results when the abduction mechanism of the hip is insufficiently strong to hold the pelvis steady when the patient is bearing weight on that hip. Instead, in an effort to stop the pelvis dropping on the weight-bearing side, the upper body leans to the side of the affected hip when it is bearing weight and the centre of gravity moves lateral to that hip, thus counteracting any tendency for the pelvis to droop on the non-weight-bearing side (Fig. 19.5). This is demonstrated by the *Trendelenburg test*; the unsupported patient lifts in turn one leg and then the other off the ground. Standing on a normal hip, the non-weight-bearing side of the pelvis rises because of the power of the abduction mechanism on the other side. When this abduction mechanism is damaged in any way by disease of the nerve/muscle unit, or if the abduction mechanism is inhibited by pain, the non-weight-bearing side of the pelvis drops. This is known as a positive Trendelenberg test. (A useful mnemonic for remembering the appearance of a unilateral positive Trendelenberg test is *sss*: 'the sound side sags'.)

Investigation

Plain radiography is the most appropriate investigation. It is important to have a system of examining hip X-rays so that nothing is overlooked (*see* box below) (Fig. 19.6 – a plain anterioposterior (AP) X-ray of the pelvis). On the AP film Shenton's line has been drawn.

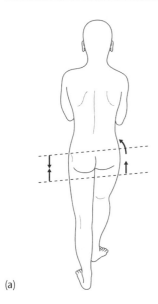 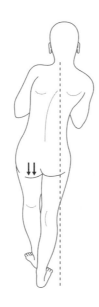

(a)   (b)

Fig. 19.5 (a) and (b) *The Trendelenburg test (see text, p. 288).*

Examining an X-ray – refer to Fig. 19.6 while reading this

- To compare both hips, the AP view of the pelvis is essential; a lateral view of the affected hip is also obtained
- The soft tissues for swelling, increased density or calcification
- The cortical outline of the femur and the pelvis for density and continuity
- The medulla of the bone for destruction or sclerosis
- The joint for narrowing of the joint space, erosion, irregularity, sclerosis or new bone formation (*osteophytes*)
- The normality of Shenton's and Trethowan's lines. Shenton's line loses its smooth arch shape in fractures of the femoral neck and in conditions such as avascular necrosis and osteoarthritis with deformity of the femoral head. (For Trethowan's line *see* Fig. 19.7.)

Acute pain

The three most likely conditions in a patient who presents with acute hip pain are fracture or dislocation following trauma, and infection.

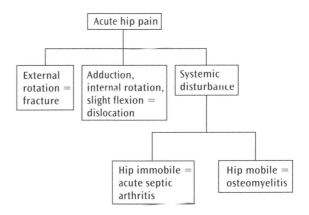

Fracture of the femoral neck is a common clinical problem in the elderly woman with post-menopausal osteoporosis, and may follow relatively minor trauma. Young people sustain these fractures in road traffic accidents. The patient presents with pain, and the leg may be externally rotated. Fractures of the intra-capsular neck of the femur, that is, the part of the neck that is within the capsule of the hip joint, can interfere with the blood supply to the head (Fig. 19.7) and need urgent attention in order to avoid avascular necrosis developing. In young people the fracture is reduced and held in position with screws, whereas in older people with displacement a quicker return to mobility is achieved by replacing the femoral head with a metal prosthesis. Extra-capsular fractures, whatever the age

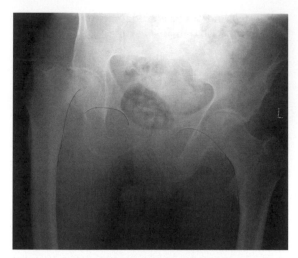

Fig. 19.6 *Anteroposterior (AP) radiograph of the pelvis. On the normal (left) side there is continuity in a smooth arch between the inferior surface of the superior pubic ramus and the medial aspect of the neck of the femur (Shenton's line: it has been accentuated with a drawn line). On the right side, Shenton's line is interrupted by displacement of the intra-capsular fractured neck of femur.*

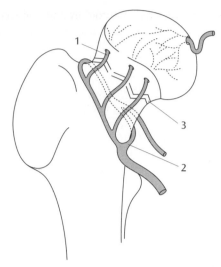

Fig. 19.7 *The main blood supply to the head of the femur arises from branches (1) of an arterial ring around the neck of the femur (2). These branches traverse the neck to perforate the head close to the margin of the cartilage. Thus intra-capsular fractures (3) damage the blood supply to the femoral head and may lead to avascular necrosis. Only about 10% of the blood supply of the head comes from vessels in the ligamentum teres.*

of the patient, heal satisfactorily as the blood supply is not interrupted, and are treated by internal fixation by a hip screw. In the absence of co-morbid factors the patient, if mobile and capable of self-care, can often leave the hospital within days. Where the medical facilities are not available, traction and bedrest give a satisfactory result despite a stay in hospital of at least 6 weeks, provided that the risks of prolonged immobility (massive pulmonary segmental collapse, deep vein thrombosis and pulmonary embolism, muscle wasting, contractures, osteoporosis and renal stones) can be prevented.

Dislocation of the hip requires significant force as the hip is a very stable joint. The limb lies in a position of adduction, internal rotation and slight flexion. The head of the femur usually dislocates posteriorly and may cause damage to the sciatic nerve. Hip dislocation is often associated with fractures of the acetabulum. The blood supply to the femoral head is compromised by dislocation which tears the capsular vessels. The hip should, therefore, be reduced as soon as possible under a general anaesthetic and muscle relaxation. If the reduction is stable, early mobilization on crutches is appropriate. If it is unstable, acetabular fractures should be fixed.

Acute septic arthritis is usually blood-borne, or may arise by local extension from adjacent infected bone, especially in children where a metaphyseal infection within the joint capsule causes inflammation of the synovium. There is intense pain on the slightest movement of the joint which is held flexed, adducted and externally rotated (position of ease) and may be tender on palpation. Pyrexia and malaise are common features. The white cell count and ESR are raised, but these changes are non-specific and an X-ray is not contributory. An ultrasound scan may show some fluid in the joint. A high index of suspicion must be maintained. Where infection is suspected, blood cultures are taken and then systemic antibiotics are commenced. Aspiration for diagnostic and therapeutic reasons is carried out under aseptic technique, and the fluid cultured. The joint is immobilized until the infection has resolved. Arthrotomy and drainage may be required if there is frank pus on aspiration. If the disease is treated early full function may be restored to the joint, but if the pathological process had involved the articular cartilage healing leaves a fibrous ankylosis.

Acute osteomyelitis is similar to septic arthritis in its clinical features, but the movement of the hip joint is not restricted. *Management* is as already described and consists of immobilization, systemic antibiotics and incision and drainage.

Chronic pain

It is important to establish whether the pain is arising from a disease of the spine or the knee, as these may contribute to pain in the hip region. Although infection of bone and joint and tumours can affect all ages, there are certain conditions that are particularly related to the age of the patient.

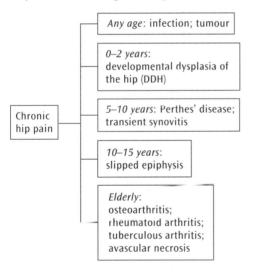

Chronic hip pain

- *Any age*: infection; tumour
- *0–2 years*: developmental dysplasia of the hip (DDH)
- *5–10 years*: Perthes' disease; transient synovitis
- *10–15 years*: slipped epiphysis
- *Elderly*: osteoarthritis; rheumatoid arthritis; tuberculous arthritis; avascular necrosis

Age-specific conditions of the hip

0–2 years. Congenital dislocation of the hip (CDH) is better called *developmental dysplasia of the hip* (DDH) to cover abnormality of the femoral head, the acetabulum or both. It occurs in two or three births per 1000, is more common in girls than boys and can be bilateral. The diagnosis is made at birth by attempting to dislocate the hip or relocate it if dislocated, and this produces a 'click' or a 'clunk'. The hip is stiff and abduction is limited. Occasionally, DDH is unrecognized until the child starts walking, when the clinical signs are shortening, asymmetrical skin creases along the adductor aspect of the thigh, limited abduction and a limp. Treatment at birth involves reduction in 45° abduction and 90° flexion and slight internal rotation. The position of reduction is confirmed by X-ray of the pelvis, and maintained in a metal splint or plaster. When diagnosed late but before walking, the hip is reduced by a period of traction, followed by open or closed manipulation before it is placed in a plaster splint for 3 months. When discovered after walking, surgery is required to deepen the acetabulum and re-angulate the femoral neck for better alignment (Fig. 19.8) but the result may not be satisfactory and secondary arthritis is a likely long-term complication.

5–10 years. Perthes' disease is an osteochondritis of the femoral head, occurs in one per 3000 children, and is of unknown aetiology. It is more common in boys than girls and in 25% is bilateral. The child presents with a painful limp and the pain is referred to the knee. The mechanism is believed to be avascular necrosis of the femoral head. Radiologically, it is initially normal in appearance or is more radio-dense

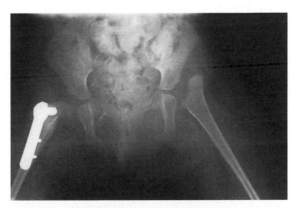

Fig. 19.8 *An anteroposterior (AP) X-ray of the pelvis in a child presenting with bilateral developmental dysplasia (congenital dislocation) of the hips. On the left side the hip is completely dislocated and the acetabulum is very shallow. On the right the femoral head has been relocated in the acetabulum and a femoral derotation osteotomy carried out; the bone fragments are held with a plate and screw.*

than the adjacent bones (Fig. 19.9) due to diminished blood supply; later, it softens and appears less dense. The head is eventually revascularized and re-ossified but is deformed. When the diagnosis is suspected, radiological changes in the appearances of the head of the femur can be observed by repeated X-rays at regular intervals. Ultrasound examination may reveal fluid in the joint. The aim of treatment is to maintain the hip within the acetabulum until the pathological process is completed. In minor degrees (up to half the head is involved) the prognosis is good without treatment but these children should remain under regular review. In children with full head involvement, although the symptoms resolve, secondary osteoarthritis develops later in life. In these patients splintage to keep the head fully contained in the acetabulum with the leg abducted, or if necessary an osteotomy of the femur to maintain this position, may help.

10–15 years. Slipped upper femoral epiphysis occurs during adolescence. The upper femoral epiphysis slips in a posterior and inferior direction. The child presents with a limp, pain which radiates to the knee and reduced range of movement. The onset may be acute or develop over several months. On examination, there is limitation of abduction, flexion and internal rotation. An X-ray must include a lateral view in order not to miss minor degrees of slippage (Fig. 19.10). Treatment is surgical if minor or moderate; progression is prevented by pinning the head in its deformed position. If the slippage is major then reduction by complicated osteotomy of the neck may be required to restore the epiphysis to its original relationship to the acetabulum, but this carries the risk of compromising the blood supply to the head

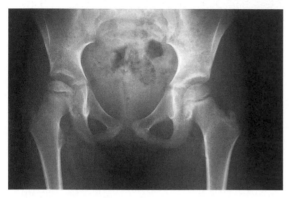

Fig. 19.9 *Perthes' disease. The anteroposterior (AP) X-ray of a pelvis and hips. There is irregularity, collapse and increased density of the right upper femoral epiphysis.*

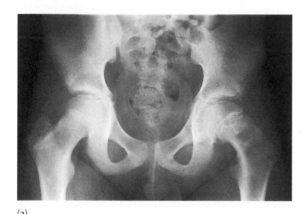

(a)

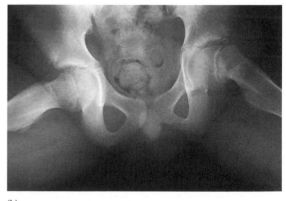

(b)

Fig. 19.10 *Slipped upper femoral epiphysis; (a) An anteroposterior (AP) X-ray of the pelvis demonstrates a left slipped upper femoral epiphysis. The direction of displacement is mainly posteriorly and only slightly inferiorly. To the untrained eye, the AP X-ray might appear normal, but on the left Trethowan's line, drawn along the upper border of the femoral neck, does not intersect with the femoral epiphysis, whereas on the normal right side, it does; (b) A lateral X-ray of the hips of the same patient confirms the significant posterior displacement of the slipped left upper femoral epiphysis.*

(*see* Fig. 19.7 above) and resulting in avascular necrosis. The other side should be watched radiologically and pinned if there is any evidence of slippage.

Transient synovitis or 'irritable hip' can be difficult to distinguish from the earliest stages of infective arthritis, Perthes' disease or slipped epiphysis. The child presents with pain and a limp and the hip is held in the position of greatest ease, but without the toxaemia or high pyrexia of septic arthritis.

Ultrasound may show a little fluid in the joint. It is usually self-limiting after a few days of bedrest and may be related to a systemic viral infection. If the symptoms persist, monthly radiographs are advisable in order to exclude Perthes' disease.

Conditions which predispose to the development of secondary osteoarthritis

- Congenital dislocation of the hip.
- Perthes' disease.
- Slipped epiphysis.
- Crystal arthropathy.
- Fracture in the joint.
- Rheumatoid arthritis.
- Septic arthritis.

In the elderly

Osteoarthritis in the elderly is commonly primary, and in the younger patient secondary to a predisposing cause. It characteristically presents with pain and stiffness, aggravated by movement and diminished with restricting activity. The reduction in range of movement can produce disturbance of function; patients may be unable to put on their socks and cut their toe nails. On examination, all movements of the hip are restricted. There is apparent shortening, and slight real shortening from loss of cartilage and flattening of the head of the femur when the disease is advanced. The diagnosis is confirmed by radiography (Fig. 19.11).

Management is aimed at pain relief and includes weight loss and use of a stick in the contralateral hand in order to reduce the load on the hip, restricting unnecessary excessive activity, but maintaining daily exercise, physiotherapy and analgesia. Non-steroidal anti-inflammatory agents (NSAIDs) are

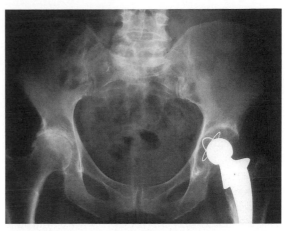

Fig. 19.11 *Anteroposterior (AP) X-ray of the pelvis and hips in an elderly patient. The right hip demonstrates narrowing of the joint space, sub-chondral sclerosis, cyst formation and osteophytes. On the left, a cemented total hip replacement has been carried out.*

prescribed for pain relief but do not alter the course of the disease. When these measures fail and pain interferes with sleep and the patient's quality of life, surgery is considered. The options are *arthroplasty*, *arthrodesis* and *osteotomy*. Arthroplasty for joint replacement is the commonly performed procedure that provides pain-free hip function. Infection early or late, and in the long term, loosening of the prosthesis are likely complications. *Arthrodesis* (surgical fusion) involves excising the femoral head and the cartilaginous surface of the acetabulum to allow the osseous ends of the joint to fuse (Girdlestone) in 30° of flexion and slight abduction; it allows pain-free gait, although it puts stress on the lumbar spine, the knee and the opposite hip. *Osteotomy* of the femur alters the femoral angle and this improves the deformity and joint alignment and provides symptomatic relief. In younger patients with a painful and limited range of movement, *arthrodesis* is probably appropriate, whereas osteotomy is suited in those with an acceptable range of movement and with relatively minimal joint degeneration, thus reserving arthroplasty for later in life.

Rheumatoid arthritis can start with hip pain. The activity of the disease tends to wax and wane, with symptomatic remissions and relapses. In the early stages the diagnosis can be difficult, especially if other joints are not involved, as there are minimal radiological changes, although the raised ESR and presence of rheumatoid factor are in sharp contrast to osteoarthritis. The radiological appearances differentiate it from osteoarthritis, although since the active rheumatoid process may remit, residual articular cartilage damage develops into secondary osteoarthritis with indistinguishable radiological changes. Treatment includes analgesics, anti-inflammatory agents, immunosuppressives and steroids. Surgery is indicated in severe cases and the only option is total replacement arthroplasty.

Tuberculous arthritis presents with a limp and pain in the joint, more often referred to the thigh or the knee, and worse on exertion but also at night. Systemic effects of the disease manifest with a low-grade temperature, malaise, weight loss and anaemia. In the early stages the leg is held in the position of ease, and as the disease progresses the hip becomes increasingly stiff, because movement is painful and is limited by adhesion formation, muscle spasm and intra-articular destruction. Initially, there is apparent shortening, because of tilting upwards of the pelvis on the affected side, but as the head of the femur becomes eroded, there is real shortening. Active and passive movements of the joint become limited and painful. There is muscle wasting of the thigh and the buttock. The presence of an effusion or an abscess may be elicited by careful palpation of the joint. Even if an abscess has formed, the overlying skin is neither red nor warm – a 'cold abscess'. Tuberculous arthritis in its early stage may be confused with infective arthritis, rheumatoid arthritis or haemarthroses complicating haemophilia.

The ESR and white cell count, mainly lymphocytes, are raised, the haemoglobin is low and a Mantoux test is strongly positive. A chest X-ray may show an active or an old lesion. An X-ray of the hip may only show decreased density of the bone adjacent to the joint and soft tissue swelling, but as the disease advances, the joint space is narrowed and bone destruction is visible. An MRI is a useful aid but if not available arthrotomy and tissue biopsy may be required. Joint aspirate, biopsy material, sputum and urine should be cultured for tubercle bacilli.

Treatment consists of immobilization of the joint in the position of function, that is, 20°–30° of flexion to allow sitting, and in neutral position as regards abduction and rotation; also antituberculous therapy, nutritional support and correction of anaemia. Surgery may be required and involves synovectomy and joint toilet or drainage of abscess followed by arthrodesis in order to provide the patient with a painless stable, although stiff joint, because the articulating bones are usually damaged.

Neoplastic disease causing persistent pain in the region of the hip joint arises from the ilium, the proximal femur or the synovial membrane of the joint. The tumours are osteosarcoma, chondrosarcoma, fibrosarcoma or synovial sarcoma. The hip bones are also common sites of secondary deposits. On radiography, usually there is bone destruction with ill-defined edges, periosteal reaction or sclerosis in the adjacent bone, and metastatic deposits appear as sclerotic or lytic. MRI scan outlines the local extent and an isotope scan shows any areas of skeletal spread. A biopsy, open or percutaneous using a hollow needle, allows histological diagnosis. Besides obvious clinical findings, a chest X-ray, a mammogram or a prostate specific antigen level will establish the primary origin of a secondary bone deposit. Management of the primary tumours is as previously described. The treatment of metastatic tumours is essentially that of symptom control with analgesics, local radiotherapy, internal fixation of pathological fractures of the femur and treatment of the primary cancer.

Avascular necrosis is associated with alcohol, long-term steroids, sickle cell disease and deep sea diving but is often idiopathic. It presents as deep pain in the hip and initially there may be no radiological changes. As it develops there is increased radiodensity and ultimately there may be collapse of a segment of the femoral head. Diagnosis of the pre-radiological stage can often be made with MRI. Core decompression of the femoral head can relieve symptoms in the early stages, but once collapse has occurred progression to osteoarthritis is almost inevitable. When a diagnosis cannot be reached and the patient is still symptomatic, a diagnostic arthroscopy or an MRI scan should identify other possibilities such as an acetabular labral tear or a synovial tumour.

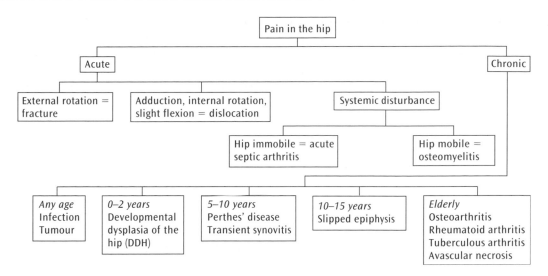

Algorithm 19.3

HIGHLIGHTS

- Intra-capsular fracture of the neck of femur requires prompt internal fixation to avoid avascular necrosis
- A diagnosis of 'irritable hip' should not be made until septic or tuberculous arthritis, slipped epiphysis and Perthes' disease have been excluded
- Lateral X-rays of the hip are essential when a slipped epiphysis or Perthes' disease is suspected
- Early diagnosis and treatment of congenital or acquired hip conditions prevent secondary osteoarthritis

PAIN IN THE KNEE

AIMS

1 Learn the important features of history-taking and examination
2 Distinguish between traumatic (acute and chronic) and atraumatic (acute and chronic) presentations
3 Understand the principles of management of the various conditions

Introduction

The knee is a major weight-bearing joint whose stability and function depend entirely on soft tissues (ligaments and muscles). The extensor apparatus of the knee comprises the quadriceps muscles, the tendinous insertion of the quadriceps muscles into the patella, the patella itself, the ligamentum patellae and the insertion of the ligamentum patellae into the tibial tubercle. This apparatus contributes to the stability of the knee joint and provides the active extension of the knee which is vital to normal gait. Its ligaments are extra-articular (medial and lateral collaterals) and intra-articular (anterior and posterior cruciate). Alone amongst the major joints it contains *menisci*. Derangement of any of these structures by injury, to which the knee joint is particularly prone, can result in disabling symptoms. Therefore, history of trauma bears particular significance to the diagnosis when assessing a patient with a knee complaint.

History

Although *pain* is the main feature, associated cardinal symptoms are *swelling*, *locking* and *giving way*. The time of onset of the swelling relative to pain or injury is important. A rapidly developing swelling is due to bleeding into the knee (*haemarthrosis*), and suggests serious intra-articular damage, whereas a progressive swelling over hours or days suggests an effusion and implies a less severe injury. A chronic swelling that may or may not fluctuate in size with activity indicates synovitis due to inflammation. Locking of the knee refers to an inability to complete extension and must be differentiated from painful stiffness occurring on movement. True locking is due to a mechanical block between the joint surfaces by a torn meniscus, a torn cruciate ligament or a loose body. The inability to complete the knee extension may last for several minutes and the patient may seek assistance to force the knee into full extension. In contrast to painful stiffness, flexion is nearly always possible in the locked knee. Giving way is noticed as an inability to maintain the knee in extension when weight is applied and without warning or pain the knee gives way and the patient may fall. Similar to locking there is loss of acute extension of the knee because of relaxation of the quadriceps muscles, caused by painful restriction of the joint movement. This should be distinguished from a stumble because of acute pain as may occur in patients with osteoarthritis.

Examination

An examination of the knee is not complete without examination of the hip because the pain in the knee can be referred from the hip.

Look

The patient is examined first in the upright position. The whole of the knee must be inspected, including its posterior aspect. The affected knee is compared with the normal. Fullness above and on either side of the patella suggests an effusion. Alignment of the joint in a varus, or valgus or fixed flexion deformity is best assessed with the patient standing. A useful sign indicative of knee pathology is wasting of the quadriceps, easily demonstrable by asking the patient to extend the leg.

The position of ease of the knee joint is in semi-flexion.

Feel

The soft tissues and bony landmarks are palpated. Points of tenderness at the insertions of ligaments, at the fibula (lateral) and at the tibia (medial) distinguishes ligamental from meniscal injury where tenderness is elicited in the joint line, the space between the tibia and femur, best examined with the knee flexed to 90°. The patello-femoral joint is examined by palpating deeply beneath the overhanging edges of the patella for tenderness, and the underlying articular surfaces of the femoral condyles by pushing the patella medially and laterally. Crepitus may be felt by moving the patella on the underlying femoral condyles.

The knee joint is also examined for crepitus when flexing and extending the knee. A knee may appear swollen because of soft tissue oedema, synovial thickening or an effusion or bleeding (or both) into the joint. The presence of fluid in the joint is demonstrated by cross-fluctuation between the suprapatellar bursa and the knee joint when the effusion is small (Fig. 19.12 (a)), by the patellar tap when moderate (Fig. 19.12 (b)) and by a fluid thrill when large. Synovial thickening gives a boggy sensation when the capsule is palpated between the finger and thumb.

Move

The patient is asked to demonstrate active movements; if there is a deficit in active movements, passive movements are carried out. There is loss of lateral and medial stability in tears of the medial and lateral collateral ligaments, and of anteroposterior stability particularly in flexion in tears of the cruciate ligaments (Fig. 19.13). Other signs involving passive movements for the diagnosis of meniscal lesions are unreliable.

Gait

The patient with a painful knee walks with an antalgic (pain-relieving) gait. The cadence is asymmetrical because the patient spends less time in the gait cycle on the affected leg than on the normal leg. A stiff knee is demonstrated by reduced knee movements.

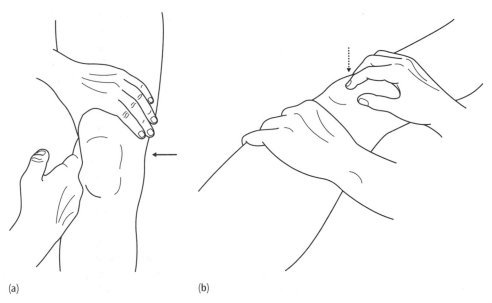

Fig. 19.12 *Detecting fluid in the knee joint; (a) The cross-fluctuation test. A small effusion can be detected by the cross-fluctuation or fluid displacement test. The supra-patellar pouch is compressed with one hand, then the medial side of the joint is stroked to displace fluid into the lateral side of the joint. Upon subsequent stroking of the lateral side of the joint, fluid will be seen to distend the medial side of the joint. This test will be negative if there is a moderate or large effusion; (b) The patellar tap. The supra-patellar pouch is compressed, the tips of the fingers of the other hand jerk the patella towards the femoral condyles. A click indicates the presence of a moderate effusion. The test may be negative if there is a tense effusion.*

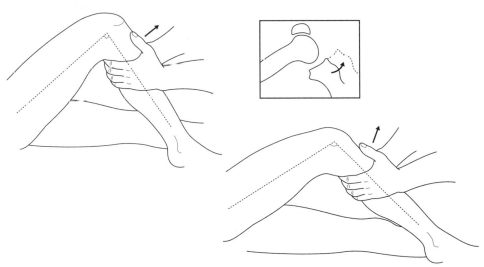

Fig. 19.13 *The anterior draw test. The knee is flexed to 90° and the foot is fixed. The upper leg is grasped firmly and pulled anteriorly. A significant displacement of the tibia will be felt and seen if the anterior cruciate ligament is ruptured.*

Radiography

The standard radiographs following acute injury are anteroposterior (AP) and lateral views with the patient recumbent. Standing (weight-bearing) views are more useful in the patient without injury in order to outline the joint space, that is, the radiolucent area between the bones occupied by cartilage which is narrowed because of loss of cartilage in osteoarthritis or inflammatory arthritides.

Presentations

There are four distinct clinical pictures: acute traumatic pain, acute atraumatic pain, chronic pain with a history of previous trauma, atraumatic chronic pain. The last contains a sub-group in which effusion into the joint is common.

Traumatic acute pain

Injuries causing damage to the extensor apparatus of the knee, fractures about and into the knee joint and ligament damage commonly occur after road traffic accidents and in sports. The acutely injured knee presents with pain, restricted movement, swelling and bruising. Examination may be limited to inspection as palpation and movement can be painful. It is essential that the popliteal circulation and nervous system are examined since fractures and dislocations of the knee can be associated with popliteal vessels or nerve injury. The swelling can be due to subcutaneous haematoma and oedema, or else to haemarthrosis when it increases rapidly after the trauma, the knee feels slightly warmer and the swelling is tense and extremely tender, a sign of intra-articular ligamentous or meniscal tear or of a fracture into the joint.

The immediate management of a patient with a knee injury is to splint the limb, treat pain and transfer the patient urgently for further assessment, including plain X-rays.

The possibility of soft tissue injuries is investigated by eliciting localized tenderness in relation to the underlying structures. If a ligament has been sprained rather than ruptured, stressing the ligament provokes pain at the injured point of insertion but does not demonstrate abnormal movement. *Ligamentous sprains* or *partial tears* are treated conservatively: pain is relieved with analgesics and if necessary local anaesthetic injections, and normal activities are restricted but the knee muscles are gradually rehabilitated with physiotherapy.

Rupture of the tendinous insertion of the quadriceps muscle into the patella, or of the ligamentum patellae, is uncommon. These injuries may not be immediately obvious because until the haematoma over the knee subsides, the gap above the patella where the muscle insertion has retracted or the gap below the patella created by the patella migrating upwards is not easily visible or palpable. Although active extension, that is, straight leg-raising is impossible, this diagnostic feature is often blamed on the pain caused by the injury. Treatment is by suture repair of the tendon or ligament with immobilization of the leg in a plaster cylinder for 6 weeks.

A rapid accumulation of liquid in the joint indicates a haemarthrosis, which is due either to rupture of the anterior cruciate ligament or to a fracture, or to a peripheral tear of a meniscus. The history often helps in that the patient often hears a popping sound when a cruciate ligament is torn. If the ligament is ruptured, the knee as a whole may be too painful to allow the ligament to be stressed. Unless there is abnormal posterior mobility (which may indicate a tear of the posterior capsule, and then liquid instilled in the joint for arthroscopy tracks into the calf and may produce a compartment syndrome), arthroscopy under anaesthesia is indicated. The knee is aspirated under aseptic technique, and is examined for ligamentous instability. A torn peripheral part of the meniscus is repaired, or a loose fragment of bone or cartilage which had been sheared off can be excised.

The treatment of *ligamentous ruptures* is controversial. The ruptured ends of cruciate and collateral ligaments usually retract, therefore if immobilization is employed the ligaments may not heal because the ends are apart. For this reason some advocate immediate exploration of the knee and primary repair, although this can be difficult with the cruciate ligaments and many surgeons do not attempt primary repair of these except when cruciate ligament is avulsed from its tibial attachment with a bone fragment which allows fixation with a screw. Following repair, the knee is immobilized in few degrees of

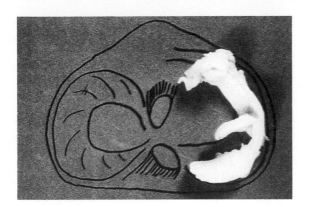

Fig. 19.14 *The photograph of a medial meniscus has been superimposed on a drawing of the articular surface of the tibia at the left knee. There is a parrot-beaked tear of the posterior part of the medial meniscus. Note the attachments of the anterior and posterior cruciate ligaments.*

flexion in a plaster cast from the groin to the metatarsal heads for 6 weeks. In most patients, conservative treatment is adopted in the hope that the soft tissue injury may heal and the patient may indeed not experience symptoms. Treatment consists of physiotherapy, in particular quadriceps and hamstring exercises, wearing a brace to prevent hyperextension; but weight-bearing is not allowed until 6 weeks after the injury when the knee is actively mobilized. If conservative management fails, and particularly if the patient is a professional sportsman, late operative repair can be undertaken.

Should there be no effusion, or only a slowly developing one, the patient is treated conservatively until the acute symptoms subside. If at this stage there are mechanical symptoms of locking or instability, arthroscopy is indicated and any lesion found, whether of a ligament or meniscus (Fig. 19.14), is dealt with. If there are no mechanical symptoms but pain and effusion are still occurring, an MR scan is requested and a decision taken in the light of the result whether to perform arthroscopy.

A *transverse fracture of the patella* presents with local tenderness, swelling or bruising: the fracture is not palpable unless the extensor apparatus is damaged sufficiently to allow the quadriceps muscles to pull the proximal fragment upwards which results in displacement and a palpable gap. Active extension of the knee is possible but painful. An X-ray outlines the fracture and degree of displacement. Treatment for undisplaced fractures is by immobilization in a plaster cylinder for 6 weeks; when displaced, open reduction and internal fixation are required. A *comminuted fracture of the patella* is treated by excision of the fragmented patella combined with reconstruction of the soft tissue components of the extensor apparatus and this should provide a satisfactory functional result. Alternatively, the fracture is treated initially by immobilization in a plaster cast, and patellectomy is reserved should the patient develop patello-femoral osteoarthritis in the long term.

A *supracondylar fracture of the femur* can show minimal displacement, but occasionally the lower fragment is rotated backwards and is pulled upwards behind the shaft and this may compress the popliteal vessels. The fracture may involve either condyle, or both condyles stretched apart by a T-shaped fracture into the joint, when there is obvious widening of the transverse diameter of the knee. These are managed by open reduction and internal fixation, with correction of the obstruction to the popliteal artery.

Tibial fractures are caused by direct and forceful impact. A fracture of the lateral condyle is common and is known as a *bumper fracture*, because of the common causative injury. The lateral tibial plateau is depressed and valgus deformity may be obvious and is associated with medial ligament tear; similarly, tear of the lateral ligament and varus deformity are associated with fracture of the medial condyle. These fractures are often open because of the thin overlying tissue and are best stabilized by internal or external fixation. Closed undisplaced tibial fractures may be managed with Plaster of Paris but unstable fractures, especially when the knee joint is involved, require careful open reduction and internal fixation.

A complication that frequently goes unrecognized is *compartment syndrome* as a result of capsular tear and leakage of blood into the calf.

Atraumatic acute pain

Acute septic arthritis or *osteomyelitis of the intra-articular bones* should be considered when pain is

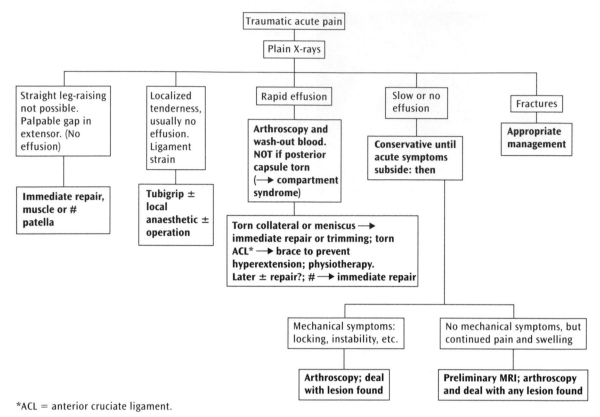

*ACL = anterior cruciate ligament.

Algorithm 19.4

accompanied by pyrexial illness and toxicity. The knee is held in the position of its greatest capacity (the position of ease) and may appear swollen. The patient allows no movement of the joint in acute suppurative arthritis, but in the 'sympathetic' effusion associated with acute osteomyelitis a certain range of painless movement can usually be obtained if the patient is examined gently. In osteomyelitis, the maximum tenderness is near the end of the bone rather than over the joint as in suppurative arthritis. As already explained, investigations are of no diagnostic value early in the disease. Blood cultures are essential before antibiotic treatment is commenced, aspiration reduces the tension within the joint, relieves the pain, and allows examination and culture of the fluid for the organism to obtain its antibiotic sensitivity. This treatment should avoid the need for arthrotomy and drainage of pus, unless there is intra-articular bone damage.

Acute suppurative pre-patellar bursitis from spreading local cellulitis can be associated with a sympathetic effusion in the knee joint, and could be confused with infective arthritis, but in the latter condition any attempt to move the joint is painful. Treatment involves antibiotic therapy and incision and drainage if there is pus collection. This condition is different from *pre-patellar* (*housemaid's knee*) or *infra-patellar bursitis* (*clergyman's knee*) where fluid gradually collects in the bursa as a result of repeated pressure. The swelling is well-circumscribed, overlies the patella, and is not tender unless infected while the knee movements are full and pain free. Aspiration, plus antibiotics when infected, can be sufficient, but persistent trouble is best resolved by excision.

In the absence of systemic infection, *crystal arthropathy* should be considered since the knee (and the hallux) are common sites. Diagnosis is made by a high concentration of uric acid in the blood and

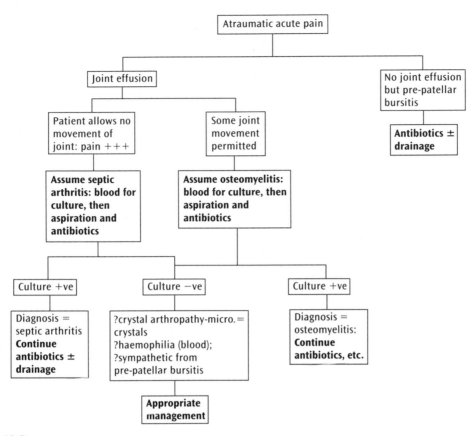

Algorithm 19.5

crystals in aspirated joint fluid. In gout, treatment during the acute episode is with indomethacin and maintenance with allopurinol. Pseudogout is caused by chemical infiltration of the intra-articular cartilage with calcium pyrophosphate and mimics gout. Anti-inflammatory agents are prescribed to control the symptoms.

Haemarthrosis may occur in *haemophilia*. The patient is usually known to suffer from the disease, and aspiration will reveal blood.

A previous injury will bear relevance to chronic and persistent knee pain, and will help to distinguish a group of patients from those with primary bone or joint disease.

Traumatic chronic knee pain

Patients with a past history of injury and with recurrent episodes of pain, locking, giving way or a combination of these symptoms probably have a torn meniscus, a torn ligament or a loose body.

Meniscal lesions. Meniscal tears are more frequent in the medial than the lateral meniscus, and in men than in women; tears can also occur in a child with a congenital discoid lateral meniscus.

The meniscus (Fig. 19.14) may be torn at one end of its peripheral attachment to the joint capsule (anterior or posterior tear) or within its substance with the attachment at both ends intact. Although the menisci are commonly torn in sports injuries or when rising from a kneeling position, as a result of rotation of the tibia on the femur in the flexed weight-bearing knee, tears of degenerate menisci occur in an osteoarthritic knee. The patient may be able to recall the injury that preceded swelling of the knee, and restricted movement that gradually improved before noticing locking and giving way. On examination, wasting of the quadriceps muscles and effusion may be evident. The distinction between a medial and a lateral meniscus

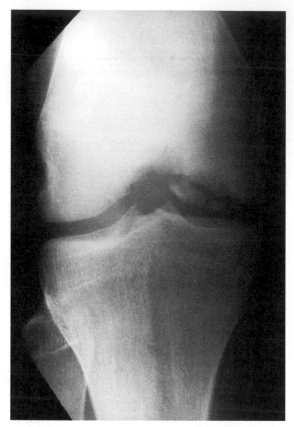

Fig. 19.15 *Osteochondritis dissecans. Anteroposterior (AP) radiograph of the right knee. Osteochondral fragments have become detached from the lateral aspect of the medial condyle. These loose bodies may give rise to mechanical symptoms.*

The acute episode may pass unnoticed since major ligament injuries are sometimes surprisingly painless in the early stages, and with complete rupture of a collateral ligament it is possible for haemarthrosis to escape from the joint and therefore not be obvious clinically.

Loss of a cruciate leads to loss of anteroposterior stability, particularly in flexion, and hence difficulty in going up or coming down stairs is a common complaint. On examination, anteroposterior or lateral movement, or attempt to invoke such movement causes localized pain in the region of the damaged ligament, and the point of tenderness should distinguish ligament from a meniscal lesion.

Loose bodies. Following a minor knee injury a fragment of cartilage and bone is sheared off into the joint and lies free in the joint. The patient may or may not recall the incident. *Osteochondritis dissecans* in male adolescents causes ischaemic necrosis and detachment of an osteochondral fragment from the articular surface of the medial condyle of the femur (Fig. 19.15). In the elderly with osteoarthritis, a detached osteophyte is the most common cause of a loose body.

When a definitive clinical diagnosis cannot be made and the patient is not sufficiently troubled, the patient is treated with quadriceps exercises while progress is observed, otherwise a full investigation is performed.

A plain X-ray is ordinarily normal in internal derangement of the knee joint, and only helpful if a loose body is osseous rather than cartilaginous, and in demonstrating the defect in the medial condyle of the femur in osteochondritis dissecans. Occasionally, fractures are seen if the cruciate ligaments avulsed their tibial attachment or if the lateral collateral ligament avulsed its fibular attachment. An MRI scan, useful in detecting subtle changes in bone and particularly in soft tissues including the menisci, is a prerequisite especially when a meniscal tear is suspected since arthroscopy may be necessary.

Arthroscopy allows removal of meniscal tears and loose bodies with the advantage of rapid recovery compared with open arthrotomy. In patients with cruciate ligament damage, treatment is offered only if symptoms interfere with daily life, which can be crucial in sportsmen. This consists of an attempt to repair or replace the torn ligament with prosthetic

injury depends on the localization of tenderness along the joint line. If the knee is locked, full range of movement cannot be obtained.

Ligamentous injury. The anterior cruciate is stressed if the knee is forcibly extended, whereas the posterior cruciate is injured if the anterior aspect of the tibia is struck when the knee is flexed. The medial collateral ligament is stressed when the tibia is abducted on the femur by a blow on the lateral side of the knee when the patient is bearing weight on the leg. The lateral collateral ligament is injured by the reverse mechanism (i.e., adduction of the tibia on the femur). Further forced abduction or adduction also stresses the cruciate ligaments.

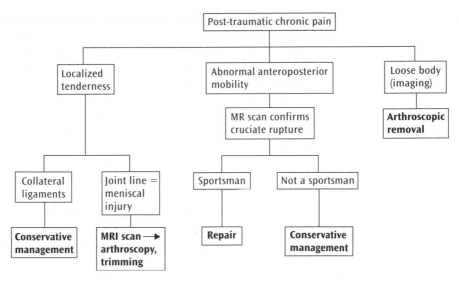

Algorithm 19.6

ligament but the long-term results are unpredictable and therefore treatment is only offered when symptoms are troublesome.

When there is no background history of injury to the knee, a discriminative feature is associated effusion which is easily noticeable by the patient as a swelling. This differentiates intra- from extra-articular disease, except that intra-articular disease is not always associated with an effusion.

Atraumatic knee pain with effusion

Rheumatoid arthritis is recognized by the presence of other stigmata of the disease. The knee is painful, stiff and swollen. In contrast to osteoarthritis, stiffness improves during the day. The patient often feels generally unwell and is mildly febrile. On palpation, there is synovial thickening and effusion. The knee movement is painful and limited and with advanced disease, there is muscle wasting and deformity especially if subluxated. The diagnosis is based on involvement of other joints, raised inflammatory markers and characteristic radiological features.

Surgery is offered if medical therapy fails, and as in osteoarthritis is aimed at pain relief, correction of deformity and functional improvement. Total knee replacement is the treatment of choice.

Tuberculous arthritis usually presents with knee swelling and moderate pain which is worse at night and on exertion. Initially, there is a reasonable range of movement, but as the disease progresses the knee joint becomes increasingly stiff and painful because of articular destruction, fibrosis and muscle spasm. The patient may have night sweats and feels unwell and febrile, especially at night. On examination, the knee is held in the position of ease and is swollen, the quadriceps muscles are markedly wasted and there is effusion and synovial thickening.

A history of tuberculosis is not always obtained. A raised ESR, lymphocytosis and a positive Mantoux test (not significant in endemic areas) are suggestive, a chest X-ray may not necessarily show an active or a healed focus, and the early radiological appearances of the knee are not dramatic.

Arthroscopy and synovial biopsy for histological examination and bacteriology are essential.

Treatment by immobilization and antituberculous therapy can arrest the progression of the disease. Surgery involves synovectomy, drainage of the joint and arthrodesis if the articulating bones are destroyed.

Bone tumours with a particular predilection to bone in the proximity of the knee joint, that is, the distal femur, proximal tibia and fibula, are osteosarcoma and giant cell tumour. Fibrosarcoma and synovial sarcoma also occur. Alone amongst the benign tumours, osteoid osteoma presents with pain which can be severe; in other benign tumours, for example osteochondroma, pain is a feature of malignant change. The radiological appearances can distinguish a malignant from a benign tumour by various features: an ill-defined osteolytic lesion with new bone formation or calcification within it, or reactive new bone formation around it with breach of the periosteum and invasion of the soft tissue; and between individual tumours, for example the sunray appearance in osteosarcoma, soap bubble appearance in giant cell tumour. Needle or open biopsy is essential. Treatment is as described for other sites.

Atraumatic knee without effusion

Osteoarthritis commonly affects the knee joint, pain is troublesome at night, with muscle spasm, reluctance to move the joint because of pain, and capsular fibrosis, the joint becomes stiff and all movements are lost. On examination, the abnormal position of ease is noticeable, swelling from effusion may be visible, and the joint is tender and its movements restricted. A crepitus can be detected in the knee or the patello-femoral joints or both. The diagnosis is confirmed on X-ray (Fig. 19.16).

Treatment consists of encouraging the patient to lose weight and use a walking stick, raise the heel, analgesia and quadriceps exercises. Should these measures fail, surgery is offered and the options are osteotomy, total replacement arthroplasty and arthrodesis, plus excision of the patella when osteoarthritis is confined to the patello-femoral joint.

Osgood–Schlatter's disease is traction epiphysitis of the patellar tendon insertion into the tubercle of the tibia. It is a fairly common condition seen in active children of both sexes, often associated with sport, characterized by a bony swelling, localized pain and tenderness in the region of the tubercle, and is worse after exercise; otherwise, knee examination is unremarkable. A plain X-ray to rule out a bone tumour shows a normal joint, the tibial tubercle may appear fluffy. It is self-limiting and usually settles with rest, although immobilization in a plaster cast is occasionally required. The symptoms cease in adolescence, when growth is complete.

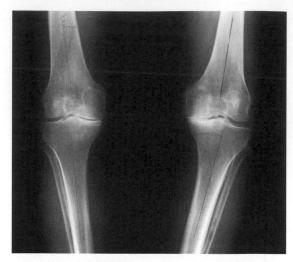

Fig. 19.16 *Osteoarthritis. A weight-bearing anteroposterior (AP) X-ray of the left knee joint showing narrowing of the medial joint space due to damage to the articular cartilage together with sclerosis and cysts. Axial lines have been drawn to show the typical varus deformity of the leg on the thigh.*

Chondromalacia patellae is an ill-understood disease which leads to fibrillation, fissuring and softening of the articular cartilage of the patella, which usually commences on its medial facet. It may follow a direct blow on the patella or recurrent dislocation of the patella, although in the majority there is no obvious cause. Often the patient is an adolescent female who presents with pain precipitated by kneeling, climbing or descending stairs, that is, when contraction of the quadriceps femoris pulls the patella against the femoral condyles. Examination will reveal localized pain on pressing the patella against the femoral condyles, usually on the medial aspect, and when the joint is moved while pressing the patella against the condyle, when a patello-femoral crepitus is apparent. A radiograph is of no value because there is no bony abnormality but helps to exclude other possibilities. The diagnosis is confirmed by arthroscopy which shows erosion of the cartilage but this is reserved only for severe cases. Conservative measures consist of pain relief and physiotherapy and are often successful as the condition resolves spontaneously in most cases. Drilling or shaving the cartilage, division of the lateral patellar retinaculum and occasionally transposition of the tibial tubercle may be necessary when symptoms persist and are severe, and are reported to be effective in pain relief. Patellectomy is a last resort but infrequently necessary.

Recurrent dislocation of the patella is associated with malformation of either the patella or the lateral condyle which allows the patella to be displaced laterally when the quadriceps muscles contract and this results in repeated locking or giving way of the knee, although the patient may not be aware of it initially. The patient exhibits apprehension when the patella is pushed laterally during examination. Treatment is based on remodelling the muscle attachments around the patella by release of the lateral patellar retinaculum and reinforcement of the medial retinaculum or resiting the patella more medially on the tibia.

Cysts of the menisci are due to myxomatous degeneration within the substance of the cartilage. The patient complains of a pain worse on exercise and relieved by rest, sufficient usually to seek advice before a swelling is obvious. As the cyst becomes larger the pain eases or may resolve. The lateral meniscus is more frequently involved than the medial meniscus, and it appears as a swelling around the posterior border of the lateral ligament. On examination, it feels hard, tender and immobile; it disappears on flexion of the joint and reappears on extension. Cysts of the menisci should be distinguished from a *semimembranosus bursa* and a *popliteal (Baker's) cyst*, which are seen in the back of the knee, but usually not painful. A semimembranosus bursa is the result of unaccustomed exercise or minor injuries to the bursa, and occurs at all ages. It lies medially, is tense when the knee is extended and flaccid when the joint is flexed, does not empty when compressed as it does not communicate with the joint and there is no crepitus on moving the joint. A Baker's cyst occurs in patients over 40 years of age, and is a herniation of the synovial membrane through the capsule associated with osteoarthritis or rheumatoid arthritis. It is situated in the mid-line and can sometimes be bilateral when it should be distinguished from a popliteal aneurysm which is also usually bilateral but pulsatile. It is more prominent when the knee is fully extended but tends to disappear when the knee is flexed, and can be emptied because it communicates with the joint, and there are signs of arthritis on examination of the joint.

A cyst of the meniscus may only require analgesia for pain relief, as it resolves spontaneously, although a menisectomy may be required for persistent symptoms. A semimembranosus bursa or Baker's cyst is not usually sufficiently troublesome to require treatment.

HIGHLIGHTS

- Always remember to examine the hip when the patient has knee problems
- In acute trauma, an immediate swelling of the joint signifies haemarthrosis and usually requires early active management
- Post-traumatic recurrent mechanical symptoms are usually due to a torn meniscus, a torn ligament or a loose body
- In chronic cases without a history of trauma, the presence of a joint effusion suggests degenerative or infective disease of the joint

---

THE BACK

AIMS

1 Recognize features associated with back pain
2 Understand the causes of back pain
3 Define the relevant physical signs and diagnostic tests
4 Understand the principles of management

Introduction

The structural elements of the vertebral column are bony, muscular and ligamentous tissue known as the *spondyls*, that encase the neurological tissue, that is, the spinal cord and its roots. Pathological processes can separately involve the spondyls (*spondylitis*) or the nerve tissue, although structural damage of the vertebral column can by compression affect the spinal cord or more commonly the nerve roots. Neurological involvement is clinically recognized by the radiation of pain and the presence of neurological disturbance.

Backache is a common complaint in the population because of the upright human posture, and is likely to be over-investigated unless patients are properly selected through careful assessment.

History

The most common symptoms related to the back are pain, stiffness and deformity. Pain is often associated with the other two symptoms, but stiffness or deformity can occur without back pain.

Pain

Pain can arise from any part of the spine from the neck to the buttocks, and patients are usually able to indicate an area rather than specify a localized point.

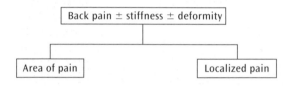

Lumbar backache descending to the buttocks and thighs may be a *referred pain* and does not necessarily imply compression of nerve roots. By contrast, lumbar backache radiating in the sciatic nerve distribution below the thigh (*sciatica*) and invariably into the foot, indicates compression of the nerve roots, as they emerge from the vertebral foramina, by direct pressure, inflammation and oedema. The sciatica is usually associated with *paraesthesiae* (abnormalities of sensation) in the same nerve root distribution, and is exacerbated by coughing and sneezing, actions that raise the intra-thecal pressure. Pain which is worse on activity usually indicates a mechanical cause, such as degenerative disorders, whereas night pain at rest is suggestive of a tumour or infection.

Claudication pain (Chapter 13) coming on after a reproducible quantity of exercise and relieved by rest is occasionally due, not to peripheral arterial disease, but to spinal stenosis. A useful differentiating feature is that the pain of spinal claudication is usually worse walking downhill rather than uphill, the reverse of the situation with peripheral arterial disease, because there is increased compression of the contents of the spinal column during flexion of the lumbar spine.

Stiffness

Like in other joints, stiffness worse early in the morning is usually due to an inflammatory disorder, whereas back stiffness that increases during the day is more likely to be due to degenerative disease. An acute onset of severe stiffness can be associated with infection, such as discitis or osteomyelitis.

Deformity

Deformity in the thoraco-lumbar spine in the coronal plane is *scoliosis*, in the sagittal plane *kyphosis*: it can be present without pain. An acute onset of scoliosis or kyphosis can be a sign of infection, a prolapsed disc or a tumour.

Examination

See Chapter 22 for acute trauma that may have produced an unstable fracture of the spine.

Look

Landmarks that outline the contour of the spine and the symmetry of the back are the *vertebra prominens*, the *spinous processes*, the *angles of the scapulae* and the *posterior iliac spines and crests*. On inspecting the lateral contour of the back there is normally a lumbar lordosis which is obliterated by spasm of the sacrospinalis muscles due to a prolapsed disc or early tuberculous (Pott's) disease of the spine. Increased lordosis is associated with spondylolisthesis. Scoliosis (Fig. 19.17) is detected by comparing the two sides of the trunk along a vertical mid-line and kyphosis by prominence beyond the normal contour of the spine. When the patient is asked to lean forwards and cross the arms over the chest so that the hands rest on the opposite shoulders, a postural deformity disappears, whereas a fixed deformity becomes more obvious. These deformities, when not due to structural abnormality of the spine, rib-cage or hips, are signs of underlying disease in the spine. The patient's posture and gait are also noted.

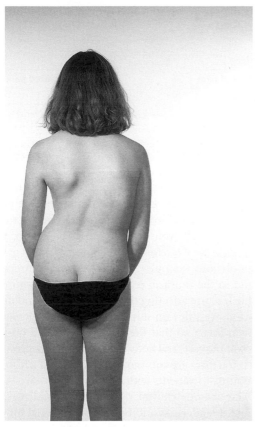

Fig. 19.17 *A photograph of a young girl with a right thoracic, left lumbar scoliosis. Note the asymmetry of the scapulae, shoulders and pelvis.*

Feel

Tenderness can be due to local disease. Muscle spasm feels firm and it causes a concavity of the spine towards the side of muscular contraction. The spinous processes and inter-spinous notches can be palpated with the index finger, and are percussed with the finger or a knee-hammer for tenderness.

Move

The standing patient is examined for mobility of the spine. Flexion, which occurs mostly in the lumbar region, is observed by asking the patient to bend forwards and touch the toes while keeping the knees straight; extension by asking the patient to lean backwards as far as possible; lateral bend as the patient

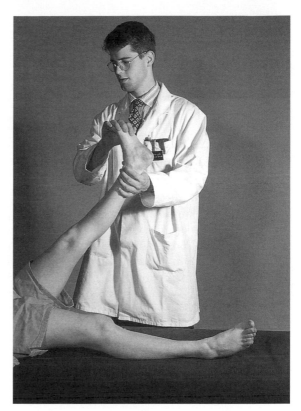

Fig. 19.18 *The Lasegue test. When the straight leg has been raised to near the point where the movement would be painful, passive dorsiflexion of the ankle stretches the sciatic nerve; production of pain with this manoeuvre confirms entrapment of the sciatic nerve.*

slides each hand in turn down the thigh. While seated on a couch with the popliteal fossae against the edge of the couch, the ranges of forward and lateral flexion, extension and rotation of the trunk are noted. Limitation of movement is usually due to pain.

With the patient supine, compensatory lordosis is ruled out by inserting the hand under the lumbar spine. Then the ankle is grasped with one hand and the other is placed on the front of the thigh to keep the leg straight while the limb is raised (*straight-leg-raising test*) until the patient experiences pain. The angle at which this occurs is recorded. Limitation of straight-leg-raising may be due to muscle spasm or nerve root entrapment. The *Lasegue test* (passive dorsiflexion of the ankle with the straight limb raised almost to its maximal position) (Fig. 19.18) stretches the sciatic nerve and pain produced by this manoeuvre confirms nerve root entrapment.

Neurological examination

A full neurological examination is mandatory in any patient with back pain as compression by a central prolapsed intervertebral disc, a tumour or Pott's disease may manifest with neurological signs. A prolapsed L4/5 disc can lead to abnormalities due to L5 nerve entrapment (decreased tone and power of extensor hallucis longus and decreased sensation in the big toe and medial aspect of the calf). A prolapsed L5/S1 disc can lead to abnormalities in tone and power of the muscles supplied by the S1 nerve root (e.g., plantar flexors of the foot), to decreased sensation in the S1 dermatome (lateral border of the foot) and to a decreased or absent ankle jerk. In patients with a cauda equina (S1–S4) compression due to a central prolapsed intervertebral disc, there is a saddle-shaped area of anaesthesia over the buttocks, anus and perineum and loss of anal sphincter tone (*see* Fig. 21.8, p. 352 for a map of the dermatomes).

Investigations

Anteroposterior and lateral radiographs are a routine preliminary investigation. In a myelogram radio-opaque contrast material is injected into the thecal space and outlines any occupying lesion. A computed tomographic (CT) scan at the same time gives added information. Magnetic Resonance Imaging (MRI) provides better tissue definition, clearly outlines soft tissue and bony deformities, and its advantages over CT scanning are the better definition of lesions without bone artefact and the fact that contrast myelography is not needed. Technetium (^{99m}Tc)-labelled compound when injected intravenously is concentrated at areas of rapid bone turnover increased by osteoblastic activity, as occurs in infection and malignancy.

Acute localized pain

This invariably follows an injury, either a direct blow or a mechanical strain. The history of the injury may be clear, but it may appear trivial or even non-apparent.

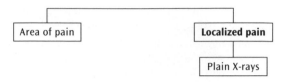

A few patients have *fractures of the vertebral appendices*, for example transverse or spinous processes, that are stable and do not constitute a threat to the spinal column: the patient may tolerate pain for some time before seeking advice. The fractures may also result from violent muscular action: the '*clay-shoveller's*' *fracture* of the spinous process of C7 is an obvious example. A *crush fracture*, commonly found in the thoracic region, is the most common stable fracture affecting the vertebral body and usually follows a flexion injury: the posterior elements remain intact so that the force is expended on the front of the vertebral body which becomes depressed. Such fractures are commonly seen without a history of trauma in patients with osteoporosis.

The obvious clinical signs in these patients are localized tenderness and restriction of spinal movements by pain. Plain X-radiographs taken in flexion and extension outline the fracture and confirm its stability.

Treatment consists of analgesia without the need for external supports or corsets, and a short period of bedrest may be required.

Area of pain, with sciatica

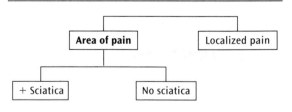

Patients who have not been involved in a traumatic incident and have back pain plus sciatica usually have a nerve root entrapment due to a prolapsed disc, or much less frequently hypertrophy of a facet joint or tumour.

Prolapse of the disc

The condition can develop spontaneously, although it commonly follows a sudden strain which results in rupture of the fibrous ring, the annulus fibrosus, of the disc, allowing the soft spongy central portion of the disc, the nucleus pulposus, to protrude into the spinal canal either in the mid-line or laterally (Fig. 19.19). The typical symptoms of low back pain with sciatica and the clinical findings for pressure on the commonly affected L5 and S1 roots have been described. In addition, the patient adopts a position of scoliosis and walks with a limping gait. The lumbar scoliosis results from muscular contraction, the convexity is usually directed to the side of the prolapsed disc, flexion and extension of the spine are normal but lateral flexion and rotation are grossly diminished. In higher (L2/3) disc lesions the pain is referred to the front of the thigh or leg. Those who have central protrusions may have compression of the cauda equina with signs and symptoms already described.

Management. The patient with a cauda equina lesion requires that the diagnosis be urgently confirmed with an MRI and urgent decompression performed to allow the maximal potential for recovery. Patients without cauda equina compression are treated with a short period of bedrest, analgesics, anti-inflammatory drugs and muscle relaxants until the pain settles. Prolonged bedrest leads to wasting of muscle and predisposes to a weakened back. If symptoms do not resolve within 6 weeks, or if pain is uncontrolled, or if weakness, sensory loss or sphincter disturbance develop, operation is considered. After imaging to confirm the diagnosis, the surgical options are percutaneous discectomy under radiological control, chymopapain injection into the disc prolapse to dissolve it or (most commonly) open discectomy. The prolapse is excised and the centre of the disc is cleared of the nucleus pulposus in order to reduce pressure within it and aid healing of the tear in the annulus fibrosus.

Every patient with backache and sciatica should be warned that the back will always be vulnerable. Patients should be taught to lift properly, and to perform back-strengthening exercises as a daily routine.

Area of pain, without sciatica

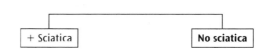

Back pain uncomplicated by sciatica is usually a self-limiting disorder. Almost everyone complains of backache at some time in their lives, but at least half have no demonstrable physical signs. Such patients, if they have no symptoms other than back pain and if no abnormality is found on physical examination,

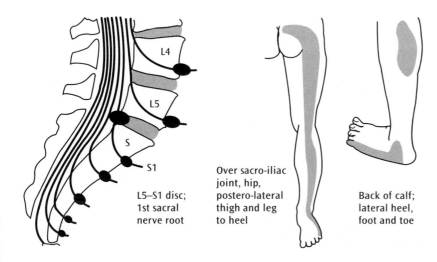

L5–S1 disc; 1st sacral nerve root

Over sacro-iliac joint, hip, postero-lateral thigh and leg to heel

Back of calf; lateral heel, foot and toe

Fig. 19.19 *Schematic drawing of an L5/S1 protruded inter-vertebral disc pressing on the S1 nerve root. Note the areas in which pain and altered sensation result.*

need no further investigation; they are reassured and referred for physiotherapy. The causative mechanism is usually obscure but probably of the nature of a sprain.

Occasionally, the patients do not respond to simple measures and further investigation becomes necessary using X-rays, MRI and appropriate blood tests including the erythrocyte sedimentation rate (ESR) as discussed below.

The difficult case

Most back problems one meets are covered by the descriptions above. The practitioner must be alert to recognize certain warning features of less common conditions (*see box below*).

Warning features of underlying disease

- The patient with backache who has no history of trauma and no physical signs, but who does not respond as expected to bedrest
- Back pain which, instead of being worse on activity (as is the case with most degenerative disorders), is worse in bed at night
- Stiffness and/or deformity of the spine without pain

Mechanical backache refers to sacro-iliac and lumbo-sacral strain, and is chronic with periods of acute exacerbation. The pain in the low back often radiates to the front and lateral aspect of the thigh, and is increased by bending forwards. Routine examination is usually negative, but there may be a slightly increased lordosis, localized spasm and tenderness of the spinal muscles during active movements, and limitation of forward bending when standing or sitting or both; straight-leg-raising is normal but produces some low backache at the extreme of elevation. Treatment includes analgesics, anti-inflammatory drugs and physiotherapy together with reassurance that the condition, although poorly understood, is benign.

Spondylolisthesis is a condition in which a lower lumbar vertebra, usually the fifth, slips forward as a result of separation of the body of the vertebra from the posterior articulation, lamina and spinous process because of a congenital or acquired defect in the pedicles that connect these two parts of the vertebra. The patient may be asymptomatic but can present with low back pain almost identical to mechanical back pain. The deformity can cause root pressure and sciatica. On examination, in a mild case the first sacral spinous process may be prominent and in a severe case there is marked lordosis with shortening of the trunk so that the lower ribs reach the iliac bones. The diagnosis is made on X-ray: oblique views better show the facets and their connecting bony bridges. X-ray studies often reveal a condition known as *spondylolysis* where slipping of the vertebra is absent or minimal, in the presence of defects in the pedicles.

The majority of these patients never require any special treatment and are managed conservatively. A lumbosacral corset may be required by some for pain relief, and in a few it is necessary to proceed to lumbosacral fusion to abolish the pain.

Ankylosing spondylitis is a process of calcification and then ossification of the ligaments and capsules of joints that results in complete bony ankylosis of the central articulations of the body. It commonly occurs in men and presents before the age of 30 years. The spine is commonly affected, and the sacro-iliac joint and the hips, the costal joints and the shoulder, may be involved. This condition is associated with or may precede inflammatory bowel disease, as well as aortic valve disease, urethritis, amyloidosis, pulmonary fibrosis and psoriasis. The patient presents with generalized back pain, tiredness and malaise. Early morning stiffness is common. In mild cases the spine may become rigid without much deformity but restricted movements, especially lateral bend, is obvious. In more severe cases the back forms a continuous curve from the base of the skull to the sacrum; often the knees are bent to maintain balance. Chest expansion is grossly and permanently reduced. Investigations show a high erythrocyte sedimentation rate and the presence of the human leucocyte antigen HLA-B27. Radiological examination shows obliteration of the sacro-iliac joints and the ossification of the spinal ligaments ('*bamboo spine*') and ankylosis of other involved joints. There is no specific treatment. *Management* includes simple analgesics and postural exercises which may help to prevent increasing deformity. Fortunately, the disease arrests spontaneously before gross spinal ankylosis and deformity develop. Osteotomy of the spine is occasionally indicated to correct severe deformity. Patients in whom the thoracic cage is ankylosed and the spine is in fixed flexion may die of pulmonary infection.

Infective spondylitis is produced by a variety of organisms, commonly *Staphylococcus aureus*, brucella and salmonella. The patient complains of deep-seated back pain that is not relieved by rest, and there may be systemic disturbance. Examination of the spine is unremarkable until later when localized tenderness and restriction of movement become evident. A raised sedimentation rate and leucocytosis are inconsistent and serological tests and blood culture frequently do not identify the organism. Plain radiology may show normal appearances since reduction in the disc space may still not be apparent when vertebral destruction and a para-vertebral collection of pus are demonstrable. MRI is particularly helpful as it demonstrates early changes.

Pott's disease (*Tuberculous spondylitis*) commences adjacent to an inter-vertebral disc in the cancellous bone of a body of a vertebra. It is rarely diagnosed until the bodies of two vertebrae and the intervertebral disc have been destroyed, with abscess formation and vertebral body collapse producing forward angulation of the spine (*kyphos*) which may damage the spinal cord. The most common site is the lower thoracic and upper lumbar vertebrae.

The patient may only complain of ache worse on exertion and at night, malaise, night fever and sweats. The only physical signs in the early stages are tenderness on percussion of the spinous processes of the involved vertebrae and minimal limitation of movement. Later a kyphos may be seen, and an abscess which has tracked down the psoas sheath to present in the right iliac fossa or in the thigh below the inguinal ligament. There may be compression of nerve roots, or paraplegia followed by exaggerated reflexes, ankle clonus and finally paralysis.

In the early stages the differential diagnosis is from osteomyelitis due to other organisms, ankylosing spondylitis, back pain due to disc prolapse and degeneration and neoplasm.

Investigations show a raised sedimentation rate and white cell count with lymphocytosis, the Mantoux test is positive and the haemoglobin is low.

Plain radiology may only show low bone density in the vertebrae involved until the disease is advanced, when there is narrowing of the disc space and lytic lesions typically in the anterior portion of the adjacent vertebral bodies. With further bone destruction and abscess formation, diseased bone is seen to lie in and around a soft tissue shadow containing fragments of bone and calcified soft tissue, and by this stage bony deformity is obvious. A chest X-ray may reveal active tuberculosis or a healed lesion. Since the clinical, haematological, immunological and radiological features are not diagnostic in the early stages, MRI is particularly valuable and histological examination of biopsy material may be essential.

Treatment consists of anti-tuberculous chemotherapy, bedrest until symptoms have subsided, and dietary and iron supplements to improve the nutritional condition of the patient. If pus has formed, it is drained via an anterior or anterolateral thoracotomy and bone grafts are packed between the involved vertebral bodies to promote healing by fusion.

Spondylosis is narrowing of the spinal canal and vertebral foramina where the nerve roots exit, as a result of osteophyte formation at the inter-vertebral joints secondary to primary osteoarthritis or disc degeneration and calcification of the para-vertebral ligaments. This may cause *spinal ischaemia* (the radicular arteries supplying the spinal cord pass through the foramina) and *compression of the spinal cord and its nerve roots*. The condition is common in the mobile areas of the spine, that is, lumbar and cervical.

The symptoms of spondylosis are progressive and common in old age, usually in patients with a history of backache. The patient develops symptoms due to nerve root irritation and leg pain radiating to the foot, with numbness and weakness exacerbated by exercise and relieved by rest. This syndrome, called *spinal claudication*, results from ischaemia of the cauda equina due to lumbar canal stenosis, and can be confused with vascular disease.

Treatment is only required in the few with severe symptoms or a progressive neurological deficit. The operation releases areas of entrapment by removal of bone and discs, and the resultant destabilization of the spine requires fusion.

Spinal tumours arise from the vertebral column or the spinal canal. *Primary tumours of the vertebral column* are rare. Chondromas, osteomas and fibromas can occur, although haemangiomas are more commonly encountered. Malignant tumours of the spine such as osteogenic sarcomas or chondrosarcomas are extremely rare and more commonly found in children and young adults. Osteocloastoma and the aneurysmal bone cyst do occur and are less aggressive. *Secondary tumours of the spine* are far more common: the majority involve both the extra-dural space and the bone, whereas 10% involve only the vertebrae. The most common primary cancer sites are the bronchus, breast, prostate, kidney and thyroid. The vertebral column is frequently involved in multiple myeloma and is often the site of the presenting symptoms. The diagnosis should always be considered in the elderly patient with persistent back pain. *Tumours of the spinal canal* are either extra-medullary, that is, within the dura but outside the cord – commonly neuromas and meningiomas; or intra-medullary, that is, within the spinal cord – astrocytomas and ependymomas are the most common. The extra-medullary are benign, whereas intra-medullary tumours tend to be slow-growing but invasive.

Patients complain of back pain that may precede or follow symptoms and signs of a neurological deficit which radiates in a band-like fashion in the affected dermatome and can be acute or progressive as a result of cord or root compression from vertebral collapse or an expanding mass or by ischaemic damage secondary to disturbance of the blood supply to the cord and nerve roots.

Examination of the spine may only elicit localized tenderness, or an angular deformity may be apparent, and rarely a mass is palpable in spinal tumours that have extended into the para-vertebral muscles. The motor and sensory signs depend on the level of the lesion and the extent of the cord damage. Diagnostic tests include raised ESR, serum calcium and alkaline phosphatase concentrations that are likely to be elevated in metastatic bone disease, serum electrophoresis studies for myeloma; plain radiographs of the spine – spinal cord tumours can produce widening of the vertebral canal with erosion or flattening of the medial pedicle margins, scalloping of the posterior margins of the vertebral bodies and thinning of the laminae, whereas metastatic neoplastic disease shows osteolytic or osteoblastic changes in the vertebral bodies, vertebral

body collapse or wedging and possibly a para-vertebral mass. A radioactive bone scan demonstrates the extent of metastasis within the vertebral column and in other bony regions; CT or CT myelography improves the visualization and shows the consistency of spinal tumours and the texture of bone; and MRI differentiates between solid and cystic lesions and can determine the shape, site and location of the tumour in the horizontal, transverse and sagittal planes while this information can be further enhanced by combining the test with a contrast agent such as gadolinium.

Treatment consists of opiate analgesia, with dexamethasone to reduce tissue oedema and slow further deterioration. Neurological deficits can be reversed by surgical decompression or local radiotherapy, but once paraplegia is established with total loss of all sensory and motor functions it becomes irreversible. In prostate and breast tumours hormonal therapy or chemotherapy can lead to regression of the spinal secondaries. Hence, acute cord compression from metastatic disease requires urgent surgical decompression, especially in the patient whose expectation of life is significant. The affected bone is excised and spinal fusion performed using bone graft and metallic fixation; this is followed with radiotherapy.

Intra-dural and extra-medullary tumours should be removed: this may involve excising bone and performing spinal fusion to allow earlier post-operative mobilization. Intra-medullary tumours, when well-circumscribed, can be excised easily; otherwise debulking followed by radiotherapy can be sufficient to give a good result in terms of survival, although neurological impairment may progress.

HIGHLIGHTS

- A plain X-ray and ESR provide helpful preliminary information
- In disc prolapse specialized imaging is only required if surgery is being considered
- Back pain with neurological deficit requires specialized imaging
- Spinal surgery is indicated mainly for nerve root or cord compression rather than for backache

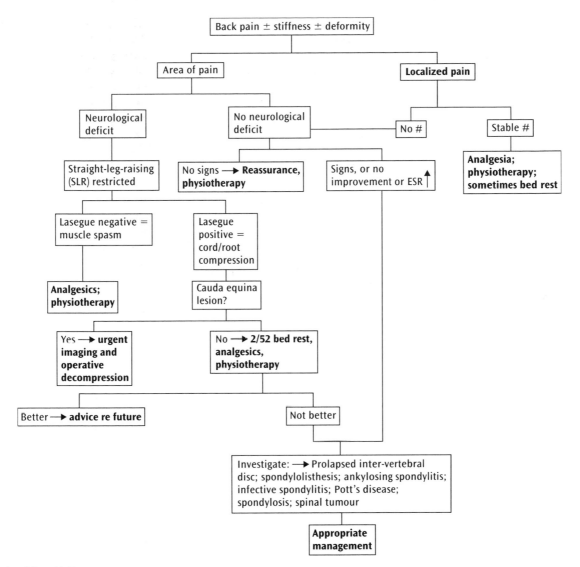

Algorithm 19.7

PART 2

Emergencies

20

Angina and cardiorespiratory arrest

REBECCA GRANT AND WILFRED PUGSLEY

INTRODUCTION

Coronary artery disease is the most common cause of death in the UK. Its management takes precedence over other disorders except emergency surgery. All surgeons at some time become involved with cardiorespiratory arrest in the course of their practice. This chapter aims to give an overview on this subject from a surgical perspective.

ANGINA

AIMS

1 Recognize the clinical features and be able to diagnose angina
2 Learn the principles of management
3 Understand the significance of the investigations used
4 Decide the optimal therapeutic option

Angina pectoris is the pain and discomfort experienced when the heart's oxygen demand exceeds its supply. The causative factors are diminished blood flow due to coronary artery stenosis, increased oxygen demand in left ventricular hypertrophy as a result of aortic stenosis or hypertension and low cardiac output because of cardiomyopathy or ischaemic cardiac damage.

Patients often describe the sensation as 'tightening', 'pressing', 'choking', or 'constricting'. The pain is retro-sternal, and often radiates to either arm, the back, the neck or the jaw. It is precipitated by physical, emotional or mental stress and by eating or cold weather. It is relieved by glyceryl trinitrate (GTN). Angina pectoris can be divided into two categories: *chronic stable* and *unstable*.

Chronic stable angina, also known as *angina of effort*, occurs after exercise. The amount of exercise required before the symptoms occur does not correlate well with the severity of coronary artery disease. *Unstable* or *crescendo angina*, and in extreme situations, *pre-infarction angina*, occurs at rest, and is also referred to when the patient's symptoms are progressing rapidly. Unstable angina is symptomatically more severe than chronic stable angina; the pain is more intense, lasts longer and is not as well-relieved by GTN. Unstable angina may progress to myocardial infarction (MI) and can be very difficult to distinguish from acute MI, unless the latter is confirmed by ECG changes (elevated ST-segments) or cardiac enzyme (CPK-MB) rises.

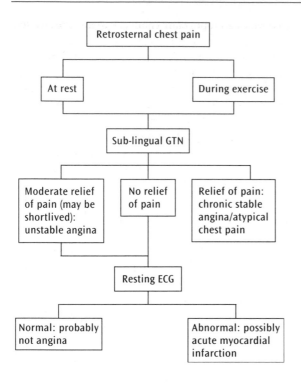

Diagnosis of angina

History

The patient's risk of coronary artery disease is assessed. The risks increase with age (>40 years for men and >60 years – post-menopausal – for women), smoking, hypercholesterolaemia, a family history of coronary artery disease, obesity and a type A (coronary prone) personality.

Examination

Important signs include xanthomata and corneal arcus indicating *hypercholesterolaemia*; evidence of associated endocrine disorders, namely diabetes and thyrotoxicosis; and precipitating factors, such as anaemia, tachycardia and hypertension. Aortic valve disease, signalled by the ejection systolic murmur of aortic stenosis and the diastolic murmur of aortic regurgitation (poor coronary perfusion) produces left ventricular hypertrophy (increased myocardial oxygen demand) and may give rise to angina-like chest pain in the absence of coronary artery disease;

these patients should not undergo exercise testing and usually do not tolerate nitrates well.

Investigations

A definitive diagnosis and assessment of severity of disease should be made, based on exercise ECG findings and other diagnostic tests. The resting ECG may indicate previous infarction or may show ischaemic changes at rest but is not diagnostic of chronic stable angina.

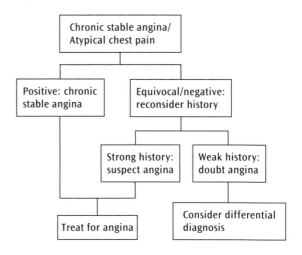

Exercise test

This is to assess the cardiac response to exercise whilst the patient is exercising on an electromechanically braked bicycle or a treadmill. Smoking, eating and drinking, and prophylactic nitrates but not β-blockers are discontinued for 2 hours prior to the test. A standard 12-lead ECG is continuously monitored at rest, during graded exercise and for at least 5 minutes after stopping the exercise. The systolic blood pressure is measured every 2 minutes; the diastolic blood pressure is only measured at rest. Exercise should be carried out until the patient reaches the predicted maximal heart rate (PMHR = 220 – age in years) calculated from the ECG. Ischaemia is indicated when typical anginal pain or arrhythmias cause the termination of the test. Angina may be accompanied by signs of ischaemia, such as a drop in systolic blood pressure of more than 10 mmHg from the resting baseline. In the

ECG, ST-segment depression of more than 1 mm from baseline suggests ischaemia of a severity proportional to the depression. Other indicators include the onset of left bundle branch block (LBBB), second- or third-degree heart block, progressive increase in R-wave amplitude and increase in the number of ventricular ectopics.

Stress echocardiography

In patients who cannot exercise, the motion in the left ventricular wall on an echocardiogram before and after cardiac stress induced by giving intravenous dobutamide or dipyridamole is compared. A change in the motion of the wall in an apparently normal segment of myocardium indicates ischaemia.

Stress thallium test

Thallium is taken up by viable cells in proportion to their blood supply. After intravenous thallium during exercise- or dobutamine- or dipyridamole-induced stress, the isotope uptake in well-perfused myocardium shows up as 'hot spots' in contrast to 'cold spots' in underperfused areas, corresponding with the diseased coronary arteries. After exercise, thallium is redistributed to viable cells through the interstitial fluid, independent of the myocardial blood supply. A scan a few hours later at rest may show isotope uptake in previously 'cold' areas if the cells are active and the myocardium is viable. The redistribution image differentiates hibernating and stunned (but living) tissue that is likely to benefit from revascularization, from dead myocardium.

Management of chronic stable angina

Preventative measures

Preventative measures aim at reducing the rate of progression of atheromatous disease and minimizing the consequences of existing disease. Patients should be informed about the cause of the chest pain they experience and advice given with regards to exercising safely within their limitations. They should become familiar with the pattern of their pain so

that they can report any change. Patients are advised to stop smoking and to take regular but gentle (not competitive or vigorous) exercise, reduce cholesterol intake and have a healthy well-balanced diet. Alcohol in moderation (e.g., one glass of red wine per day) may have a beneficial effect. Weight reduction measures are instigated, and hypertension is controlled medically. Attempts to reduce stress and anxiety may involve altering work habits and ensuring adequate rest and leisure time. Types of employment not permitted include driving heavy goods or public service vehicles and flying aeroplanes. Associated endocrine disease, such as diabetes or hyperthyroidism, is controlled with specialist help.

If a random serum cholesterol concentration exceeds 6.5 mmol/l, fasting cholesterol, and high- and low-density lipoprotein (HDL and LDL), are measured. Therapy aims to reduce cholesterol to below 5 mmol/l and LDL to below 2.5 mmol/l. Should diet alone fail, drug therapy should be considered, especially in patients under 70 years of age. HMG Co-A reductase inhibitors, known as the *statins* (e.g., imvastatin) are the first-line therapy.

Therapeutic measures

The medical management of chronic stable angina utilizes drugs that reduce oxygen demand, increase oxygen supply to the heart and prevent occlusion of diseased coronary arteries.

Antiplatelet drugs inhibit platelet aggregation and reduce the risk of coronary artery thrombosis. Aspirin is recommended at a dose of 150 mg daily, although half this dose is effective. Gastrointestinal symptoms and peptic ulceration are common side-effects.

Nitrates are systemic vasodilators that act by decreasing myocardial oxygen demand. They lower venous pressure, thereby reducing pre-load on the heart. Coronary perfusion may also be improved with the dilatation of coronary vessels. GTN administered sub-lingually, either in aerosol or tablet form, should relieve anginal pain within a few minutes. Common side-effects include headache and faintness. GTN can be used prophylactically, before starting exercise. If angina occurs regularly and nitrates are well-tolerated then long-acting nitrates, such as isosorbide mononitrate, are prescribed.

Beta-adrenoreceptor antagonists (β-blockers, e.g., propranolol) act by slowing the heart and reducing myocardial contraction, thereby reducing the oxygen demand of the myocardium. They are administered prophylactically for the symptoms of angina, especially when hypertension is also present. Beta-blockers cause bradycardia and may precipitate heart failure. Side-effects include broncho-constriction, lethargy, depression and impotence.

Calcium antagonists (e.g., nifedipine, verapamil and diltiazem) act by inhibiting the transmembrane influx of calcium ions through the slow channels of active cell membranes. They relieve angina by reducing the contractility of the myocardium and by reducing peripheral vascular resistance, thereby lowering the after-load. The specialized conducting tissue of the myocardium may be affected, leading to depression of electrical activity in the heart. Side-effects are related to their vasodilator action and include headaches, flushes, dizziness and ankle oedema. The negative inotropic effect may lead to left ventricular failure in patients with coronary artery disease and impaired left ventricular function.

The potassium channel openers (e.g., nicorandil) cause relaxation of vascular smooth muscle, both in the systemic veins and large coronary arteries, and in the peripheral and small coronary resistance arterioles. They therefore reduce pre-load and after-load and also increase coronary blood flow. Side-effects include headaches, dizziness, flushing and vomiting.

Even if angina appears well-controlled, the patient's management may need altering if the side-effects of drug therapy affect his or her quality of life adversely.

Management of unstable angina

The aim is to stabilize the patient. Bedrest is mandatory. Visitors are denied access. The patient is given analgesia to relieve the pain; opiates may be needed. If the patient is not on maximal medical therapy (i.e., nitrates, β-blockers and calcium antagonists) then this is started, provided there are no contraindications to the use of any of the drugs. If the patient is already on this triple therapy then intravenous nitrates are commenced and the rate of infusion is gradually increased until the patient's angina is relieved or hypotension occurs. The addition of a potassium channel opener should also be considered. Aspirin is prescribed to reduce platelet adhesiveness and low molecular weight heparin (Fragmin) is given subcutaneously.

Once the symptoms have settled urgent coronary angiography is arranged. If pain persists, especially in the presence of ST-segment changes on ECG, an intra-aortic balloon pump (IABP) may be used in order to stabilize the patient during and after angiography.

Intra-aortic balloon pump (IABP)

This is a 40 cc balloon, inserted over a guide wire from the femoral artery into the descending aorta, just at the level of the left subclavian artery.

```
                Chronic stable angina
                        |
                 Sub-lingual GTN
                   /         \
        Angina subsides    Angina is persistent
        in 2–3 minutes     or recurring regularly
                                |
                          Long-acting
                          nitrates (ISMN)
                                |
                         Angina worsening
                                |
                      Calcium antagonists/
                         β-blockers
                        /           \
        Angina worsening/          Angina
        intolerance to             controlled
        therapy/strongly              |
        positive                  Continue
        exercise test             medical
            |                      therapy
        Coronary angiography
```

The balloon is inflated with helium and inflation is timed to coincide with closure of the aortic valve at the end of systole. By inflating after valve closure, the balloon increases coronary perfusion and also the systemic arterial flow. By deflating, just before systole, the balloon reduces after-load and thereby the work of the heart.

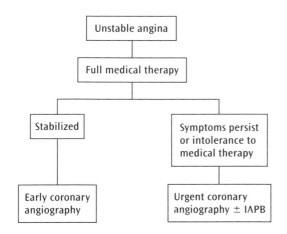

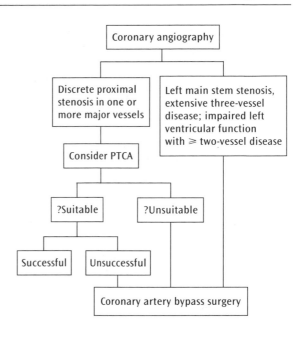

Coronary angiography

The coronary vessels are visualized by injecting radio-opaque contrast medium into the coronary ostia through a specialized cardiac catheter under X-ray control. Access is via a brachial artery, which requires arteriotomy, or more commonly via a percutaneous puncture of the femoral artery. A guide wire is passed along the lumen of the vessel into the aorta, until its end lies in the aortic root, above the aortic valve. Pig-tailed catheters are then threaded over the guide wire and made to engage first in the left and then in the right coronary ostium. Contrast is injected and the coronary circulation is observed on the X-ray screen. The images are recorded on videotape or CD-ROM. A stenosis causing more than 50% narrowing of the vessel lumen is considered significant, and when 95% or more of the lumen is occluded it is critical. Contrast is also injected into the left ventricle during diastole: the proportion of contrast ejected during ventricular systole, the left ventricular ejection fraction, is a measure of left ventricular function. Coronary angiography outlines the sites and severity of the disease and determines future management.

Percutaneous trans-luminal coronary angioplasty (PTCA) and coronary stenting

With one- or two-vessel disease not involving the left main stem, angioplasty (if technically feasible) is recommended if medical therapy fails.

Coronary angioplasty (PTCA) is carried out under local anaesthesia. As in coronary angiography, a guide wire is floated into the coronary artery and positioned across the lesion as confirmed by injection of contrast. A balloon angioplasty catheter is then threaded over the guide wire until the balloon is positioned within the narrowed segment of the artery. The balloon is then inflated for 2–3 minutes and the stenosis is dilated. Re-stenosis occurs in 20–30% of patients within 6 months. In order to reduce the incidence of re-stenosis an expanding mesh cage or coil (*stent*) can be inserted over the angioplasty balloon. When the balloon is inflated at high pressures, 16–20 atms, the stent is expanded into place; the balloon is deflated and removed and the stent is left at the site of stenosis to allow continued blood flow through the vessel. The possible thrombotic effects of the early stents were a problem and a strict anticoagulant protocol was followed. The newer stents are coated with special materials to try to reduce the thrombotic effects.

Surgical treatment

Coronary artery bypass grafting (CABG) is indicated in patients who have satisfactory distal vessels with an obstructive proximal lesion. It is recommended for symptomatic relief in patients intolerant of, or with angina refractory to, medical therapy. It is also of prognostic benefit in patients with left main stem stenosis before it bifurcates into anterior descending and circumflex arteries, in triple-vessel disease (right, left anterior descending and circumflex) and double-vessel disease involving the left anterior descending artery; in those with a positive exercise test after myocardial infarction in the presence of operable coronary artery disease and patients with chronic ischaemia and left ventricular dysfunction.

In cardiac operations the heart is arrested to allow performing the required procedure, while the function of the heart and lungs is replaced by a cardiopulmonary bypass (CPB). During the operation the heart is not perfused, and must therefore be protected from ischaemia.

Cardiopulmonary bypass

A cannula is positioned in the ascending aorta and a venous drainage cannula in the right atrium. The two cannulae are then attached to the (CPB) circuit (Fig. 20.1), the essentials of which are an oxygenator and a pump. Blood is drained from the right atrium to the oxygenator where oxygen is delivered to the blood and carbon dioxide is eliminated. The oxygenated blood is returned to the systemic circulation by a roller pump via the aortic cannula. The blood passes through a heat exchanger for cooling during, and re-warming at the end of, the bypass. By cooling the blood the body temperature is lowered, reducing the metabolic rate of the tissues and protecting the cells from hypoxic damage. The clotting cascade is activated during bypass and coagulation is prevented by heparin, which is reversed with protamine at the end of the procedure. Coagulopathy may persist because the platelets and other clotting factors are consumed during bypass; blood products may be necessary.

Myocardial protection

Once a circulation to the rest of the body, in particular the brain, has been established by CPB, the heart is isolated and stopped by applying a cross-clamp between the aortic valve and the arterial cannula. The heart is thus deprived of its blood supply. Ischaemic damage to the heart is limited by two methods:

- *Defibrillation*. The heart is fibrillated by use of an electric fibrillator to arrest its movements which allows a safe period of 15 minutes before its sinus rhythm is restored with a defibrillator and the aortic clamp removed to re-perfuse the heart.
- *Cardioplegia*. The heart is arrested in diastole by infusing a cold (4°C) crystalloid solution containing high concentrations (10–15 mmol) of potassium into the coronary arteries via a cannula in the aortic root below the clamp. The cold temperature protects the myocardium from ischaemic damage and provides about 30 minutes of safety for a litre of solution infused. Blood, either warm or cold, has also been used to perfuse the coronary arteries with high concentrations of potassium.

Coronary artery bypass grafts

Veins. The long saphenous vein, or alternatively, the short saphenous or an arm vein, is widely used. However, vein grafts are prone to occlusion at a rate of 2–3% per year, and by 10 years nearly 90% are occluded.

Internal mammary artery. The left internal mammary artery (LIMA) is commonly used to bypass occlusion in the left anterior descending (LAD) coronary artery. Its patency rate is 90% at 10 years, and it therefore offers better long-term protection against subsequent ischaemic complications.

Other arteries have been used, including the right internal mammary artery (RIMA), the gastro-epiploic artery from the stomach and the inferior epigastric artery.

With the heart arrested and relatively bloodless, an arteriotomy is made distal to the coronary artery

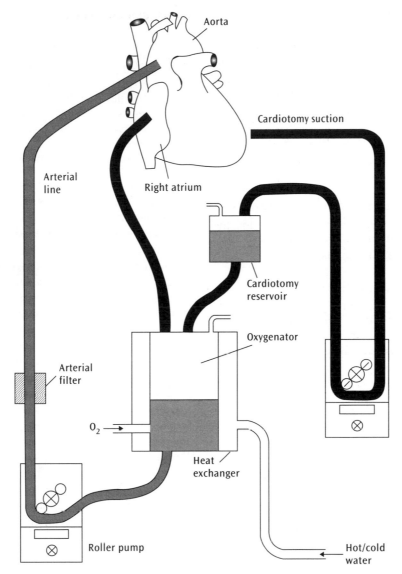

Fig. 20.1 *Cardiopulmonary bypass circuit. (Reproduced with the kind permission of the Resuscitation Council (UK) from the* Advanced Life Support Manual.*)*

stenosis. The long saphenous vein is reversed, and the top (*inguinal*) end is anastomosed to the coronary artery. If the internal mammary artery is being used, it is anastomosed last. When all the distal anastomoses are completed, the aortic cross-clamp is released to re-perfuse the heart while the proximal anastomoses to the aorta are performed.

Results. The operation has a 1–5% mortality rate, with a lower level of risk in elective cases, younger, lean patients with chronic stable angina, with satisfactory left ventricular function, and without associated illness. There is a 2% chance of stroke, related to micro-emboli of air and other material during bypass or to pre-existing carotid disease. Although

90% of patients are relieved of their angina, it is likely to recur within the first year after surgery. The long-term outlook is related to the graft used and about 10% of patients require another operation within 10 years. Re-operation is restricted to refractory symptoms as there is an increased operative mortality.

Off-pump surgery. In view of the morbidity and mortality associated with surgery using cardiopulmonary bypass, much attention has focused on performing CABG on the beating heart. This is effected by means of 'stabilizing' retractors which hold the beating heart in position whilst the surgeon performs the graft anastomoses, without using cardiopulmonary bypass. This technique, although gaining popularity, is still under evaluation.

Management of myocardial infarction

Patients with angina, including those with asymptomatic ischaemia, are at risk of myocardial infarction. When admitted with continuing chest pain and an ECG at rest showing elevation of the ST-segment, patients are treated with thrombolytic therapy (e.g., streptokinase) in an attempt to open up an acutely thrombosed artery. This therapy may cause haemorrhage.

The major causes of sudden death following myocardial infarction are cardiac rupture and ventricular fibrillation. Cardiac rupture may occur along the free wall of the left ventricle and is fatal. However, rupture may be confined to the ventricular septum, causing a ventricular septal defect, or to the papillary muscles, resulting in acute mitral regurgitation. Both these complications carry a high mortality but surgical correction of the mechanical defect can be life-saving. Ventricular fibrillation is a form of cardiac arrest and resuscitative measures should be undertaken as described below. ECG and echocardiography demonstrate the presence and extent of an infarct. Cardiogenic shock is treated with inotropic drugs, vasodilators and diuretics. IABP may be required, and if the patient is stable angiography is performed before revascularization and other corrective procedures are carried out.

HIGHLIGHTS

- Treatment of unstable angina is more demanding than that of stable angina
- Exercise tests and coronary angiography are specific diagnostic investigations of angina
- Angiography determines management by outlining the sites and severity of coronary artery disease
- Consideration of CABG takes into account myocardial function determined by left-ventricular ejection fraction and a thallium scan
- Surgery is required for the complications of myocardial infarction

---

CARDIORESPIRATORY ARREST

This is defined as 'collapse with cessation of a viable circulation'. Respiration may cease or become ineffectual. If intervention is delayed the inevitable consequences are brain ischaemia and major organ failure. Irreversible cerebral damage may occur in as little as 2 minutes.

Cardiorespiratory arrest is recognized by unconsciousness and the absence of a central pulse (carotid or femoral). Ventilatory movements may be absent or there may be ineffectual gasps. Wherever cardiorespiratory arrest occurs, the emphasis is on rapid institution of basic life support and early access to help. In the operating theatre or intensive care unit all the necessary apparatus and personnel may be at hand, but in other parts of the hospital or outside early access to emergency services is of vital importance. Guidelines issued by the Resuscitation Council (UK) describe the treatment of those suffering cardiorespiratory arrest in terms of a chain of survival. The chain links are:

- Early access to emergency services (in hospital, calling for the cardiac arrest team).
- Early basic life support.
- Early defibrillation.
- Early advanced life support.

Basic life support

Cardiorespiratory arrest is confirmed by gently shaking, squeezing and shouting at the subject to

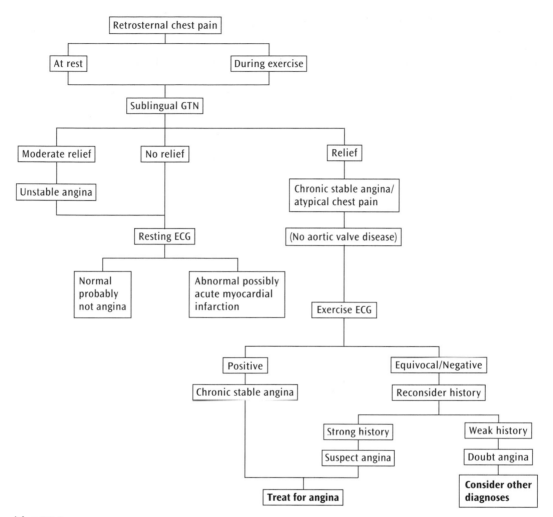

Algorithm 20.1

elicit any response. If there is no response help should be summoned urgently.

Airway assessment and artificial ventilation

The airway is opened by tilting the head backwards and lifting the chin. (If there is a suspicion of an associated neck injury the jaw is instead thrust forward by pressure behind the angle of the mandible.) The airway is cleared of any visible obstruction – blood, vomit or foreign bodies – although well-fitting dentures should be left in place. Signs of breathing are checked by looking for rising and falling chest movements, feeling for expired air and listening for breath sounds for 10 seconds.

If there is no regular breathing, *expired air ventilation* is commenced. Whilst maintaining an open and cleared airway, expired air ventilation is best performed by use of a barrier method, typically the pocket mask. If the mouth-to-mouth technique is indicated, the nose is pinched and the lungs are inflated by blowing steadily into the subject's mouth for 1–2 seconds whilst checking to see the chest rising. This is repeated up to five times to achieve two effective breaths.

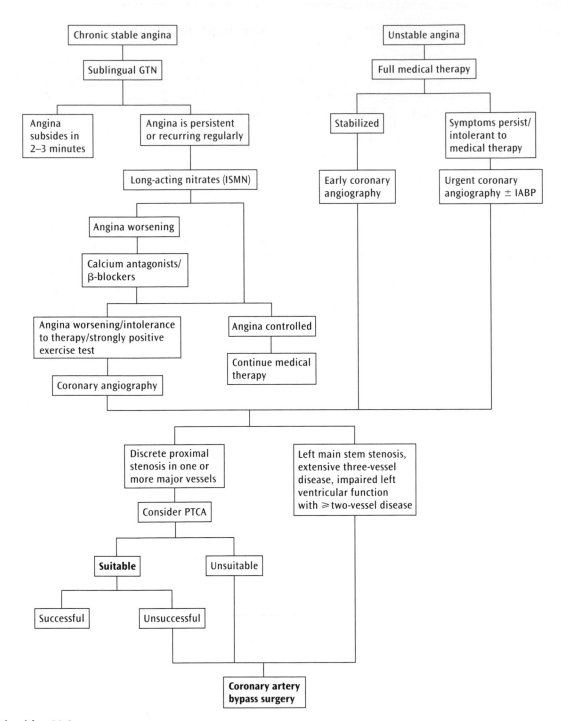

Algorithm 20.2

Chest compressions

If there is no palpable central pulse after a 10-second pulse check, chest compressions are commenced. The aim is to create a thoracic pump, drawing blood from the venous circulation into the thorax and pumping it into the arterial circulation to supply the major organs, in particular the heart and brain. The heel of one hand, with the other hand on top and the fingers of both hands interlocked, is placed over the middle of the lower-third of the sternum (two finger breadths upwards from the xiphisternum). With the arms extended, the sternum is pressed down and released at a rate of about 100 times per minute, moving the chest wall 2–5 cm with each compression.

If cardiopulmonary resuscitation (CPR) is being undertaken single-handed, artificial ventilation and chest compression should be carried out in the ratio of 15 compressions per two breaths. When help is available the ratio should be five compressions per breath. The femoral or carotid pulse is felt during CPR to ensure that an adequate circulation is being achieved (*see* Fig. 20.2).

Advanced life support

CPR should be continued until expert help and necessary equipment are available. The heart rhythm should be displayed at the earliest opportunity to distinguish shockable from non-shockable rhythms. This distinction determines subsequent management.

Defibrillation

The most common cause of cardiac arrest in hospital is ventricular fibrillation (VF) or pulseless ventricular tachycardia (VT) for which the definitive treatment is a direct current (DC) shock. The chances of successful restoration of rhythm and output decrease with time, so early recognition and defibrillation are vital to success.

The defibrillation paddles must make adequate contact with the chest wall. One is positioned to the right of the upper part of the sternum below the clavicle and the other just outside the cardiac apex. Gel pads are used to aid the flow of current between

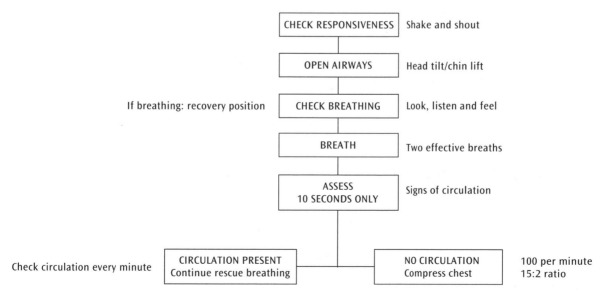

Send or go for help as soon as possible according to guidelines

Fig. 20.2 *Adult basic life support. (Reproduced with the kind permission of the Resuscitation Council (UK) from the* Advanced Life Support Manual.*)*

the paddles and the chest wall. For the first shock 200 J is used; this may be repeated and then a third shock of 360 J is given if the dysrhythmia persists. If at any time the ECG shows return to a rhythm compatible with an output the pulse should be checked. If VF persists after three shocks, 1 minute of CPR is performed (i.e., 10 cycles of 5:1 compressions to breaths) before three further shocks of 360 J are administered.

This pattern is repeated while VF or pulseless VT persists. During this time attention should be focused towards possible causes of intractable VF (e.g., hyperkalaemia) and to the quality of defibrillation, including positioning of the paddles and electrical contact. Once 12 shocks have been delivered (i.e, four loops of the algorithm) an anti-arrythmic agent is given, for example bretyllium (Fig. 20.3).

Respiratory support

The aim of advanced respiratory support is to inflate the lungs with a high concentration of oxygen. This may be achieved using a self-inflating bag with a one-way valve attached to a high flow of oxygen and a variety of airway adjuncts, including guedel airways, laryngeal mask airways or ultimately endotracheal intubation.

Circulatory support

During advanced life support, circulation is maintained by good-quality chest compressions, augmented by the administration of 1 mg of adrenaline every 3 minutes to increase perfusion pressure of the vital organs. Intravenous access, either peripheral or central, should be gained to enable drugs and fluids to be administered. If access is not successful, adrenaline and atropine may be given via the endotracheal route at twice the intravenous dose.

Asystole/electromechanical dissociation

Non-shockable rhythms are asystole and electromechanical dissociation (EMD). However, it is vital that fine VF is excluded before asystole is diagnosed. Electrode contact to the patient, the selected lead and the gain of the ECG machine (to enlarge the trace) should be checked.

Treatment of asystole/EMD comprises full respiratory and circulatory support; in asystole 3 mg atropine is given once only to block vagal tone. During the cardiorespiratory support, investigation of the underlying cause of the arrest and its treatment are pursued. Any relevant history is obtained, the patient is examined and relevant investigations performed, including arterial blood gases and electrolyte measurements (Fig. 20.4).

Causes of cardiac arrest

The cause of cardiac arrest should be sought early and potentially reversible causes treated. They may be remembered as 'the four H's and four T's' (Table 20.1).

Hyperkalaemia, hypocalcaemia or toxicity due to calcium antagonists is treated with 10 ml 10% calcium chloride given intravenously. Severe acidosis (pH < 7.1) despite effective ventilation and chest compressions may be treated with small doses (20–50 ml)

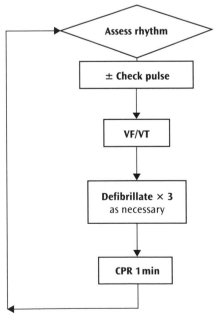

Fig. 20.3 *The 'shockable algorithm'. (Reproduced with the kind permission of the Resuscitation Council (UK) from the* Advanced Life Support Manual.*)*

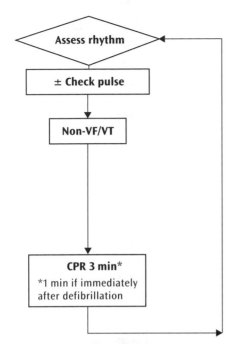

Fig. 20.4 *The 'non-shockable algorithm'. (Reproduced with the kind permission of the Resuscitation Council (UK) from the* Advanced Life Support Manual.*)*

Table 20.1 *Potentially reversible causes of cardiac arrest*

Hypoxia
Hypovolaemia
Hyper-/hypokalaemia
Hypothermia
Tension pneumothorax
Tamponade
Toxic/therapeutic disturbances
Thromboembolic/mechanical obstruction

of 8.4% sodium bicarbonate guided by blood gas analysis, although this may actually worsen cellular acidosis.

Ethical considerations

The decision to initiate and to discontinue CPR rests with the team present on site and each case should be judged in light of the underlying medical condition of the patient. If the diagnosis is not established or the arrest is unexpected then full resuscitative measures should be attempted whilst further information is obtained.

HIGHLIGHTS

- Resuscitation is necessary when cardiorespiratory arrest is unexpected or its cause is unknown
- Treatment of recognized causes of cardiac arrest is a priority in management
- Airway maintenance, expired air ventilation and chest compression are the essentials of basic life support
- Mechanical ventilation is required for respiratory support
- Ventricular fibrillation or tachycardia should be distinguished from asystole

21

The severely injured patient

CHRISTOPHER BD LAVY AND PAUL B BOULOS

> **AIMS**
>
> 1 Learn the principles of management of the severely injured patient
> 2 Recognize life-threatening injuries and learn their management

INTRODUCTION

The scale of the problem

Injury has been described as the forgotten epidemic and many are not aware of the scale of the problem. In the UK, injury is the most common killer in those aged under 35 years, exceeding the combined total of deaths from cardiovascular disease and cancer. Injuries commonly result from blunt trauma in road traffic accidents; less frequently from stab wounds; and rarely from bullet wounds. Blast injuries are rare in civilian life but may occur as a result of gas leakage or chemical explosions in industry. There are approximately 40 deaths per day from accidents, mostly on the roads, with 500,000 trauma admissions to hospital and between 10,000 and 16,000 patients suffering multiple injuries each year. At any single time patients with trauma occupy 13,500 beds. In the USA there are 60 million injuries per year, of which 3.6 million are admitted to hospital, 145,000 people per year die and 300,000 are permanently disabled.

Tri-modal distribution of deaths

Deaths following major trauma occur at three different times following the initial injury. Half occur within the first few minutes, due to major fatal injuries to the brain, the spinal cord, the intra-thoracic structures and the major vessels. There is little that medical services can do and responsibility falls on legislators to improve road safety and working conditions. However, over one-third of all the deaths that occur within hours of the injury are caused by corrigible hypoxia and inadequate blood replacement that is preventable by optimal resuscitation at the scene of the accident and by early transfer to hospital. Prompt and efficient resuscitation would prevent deaths occurring days or weeks following the injury in the remaining 20% of patients, as a result of secondary complications due to sepsis and multiple organ failure. It is for this reason that the concept has been formulated of the 'golden hour' which is the most important period in management that determines the overall outcome.

Definition of severely injured

Severity is not necessarily related to the extent of tissue injury but also to a cascade of complicating pathophysiological changes that threaten the patient's life. An example where extent parallels severity is a burn but for many forms of injury this parallelism does not hold. A patient with superficial lacerations over a wide area of the body surface will be distressed but not in danger, whereas a patient with a minute puncture in the lung complicated by a tension pneumothorax is in grave danger. An injury is best regarded as severe when it threatens life.

Basic goals of management

Since a severe injury threatens life, the first goal is to *save life*. Ideally, all injuries should heal with treatment, restoring normal structure and function, in order to achieve a desirable quality of life. Thus, the second goal is expressed as *repair damage*. A corollary is that from the moment the patient is first seen, every effort must be made to prevent further damage; thus, the second goal may be expanded to *limit damage; repair damage*. The third goal is to *relieve symptoms*, a principle that may seem self-evident, but in the heat of the moment can easily be overlooked. The fourth goal is *rehabilitation* which is crucial in the long term but is not covered in this chapter. The surgeon is only one member of a team that includes physiotherapist, occupational therapist, psychologist and counsellor, all of whom help to restore the patient to pre-injury activities.

PROTOCOL OF MANAGEMENT OF THE SEVERELY INJURED

A team approach is especially important in the acute situation where time is vital and several measures need implementing. An effective team needs a leader who takes overall responsibility for the continuing care of the patient until a management plan is formulated and until the transfer of the patient to the care of one of the inpatient surgical teams or to another hospital. The trauma team leader should allocate roles to each member of the team who should be familiar with *advanced trauma life support* (ATLS) guidance in resuscitation, which is now being universally adopted. The management protocol on arrival at hospital is rapid *primary survey* combined with *resuscitation*, followed by a *secondary survey* to determine the potential for developing further complications, identify other existing injuries and prioritize the treatment of individual injuries.

Primary survey and resuscitation

This includes simultaneous assessment, identification and management of life-threatening problems. A brief history is obtained, from the patient (*direct*) if possible or from witnesses (*collateral*), about the time and details of the accident, the conscious level of the patient at the time and subsequent changes after the injury, an estimate of blood loss and details of medications and fluids administered, and past medical illnesses, including drug history and drug allergies. The time since the last meal or drink is determined. A rapid survey includes evidence of pain, signs of distress, state of consciousness, airway, breathing, pallor, cyanosis, respiratory pattern, pulse rate and blood pressure, ability to move all limbs and the presence of any obvious gross injuries.

Resuscitation and support of cardiovascular and respiratory function

Hypoxia or lack of oxygen is immediately life-threatening if left uncorrected for more than a few minutes since it will cause cardiac arrest and brain ischaemia leading to brain death, or to permanent mental disability should the patient survive. The clinical signs of hypoxia are confusion, anxiety and restlessness; the patient is cyanosed and the breathing is rapid or slow or the patient may be apnoeic.

The causes of hypoxia in the injured patient are airway obstruction, impaired breathing or circulatory failure.

Airway obstruction. Depression of the respiratory centre as may follow head injuries, and in patients with impaired level of consciousness the loss of the gag and cough reflexes, result in aspiration of foreign material into the bronchial tree; the tongue musculature may fail to lift the tongue forwards and the position of the head in flexion further narrows the pharynx. Facial fractures cause laryngeal obstruction by the tongue falling backwards if the mandible which supports its musculature is fractured or the maxillae are displaced posteriorly over the larynx. The aspiration of blood, vomit or gastric juice causes laryngeal and bronchial spasm with retention of secretions leading to pulmonary oedema and acute respiratory distress syndrome.

The measures adopted to ensure a clear airway are: the mouth and nose are inspected for external signs of injury or bleeding; the neck is extended, the mandible is pulled forward in order to correct oropharyngeal obstruction; any secretions, vomit or blood in the mouth or pharynx are removed by suction and with the gloved fingers foreign bodies, including broken teeth or dentures, are removed. If the patient is unconscious a nasopharyngeal or oropharyngeal airway is inserted. If the upper airway is blocked, the pharynx is cleared with a laryngoscope and an endotracheal tube is passed. If this fails cricothyrotomy or mini-tracheostomy may be required.

At this stage in resuscitation it is important to take care of the cervical spine, especially in the unconscious patient since manipulation of the neck in the course of maintaining the airway may aggravate an unrecognized underlying injury of the cervical spine. A member of the team should be assigned to stabilize the head in line with the trunk until the cervical spine can be cleared of injury.

Impaired breathing. Ventilation is impaired because of pain from direct trauma to the chest wall or fractured ribs and by diminished lung expansion because of a flail chest, pneumothorax or haemothorax. It is therefore essential to ensure that breathing is spontaneous and is normal. The respiratory system is examined by inspection of the chest wall for injuries, expansion and paradoxical movement, that is, the chest wall moves in with inspiration and out with expiration; by auscultation for air entry to both lungs, for the presence of bronchial breathing and crepitations indicative of consolidation due to parenchymal oedema or haematoma; and percussion if air entry is absent will determine whether the affected side is hyper-resonant (air in the pleural cavity), dull (pneumonic consolidation) or stony dull (fluid in the pleural cavity).

The immediate management, especially if there is gross respiratory embarrassment, is to maintain breathing by mouth-to-mouth breathing, and if there is obstruction mouth-to-nose ventilation is tried until an oxygen delivery system is available. After an airway has been introduced, mouth-to-airway ventilation can be commenced. A self-refilling bag valve unit is particularly effective once the patient has been intubated and if the patient is likely to require long-term support mechanical ventilation is indicated. The management of a chest injury is described later.

Circulatory failure. Arterial oxygenation and tissue perfusion are dependent on an adequate circulation. Circulatory failure is usually due to acute blood loss and should be obvious if external from surface injuries, but the bleeding may be internal from a ruptured viscus or fractures of long bones. Trauma may compromise cardiac function if there is a pre-existing heart disease, but bleeding into the pericardial sac or myocardial damage following blunt or penetrating chest injuries are possible causes of diminished cardiac output and circulatory failure.

A patient in hypovolaemic shock is pale, cold and sweaty. If the peripheral pulse is absent, no pulse is palpable in the carotid or femoral arteries, and the patient is apnoeic, CPR should be instituted immediately. If the pulse is fast and weak and the blood pressure is low, a venous cannula is placed and blood samples obtained for measuring haemoglobin, haematocrit, urea and electrolytes and for grouping and cross-matching. Lost fluid is then replaced, monitored by central venous pressure (CVP) and urine output measured hourly after catheterizing the bladder. Haemorrhage should be controlled once the patient's condition is stable, and for external bleeding compression or a tourniquet is a temporary measure.

Cardiac tamponade, recognized by neck distension and inaudible heart sounds, is decompressed by long needle aspiration.

Secondary survey

Once the critical situation is under control, a secondary survey follows. Further history-taking may become relevant, and a detailed 'head to toe' examination is performed for signs of serious head, spine, chest and abdominal, pelvic and limb injuries.

In seriously injured patients, X-rays are obtained of the skull, cervical spine, chest and pelvis as well as of any other obvious bony injuries. Blood tests if already requested may have to be repeated to monitor the effect of the corrective measures undertaken. The tests include haemoglobin, haematocrit, urea and electrolytes, liver function tests, clotting screen, blood grouping and cross-matching; and an appropriate number of units of blood are ordered. Arterial blood gases are measured as a baseline to monitor any changes in the cardiovascular or respiratory status.

Further investigations are dependent on the nature of the individual injuries which are dicussed in this and other chapters.

HIGHLIGHTS

- Correction of hypoxia and adequate blood transfusion significantly diminishes death following injury
- Secondary survey to determine the extent of injuries should follow primary survey and resuscitation

HEAD INJURIES

See Chapter 22.

CHEST INJURIES

AIMS

1 Recognize the clinical features of chest injuries caused by trauma
2 Understand the management of chest injuries

Introduction

Although minor injuries involve only the chest wall, major injuries are associated with injury to the vital intra-thoracic organs.

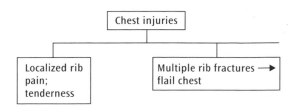

Fractured ribs is the most common chest injury, recognized by localized pain on breathing or coughing, tenderness over the fracture and chest X-ray appearances. Multiple fractures result in a flail segment of the chest wall which causes respiratory embarrassment, because of paradoxical movement: on inspiration, the flail segment is sucked inwards while the rest of the chest wall moves outwards, and on expiration, the flail segment moves outwards while the chest wall moves inwards. *Fractured sternum* occurs at the manubriosternal junction as a result of severe impact and is associated with flail chest and major intra-thoracic, abdominal and spinal injury.

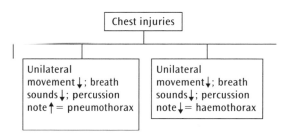

Pneumothorax, air in the pleural cavity causing lung collapse, may only be evident radiologically. However, when large the patient is breathless and may be cyanosed, and there are unilateral chest signs: loss of chest movements and of breath sounds, a resonant percussion note and sometimes chest wall emphysema confirmed by chest X-ray. *Tension pneumothorax* arises when a lung laceration or a wound in the chest wall acts as a one-way valve, allowing air into the pleural cavity with inspiration but closing during expiration, with progressive accumulation of air and rise in pleural pressure resulting in lung collapse and shift to the opposite side of the mediastinum, including the heart and great vessels, leading to cardiovascular collapse. The clinical features are of pneumothorax with tachypnoea, tachycardia and hypotension, tracheal deviation, resonant percussion note and absent breath sounds on the affected side.

Open pneumothorax results from a sucking chest which allows air flow with free movement of the mediastinum from side to side with respiration. It presents with gross respiratory embarrassment and audible sucking of air through the chest wall.

Haemothorax, blood in the pleural cavity, usually results from ruptured inter-costal or internal mammary vessels. The accumulation of blood produces pulmonary collapse and breathlessness depending on the volume of bleeding. The clinical signs are diminished chest movements, dull percussion note and absent breath sounds on the side of the injury as well as tachycardia and hypotension due to blood loss.

Lung injuries include pulmonary contusion or haematoma usually associated with haemoptysis and hypoxaemia, or pulmonary laceration caused by fractured ribs or penetrating trauma resulting in a pneumothorax. A chest X-ray will show opacification of the affected lung field, and associated pneumo- or haemothorax.

Trans-bronchial disruption commonly occurs near the carina and manifests clinically with respiratory distress and a large pneumothorax with mediastinal and subcutaneous emphysema.

Rupture of the oesophagus may present with surgical emphysema in the neck and pneumomediastinum on chest X-ray but the diagnosis is often missed until mediastinitis or empyema develop.

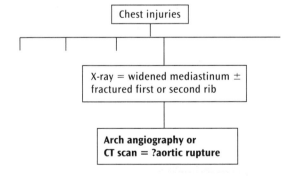

Rupture of the aorta results from a deceleration injury and is usually fatal, unless the rupture is contained within the mediastinum to form a false aneurysm. The clinical features are back pain, hypotension, systolic murmur or signs of cardiac tamponade. A chest X-ray shows widening of the mediastinum and the diagnosis is confirmed by arteriography.

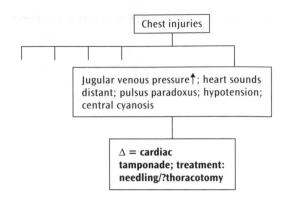

Cardiac injuries result from penetrating or from blunt trauma associated with fractures of the first and second ribs or the sternum causing myocardial contusion. Cardiac tamponade develops after only 100–150 ml of blood collects in the pericardial sac. The classical features are jugular venous distension, distant heart sounds, hypotension, pulsus paradoxus and central cyanosis. A chest X-ray may be normal and an ECG may show decreased voltage.

Diaphragmatic rupture, usually a linear split in the left diaphragm as the right side is protected by the liver, is associated with gut herniation into the pleural cavity, evident on a chest X-ray. It may be a minor tear and asymptomatic, and not diagnosed until later in life when weakness in the diaphragm allows herniation of intra-abdominal viscera.

Management of chest injuries

The initial management follows the principles of ensuring the patency of the airway, maintaining respiration and the circulation, and treating individual injuries. These can easily be recognized by a thorough physical examination of the chest wall and respiratory tract, without necessarily the need for a chest X-ray which, if not immediately available and especially if the patient is hypoxic, can be deferred until specific life-saving resuscitation treatment has been instituted. The chest radiograph is an adequate diagnostic aid in most injuries but a contrast-enhanced CT scan must be considered when there is widening of the mediastinum.

Rib fractures are treated by oral or parenteral analgesics, and when these are ineffective, by intercostal block, injecting local anaesthetic agent at the angle of the fractured rib and the normal rib above and below it. In patients with chronic bronchitis, physiotherapy and antibiotics are recommended. Complicating pneumo- or haemothorax is treated accordingly.

Caution is necessary in fractures of the first and second ribs; the frequently associated aortic or oesophageal injury should be suspected if the chest X-ray shows a widened mediastinum or fluid in the chest and the patient is haemodynamically unstable. A CT scan of the chest or arch arteriography is always advisable. A water-soluble contrast swallow will rule out an oesophageal rupture.

When there are multiple fractures with a flail chest, the immediate management is to apply pressure with the palm or place a sandbag on the flail segment. Pain and respiratory difficulty, especially with measured hypoxemia, are indications for endotracheal intubation and positive pressure ventilation until the chest stabilizes, as assessed by ease of spontaneous breathing when off the ventilator. Open surgical fixation is only performed in patients who require a thoracotomy for a major intra-thoracic injury.

The presence of a pneumothorax or haemothorax, or both, is established by chest radiography, although when substantial, the physical signs are evident. If the lungs appear fully expanded, the patient is monitored by regular clinical examination of the chest and assessment of dyspnoea, tachypnoea and tachycardia. At the earliest indication of an increasing pneumo- or haemothorax with compression of the lung the chest is drained. For progressive tachypnoea and cyanosis, as occurs in tension pneumothorax, drainage by the insertion of a large-bore hypodermic needle into the affected side via the second inter-costal space in the mid-clavicular line is a life-saving measure. An open pneumothorax, if due to a penetrating wound, will in addition to drainage, require immediate secure sealing of the open wound in the chest wall, initially with a pressure dressing, until suture closure can be carried out.

The pleural cavity is decompressed by an intercostal drain, placed in the fourth inter-costal space for a pneumothorax or the fifth for a haemothorax in the mid-axillary line, through a stab incision near the upper border of the rib and by blunt dissection, using artery forceps, the pleural cavity is entered and a chest drain (28 French gauge) is positioned in the apex for a pneumothorax or in the base for a haemothorax. When both pneumo- and haemothorax are present, apical and basal drains are required. The drain is attached to the chest wall with a purse string around the wound. Satisfactory positioning of the drain is confirmed by a chest X-ray.

The drainage tube is connected to a rigid tube whose end is situated under water contained in a bottle with an exit tube lying above the water level (Fig. 21.1). The exit tube is exposed to atmospheric pressure, or low pressure suction may be applied to it. When the pressure in the pleural cavity is greater than atmospheric pressure, air or blood will drain out through the water-immersed tube, whilst

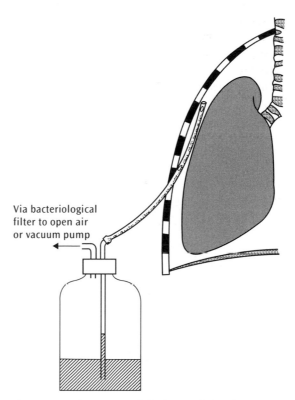

Via bacteriological filter to open air or vacuum pump

Fig. 21.1 *Underwater-seal drainage of the pleura. Note the two side holes in the drain near apex and base of the thorax. The meniscus of the liquid in the seal is drawn up the tube leading from the pleura by the negative intra-pleural pressure. When the patient coughs, air or blood in the pleura is expelled through the trap. To cope with excessive drainage of air or blood, the shorter tube can be connected to suction.*

atmospheric air is prevented by the water level from being sucked into the pleural cavity when the pleural pressure is negative. The under-water seal should always remain at a lower level than the chest, and when transporting the patient or emptying the bottle, the drainage tube must be clamped to avoid water or air being sucked into the pleural cavity.

Drainage of air or blood through the inter-costal drain is enhanced by deep inspirations to expand the lung and increase the pleural pressure, and physiotherapy is maintained until the lung is fully expanded. This is recognized by the cessation of movement of the fluid column in the water bottle and confirmed by a chest radiograph. When it is time to remove the tube, 24 hours after all air- or blood-leakage has ceased, it is clamped for several hours and if there are no signs of respiratory distress, and the lungs remain expanded both clinically and on a repeat chest X-ray, the drain is removed while the patient takes a deep inspiration to prevent atmospheric air being sucked into the pleural cavity while pulling on the purse string to close the wound in the chest wall.

Indications for thoracotomy

A persistent and/or excessive air leak recognized by bubbling through the water of the underwater seal, and made worse by inspiration or coughing, especially when associated with significant pneumothorax or surgical emphysema and failure of the lung to expand, suggests a pulmonary laceration or bronchial damage, and a thoracotomy should be considered. This may be obvious instantly following the injury or days after chest drainage. A fibre-optic bronchoscopy is helpful to confirm a bronchial tear when suspected.

Drainage of more than a litre of blood at the time of insertion of the inter-costal drain, or continuous bleeding of more than 200 ml/hour for 2–4 hours or 100 ml/hour for 6–8 hours or more than 1 l within 24 hours, requires a thoracotomy to suture/ligate bleeding vessels, resect lacerated lung or, if the hilar vessels are damaged, perform a pneumonectomy. The possibility of disruption of the aortic root should always be considered, especially in deceleration injury and if the mediastinum is widened on a chest X-ray. A CT scan or arch arteriography is urgently arranged to allow early transfer to a specialist unit where facilities for cardiopulmonary bypass are available for major arterial repair.

Although long needle aspiration via the epigastrium as the sole therapy for cardiac tamponade is successful in half the cases, thoracotomy should be considered if after a dry tap tamponade is still suspected or there are signs of continuous bleeding.

Pyrexia, chest pain and dyspnoea following chest injuries can be due to complicating chest infection which is treated with antibiotics and physiotherapy. However, one should always suspect an empyema demonstrable on a chest X-ray or by ultrasound examination as a result of residual infected material. If inter-costal drainage is inadequate open drainage may be necessary. The possibility of oesophageal perforation should always be considered and ruled out, by a CT scan and a water-soluble contrast swallow as early surgical repair with drainage and broad spectrum antibiotics will reduce the morbidity associated with mediastinitis due to delayed diagnosis.

HIGHLIGHTS

- Pericardiocentesis and thoracocentesis are life saving measures for cardiac tamponade and tension pneumothorax
- Major intra-thoracic injuries should be considered with fractures of the first and second ribs or the sternum
- An arch aortogram or CT scan is essential if the mediastinum is wide on a chest X-ray
- Excessive and persistent blood or air after chest decompression is an indication for thoracotomy
- A missed oesophageal tear is a likely cause of mediastinitis following a chest injury

---

VASCULAR INJURIES

AIMS

1 Recognize the type of injury that is likely to cause vascular damage
2 Learn the principles of management of vascular injuries

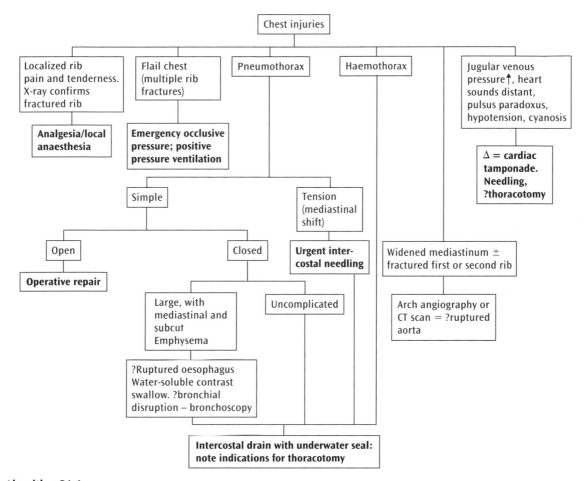

Algorithm 21.1

Introduction

Severe vascular injuries are a rare component of major blunt injuries. Penetrating injuries carry a higher risk. Severe limb injuries, especially joint dislocations and fractures adjacent to joints, carry a high risk of associated vascular damage. Ischaemia due to intimal damage and thrombosis or compression by a fracture, a dislocation or an expanding haematoma can present a threat to a limb, whereas haemorrhage from a vascular injury is a threat to life.

Management of vascular injuries

After primary care, haemorrhage must be controlled at the site of the accident by local pressure on an artery, and by elevation followed by firm bandaging for venous control. A tourniquet should be used with care because of the danger of converting partial to total ischaemia. It has a place when transporting a patient with severe arterial haemorrhage, provided it is released every hour if definitive treatment is delayed. Fractured limbs are straightened and splinted, dislocations reduced (Fig. 21.2). All patients with injuries, especially when adjacent to major vessels, should have full distal neurological and vascular examination, with careful observation of skin pallor, pulse volume and symmetry, and skin temperature, sensation and capillary perfusion, although these features may be masked by associated injuries. Comparison with the contralateral side may demonstrate an ischaemic limb, even in a shocked patient. Re-assessment is

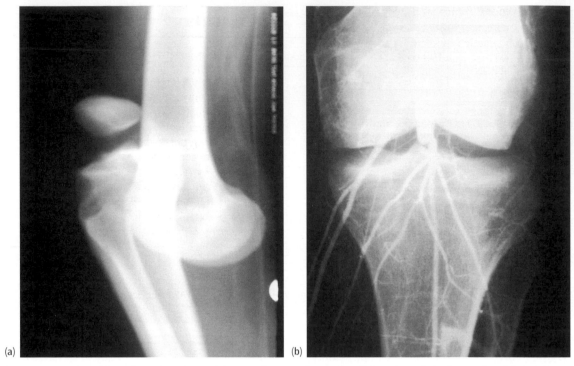

(a) (b)

Fig. 21.2 *Anterior dislocation of the knee; (a) Lateral X-ray of anterior dislocation of the knee. The tibia has been forced up in front of the femur; (b) Arteriogram of the same knee after reduction. The popliteal artery has been interrupted at the level of the joint by an intimal tear.*

repeated at intervals as in the initial phase the pulses can be present in spite of stretching or compression of the vessel wall until later when thrombosis or compartment syndrome develops. Re-assessment allows early treatment before irreversible ischaemia, identified by skin staining and muscle rigidity, ensues.

Doppler ultrasonography demonstrates the presence, reduction or absence of an arterial signal and pressure measurement provides a baseline for future comparison. Arteriography is essential and even in the absence of reduced distal perfusion it is mandatory in dislocations of the knee and other joint injuries but should not delay transfer to a specialist unit or exploration, as a per-operative study can be performed.

When haemorrhage or ischaemia is present in a limb, and resuscitative measures are completed, treatment aims at obtaining reperfusion of the limb within

6 hours of injury. The vascular injury is explored usually under general anaesthesia. Digital pressure is applied over the bleeding point while normal vessel wall is exposed proximal and distal to the injury so that vascular clamps can be applied. Partial or complete vascular lacerations are sutured after trimming damaged edges. When there is loss or extensive damage, the vessel is sufficiently mobilized to allow resection and anastomosis, whereas a larger defect is bridged with autogenous vein. Ligation of a bleeding vessel may be possible when there is cross-circulation. In the presence of spasm, the vessel is distended gently by direct injection of heparinized saline or with a metal dilator through an arteriotomy. Although spasm is more common in children, in an adult reduced flow is more likely to be caused by thrombosis which can be distinguished by peri-operative arteriography.

Major vein damage requires reconstruction since this will influence the outcome of arterial repair by improving venous return and reducing oedema. Oedema following revascularization can be considerable and prophylactic fasciotomies are undertaken. In open wounds thorough debridement is carried out excising devitalized tissue and, if possible, the vascular repair is covered with viable muscle. Contaminated wounds are gently packed and delayed primary closure is carried out a few days later. Antibiotics and tetanus prophylaxis are prescribed.

Primary amputation may be required if revascularization is delayed beyond 6 hours since muscle ischaemia is accompanied by renal failure, metabolic acidosis and terminal sepsis. Amputation may also be more appropriate if the injury to a limb by vascular damage, ischaemia or soft tissue and/or bone damage is extensive.

HIGHLIGHTS

1 Other than penetrating injuries, dislocations and fractures adjacent to joints carry the risk of causing vascular injury
2 Arteriography is mandatory in dislocations of the knee joint and other joints
3 A tourniquet for controlling arterial bleeding should be applied with care
4 The risk of compartment syndrome is reduced by venous reconstruction and prophylactic fasciotomies after arterial repair
5 Amputation is more appropriate for prolonged (>6 hours) ischaemia and extensive soft tissue and bone damage

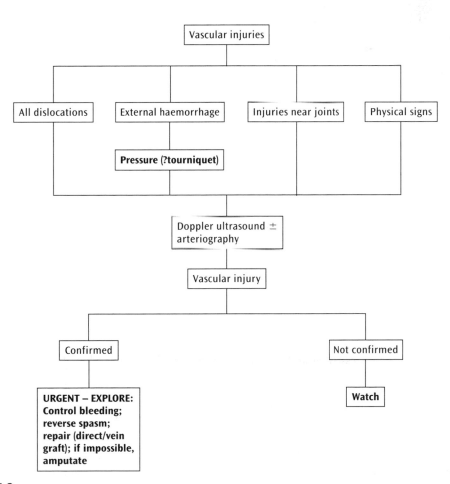

Algorithm 21.2

ABDOMINAL INJURIES

AIMS

1 Recognize the clinical features of intra-abdominal injuries
2 Identify specific organ injuries
3 Understand the management approach of penetrating and blunt trauma
4 Learn the surgical management of visceral injuries

Introduction

The abdominal injury may be solitary or one of multiple injuries. An intra-abdominal injury should be suspected particularly with fractures of the lower ribs or the pelvis. While the mortality can be low if managed promptly and adequately, uncontrolled bleeding from the liver or spleen or major arteries can be fatal. The immediate priority is resuscitation while assessment is being carried out and the degree of investigation is dependent on the stability of the patient.

Management of abdominal injuries

The initial management focuses on the airway, breathing and circulation. Fluid replacement is commenced while blood is cross-matched and monitoring is performed with a central venous line and urinary catheter. The patient's clinical picture is assessed while resuscitation is being carried out, and depending on the response to the resuscitative measures and the findings on history and examination, a decision on the need for and urgency of a laparotomy is made.

Assessment: history and examination

The nature and extent of the trauma gives an indication of the damage, although patients are often vague in recollecting the incident or may not be fully conscious. A detailed physical examination looking for relevant signs associated with recognized common injuries is fairly reliable. Generalized abdominal distension and pain with tenderness, although difficult to assess in the presence of abdominal wall bruising, is suggestive of a perforated viscus, free intra-peritoneal blood or urine. Contusions or subcutaneous haematoma may indicate deeper injuries to the pelvis or retro-peritoneum, and a characteristic seat belt bruise suggests impact of sufficient force to cause internal damage. Lateral lower rib fractures may be associated with injury to the spleen, liver or kidney. Blunt trauma to the lower abdomen can result in bladder injury. Pelvic fractures are often associated with bladder or urethral injuries suggested by abdominal pain and signs of peritonism, difficulty in voiding urine, bruising and evidence of urinary extravasation, that is, bruising and swelling of the perineum, external genitalia and lower abdomen and the presence of blood at the external meatus. Gross or microscopic haematuria suggests genitourinary tract injury.

The unstable patient

A patient with intra-abdominal haemorrhage shows progressive abdominal distension, and either requires rapid fluid infusion to maintain the blood pressure or remains hypotensive despite massive fluid replacement. The likely cause of the bleeding is either organ injury (liver, spleen), a major vascular injury (vena cava, aorta, iliac artery) or fracture of the pelvis.

Having established intravenous lines and ensuring that sufficient blood and coagulation factors are available, immediate laparotomy is essential. In patients with profound hypotension and gross tense abdominal distension associated with blotchiness of the lower limbs due to compression of the iliac veins, the tamponade effect of the abdominal wall is lost with the sudden decompression induced by muscle relaxants and laparotomy and can result in fatal and uncontrollable bleeding. In these patients preliminary aortic clamping through a lower left anterolateral thoracotomy or through the abdomen at the level of the diaphragm reduces the bleeding, provides a better view and may be life-saving.

The stable patient

A patient with convincing abdominal signs following a blunt or penetrating injury is optimized in preparation for a laparotomy, whereas a patient with equivocal abdominal signs is observed. A patient with a penetrating injury, in the absence of abdominal signs, can also be managed expectantly, especially if unfit or with other injuries. The patient with multiple injuries should be assessed carefully and monitored regularly as, in the absence of abdominal signs, systemic disturbances such as pyrexia or a change in blood pressure, pulse or respiratory rate may not necessarily be related to the abdominal injury. Sedation, impaired consciousness or mechanical ventilation make interpretation of abdominal findings difficult. The decision for a laparotomy should be made with caution in the unconscious or severely injured patient as an unnecessary laparotomy may jeopordize the patient's recovery. In these patients, relevant investigations provide information that could spare the need for a laparotomy.

Management of the penetrating wound

Stab wounds may or may not penetrate the peritoneum, and therefore unless the wound is obviously superficial, the abdomen may have to be explored by laparotomy or laparoscopy. In case of uncertainty about the depth of penetration and in order to determine whether the peritoneum has been penetrated it is advisable that the wound is explored. This is performed under local anaesthesia when conservative treatment is planned because the patient is considered unfit due to co-morbidity from other injuries or medical illness, or alternatively under general anaesthesia with the plan to proceed to laparotomy if the injury has penetrated the peritoneum. However, the latter exposes the patient to an unnecessary general anaesthetic if the wound proves to be superficial. It is more logical to explore the wound under local anaesthesia and proceed with a laparotomy under general anaesthesia only if indicated.

Exploration of the stab wound is more precise than relying on the depth a metal probe can be passed through the wound, as it may not follow the penetration track and can be unreliable particularly in the obese abdomen.

Even if the injury has obviously penetrated the peritoneum, the need for exploration is controversial, especially in the absence of systemic disturbance and abdominal signs, since a laparotomy may prove to be of no benefit. For this reason it is preferable to observe the patient for signs of deterioration (i.e., pyrexia, tachycardia, drop in blood pressure, abdominal pain, distension, tenderness and guarding) particularly in those with depressed consciousness from head injury or alcohol, or with other more pressing injuries that require attention. An ultrasound or CT scan and peritoneal lavage are employed to ensure the safety of this line of management. Alternatively, laparoscopy under intravenous sedation and local anaesthesia can reliably exclude intra-abdominal injury and minor lacerations which do not require laparotomy.

However, in patients with persistent hypovolaemia or requiring intensive resuscitation, or with abdominal signs, that is, distension or tenderness, those with eviscerated omentum or viscera, with extensive or potentially contaminated penetrating wounds, and all gunshot wounds, laparotomy to examine for visceral damage is mandatory.

Investigations

In the absence of convincing abdominal signs, chest X-rays may show free intraperitoneal gas due to a perforated viscus (not significant in penetrating injury as this is atmospheric air). Abdominal X-rays show fractures of the ribs, transverse processes of the vertebrae and pelvis; the renal outline, loss of the psoas shadow or displacement of bowel gas by retroperitoneal haematoma.

Ultrasound and especially contrast-enhanced CT scanning are useful in detecting lesions of the liver, spleen and kidneys as well as a haematoma or haemoperitoneum. In the emergency situation intravenous urography is adequate in defining renal injuries.

Peritoneal lavage is useful in equivocal cases and is performed by inserting a dialysis catheter under local anaesthetic into the peritoneal cavity through a small incision made in the mid-line below the umbilicus. A litre of normal saline is infused over 5–10 minutes, and is then drained by placing the empty bag below the level of the patient's bed. The siphoned perfusate is examined for the following positive criteria: red blood cells $> 100,000/ml$; white

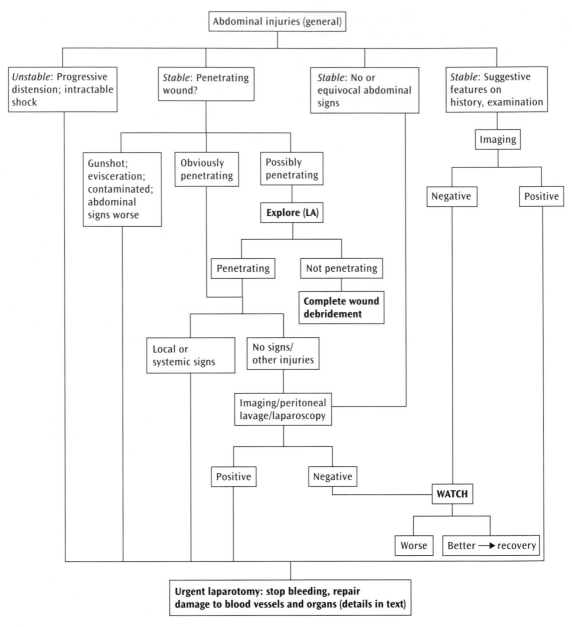

LA: local anaesthetic

Algorithm 21.3

blood cells > 500/ml; amylase > 110 u/100 ml; the presence of bile, bacteria or intestinal contents. This test has a high false positive rate, due to minor lesions which stop bleeding by the time laparotomy is performed.

Management of specific visceral injuries

Diaphragmatic injuries occur following blunt forceful trauma to the abdomen. Herniation of intra-abdominal viscera results from large tears, commonly in the left hemidiaphragm, which by deforming the lungs and mediastinum cause respiratory distress and hypotension from reduced cardiac output. A chest radiograph shows soft tissue shadowing and some-times a fluid level overlying the cardiac shadow, fur-ther demonstrated on lateral films. This requires a laparotomy and urgent repair of the diaphragm.

Hepatic injuries are clearly defined by CT scans. Minor lacerations in a stable patient do not require surgical intervention. The patient is monitored and scans are repeated to ensure resolution. Laparotomy is required for persistent signs of bleeding from deep lacerations or tears which are managed by suturing or resection. Severe hepatic bleeding can be con-trolled by bimanual compression or compression of the liver against packs placed between it and the posterior abdominal wall, or by clamping the portal triad. The possibility of tears in the inferior vena cava or hepatic veins should be considered in these situations and the patient is transferred to a special-ist unit.

Splenic injuries should be suspected in patients with left lower rib fractures and upper abdominal tenderness. The extent of the injury and any associ-ated renal injury are demonstrated on a CT scan. In a stable patient, a sub-capsular laceration or haematoma with little free intra-peritoneal fluid is managed conservatively with careful observation for signs of bleeding. Parenchymal or hilar lacerations present with abdominal signs of peritonism and hypotension. Laparotomy is carried out with attempt at splenic preservation especially in children, unless the spleen is not salvagable because it is fragmented or the hilar vessels are damaged.

Because of the risk of post-splenectomy infection and septicaemia, prophylactic vaccination against *Streptococcus pneumoniae*, *Haemophilus influenzae* and meningococcal groups A and C is essential and should be administered before or soon after splenec-tomy. Antibiotic prophylaxis should be given to children (amoxycillin 250 mg daily) until the age of 16 and to adults (500 mg daily) for 2 years after splenectomy, although antibiotic prophylaxis for life has been recommended. Anti-malarial prophylaxis is required when travelling to endemic areas.

Pancreatico-duodenal injuries show signs of peri-tonitis or there is bile in the effluent after peritoneal lavage. Duodenal perforations are repaired, tears in

the pancreas when minor are sutured while lacera-tions may require partial resection with drainage. In severe injuries pancreatico-duodenectomy may be necessary. Total parenteral nutrition and somato-statin promote healing of pancreatic fistulas that may complicate pancreatic injuries.

Intestinal injuries involve the small bowel, more commonly than the large bowel and a pre-operative diagnosis is made by signs of peritonitis or on peri-toneal lavage.

A small intestinal perforation or a tear is repaired by primary closure, but if the intestine is devitalized or is severed from its mesenteric attachment, it is resected and primary anastomosis is carried out.

Colonic injuries include seromuscular tears, haematomas and lacerations with involvement of the adjacent mesentery or omentum. A minor injury is closed with primary suture, whereas severe lacera-tions are treated by resection and primary anastomo-sis, with or without a proximal defunctioning stoma depending on the extent of faecal contamination and colonic loading. The stoma is closed a few months later. Alternatively, the bowel ends are exteriorized as a proximal colostomy and a mucous fistula and intestinal continuity restored months later by sec-ondary anastomosis. Injuries to the right colon are usually safely managed by primary anastomosis.

Incisions in the mesenteric leaf are used to decompress large mesenteric haematomas that may progress and jeopardize the blood supply to the intestine.

In the presence of significant contamination, the skin and subcutaneous tissues are better left unsutured and packed with antiseptic-soaked gauze. Secondary suture is performed 5–7 days later.

Renal injuries should be suspected in all penetrat-ing or blunt injuries to the loin, especially when asso-ciated with fractures of the lower ribs or vertebral transverse processes. Bruising over the flank, swelling and tenderness are not necessarily indicative of a renal injury. Haematuria, gross or microscopic, is highly suggestive but does not correlate with the degree of injury. If a CT scan is not available, an intravenous urogram is carried out to establish the presence of both kidneys and their function. If extravasation of the dye is noted, nephrotomograms are required to define further the extent of the dam-age to the kidney, whereas absent perfusion suggests renal vascular injury when urgent arteriography is required. A contrast-enhanced CT scan better defines the renal injury and identifies other injuries. According to the radiological appearances the renal injury can be classified as:

- *Minor*, which includes renal contusion, sub-capsular haematoma or superficial laceration not involving the collecting system.
- *Major*, which is a deep laceration with partial or complete disruption of the kidney extending to the collecting system with urine extravasation and associated with peri-nephric and retro-peritoneal haematoma.
- *Renal vascular injury* if the kidney is not opacified through lack of perfusion because of intimal tear or thrombosis or avulsion of the segmental arteries or veins or of the main renal pedicle. This requires urgent arteriography for confirmation.

The patient with minor injury is managed by bedrest and observation of the vital signs, the haematocrit, and the presence of blood in the urine. A major injury is treated similarly unless there are signs of continued or significant bleeding, suggested by tachycardia, hypotension, a falling haematocrit or increasing size of peri-nephric or retro-peritoneal haematoma, or evidence of renal vascular injury. After successful conservative treatment, a repeat examination of the kidney by CT or ultrasound scan is required as a large urine collection (*urinoma*) or abscess may necessitate percutaneous or open drainage.

When exploration is necessary, the presence and function of both kidneys should be established pre-operatively from the intravenous urogram or CT scan. Unless the kidney is severely lacerated or avulsed at its pedicle, segmental or partial nephrectomy avoids the loss of a kidney.

Bladder and urethral injuries result from blunt trauma to the abdomen with a full bladder causing rupture at its dome and extravasation of urine into the peritoneal cavity, but more commonly from perforation by a bone fragment and extravasation of urine into the retropubic space, following a comminuted or displaced pelvic fracture. Simultaneous injury of the posterior urethra occurs in 10–20% of patients with a fractured pelvis, and is more common in males because the female urethra is short, mobile

and without significant attachments to the pubic bones. In a stable fracture, all four fractured pubic rami and the prostate, which is fixed to the back of the pubic bone, are forced backwards, shearing the membranous urethra as it passes through the perineal membrane. Unstable fractures that involve the anterior part of the pubic ring and the sacro-iliac joint cause injuries to the posterior urethra by fractured bones or by shearing of the urethra by opposing traction of the puboprostatic ligament and the urogenital diaphragm, as a result of distortion of the bony pelvis.

Injury to the bladder and urethra should be considered in all patients with pelvic fracture and is suspected when a patient is unable to urinate and there is gross or microscopic haematuria. Abdominal pain with tenderness and guarding suggests free intra-peritoneal urine but can be due to a perforated viscus since one in five patients with a bladder injury has another intra-abdominal injury, and these signs may not be apparent in the inebriated or unconscious patient. There may be bruising and swelling in the lower abdomen, perineum and external genitalia from extravasation of urine or blood. The presence of blood at the external urethral meatus is a cardinal sign of urethral or bladder injury. When associated with inability to void and a palpable distended bladder, complete urethral disruption is the logical possibility to pursue, although these features may be related to sphincter spasm due to pain. Rectal examination is carried out to palpate the prostate since with posterior urethral disruption it is displaced posteriorly although this may be difficult to ascertain because of swelling and oedema. The rectum is examined digitally and by proctosigmoidoscopy as rectal injuries can also complicate pelvic fractures. Blood on the examination finger is highly suggestive of such an injury.

Urine must be obtained for testing, and if haematuria is present, a bladder or urethral injury is likely, but a renal injury may also co-exist and if this is suggested by the nature of the injury an intravenous urogram or a contrast-enhanced CT scan is essential. The latter further outlines bony and soft tissue disruption with a pelvic fracture, free intra-peritoneal fluid or pelvic collection and other intra-abdominal injuries. When a CT scan is not available an ultrasound may be useful in demonstrating free fluid in the abdomen, a pelvic collection, a full bladder, irregularities in the bladder wall and associated intra-abdominal injury. A plain radiograph of the pelvis determines the extent of the bony injury. A rise in blood urea without a corresponding rise in creatinine levels, due to reabsorption of urea by the peritoneal membrane, is suggestive of extravasation of urine. If there is blood at the external urinary meatus or difficulty in passing a catheter or any other reason to suspect a urethral injury, no attempt should be made to pass a catheter into the bladder. First, a retrograde urethrogram is obtained by placing a 12F Foley catheter in the penile urethra and water-soluble contrast is gently injected to outline the urethra. If the urethra is normal, the catheter is advanced to the bladder and a retrograde cystogram is carried out. A film of the bladder distended with at least 250 ml of contrast is obtained and a second film is taken as the bladder is drained, to detect any extravasation either intra- or extra-peritoneal. If the patient is in urinary retention and a urethral injury cannot be excluded, a supra-pubic catheter is inserted and simultaneous urethrography and cystography can be performed later.

Intra-peritoneal rupture requires surgical exploration by a trans-peritoneal approach, and the bladder is repaired with absorbable suture material. The peritoneal cavity is washed out and prophylactic antibiotics prescribed. The bladder is drained with a supra-pubic catheter as well as a urethral catheter. A cystogram is performed at 10 days to establish the bladder integrity, when the urethral catheter is removed, whilst the supra-pubic catheter is retained to confirm adequate bladder emptying by measuring post-voiding residue before it is removed.

Extra-peritoneal rupture can be treated conservatively by adequate bladder drainage and antibiotic cover for Gram-negative and Gram-positive aerobic and anaerobic organisms while observing for signs of sepsis as a pelvic haematoma may develop into an abscess. A cystogram is performed after about 1 week of bladder drainage. Contraindications to conservative treatment are severe haematuria requiring repeated bladder washouts or irrigation, pelvic haematomas and persistent extravesical leakage on cystography despite prolonged catheterization. The bladder is opened and the perforation is closed intra-vesically using absorbable suture material. The extra-peritoneal space and bladder are drained.

Urethral injury is managed initially by draining the bladder to prevent further extravasation, by a supra-pubic cystotomy by the percutaneous or open route if there is an associated bladder injury that requires repair. If there is definite evidence of a complete urethral rupture with an expanding pelvic haematoma, and if surgery for other associated injuries is planned, urethral re-alignment may be considered. The bladder is opened, and 'railroading' of the urethra is undertaken by use of two urethral catheters, one each from above and below; these are tied together at their tips and the penile urethral catheter is pulled through into the bladder. This should limit the extent of urethral disruption and re-aligns the urethra so that the resultant stricture is shorter and easier to repair. Open and penetrating contaminated injuries are managed by debridement of necrotic tissue and supra-pubic cystotomy and diverting colostomy if there is an associated rectal injury. The supra-pubic catheter is left for a few weeks and a micturating cystourethrogram is performed prior to its removal to ensure that the injury has healed. Delayed repair may be necessary for defects with long strictures when the perineal haematoma and swelling or infection have resolved. Immediate repair of urethral injuries is only attempted if the patient is stable, the wound is clean and haematoma is minimal.

HIGHLIGHTS

- Fractured lower ribs and pelvis are usually associated with injuries to the spleen or liver and of the bladder and urethra
- An unstable patient requires urgent laparotomy after clamping the aorta via a thoracotomy
- A laparotomy is not mandatory in a stable patient with no abdominal signs even if the injury is penetrating
- A CT scan, peritoneal lavage and laparoscopy are useful investigations when there is no clear indication for a laparotomy
- A CT scan is particularly helpful in the management of liver, spleen and kidney injuries
- A urinary catheter should never be passed when there is blood at the external meatus, before a urethrogram and cystogram are performed

SOFT TISSUE INJURIES

> **AIMS**
>
> 1 Recognize nerve and tendon injuries
> 2 Learn the principles of management of soft tissue injuries

Management of soft tissue injuries

This should take into account the site, the extent of tissue damage, the degree of contamination and the presence of foreign material in the wound. The wound is carefully cleansed of all foreign material and dead tissue is excised (*debrided*). Provided that the wound is not heavily contaminated and not more than 6 hours have elapsed since the injury, the wound is sutured immediately and can be expected to heal with minimal risk of infection, especially when on the face or the scalp because of the rich blood supply. Otherwise, the wound is left open, covered with a sterile dressing, and is examined 5 days later when a delayed primary suture is carried out if it is clean and there is no sign of infection, or else left to heal by secondary intention, that is, granulation tissue, scarring and contracture.

With limb injuries, the possibility of nerve, tendon or vascular damage should be considered and assessment should include a documented examination for sensation, movement, distal pulses and tissue perfusion, that is, warmth, colour and capillary refilling after blanching. Vascular injuries are managed as discussed already. Tendons and divided nerves usually require repair using fine sutures and magnification. Rest and elevation of the affected limb limit the swelling and also help to reduce pain.

The risk of infection, especially in injuries of the fingers and hands which are vulnerable to infection of the pulp and palmar spaces, requires antibiotic prophylaxis against staphylococci and streptococci with, for example, flucloxacillin and amoxycillin. The risk of gas gangrene must also be considered in contaminated and contused wounds when, besides thorough cleansing, benzylpenicillin is given prophylactically. Tetanus prophylaxis should also be provided with a booster dose if the patient had previously been fully immunized, but if not, passive immunization with human anti-tetanus immunoglobulin is given and a full course of active immunization with toxoid is commenced.

Nerve injuries

Nerves are crushed, stretched or severed as result of crushing or penetrating injuries, fractures or dislocations. A common example of a fracture-induced nerve injury is a radial nerve palsy following a humeral shaft fracture. It is important that any neurological deficit observed with an injury is documented prior to treatment. In a penetrating or open wound, nerve division (*neurotmesis*) should be suspected, especially in vulnerable sites; the wound should be explored and if the injury is confirmed the nerve is repaired. If the wound is clean and the surgeon is experienced then the procedure can be undertaken instantly, otherwise it is deferred and carried out electively. The best results are obtained if this is done preferably within 2 weeks, but the outcome is often disappointing. The nerve is repaired, if possible by direct suturing without tension, but if there is a defect, this is bridged with a nerve graft using a nerve such as the sural nerve of the leg that is unlikely to leave a significant disability in the area it supplies when removed. Mixed sensory and motor nerves have a particularly poor prognosis, whereas sensory nerves such as those in the fingers are most likely to recover.

Non-penetrating injuries such as a fracture or a direct blow may result in stretching or crushing of adjacent nerves causing sensory loss, paraesthesia and weakness of muscle groups. The resultant damage to the nerve is likely to be either a neurapraxia or axonotmesis. In neurapraxia, the nerve fibres and sheath are intact, whereas in axonotmesis the sheath remains intact but the nerve fibres are damaged to a variable degree. These are distinguished clinically by the rate of return of motor and sensory functions; provided the causative factor is treated, sensation recovers in the whole limb within a period of hours in a neurapraxic injury while in axonotmesis there is a gradual return of sensation and movement according to the proportion of nerve fibres that have remained intact, but recovery is not complete. Physiotherapy to maintain the mobility of the muscles and joints in the area of damage will enhance rehabilitation once the nerve recovers. Electromyography and nerve conduction studies are helpful in establishing the nature and level of the nerve damage, and the prognosis.

Tendon injury

This arises from penetrating or crushing injury. The flexor tendons of the hands are commonly injured. Examination for movements of the involved joints give an indication and the damage is recognized on exploring the wound. Tendon injury usually requires surgical repair, followed by physiotherapy with controlled movement in order to discourage adhesions and joint stiffness without jeopardizing the repair.

Replantation

This is indicated in clean-cut injuries of whole upper limb or hand, for loss of thumb as this results in considerable disability but not for loss of a single finger, and for loss of all digits when the thumb and not more than two fingers are replanted. The severed part is preserved by washing it and placing it in a wet towel and then in a plastic bag immersed in ice-cold water, and should be replanted within 12 hours. The amputated part is reattached by bone fixation using microsurgery for vascular reconstruction and repair of nerves. This treatment is not employed in crush or avulsion injuries.

HIGHLIGHTS

- Primary closure of a wound should be avoided if the wound is contaminated or more than 6 hours old
- Antibiotics against infection, including gas gangrene, and tetanus prophylaxis are essential in contaminated and contused wounds
- In limb injuries, vascular, nerve and tendon damage must be checked
- Primary repair of a severed nerve or tendon is desirable provided there is no contamination
- Neurapraxia is distinguished from axonotmesis by the rapid recovery of sensory and motor function
- Replantation is not employed in crush or avulsion injuries

FRACTURES

AIMS

1 Define fractures and dislocations; recognize their clinical features
2 Learn the principles of management of fractures and dislocations
3 Recognize the complications associated with fractures and dislocations

---

Introduction

The signs of a fracture are deformity, tenderness, swelling, loss of function and crepitus. In any fracture, injuries to neighbouring skin, muscle, vessels and nerves should be sought. If the skin has been breached the fracture is regarded as *open*, but if not as *closed*. A swelling causing deformity can be due to soft tissue oedema as a result of damage to the subcutaneous fat and muscle without underlying bony displacement. The latter is identified by crepitus due to grinding of the broken ends. This may not be easy to elicit because it may cause the patient severe pain.

Management of fractures

Immediate management is to relieve pain with opiates, given intravenously rather than intramuscularly, although they should be used cautiously when serious head injury is suspected. Splintage by restricting movement of the fractured bones is effective in relieving the pain, especially when transporting the patient before definitive treatment is instituted. A splint should encompass the joint above and below the fracture, using a slab, although binding the arm to the chest wall or the legs together is sufficient. Traction serves a similar purpose and is particularly useful for fractures of the femoral neck where splintage is not possible. Patients with pelvic or long bone fractures should be cross-matched for blood and venous lines established as the blood loss can be substantial. Once the patient is relatively comfortable, two plain X-ray views are taken at right angles, usually anteroposterior and lateral views, and oblique views are also sometimes obtained.

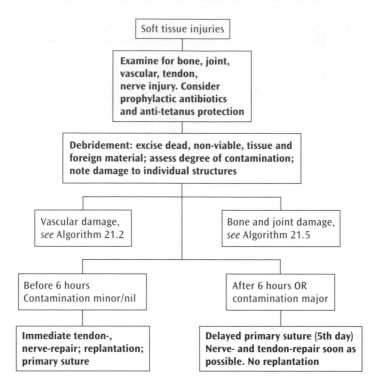

Soft tissue injuries

Examine for bone, joint,
vascular, tendon,
nerve injury. Consider
prophylactic antibiotics
and anti-tetanus protection

Debridement: excise dead, non-viable, tissue and
foreign material; assess degree of contamination;
note damage to individual structures

Vascular damage,
see Algorithm 21.2

Bone and joint damage,
see Algorithm 21.5

Before 6 hours
Contamination minor/nil

After 6 hours OR
contamination major

Immediate tendon-,
nerve-repair; replantation;
primary suture

Delayed primary suture (5th day)
Nerve- and tendon-repair soon as
possible. No replantation

Algorithm 21.4

In fractures of long bones, the joint above and below the fracture should be included. The radiological appearances are lucency at the fracture and discontinuity in the cortex or surface of a bone or joint.

Closed (simple) fractures are treated by reduction and immobilization. Closed reduction is achieved by traction on the distal fragment, then relocating it back on to the proximal fragment by manipulation, carried out under general or regional anaesthesia. If unsuccessful, open reduction is required: the fracture site is explored surgically and reduction performed under vision. The final position of the fracture is checked by a repeat X-ray. Once the fracture is re-aligned, immobilization, which should include the joint above and below the fracture, is achieved with a Plaster of Paris, glassfibre or polyurethane cast, but for unstable fractures re-alignment and stabilization of the fracture require internal fixation using wires, screws or plates depending on the site and type of fracture (Figs 21.3 and 21.4). Immobilization is maintained on average for nearly 6 weeks for upper limb fractures, and 12 weeks for

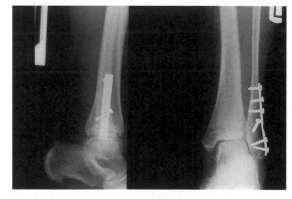

Fig. 21.3 *A displaced intra-articular ankle fracture has been reduced and fixed with a plate and screws. All intra-articular fractures need anatomical reduction: rigid fixation allows earlier mobilization, and reduces joint stiffness and any future tendency to osteoarthritis.*

lower limb fractures, until the fracture is deemed united as verified clinically by restoration of pain-free movements. During this time the patients are encouraged to use their joints and exercise their limb

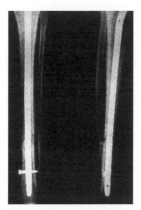

Fig. 21.4 *A fracture of the shaft of the tibia treated by immobilization with an intra-medullary nail. The locked screws control rotation.*

muscles, in order to minimize muscle atrophy and joint stiffness that may lead to contracture and post-traumatic sympathetic dystrophy.

Open (compound) fractures are serious injuries because the breach in the skin permits bacterial contamination of the bone. The wound is thoroughly cleansed and covered with sterile dressing until formal surgical debridement is carried out. After debridement, the wound is left open, especially if closure cannot be achieved without tension on the tissues. These patients require broad-spectrum antibiotics and tetanus prophylaxis; toxoid booster to those who had previously been immunized or human anti-tetanus globulin for those who had not received immunization.

The subsequent management of the fracture is along the principles already described; in general stable fractures are treated by reduction and immobilization in a cast, whereas unstable fractures, especially when soft tissue damage is extensive, will require either internal fixation or external fixation. External fixation (Fig. 21.5) comprises strong metal rods which are placed parallel to the fracture and are attached to the bone by a series of pins. Its advantage is that it allows access to inspect the wound for dressings and secondary surgery, such as further debridement or skin grafting if required, but there is the risk of infection at the pin sites.

Pelvic and *acetabular fractures* are most demanding, as they often are associated with more pressing injuries, requiring the involvement of several

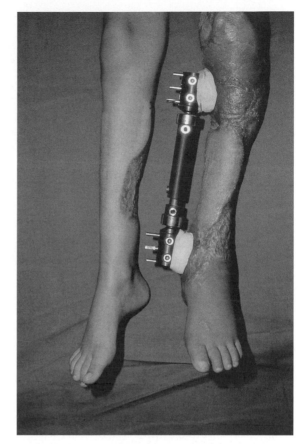

Fig. 21.5 *An external fixator has been used to immobilize an open fracture of the shaft of the tibia. A free musculocutaneous flap has been performed to cover the exposed bone. The skin graft on the other leg marks the donor site.*

specialist teams. The immediate application of a pelvic external fixator is indicated when there is haemodynamic and mechanical instability. For open pelvic fractures with wounds in the perineum, buttock, vagina, bladder, urethra or rectum, a defunctioning colostomy and washout is mandatory. The colostomy is better sited in an upper quadrant if the lower abdomen is damaged or pelvic surgical approaches are anticipated. A supra-pubic cystostomy may also be necessary. The soft tissue injuries are treated by cleansing, irrigation and debridement. Radiographs and CT scans are required for pelvic disruptions. Any necessary definitive reconstructive surgery should be performed within 10 days of the injury.

Complications that may follow fractures should be recognized and treated promptly. Pain at the fracture site can be due either to infection or to compartment syndrome. *Infection* may occur after open fractures or internal fixation, resulting in osteomyelitis. A rise in temperature, swelling and redness at the fracture site if accessible to inspection or a complaint of throbbing pain if in a cast, should raise suspicion. The cast is removed to examine the limb. A raised white cell count or C-reactive protein is suggestive. Radiography does not provide information at this early stage, and unless blood culture is positive, the diagnosis is based on circumstantial evidence unless the physical signs are obvious. An MRI or radio-isotope scan demonstrates early changes due to osteomyelitis. Intravenous broad-spectrum antibiotics are administered, and pus if present is drained. Provided the fracture is stable, it will unite despite infection. *Compartment syndrome* occurs as a result of increased pressure due to soft tissue swelling within a closed anatomical space, such as the flexor osseofascial compartment of the forearm or the leg (compartment bounded by bone and fascia). The rise in pressure will initially impede venous flow, whereas arterial inflow is uninterrupted causing further swelling and rise in pressure until it is greater than the capillary perfusion pressure, leading to ischaemia. Compartment syndrome should be suspected in any closed limb injury even if the distal pulses are present. The clinical features are tenderness over the arm or leg and pain on passive stretching of the intercompartmental muscles, for example in the flexor compartment of the forearm, extending the fingers to stretch the flexor digitorum muscles. The intercompartmental pressure can be directly measured by use of a needle probe connected to a manometer, but this should not delay treatment which consists of relieving the pressure by dividing the fascia and allowing the muscles to expand.

Fat embolism may complicate fractures of long bones and usually occurs in men under the age of 20, and should therefore be considered in these young patients and not mistaken for respiratory infection. It is believed to be due to fat embolization from the marrow of the fractured bone to the lungs, or precipitation in the lungs of fatty acids from tissue fats. The patient develops tachypnoea within a few days of the injury; an associated petechial rash on the chest, neck and conjuctiva is strongly suggestive but not always present. Blood gases show hypoxaemia and respiratory alkalosis from hyperventilation, and a chest radiograph shows diffuse opacities. The presence of fat globules in the sputum and urine or in the retinal vessels at fundoscopy is diagnostic. However, having ruled out infection, early diagnosis is based on suspicion. Treatment is with oxygen therapy and physiotherapy and in severe respiratory distress mechanical ventilation is required.

Acute renal failure should be anticipated and prevented by early measures to maintain the circulation and encourage diuresis by adequate hydration, as blood loss, infection and precipitation of myoglobin in the renal tubules following crush injuries causing massive soft tissue and muscle damage are the main contributing factors.

DISLOCATIONS

A *dislocation* implies complete, a *subluxation* implies partial loss of contact between the articular surfaces in a joint (Figs 21.6 and 21.7). Dislocations are more prone than fractures to cause damage to neurovascular and soft tissue. Any joint may be dislocated after major trauma and dislocation should be recognized by deformity and loss of movement of the joint. Considerable force is required to dislocate the hip joint or the sacro-iliac joint which should be reduced and placed in skeletal traction as an emergency.

HIGHLIGHTS

- Dislocations are more likely to be associated with neurovascular and soft tissue injuries than fractures
- An unstable fracture is better immobilized by internal fixation, whereas external fixation in open fractures allows access to the wound
- Pelvic fractures can be associated with extensive soft tissue damage

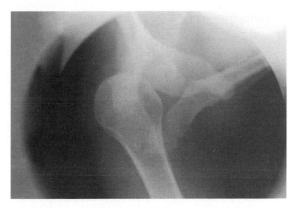

Fig. 21.7 *Lateral X-ray of the same case as Fig. 21.6 confirms that the head of the humerus is displaced posteriorly with respect to the glenoid fossa of the scapula.*

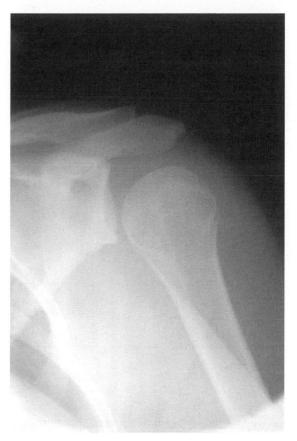

Fig. 21.6 *Anteroposterior (AP) X-ray of a posterior dislocation of the right shoulder. This view gives the false impression that the joint is congruent. However, the accompanying internal rotation of the shoulder decreases the prominence of the greater tuberosity so that the head of the humerus has a smooth contour reminiscent of an upturned lightbulb.*

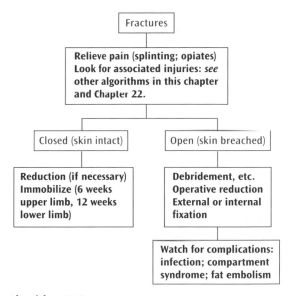

```
                    ┌──────────────┐
                    │  Fractures   │
                    └──────────────┘
                            │
       ┌────────────────────────────────────────┐
       │ Relieve pain (splinting; opiates)       │
       │ Look for associated injuries: see       │
       │ other algorithms in this chapter        │
       │ and Chapter 22.                         │
       └────────────────────────────────────────┘
              │                        │
   ┌────────────────────┐   ┌────────────────────┐
   │ Closed (skin intact)│   │ Open (skin breached)│
   └────────────────────┘   └────────────────────┘
              │                        │
   ┌────────────────────┐   ┌────────────────────┐
   │ Reduction (if       │   │ Debridement, etc.   │
   │ necessary)          │   │ Operative reduction │
   │ Immobilize (6 weeks │   │ External or internal│
   │ upper limb, 12 weeks│   │ fixation            │
   │ lower limb)         │   └────────────────────┘
   └────────────────────┘             │
                          ┌────────────────────────┐
                          │ Watch for complications:│
                          │ infection; compartment  │
                          │ syndrome; fat embolism   │
                          └────────────────────────┘
```

Algorithm 21.5

SPINAL INJURIES

AIMS

1 Recognize the clinical features of spinal cord injury
2 Learn the principles of management

Introduction

The spine is best considered as composed of three columns rather than one: an *anterior* consisting of the anterior two-thirds of the vertebral bodies; an *intermediate* consisting of the posterior third of the vertebral bodies; and a *posterior* consisting of the facet joints, the spinous processes and their ligaments. When two of the three columns are disrupted

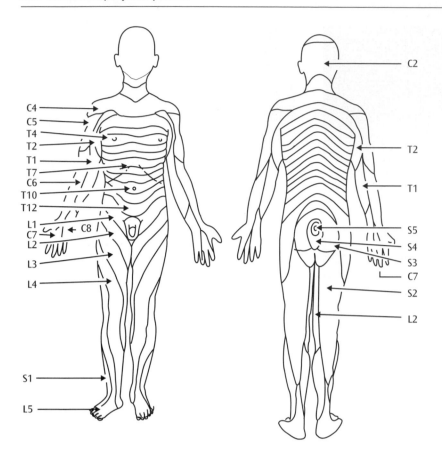

Fig. 21.8 *The dermatomes allow recognition of the level of spinal cord injury.*

Diagnosis of spinal injuries

All patients with a spinal injury should be handled carefully until spinal cord injury is ruled out.

Management involves determining the level of the injury, the extent of the cord lesion and the stability of the spine. A spinal cord injury should be suspected in patients with neck or back pain, sensory disturbance in the hands or feet and weakness or paralysis in the limbs, although these features can be difficult to ascertain in the inebriated patient or one with a head injury. The force of an injury sufficient to cause unconsciousness is also transmitted to the neck. In high lesions, paradoxical movement of the fracture is unstable and carries the risk of compressing the spinal cord, but if only one column is disrupted the spine remains stable.

the chest wall with diaphragmatic breathing or the presence of priapism in men are helpful clues. The plantar response (*Babinski's reflex*) if present may be down-going and in the acute stage is unreliable evidence of an upper motor neurone lesion.

The sensations in the limbs, chest wall, trunk and perineum are tested with a pin (Fig. 21.8). The lowest normal sensory segment is considered to be the level of neurological injury.

Changes in muscle power generally follow the pattern of pain and temperature loss. Flaccid paraplegia or quadriplegia with loss of sensation usually indicates a complete lesion (Fig. 21.9). Incomplete injury shows selective involvement of part of the cord with corresponding neurological signs (*central cord syndrome, anterior cord syndrome* or *Brown–Séquard syndrome*).

Anteroposterior and lateral radiographs of the suspected site and the whole spine should be obtained,

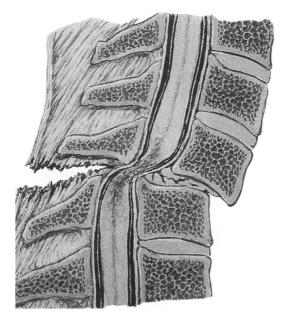

Fig. 21.9 *Diagram of a complete transection of the cord. The X-rays might appear normal in this unstable ligamentous injury.*

in order to determine whether or not the fracture is likely to be stable. CT scanning or MRI should include the first normal vertebra above and below the fracture and provides information on the integrity of the posterior elements and degree of encroachment of bone in the spinal canal.

Acute management

Injury to the spinal cord, especially high lesions, is associated with autonomic disturbance (*neurogenic shock*). Loss of sympathetic tone results in peripheral vasodilatation which makes the patient vulnerable to hypotension and hypothermia. Where sympathetic outflow to the heart is also involved, there is often associated bradycardia that may lead to cardiac arrest precipitated by procedures that stimulate the vagus. Therefore, oropharyngeal suction or endotracheal intubation should not be carried out unless atropine has been administered or is immediately available. Hypotension should not be regarded as solely due to the injury unless acute blood loss has been ruled out.

Respiration is not disturbed in patients with lesions below the level of C5 unless there is associated chest injury. Patients with a mid-thoracic spinal lesion and inter-costal muscle paralysis have para-doxical movements of the chest wall with indrawing of the inter-costal spaces during inspiration. These patients are dependent on diaphragmatic breathing, and have a reduced vital capacity. In cervical lesions, there is diaphragmatic paralysis and higher lesions involve the respiratory centre. Therefore, monitoring the respiratory rate and oxygen saturation should provide early warning of respiratory insufficiency. Physiotherapy and if necessary a mini-tracheostomy to aid clearance of secretions, with oxygen therapy or mechanical ventilation depending on the severity of respiratory embarrassment, should be provided.

The bladder is drained with an indwelling catheter until the patient is stable, then intermittent catheterization every 4–6 hours is commenced in those who develop a flaccid bladder. Men with supra-conal cord lesions are established on reflex bladder emptying into a condom urinal system. The rectum in the initial stages requires manual evacuation, but with return of reflex anal activity evacuation can be achieved with suppositories or micro-enemas until regular bowel function is established with the aid of bulking agents, stool softeners and aperients.

These patients require careful nursing in order to maintain alignment and prevent damage to the skin. Special beds, appropriate positioning of the patient, supporting pillows and keeping the skin clean and dry are the important features.

Fracture management

Stable fractures do not require any specific treatment besides analgesia and bedrest if necessary.

Unstable cervical spine fractures are treated by skull traction by use of skin calipers or halo-body or halo-vest to establish and maintain alignment, and internal fixation is required in certain fractures.

Thoracolumbar injuries may be treated conservatively by bedrest for 6–10 weeks followed by immobilization in a spinal brace. However, operative treatment with rigid internal fixation allows early mobilization and prevents chest complications and deep vein thrombosis.

Prevention of complications

The efficacy of corticosteroids in acute spinal cord injuries, administered within the first 8 hours, is controversial. The advantages of anticoagulation (decreased risk of deep vein thrombosis and death from pulmonary embolism) must be weighed against the potential disadvantage of causing further cord damage due to the increased risk of bleeding. Most centres now use anticoagulation. When possible, compression stockings should be worn. H_2 receptor antagonists given parenterally for the first few days, then orally, prevent stress peptic ulceration with perforation and haemorrhage which is another common complication.

HIGHLIGHTS

- Caution must be exercised in avoiding cardiac arrest because of autonomic disturbance
- Respiratory function must be monitored carefully, especially in lesions above the level of C5
- Careful nursing is required to maintain alignment and prevent skin damage
- Internal fixation is preferable to conservative treatment in thoracolumbar injuries as it allows early mobilization and prevents chest complications and deep vein thrombosis

---

TRIAGE

This term refers to the task of sorting patients into management groups depending on the availability of resources and manpower. The triage categories are:

- *Critical*: requires immediate surgery.
- *Serious*: requires surgery but can wait.
- *Minor injury*: expectant.
- Severely injured and unlikely to survive even with aggressive treatment.
- Dead.

There are two triage situations. When resources are adequate but manpower is limited patients with life-threatening and multi-system injuries are offered priority treatment. When resources are insufficient those patients with the best prospect of survival with the minimal resources and personnel are treated first.

Trauma scores

It is important to quantify the degree or seriousness of an illness, for better evaluation of treatment outcomes. Several scoring systems for trauma have been designed but the revised trauma score is the most commonly used (Table 21.1). The scores for the respiratory rate, the systolic blood pressure and the Glasgow Coma Scale, measured independently, are summed to give a total range between zero and 12. Further refinements can be made, for example, it can be combined with an 'injury severity score' which depends on the degree of injury of six main anatomical sites: this provides a statistical probability of survival based on large data from the USA on the outcome of injuries.

Table 21.1 *Revised trauma score*

Respiratory rate	Systolic blood pressure (mmHg)	Glasgow Coma Scale	Score
10–24	>89	13–15	4
25–35	70–89	9–12	3
>35	50–69	6–8	2
1–9	1–49	4–5	1
0	0	<4	0

22

Head injuries

MICHAEL HOBSLEY AND JASMIN HUSSEIN

AIMS

1 Relate the management to the pathophysiology
2 Distinguish between minor and major head injuries
3 Define criteria for hospital admission and observation
4 Recognize salvageable severe injuries and apply measures to minimize secondary effects
5 Recognize the clinical indications for referral to a neurosurgical unit

INTRODUCTION

Head injuries are common. About 2000 patients per 100,000 present to Accident and Emergency departments in the UK each year with head injury; 250 patients per 100,000 require admission and nine per 100,000 patients do not survive the injury. Over half of the patients who sustain head injuries are less than 30 years of age and it is the most common cause of death in the 15–24-year-old population.

The principal causes of head injury include road traffic accidents, assaults, falls and accidents at work and during sports. The most common factor associated with trauma is excessive alcohol ingestion. Occasionally, a medical illness precipitates a fall with trauma to the head.

The picture is one of a large number of relatively minor injuries which do not require any specific treatment, a small number that will cause death despite any form of treatment and a few cases whose management, especially in the first few hours, determines survival or the degree of permanent disability.

There are many aspects to the care of head injuries related to surgical management, rehabilitation, psychological and social support. This chapter deals with the immediate care of head injuries, which is better appreciated by understanding the pathophysiological mechanisms involved.

PATHOPHYSIOLOGY

There is a variable amount of damage which can occur to the coverings of the brain, skull and scalp, with associated cranio-facial fractures; damage to the base of the skull, in particular the cribriform plate and tegmen tympani, results in cerebrospinal fluid (CSF) fistulae. A skull fracture indicates the degree of force applied to the skull, therefore is often associated with scalp bruising, swelling or laceration, and primary brain damage is more likely than when there is no fracture. Depressed fractures rarely produce serious primary brain injury, but may tear the dura. The fracture itself is of no consequence unless it is compound.

Damage to the brain occurs as a result of direct impact or deceleration as in whip-lash injuries or in a high-speed car crash or in a fall from a height in which the body decelerates rapidly; the brain, by its movement within the cranium, is injured by the dural edges and sharp bony prominences. Blood vessels, being relatively stronger than neural tissue, act as 'cheese cutters'. There are also generalized shear and rotational forces causing the tearing of axons. With ageing the brain shrinks allowing greater mobility and hence brain injury can be more pronounced in elderly patients.

Pathological damage to the brain is classified as *primary* or *secondary*.

Primary damage occurs at the moment of impact and is irreversible. *Concussion* or loss of consciousness, may or may not be associated with a period of amnesia, temporary or permanent, for the period prior to this. It may be due to dysfunction of the subcortical white matter, including that of the brainstem. *Diffuse axonal injury* (DAI) results from mechanical shearing following deceleration and can occur even when the injury is trivial: the characteristic histological appearance is of petechiae. This does not cause an increase in intra-cranial pressure unless there is associated haematoma. *Focal brain damage* occurs in localized areas and results in cerebral contusions, or laceration, haemorrhage and haematoma which usually occur beneath the area of impact (*coup*) or at the frontal, temporal and occipital poles away from the site of injury (*contre-coup*), when the brain moves within the cranium and hits the opposite side of the skull. Focal injuries may cause secondary brain injury by mass effect. Diffuse or focal brain injury is associated with a varied degree of disturbance of, and recovery from, consciousness, related to the extent of injury.

Secondary damage which exacerbates the primary damage is caused by cerebral hypoxia, cerebral oedema, intra-cranial bleeding, infection and hydrocephalus. *Cerebral hypoxia* is due to central respiratory depression, airway obstruction, haemo- or pneumothorax, aspiration pneumonia, or alcohol- or drug-abuse related to the accident. *Hypotension* from hypovolaemia, usually due to other injury, may contribute to cerebral hypoxia by reducing cerebral perfusion. Epileptic fits are common in head injury and cause ischaemia during a fit. *Cerebral oedema*, due initially to an increase in intra-cranial blood volume as a result of loss in cerebral autoregulation, and in the ensuing days to an increase in interstitial fluid from tissue injury, causes a rise in intra-cranial pressure (ICP) which impedes cerebral perfusion. This leads to ischaemia and a vicious circle of further brain swelling and rise in ICP. *Intra-cranial bleeding* results in haematomas outside (*extra-dural*) or within the dura (*sub-dural* and *intra-cerebral*) which by compressing the brain cause focal neurological effects, and also a rise in ICP with secondary cerebral hypoxia and oedema, leading to temporal lobe herniation under the tentorium cerebelli or coning of the brain stem through the foramen magnum or both. Whereas intra-cerebral and acute sub-dural haematomas are usually associated with severe primary injury, extradural and chronic sub-dural haematomas are not, and the haematoma spreads slowly over a few hours or days so that its evacuation before the ICP rises allows complete recovery. *Infection* leading to meningitis or a brain abscess complicates compound fractures of the skull vault, or basal skull fractures that may communicate with the sphenoid or ethmoid sinuses, the nasal cavity or the external auditory canal. *Hydrocephalus* develops as a result of diminished absorption of the CSF by the arachnoid granulation over the surface of the hemispheres, because of high protein content of the CSF caused by the injury, sub-arachnoid haemorrhage or infection.

Primary brain damage is irreversible because of the poor regenerative capacity of the brain, so management is aimed at maintaining the patient during natural spontaneous recovery and preventing secondary damage by the appropriate prophylactic and interventional measures.

ASSESSMENT

History

The history about the events preceding the injury, for example epileptic fit, fainting, alcohol consumption or medications, medical illnesses such as anaemia, diabetes and myocardial infarction or cerebrovascular accidents, is taken from the patient or a witness. Retrograde amnesia, that is, for events before the accident, bears no relation to the severity of the injury and may improve with time. The duration of unconsciousness and *post-grade amnesia*, that is, for events after the accident, are related to the severity of head injury.

Examination

A general examination is carried out to exclude multiple injury; with care to prevent further damage at the site of any spinal injury, especially the neck. The examination focuses in particular on the level of consciousness, signs in the head and face, pupillary and eye movements, and limb responses.

Level of consciousness

This is assessed after resuscitation by the Glasgow Coma Scale (GCS) (Table 22.1), taking into account sedative drugs or alcohol intoxication and any direct orbital injury as these may interfere with the interpretation of the findings. If eye and verbal responses cannot be employed, the motor response is an important observation. The GCS classifies patients into *severe* (3–8), *moderate* (9–12) and *mild* (13–15).

The head and face

The scalp is examined for swelling or bruising, and if there is a deep laceration or history of penetrating injury the scalp is probed with the gloved finger for a defect or a depression.

Facial bruises and haematomas can be features of fractures to the base of the skull: peri-orbital haematoma, usually bilateral and limited by the margins of the orbicularis oculi (*panda eyes*) and sub-conjuctival haemorrhage, with no posterior limit

as blood tracks from behind forward unlike a sub-conjuctival haematoma from direct trauma to the eye, are signs of anterior fossa fractures; bruising over the mastoid area behind the ear (*Battle's sign*) is a sign of middle fossa fracture. These fractures are also associated with clear fluid or blood-stained discharge from the nose (*rhinorrhoea*) or the ear (*otorrhoea*), respectively, because of leakage of CSF and if present must be differentiated from a local tissue injury.

Eye signs

Pupillary responses and eye movements are dependent on intact IInd and IIIrd cranial nerves and pupillary inequalities or abnormal responses to light are indicative of increased intra-cranial pressure, usually from intra-cranial bleeding. *Pupil asymmetry* is common in the population, although it may not be possible to establish if this existed beforehand, and *pupillary dilatation* may be the result of alcohol, drugs and direct trauma to the eye (*traumatic mydriasis*), when there is usually another obvious injury such as a sub-conjuctival haematoma or a hyphema (bleeding into the anterior chamber). *Unilateral pupillary dilatation* and loss of constriction to light result from compression of the brain and traction on the IIIrd nerve in its long intra-cranial course on the same side. *Bilateral pupillary dilatation* and loss of the light reflex are signs of brainstem injury from coning, as a result of increased ICP.

Neurological examination

A full neurological examination is essential, to establish the presence or absence of focal signs but this may not be feasible in the drowsy or unconscious

Table 22.1 *The Glasgow Coma Scale (GCS)*

Eye-opening		Best motor response		Verbal response	
Spontaneous	4	Obeys command	6	Oriented	5
To speech	3	Localizes pain	5	Confused conversation	4
To pain	2	Flexion withdrawal to pain	4	Inappropriate words	3
		Abnormal flexion	3		
		Extends to pain	2	Incomprehensible sounds	2
None	1	None	1	None	1

Glasgow Coma Score = sum of the scores in the three columns, 3–15.

Table 22.2 *Factors suggesting major head injury*

Disturbance of consciousness/amnesia, known or
  suspected
Sero-sanguinous discharge from nose or ear
Headache, vomiting, neurological signs
Suspected penetrating injury or scalp laceration
  >5 cm or reaching bone
Skull fracture
Inadequate history or difficulty in assessing the
  patient
In infants and children under 5 years:
  tense fontanelle
  suspected non-accidental injury

patient. The limbs, tone, power, co-ordination and
sensation are regarded as useful measurements of
neurological deficit. Hemiparesis or hemiplegia
usually occurs in the limbs contralateral to the side
of the lesion, but may occur in the ipsilateral limbs
due to indentation of the contralateral cerebral
peduncle by the edge of the tentorium cerebelli.
Therefore, limb deficits are of limited value in localizing the site of the lesion.

   At the end of assessment, the decisions to be
made are whether the patient has a *minor* or *major*
head injury (*see* Table 22.2).

Management of minor head injury

In the absence of such suggestive features, small lacerations of scalp are sutured and the patient can be
sent home with a responsible adult and advice to
return immediately if unwell. However, should no
such responsible adult be available, the patient should
be admitted for 24 hours' observation.

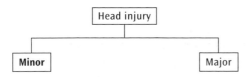

   An admitted patient undergoes routine neurological observations recorded by the nursing staff on
a *head injury chart* which includes: conscious level
(GCS), pupil size and light response, respiratory
pattern and rate, pulse rate and blood pressure.
These are reliable parameters that provide early
indication of deterioration.

   If any one (or more) of the factors is present, the
minimal requirement is for skull X-rays.

Skull radiography or CT scan

The risk of significant intra-cranial haematoma after
head injury is one in 6000 among alert patients with
no skull fracture, one in 120 among alert patients
with a fracture, one in four among drowsy patients
with a fracture, and one in 12 in children. A *routine*
CT scan is therefore not cost-effective. A skull X-ray
consists of anteroposterior (AP), lateral and (for the
skull base) *Towne's view* and the films are examined
for fractures, pineal shift and fluid levels in the
sphenoid and frontal sinuses indicative of basal skull
fracture.

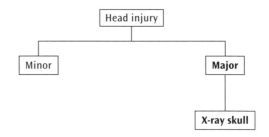

Management of major head injury

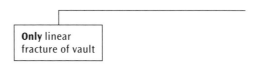

A patient who has been admitted because of a *brief
period of unconsciousness* or suspected unconsciousness, or for lack of an attendant responsible adult,
and remains stable for 24 hours is allowed home
even if there is a simple linear skull fracture of the
vault, and is advised to rest for about a week as the
post-concussion syndrome (p. 363), if it develops,
may limit the ability to resume work.

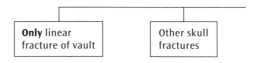

Fractures of the vault, when linear, require no
treatment. A *depressed fracture* is unlikely to cause

primary brain injury unless the depression is more than the thickness of the skull vault or it has lacerated the dura which can be demonstrated on a CT scan, when elevation of the depression is indicated. A penetrating injury may cause a *compound fracture*, with fragments of bone or foreign body penetrating the meninges and the brain. This requires wound debridement and repairing the dura under antibiotic cover. *Basal skull fractures* are regarded as compound as they may communicate with the exterior, with the risk of infection, and are assumed to be present if there is evidence of a CSF leak, even without confirmatory X-ray evidence. Antibiotics are given until the CSF leak stops but a formal repair to close the dural tear should be considered if the leak persists more than a week when from the nose, or more than 3 weeks when from the ear.

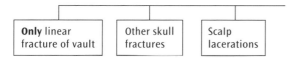

Scalp lacerations longer than 5 cm are frequently associated with skull fractures and it is therefore important to ensure that the fracture is not compound. The wound is cleared of foreign debris, the hair is shaved around the wound, the skin edges are debrided and the scalp is sutured in a single layer under local anaesthesia using lignocaine with adrenaline.

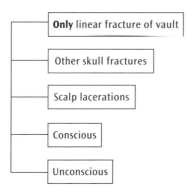

The *conscious* patient who has been admitted because of a history of an appreciable period of unconsciousness with or without post-traumatic amnesia, but without any other of the features of major injury, is observed until judged to have

Table 22.3 *Criteria for neurosurgical consultation and CT scan*

Fractured skull in combination with confusion or depression of conscious level or focal neurological signs or fits

Confusion or other neurological disturbances persisting for >12 hours even if there is no skull fracture

Coma continuing after resuscitation

Suspected open injury of the vault or base of the skull

Depressed fracture of the skull

Deterioration of conscious level or other neurological signs

improved sufficiently to be allowed to leave hospital with the usual instructions about returning should deterioration ensue.

A patient *unconscious* or *with a depressed conscious level* (GCS < 12) may have neurological signs or show signs of deterioration on admission, although a history of alcohol or drug intake may confuse the picture and should be taken into account. The management consists of resuscitation, assessment and definitive treatment with the objective of preventing secondary damage to the brain conducted with an intensity depending on the severity of the injury. This treatment is better undertaken in a neurosurgical unit once the immediate life-saving resuscitative measures are completed and the patient is stable for transfer. The criteria for requesting a neurosurgical consultation and CT scan are summarized in Table 22.3.

Resuscitation

The care of the airway is of utmost importance, simple measures employed are sucking out secretions or vomit and keeping the tongue forward, but the airway is best secured by intubation and ventilation, especially if the patient is in coma or if the blood gases are inadequate ($pO_2 < 13\,kPa$ or $pCO_2 > 6\,kPa$), ensuring that there is no haemo- or pneumothorax. An elective tracheostomy to replace intubation is not considered before 5–7 days. A naso-gastric tube is placed to prevent inhalation of stomach contents and antacids (H_2 antagonists or proton pump inhibitors) are prescribed to reduce gastric secretion and the risk of stress ulceration. One or more large-bore cannulae, a central venous pressure line and a urinary catheter are inserted. Hartmann's or dextrose-saline is administered as hypovolaemia should be avoided, after samples of blood have been taken for grouping, cross-matching and arterial blood gas analysis. Unless there is hypotension, fluid is administered cautiously in order not to induce cerebral and pulmonary oedema. An input and output fluid balance chart and a head injury chart provide essential observations in monitoring progress. If the patient's conscious level is deteriorating, an intravenous bolus infusion of 100 ml of 20% mannitol should 'buy time' by temporarily reducing the intra-cranial pressure until definitive planned investigation or treatment can be carried out. Routine prophylactic antibiotics are only administered if there is pulmonary soiling, compound skull injury or CSF leak. Anticonvulsants are not prescribed routinely unless there is an extensive open wound when it is a wise precaution to commence therapy. Phenytoin 300 mg a day and phenobarbitone 60 mg three times a day orally is the standard dose. Acute epilepsy is not controlled by these measures and requires intravenous diazepam or barbiturate; status epilepticus is best managed by controlled ventilation.

Assessment

The level of consciousness is better assessed following resuscitation and adequate oxygenation. Pupillary inequalities or abnormality of the light reflex, focal neurological signs, nausea and vomiting may suggest intra-cranial compression. An epileptic seizure may also indicate a brain contusion or a laceration. The unconscious patient with fixed dilated pupils unresponsive to light noted from the time of injury has severe primary brain damage, and if there is no response to painful stimuli is unlikely to survive, an important consideration for withholding active treatment. The patient must be stable and sedated before transfer to a radiology department. Skull, cervical spine and chest X-rays are mandatory. A CT scan is crucial in planning the subsequent management of the brain injury.

A thorough examination is conducted for other injuries, particularly in the chest, the viscera, the limbs and the spine, although in the unconscious patient meaningful abdominal signs can be difficult to elicit.

If the patient has multiple injuries, radiographs of the thoracic and lumbar spines, abdomen, pelvis and any suspected fractures should be obtained, and a CT scan of the chest and abdomen are of added value.

Definitive treatment

In multiple injuries, careful definition of priorities in a team approach is demanded.

A head injury takes precedence over other injuries if it is life-threatening, that is, compromising airway, breathing or circulation (ABC) (*see* Chapter 21). CT scan is a crucial investigation in determining the nature of the damage and in deciding on either an interventional or a conservative approach as illustrated in the following clinical situations.

Surgical treatment

Extra-dural haemorrhage (Fig. 22.1) occurs in about 10% of severe head injuries, commonly associated

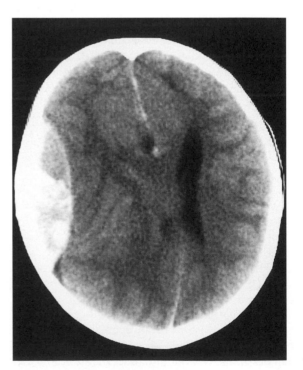

Fig. 22.1 *An extra-dural haematoma.*

with fractures that cross the middle temporal artery in the temporal region, and occasionally with a ruptured sagittal or transverse sinus. A haematoma forms rapidly between the skull and dura, compressing the brain. It is suspected when there is loss of consciousness after a lucid period of drowsiness or headache, a fixed dilated pupil on the side of the injury, or hemiparesis on the opposite side. The signs of increased intra-cranial pressure develop rapidly, with a rise in blood pressure, a fall in pulse rate and slow respiration. This requires urgent decompression: performed ideally within 2 hours from the time of deterioration complete recovery is likely, but if delayed to more than 6 hours the mortality is 90%. The signs of deterioration may be so rapid as not to allow time for a CT scan or transfer to a neurosurgical unit. Evacuation of the haematoma via burrholes in the temporal region on the side of the injury is a life-saving measure. Otherwise, the haematoma is localized by CT scan, and a 'horse-shoe' craniotomy flap is used to allow complete evacuation of the haematoma.

Acute sub-dural haematoma (Fig. 22.2) is four times more common than extra-dural haematoma and tends to occur in older patients because of the increased mobility of the brain within the cranium. The bleeding is the result of tearing of the veins running from the cortical surface to the venous sinuses. There is invariably primary brain injury. Contusions in the frontal and temporal lobes cause intra-cerebral haematoma which may expand and track into the sub-dural space (*'burst lobe'*). The patient is therefore confused or unconscious from the time of the injury, and shows deterioration as the haematoma spreads. A 'question mark' flap sited according to the CT scan findings permits access to both frontal and temporal lobes and evacuation of the haematoma and any necrotic brain. This may stop further deterioration, but recovery is incomplete or slow and the mortality is high because of the underlying brain injury.

Chronic sub-dural haematoma does not become manifest until weeks or months after a trivial head injury as the haematoma enlarges because of osmotic absorption of the CSF into the clot. The patient may complain of headache, drowsiness or confusion, or show non-specific neurological symptoms. These symptoms should arouse suspicion after any form of head injury. The diagnosis is made by CT scan. Burr holes are usually adequate to drain the haematoma but a craniotomy may be required when the clot is solid.

Not all patients with intra-cranial haematoma will necessarily require surgical treatment. In some, the haematoma is small. In others the CT scan may reveal a moderate sized haematoma with minimal or no mass effect and the patient is conscious but confused. In this group of patients, intra-cranial pressure monitoring is a useful guide: when it exceeds 30 mmHg, the prospect of recovery without intervention is unlikely.

Hydrocephalus is a late complication and should be considered if recovery is prolonged. It is treated by draining the CSF via a silicone tube with a one-way pressure-regulating valve into the peritoneum where it is re-absorbed into the circulation (=VP shunt).

Conservative treatment

Intra-cerebral haemorrhage and *focal brain injuries* are often associated with diffuse axonal injury, and cause irreversible damage. The patient is likely to be unconscious on presentation with a neurological deficit dependent on the extent and location of the

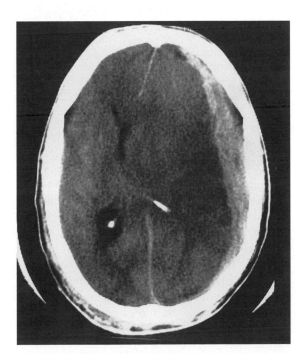

Fig. 22.2 *A sub-dural haematoma.*

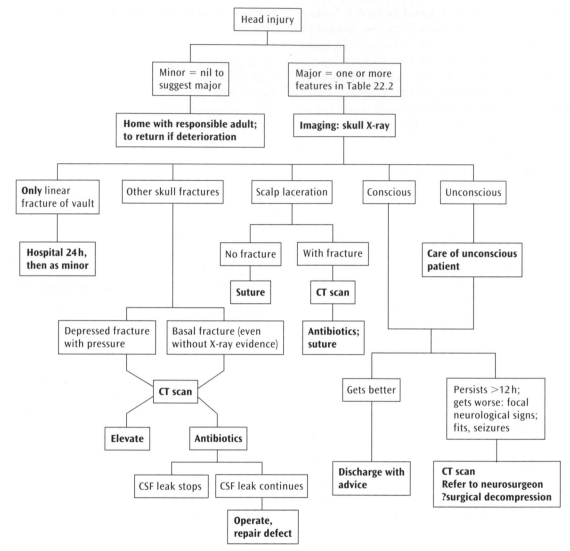

Algorithm 22.1

damage. The diagnosis is established by CT. This group of patients are treated expectantly. Mechanical ventilation may become necessary, especially if the blood gases are unsatisfactory. In those who are having epileptic fits or decerebrate spasms and in those who are not showing improvement in the level of consciousness after 24 hours, ventilation is desirable and should be instituted earlier if there are signs of respiratory complications. Ventilation may also be necessary in patients who have undergone surgery.

Ventilation, with sedation using propofol as the first-line agent, is indicated to control intra-cranial pressure (ICP), by reducing P_{CO_2} which, in turn, reduces cerebral blood flow. Light head-up tilt with the neck in the neutral position allows maximal venous drainage and a reduction in ICP. Hyperventilation to a therapeutic level of a P_{CO_2} between 4.0 and 4.5 kPa, causes cerebral vasoconstriction and diminished cerebral blood flow and has been employed to reduce ICP. By contrast, hypoventilation should be avoided as it reduces cerebral blood flow to critical levels and precipitates cerebral ischaemia. Furthermore, placement of a ventricular drain allows drainage of CSF to reduce ICP.

ICP is measured by making a small drill hole in the skull, just penetrating the dura, and inserting a ventricular catheter or a metal bolt filled with saline and connected to a transducer. Normal ICP is $<10\,$mmHg, and if $>30\,$mmHg, it requires treatment.

Each neurosurgical unit is likely to adopt its own policy for monitoring ICP and cerebral perfusion pressure (CPP) which is the difference between the mean systemic blood pressure and ICP.

Future brain protective agents include free radical scavengers (e.g., α-tocopherol), calcium channel blockers (e.g., nimodipine) and glutamate and aspartate antagonists (e.g., dizolcipine). It is important to prevent hyperglycaemia because it leads to high levels of lactate locally in ischaemic areas and this correlates with poor neurological outcome.

The supportive measures already described above when resuscitating these patients on admission would have been implemented. Furthermore, whilst in coma, patient care includes: suction to clear the airway, chest physiotherapy when not ventilated, oral hygiene, gelatin pads to protect the cornea, skin care at pressure points to avoid bed sores, enteral or parenteral feeding to maintain nutrition, bladder catheter or penile sheath to avoid wetness, regular laxatives or enema to prevent constipation.

The longer the period of unconsciousness, the less likelihood of recovery, especially in the elderly. Fixity of the pupils for more than 48 hours, decerebrate rigidity with paralysis of all four limbs or absence of any signs of improvement for more than 1 month are unfavourable indicators. Regular ICP recordings and CT scans may identify hydrocephalus, infection or a chronic sub-dural haematoma which must be considered as possible causes for failure of recovery.

Outcome of head injury

Mortality is related to the level of consciousness on admission which reflects the severity of the injury: the mortality for a GCS score of 15 is less than 1%, and for 8–12 it is 5%. Of those admitted in coma (GCS $<$ 8), 40% die, 30% fully recover, 20% have some residual disability but are semi-dependent, and the remaining 10% will be severely disabled requiring care, or in a persistent vegetative state.

HIGHLIGHTS

- Patients with skull fracture require admission as they are more likely to have an intra-cranial haematoma
- A CT scan is crucial in outlining the extent of injury and planning treatment
- Not all intra-cranial haematomas require evacuation and recovery after decompression is dependent on the extent of primary brain damage
- The main objectives in resuscitation are to avoid hypovolaemia and hypoxaemia in order to prevent secondary brain damage
- Complications of head injury: hydrocephalus, infection and chronic sub-dural haematoma may be responsible for delayed recovery

23

Burns; loss of skin cover

DA McGROUTHER

BURNS

AIMS

1 Learn first aid measures
2 Distinguish between major (life-threatening) and minor burns
3 Learn the overall management of burns

A burn is usually regarded as an inflammatory response of the skin and subcutaneous tissues to thermal injury due to exposure to heat, either *dry,* by direct contact with a hot object, or *moist,* caused by hot liquid or vapour. Other physical agents, including electric current in domestic or industrial accidents, radiation overdosage in radiotherapy or after accidents in nuclear power stations, and chemicals such as caustic alkalis and acids, produce similar damage. The distinguishing characteristic of a burn is the rapid destruction of an area of the superficial tissues (skin or mucous membrane) which initially is large compared to the depth to which the agent penetrates. However, burns due to an electric current may be small in area and do not show an area of demarcation but are always deep. Electrical energy is converted into heat and the severity of burning is proportional to the electrical resistance of the tissue through which the current is transmitted.

Management

Since the prognosis is influenced by the depth of the injury, urgent steps to limit the action of the agent are required. In the common burn due to heat, the first aid measure should be immersion of the part involved in cold water or cooling by other means as quickly as possible and without waiting for the area of the burn to become visible. In chemical burns, the substance should be thoroughly washed off the burned surface under tap water, and this is probably much more effective than a chemical antidote, such as a weak alkali for acid burns, especially if one has to wait for the antidote. Radiation burns do not become apparent until days after the exposure, and like thermal burns, show erythema and blistering of the skin which is left as it heals spontaneously, though slowly.

Criteria for admission to hospital

- *Partial thickness burns*: >15% of body surface in adults; >10% in children
- *Full thickness burns*: >2%
- Circumferential burns in the limbs
- Suspicion of inhalation of gas or smoke
- *Burn-sensitive areas*: hands, feet, face, eyes, perineum
- Electrical burns
- Radiation injury

Threats to life – systemic effects

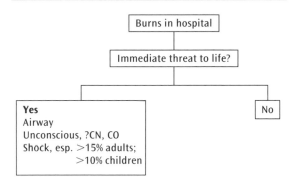

The burns may be associated with other forms of injury which constitute a threat to life. Inhalation of hot air, smoke and toxic gases may cause acute inflammatory oedema of the respiratory tract and acute anoxia, requiring intubation, or rarely, a tracheostomy. In addition, noxious agents may also cause pulmonary injury, resulting in pulmonary oedema, atelectasis and secondary pneumonias. Where inhalation injury is suspected, the patient is carefully examined for evidence of soot or skin burn around the mouth, nostrils and throat. Investigations include chest X-ray, estimation of blood gases and carbon monoxide, and flexible bronchoscopy. Poisoning by carbon monoxide or cyanide from burning of upholstery should be suspected in the unconscious patient.

Acute disturbance of the body fluids can follow burns. One of the functions of the skin is to limit the loss of water by evaporation from the surface, so there is an increased loss of water through the damaged area. In addition, beneath and around the area of

thermal injury there is a zone of cellular injury which results in inflammation, oedema, increased capillary permeability and the exudation of a fluid that is similar in composition to plasma. The loss into the tissues can be greater than in the damaged integument and depends primarily on the area of the burn, and to a lesser extent upon the depth of the burn. The rate of loss can be considerable, and oligaemic shock can develop rapidly. On presentation, the patient appears to be in good condition, but unless resuscitated immediately develops 'burn shock'.

It is therefore important to estimate the area of the burn with speed and reasonable accuracy. The 'rule of nines' (Fig. 23.1) is the usual method. The head and neck, each upper limb and – separately – the front half and the back half of each lower limb, each represent 9% of the total surface area, whereas the trunk represents $4 \times 9 = 36\%$. This estimate leaves 1% for the perineum and external genitalia. Any burn affecting as much as 15% of the surface area of an adult, or 10% of the surface area of an infant, is regarded as a major burn, and will require urgent intravenous resuscitation and other emergency procedures.

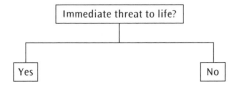

In a minor burn, it is usually sufficient to ensure that the patient increases oral intake of fluids above the normal and takes a nourishing diet. In major burns, the nature and quantity of replacement by the intravenous route can be worked out from first principles (Chapter 16). Most fluid is lost in the first 12 hours, but considerable losses continue for at least 36 hours. Several regimes consist of varying proportions of crystalloids (e.g., *Ringer lactate* or *Hartmann's solution*) and colloids (*human albumin solutions*). Various formulae have been designed to aid assessment and replacement of fluid losses, for example *Muir and Barclay's formula*, which estimates that the fluid loss in millilitres in each of the first three 4-hour periods immediately after the burn is, in an adult patient, half the product of the percentage surface

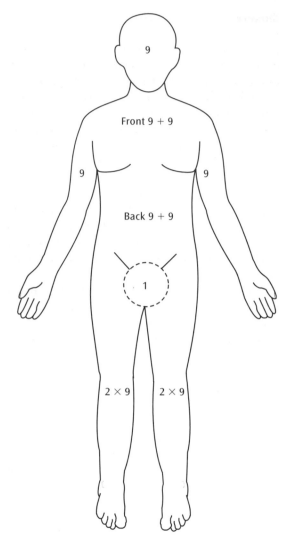

Fig. 23.1 *The 'rule of nines' helps the surgeon to estimate the percentage of body surface area burned.*

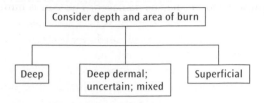

The problem of infection

The dead burned tissue is a medium for the growth of micro-organisms, and once infection has become established, superficial burns can become converted into full-thickness burns, skin grafts can be destroyed and systemic infection can be life-threatening, and the patient lives with the ever-present threat of septicaemia. Organisms of particular relevance are β-haemolytic streptococcus, *Pseudomonas aeruginosa* and the coagulase-positive staphylococcus. Inspections and culture swabs of the wounds, topical antimicrobial agents, prophylactic oral or systemic antibiotics or, when there is evidence of invasive infection, early surgical excision and skin grafting are general measures that are adopted to minimize the risk and promote healing.

Local management of the burn site

The depth of the burn is of crucial importance to the healing process and influences the line of management. In a *superficial dermal (partial thickness)* burn there is erythema with blanching on finger-pressure, and blistering, but the sensation is intact. Pin-prick is used to determine whether the nerve-endings have (*full-thickness*) or have not (*partial thickness*) been damaged. The dermal elements are spared and therefore healing is spontaneous without scarring. In a *deep dermal partial thickness* burn, if all sources of epithelium have been destroyed, the damage extends into the dermis. Such a burn has a whitish appearance which sloughs days later exposing new skin underneath. Healing from the deeper residual epithelial elements, the sweat and sebaceous glands and hair follicles, will take place but is slow and with scarring. Some form of skin grafting is therefore essential. A *full-thickness burn* involves the whole epidermis and dermis, and deeper structures such as

area of the burns and the body weight in kilograms. Thereafter, the same volume is administered in each of the next two 6-hour periods, and again in the following 12-hour period. However, clinicians should rely on standard clinical observations, that is, the state of hydration, pulse, blood pressure, urine output and haematocrit. The resuscitation challenge in the burned patient is very similar to that in other forms of hypovolaemic shock and requires the same approach.

muscle and fat may be damaged. The skin is numb, charred, hard and leathery with thrombosed skin vessels. Unless the area is small, excision and skin grafting are essential.

The main objective of local management is to encourage healing of the burn site by preventing infection and by excision of full-thickness burns and deep dermal burns followed by the application of a suitable skin graft. It may not be possible to determine the depth of the burn in the early stages, and many burns become deeper with time. A pin-prick test is not always reliable for determining burn depth.

After local cleansing, loose tissue and blisters are debrided, and the area of the burn is treated by exposure or dressings.

Exposure

This requires a clean environment, which may necessitate admission to a special bed in a burns unit. Exposure of the burn rapidly leads to the formation of a solid coagulum of dead tissue and exudate. Although the coagulum is not sterile, its dryness prevents too free a penetration of organisms into the deeper tissues. Burns of the face and the perineum are treated in this way. So are children and elderly patients, who may be restless and unco-operative about keeping dressings in place.

Dressings

These are applied to absorb wound exudate and lower bacterial contamination by their content of antiseptic or antibiotic agents, and act as a mechanical barrier to infection. The dressings commonly used are tulle gras impregnated with chlorhexidine or povidone-iodine and silver sulphadiazine cream (*Flamazine*). The dressing is then covered with a thick absorbent layer of gauze and wool. The outer layers can be changed as necessary when they get soaked with exudate. Burns of the hands and feet are treated by coating with silver sulphadiazine and placing the extremity in a plastic bag. Although the dressings provide some pain relief, burns are painful and suitable analgesia is necessary. Opiates will often be required, and in shocked patients are administered intravenously.

Surgery

Areas of full-thickness or deep partial-thickness burns are debrided as soon as possible, using a skin knife or dermatome and then a split-skin graft is applied.

The majority of burns consist of areas of both partial- and full-thickness injury (*mixed-thickness burns*) and are usually treated conservatively for 2–3 weeks, to allow the areas of superficial burns to re-epithelialize, whereas the deeper burns demarcate by forming a solid eschar. This policy minimizes the excision of potentially viable tissue. Where early excision has not been performed, spontaneous desloughing can be assisted enzymatically, for example with Varidase. The modern tendency seems to be towards early surgery in the form of *tangential excision* (Fig. 23.2) and skin grafting. Progressively larger tangential slices are cut from the region of the centre of the burn until tissue that will support a skin graft is reached. The advantages of this approach to conservative treatment are a reduced healing time and hospital stay and a better cosmetic result.

In the case of *deep circumferential burns* of a limb or digit or the thorax, the rigidity of the contracting eschar may constrict the tissues, reducing blood flow and respiratory movements. In such cases it is necessary to slit the eschar longitudinally down to bleeding tissues – a relatively painless procedure known as *escharotomy*.

Physiotherapy should be instituted immediately after the burn so that function is maintained and contractures are avoided, especially with burns across joints.

HIGHLIGHTS

- Identify inhalation burn and ensure adequate oxygenation
- Administer intravenous fluids, including sufficient colloid
- Early excision of deep burns and provision of skin cover prevents infection
- Escharotomy is an emergency measure to prevent limb ischaemia
- Physiotherapy prevents contractures

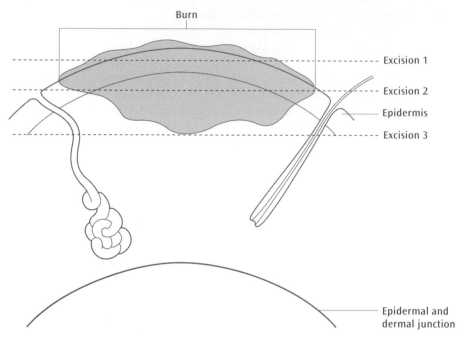

Fig. 23.2 *Layers are excised tangentially to remove coagulated tissue until the bleeding points are encountered throughout the area. In the diagram, healthy skin is not reached until the excision level 3, and this leaves intact the epidermal–dermal junction and the adnexel structures (hair follicles and sweat and sebaceous glands) which provide stem cells for re-epithelialization. If the burn extends deeper than the adnexal structures, a split-skin graft is applied.*

LOSS OF SKIN COVER

AIMS

---

1 Distinguish acute and chronic skin loss
2 Understand the importance of control of sepsis
3 Appreciate the importance of early skin cover
4 Know the principles of the various skin grafts and flaps and their indications

---

Acute skin loss is a common surgical challenge and can result from a broad spectrum of diseases, injuries and operations.

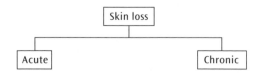

Causes of loss of skin

Acute

The most common cause of skin loss is traumatic loss, referred to as *primary* when due to the injury itself and *secondary* when surgical excision of damaged tissue (debridement) is necessary. Skin loss may be associated with wounds caused by sharp instruments, such as a knife, glass or tin can. Prominent anatomical parts are most vulnerable, such as fingertips, elbows, knees, nose and ears. *Blunt trauma* can also cause skin loss through avulsion of tissue, for example by machinery or crushing.

A frequent example of secondary traumatic loss is a compound leg fracture. Wounds will not heal if they contain foreign bodies or dead tissue because such materials promote infection. It is therefore necessary to remove foreign matter, and to excise

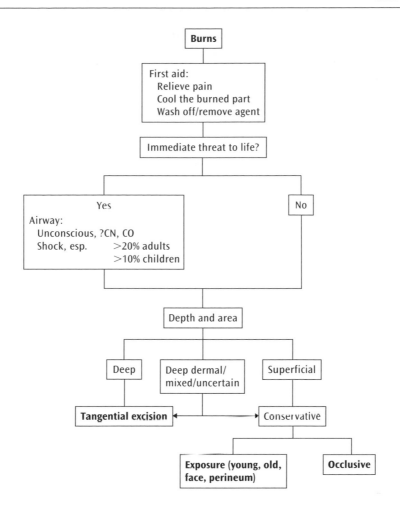

Algorithm 23.1

and replace crushed and devitalized tissue, including fragments of bone, dead muscle and skin.

Skin cover in trauma may be required to replace not only skin but also lost anatomical parts, such as an amputated digit or limb or a muscle compartment in a limb. Open wounds heal by granulation followed by contraction and epithelialization, but these are slow processes and may lead to considerable loss of function. Moreover, granulation tissue will not develop across bone, cartilage or tendon and therefore skin grafts will not take on these sites, making more complex types of wound cover appropriate.

Skin loss may result from *surgical excision*, required as part of debridement, or else as part of the elective treatment of benign or malignant skin tumours or in the radical resection of deeper malignancies as in breast cancer.

Skin can also be lost in *local infections*. β-haemolytic streptococci can cause *cellulitis* or the more severe *necrotizing fasciitis* with progressive skin necrosis and spread of the infection along fascial planes. Aggressive drainage and often extensive excision of infected skin and subcutaneous tissue are necessary to control infection; antibiotics are not effective without adequate drainage. Spreading infection with skin loss also occurs in ischaemic tissue, such as a gangrenous limb or the rare anaerobic infection of the scrotum, *Fournier's synergistic gangrene*.

Generalized infections can also result in skin loss. Meningococcal septicaemia causes infarctions of skin resulting in deep punched-out ulcers, and the associated *diffuse intravascular coagulation* (DIC) can cause gangrene of fingers, feet and the nose.

Burns have already been considered.

Chronic

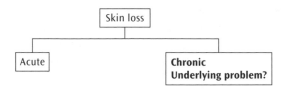

Loss of skin in chronic wounds can be due to arterial or *venous insufficiency*, *pressure sores*, *infections* or many other causes. The main therapeutic focus should be the management of the underlying problem, but it may be necessary to replace skin cover as part of the management.

Management

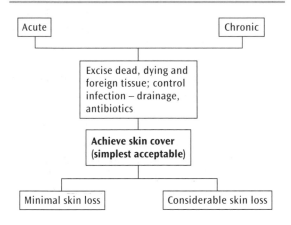

Objectives of skin cover

- Encourage wound healing, achieving complete epithelialization of the raw surface.
- Provide functional cover with sensation and mechanical durability as similar to the original skin cover as possible.
- Produce the best possible appearance (*cosmesis*).
- Leave minimal scarring or functional loss at the donor site.

Priorities

These depend upon the *patient*, the *pathology* and the *site*. The dominant patient factor is *age*; for the older patient, simplicity and safety of the surgical technique are the foremost considerations, whereas for the younger patient the best possible restoration of function is important. This is also likely to result in the best appearance. *Pathology* is also important. A surgeon may choose to apply a thin skin graft after excision of a tumour in order to watch for recurrence, or a thick flap may be used in order to allow radiotherapy. In resurfacing a specialized *site*, such as the sole of the foot, it is desirable to reconstruct like with like and a flap from the other foot may be chosen.

Techniques of skin replacement – the ladder of reconstruction

The ladder extends from simple to more complex techniques. The principle is to use the simplest technique that fulfils the aims in that patient. The more complex the technique, the higher the risk of failure. The surgeon must always have a plan in reserve, in case the first treatment fails.

Simple wound closure

It may be possible to close the wound directly where there has been minimal skin loss. Wounds must not be closed under undue tension. Primary closure is used for surgical incisions and clean wounds caused by trauma. Delayed primary closure is used for a contaminated wound after debridement and dressings until the wound is clean.

Split skin grafting

A sheet of the superficial layers of the epidermis is harvested by a guarded (*Watson* or *Cobbett*) knife to allow cutting to a pre-determined fixed thickness so that only part of the dermis is removed. An electric dermatome is more accurate. The residual donor site, usually the arm or thigh, will heal spontaneously. A split-skin graft must only be applied on sites that produce granulations, therefore inappropriate sites are bone, cartilage, tendon and cavities. The sheets of graft can be *meshed* (passed through a machine which makes multiple parallel cuts so that the sheet can be opened out like a string vest) to increase the area covered. This technique is employed to provide large areas of autograft for covering large wounds, such as burns, or contaminated wounds, for example chronic ulcers, or muscle which tends to produce serous fluid causing grafts to separate. Allograft skin from donors can be used as temporary cover in a patient unfit for anaesthetic.

Full thickness skin grafting

This provides usually small pieces of skin from sites such as the post-auricular for resurfacing small facial defects or the naso-labial fold for application to the nose. Large areas of full-thickness skin will take on a healthy bed, such as well-vascularized fascia. A common example is the replacement of de-gloved skin which should be completely detached, cleaned of subcutaneous tissue and re-applied as a full-thickness skin graft. Curiously, the graft is more likely to survive when completely detached than if there is a persistent venous attachment because congestion ensues. The defect at the donor site requires closure by suturing. A full-thickness graft is less likely to contract than a split-skin graft, and because it is taken close to the recipient site it has the same colour and texture; however, because it is thicker it takes longer to 'take'.

Skin flaps

Where more than skin is required a flap is used. This may be defined as a transfer of tissue which retains a blood supply during transfer, whereas a graft is totally detached and is revascularized by the angiogenesis of the wound healing process. The simplest flap is a local (*random pattern*) flap which is tissue transferred from the margins of the defect by cutting in one of a number of patterns. Such flaps are classified as *advancement, rotation, transposition* and *island* varieties. Because the blood supply is not defined, the flap should not be large and its length should not exceed its width. These flaps are used in the head and neck.

Complex skin flaps

More complex flaps consist of a piece of skin or other tissue, elevated with the artery and vein supplying the area of the flap. Many types are available, all having in common the artery and vein:

- The *axial pattern* skin flap has skin and subcutaneous fat and the appropriate artery and vein, which run along the long axis of the flap. Thus, a large flap with a high length-to-width ratio can be safely fashioned. Examples are the groin flap, forehead and deltopectoral flaps.
- A *muscle* can be raised as the basis for the flap, and transferred with a split-skin graft to provide epithelialization, or the muscle can be transferred with its overlying skin as a musculocutaneous flap. An example is the *latissimus dorsi/pectoralis major/transversus rectus abdominis muscle* (TRAM) *musculocutaneous flap* widely used for breast, head and neck, or trunk reconstructions.
- A *sheet of fascia* is raised with its blood supply, with or without overlying skin. The radial artery (*Chinese*) flap contains the radial artery elevated in the flap, the ulnar artery being adequate to perfuse the arm.
- The *elevated flap* (*axial, muscle, musculocutaneous* or *fasciocutaneous*) may be completely detached by isolating and ligating the artery and vein, allowing transfer of the tissue to another part of the body where the vessels are anastomosed to appropriate local vessels using the techniques of microvascular anastomosis. This type of flap, the free tissue transfer or 'free flap', is a rapidly evolving area of surgery.

For examples of grafts and flaps, *see* Figs 23.3 and 23.4.

Aftercare of grafts and flaps

Split-skin grafts

Split-skin grafts are applied to the wound bed with pressure, in order to *immobilize* the graft and minimize collection of fluid, thereby facilitating revascularization. To assist with this immobilization of

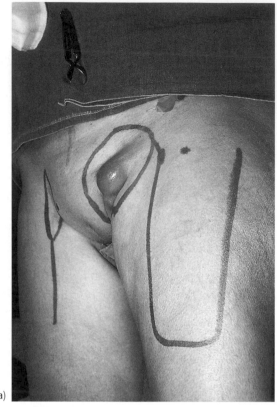
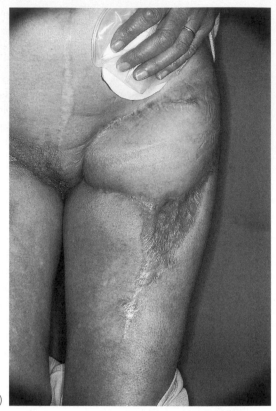

(a)　　　　　　　　　　　　　　　　　　　(b)

Fig. 23.3 *(a) Metastatic malignant melanoma in left groin nodes. A tensor fascia lata musculocutaneous flap is marked out for transposition; (b) The flap has been transposed medially after radical lymph node dissection. The flap donor site has been partly closed and partly skin-grafted. The patient, incidentally, had a colostomy.*

the graft–wound interface, it may be necessary to immobilize the part involved or even the whole patient, especially in children and restless unco-operative patients.

The wound is inspected at 5–7 days unless there is suspicion of infection, such as discharge or increase in pain. If vascularization is satisfactory, the ideal management at that stage is to expose the area at the earliest possible time, although some mechanical protection may be deemed appropriate until healing is complete.

The *donor site* is dressed at 10–14 days.

Full-thickness skin grafts

The principles of *immobilization* and *avoidance of early inspection* are the same as for grafts, except that

the first inspection should not be carried out until 10 days. The donor site has usually been closed by primary suture, and care does not differ from that of any surgical incision.

Flaps

Flaps are vulnerable to deficiencies of circulation, whether arterial or venous. The usual causes are kinking and tension, leading to thrombosis. Therefore, the circulation in the flap must be observable and monitored, so dressings must be as small as possible. The first 48–72 hours are critical. A useful routine is to prepare a chart for the nursing staff to record the colour and temperature of the flap hourly, and to alert the medical staff at the first sign of insufficiency.

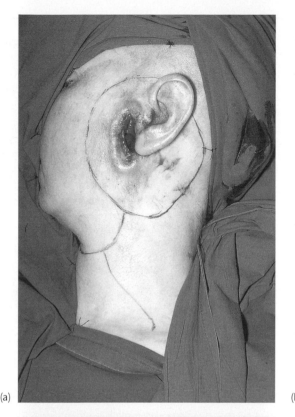

(a)

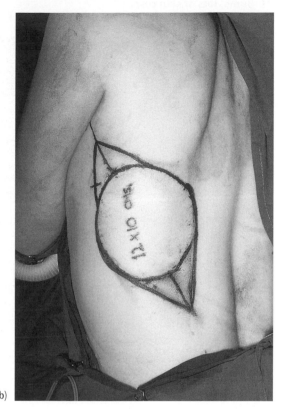

(b)

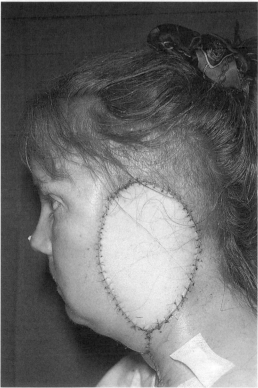

(c)

Fig. 23.4 *(a) A maligant parotid tumour has ulcerated in the pre-auricular area. This was treated by radical parotidectomy and facial nerve grafting; (b) A latissimus dorsi musculocutaneous flap is marked out; (c) The muscle has been transferred as a free microvascular flap. The latissimus dorsi vessels have been anastomosed to vessels in the neck.*

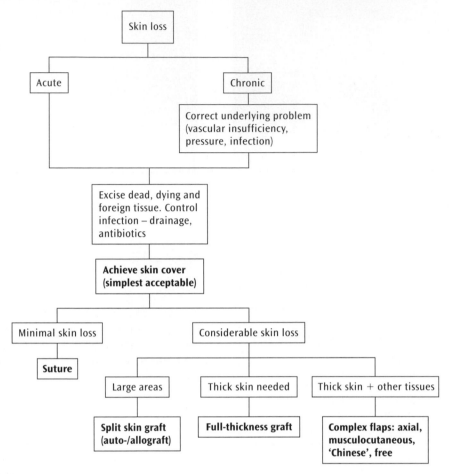

Algorithm 23.2

After this period, care becomes that of an ordinary surgical wound. The stitches are not removed until the tenth day.

HIGHLIGHTS

- Acute skin loss requires adequate cleansing (**debridement**) and early skin cover
- Chronic skin loss requires identification and treatment of the underlying disease
- The simplest technique that will restore function and appearance should be used
- In grafts or flaps, the crucial importance of minimizing scarring at the donor site must be remembered
- The surgeon must always have a reserve plan in case of failure of wound healing

24

Intensive care

MERVYN SINGER

AIMS

1 Recognition of a sick patient
2 Principles of basic resuscitation
3 Criteria for referral to intensive or high dependency care
4 Description of intensive care unit (ICU) monitoring and therapeutic techniques

INTRODUCTION

Although the intensive care unit (ICU) is a highly specialized, high-technology area, the general principles of patient management are similar to those that can and should be employed in the casualty department, operating theatre, ward, the 'field' and the community. The major distinction between intensive care and other locations is the higher intensity of monitoring, organ support technology and nursing available. The physiological, biochemical and anatomical derangements afflicting the critically ill patient are identical to any other patient, although usually magnified and often multiple. However, patients will often reveal features of critical illness before being admitted to the ICU. The onus is on clinicians to recognize these features at an early stage, and to act

promptly and effectively in terms of life-saving or organ-sparing therapies or procedures. Where necessary, this includes referral to senior colleagues or transfer to the ICU. The *intensivist* is also available for advice or assistance on the ward and utilization of this resource is encouraged.

This chapter covers identification of the sick patient, when referral to the ICU is appropriate, the facilities and techniques that are offered, and the philosophy behind patient management on the ICU, dealing both with specific organ systems and general support issues, such as nutrition, infection control and skin care. Current thinking into mechanisms underlying the pathophysiology of systemic inflammation, including sepsis, are discussed and, finally, the chapter alludes to new ideas and therapeutic approaches.

IDENTIFYING A SICK PATIENT

What is a sick patient? First impressions are both useful and important. They guide both the speed of thought and the rapidity of therapeutic intervention. They should propel the clinician towards determining priorities quickly, of which life-saving manoeuvres obviously assume first claims. Unfortunately, and not infrequently, these priorities are not clear-cut, often to the detriment of the patient. A shocked patient need not necessarily be hypotensive to have significant organ hypoperfusion.

Causes of shock are:

- *Hypovolaemic*: e.g. haemorrhage, severe diarrhoea.
- *Cardiogenic*: e.g. extensive myocardial infarction.
- *Inflammatory*: e.g. sepsis.
- *Obstructive*: massive pulmonary embolus, pericardial tamponade.
- *Anaphylactoid*: e.g. adverse drug reaction, bee sting.
- *Neurogenic*: following spinal cord injury.

First impressions

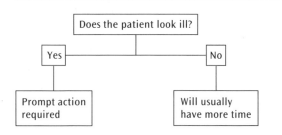

On first sight, does the patient look ill? This is determined by some essential observations:

- The patient's level of consciousness, whether the patient is *compos mentis*, comfortable, agitated, in pain or obtunded, immobile or active, showing a glint in the eye or a dull, disinterested torpor.
- Is the patient centrally cyanosed? Is breathing adequate, poor or absent?
- Whether the breathing involves great, laboured efforts or shallow, distressed respirations.
- Whether the patient exhibits signs of an inadequate circulation manifested by depressed or disordered conscious level, peripheral shut-down and/or cyanosis, a weak/absent pulse and/or blood pressure.
- The presence of any obvious deformities or evidence of external blood loss.
- Whether the patient is excessively hot or cold.

Initial resuscitation – 'ABC'

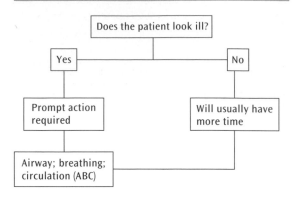

Positive answers to any of the above first worrying impressions should prompt the taking of a rapid yet concise history whilst instituting initial ABC management, namely, securing and protecting the *Airway*, if necessary by endotracheal intubation or, rarely, by cricothyroidotomy; ensuring *Breathing* and gas exchange are adequate by administration of high-flow, high concentration of oxygen with drugs (e.g., β_2 agonists) as required, or mechanical ventilatory support (e.g., positive pressure ventilation); and restoring the *Circulation* to provide adequate organ perfusion with insertion of adequately sized venous cannulae, administration of fluid and/or vasoactive drugs, and institution of mechanical support, for example mechanical ventilation, aortic balloon counter-pulsation.

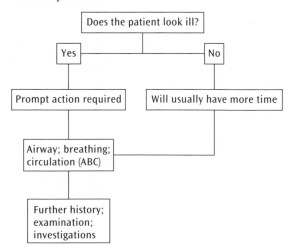

Once the airway, breathing and circulation are secure, or at least any abnormalities present are being corrected actively, then a full examination, detailed history and appropriate investigations should be performed to elicit causative factors, any relevant past medical history and coincident pathological findings.

Further signs of critical illness

The body's homeostatic mechanisms compensate for cardiorespiratory or metabolic derangements so that any deficiency may not be readily apparent – and may be at risk of being missed or ignored – until the process is fairly advanced. For example, 30–40% of circulating blood volume needs to be lost in a young, healthy person before the blood pressure falls. Indeed, the blood pressure often rises initially due to compensatory vasoconstriction. Postural hypotension, where blood pressure falls by 10–15 mmHg or more on sitting upright, is an earlier sign of hypovolaemia compared with supine pressure measurement alone. Similarly, the central venous pressure may also be maintained in the face of progressive hypovolaemia by compensatory vasoconstriction and will only fall when this reflex fails.

Early symptoms and signs of cardiovascular or respiratory distress are:

- *Thirst*: a symptom of hypovolaemia.
- *Postural hypotension*: indicative of early hypovolaemia.
- *Tachycardia*: should not be ascribed simply to pain or anxiety but suggests increased sympathetic activation.
- *Tachypnoea*: may be indicative of a respiratory pathology but may also be the clinical manifestation of the body's attempt to compensate for a metabolic acidosis by hyperventilating.
- *Urine output*: increasing oliguria is usually suggestive of renal hypoperfusion and/or hypovolaemia. In the latter, the kidney attempts to compensate by increasing re-absorption of filtered salt and water. As diuretics mask this useful sign in the short term, these drugs should only be considered when the intra-vascular volume compartment is repleted.
- *Tissue turgor*: an unreliable sign of hypovolaemia as it primarily reflects contraction of the extra-cellular space rather than a reduction in intra-vascular volume.

The severity of the illness is better determined by a few blood tests:

- *Metabolic (lactic) acidosis*: a rapidly increasing arterial blood base deficit is a good marker of increasingly *severe organ hypoperfusion* (e.g., severe hypovolaemic or cardiogenic shock) or *tissue necrosis* (e.g., infarcted bowel). This rapid rise in base deficit occurs in the absence of acid ingestion, for example aspirin overdose. A metabolic acidosis secondary to acute renal failure or diabetic ketoacidosis takes several days to develop. The change in base deficit is used as an indicator of the efficacy of the treatment.
- *PaO$_2$*: as a rough guide, the arterial oxygen tension measured in kPa should be approximately 10 less than the inspired oxygen concentration (FiO$_2$). Thus, 60% oxygen should produce a PaO$_2$ of 50 kPa in a patient with a normal cardiorespiratory system. This should be used as a reference point rather than removing the oxygen mask to measure the PaO$_2$ in air, thereby possibly making the patient hypoxaemic in the process! The PaO$_2$:FiO$_2$ ratio may also be used as an index of the degree of abnormality of gas exchange; ratio values falling below 40 kPa have been defined as indicative of acute lung injury.
- *PaCO$_2$*: a value within the normal range, or a rising level, in the face of an increasing metabolic acidosis and/or hypoxaemia suggests respiratory muscle fatigue and is an indication that mechanical ventilatory support may shortly be needed.
- *A low or falling platelet count (in the absence of bleeding)*: suggestive of an acute ongoing systemic inflammatory process.

Arterial base deficit

- -2 to $+2$ mmol/l: normal
- -2 to -5 mmol/l: cause for concern
- -5 to -10 mmol/l: worrying
- > -10 mmol/l: extremely worrying

WHEN DOES A PATIENT NEED INTENSIVE CARE?

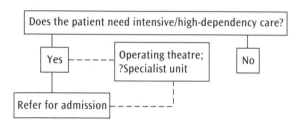

Indications for transfer of a patient to intensive care include the following:

- *An airway requiring protection by an endotracheal tube,* that is, there is concern that the patient is at risk of aspirating gastric contents (depressed gag reflex) or is so deeply comatose that passive changes in head and neck posture will obstruct the airway. Patients undergoing tracheostomy should also be managed post-operatively in an ICU unless trained staff are available in the general ward.
- *Patients who are at risk of losing their gag reflex,* for example patients with severe alcohol withdrawal receiving large doses of sedation, such as chlormethiazole or similar agent, or following head injury. At the very least, such patients should be monitored and nursed on a high dependency unit.
- *Requirement for mechanical ventilation.* This may be 'invasive', that is, requiring endotracheal intubation, or 'non-invasive' by tight-fitting face or nasal mask (e.g., for continuous positive pressure ventilation, CPAP).
- *Haemodynamic instability,* requiring use of inotropic or pressor drugs or large volumes of fluid. A coronary care or high dependency unit may be suitable provided there is the monitoring necessary to manage such patients. If an illness is severe enough to warrant powerful vasoactive drugs then monitoring of stroke volume and cardiac output is mandated as blind treatment may well be deleterious.
- *Multiple organ dysfunction,* if homeostasis is compromised, management should be optimized at *an early stage* using a more sophisticated and intensive level of monitoring and equipment, and a higher nursing input.

- *Severe metabolic abnormalities,* including diabetic crises, renal failure, hepatic failure, hypo- or hypernatraemia and hyperkalaemia, etc.
- *Severe thermoregulatory abnormalities,* for example hyperpyrexia, hypothermia.
- *Neurological instability,* for example recurrent seizures, raised intra-cranial pressure.

Many patients fitting the above categories could equally well be managed in a properly equipped and staffed high dependency unit. However, this facility is not yet widely available, the monitoring capability and medical or nursing expertise vary considerably, and no hard and fast, validated admission criteria exist. Nevertheless, patients suitable for a high dependency unit encompass a requirement for nursing and monitoring over and above that available on a general ward, although mechanical ventilation would normally be considered inappropriate.

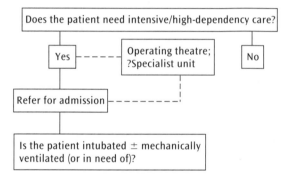

Indications for mechanical ventilation

- Respiratory muscle fatigue and inability to maintain adequate gas exchange resulting in hypoxaemia and/or hypercapnia. Causes include lung parenchymal, respiratory muscle and cardiac disorders.
- Ongoing depression of ventilatory drive or respiratory muscle paralysis (e.g., following sedative drug overdose, post-operatively).
- Neuroprotection to lower raised intra-cranial pressure.

Note: patients can be intubated to protect their airway but remain breathing spontaneously with no mechanical ventilatory support.

MONITORING TECHNOLOGY

Many devices used in the ICU are invasive and thus carry a risk of complications, both as a consequence of insertion of catheters into veins, arteries or the heart, and by virtue of being indwelling, often for long periods. Bleeding, damage to viscera, infection and arrhythmias are common complications of such invasive procedures. This is the reason for concentrating resources and expertise in a specialized area. Despite many of these procedures being commonplace, the risk:benefit ratio has to be carefully weighed for each device. Adequate medical and nursing expertise are therefore essential prerequisites.

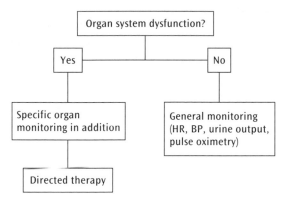

Haemodynamic

'Routine' cardiovascular monitoring in an ICU patient consists of heart rate, ECG (usually lead II), arterial blood pressure, central venous pressure and urine output. Systemic blood pressure can be monitored by a sphygmomanometer but, for accuracy and continuous measurement, it is more usual to use an electronic pressure transducer connected to a small intra-arterial cannula placed in a radial artery or occasionally in other sites, including femoral, dorsalis pedis and ulnar arteries. An added advantage of arterial cannulation is the facility to draw frequent blood samples for biochemical analysis without repeated arterial punctures.

Central venous pressure (CVP) is measured with a catheter usually inserted via a jugular or subclavian vein and advanced so that the catheter tip is located at the junction of the vena cava and the right atrium. The CVP is thus a measure of right atrial pressure and an indirect measure of right ventricular end-diastolic pressure. As for arterial pressure, the central venous catheter is connected to a pressure transducer for continuous monitoring. Many central venous catheters now incorporate multiple lumens (up to four) to enable continuous pressure monitoring and administration of drug infusions.

The pulmonary artery (*Swan–Ganz*) balloon flotation catheter (PAC) is a specialized type of intravascular catheter which, with the aid of an inflated balloon sited near the catheter tip, is 'floated' through the right side of the heart so its tip lies in a main branch of the pulmonary artery. The catheter is slowly advanced to the point where the inflated balloon occludes forward blood flow; the pressure measured at the tip by an external pressure transducer and displayed on a bedside monitor loses its characteristic pulmonary artery pattern and becomes flattened. This represents the pressure ahead of the catheter which is assumed to be in continuity with left atrial and left ventricular end-diastolic pressure and is known as the *pulmonary artery wedge* (or *occlusion*) *pressure*. The inflated balloon in this position represents an iatrogenic pulmonary embolus so it should be deflated after 10 seconds in order to regain the pulmonary arterial waveform trace and allow normal flow. For this safety reason, the pulmonary artery pressure waveform should be monitored continually.

PAC can also be used to measure cardiac output by the thermodilution method. A bolus of 5% glucose is injected through a lumen which emerges 30 cm proximal to the tip; a thermistor at the tip measures the change in blood temperature during the passage of the bolus which is used by an online computer to calculate the cardiac output.

Blood drawn from the distal lumen of the catheter which opens in the pulmonary artery allows measurement of the mixed venous oxygen saturation (SvO_2). Normal values are 70–75%; a fall in SvO_2 indicates increased extraction of oxygen by the body tissues in an attempt to compensate for a decreased supply, for example in acute heart failure. A modified pulmonary artery catheter with a fibre-optic probe can measure SvO_2 continuously. Other catheter modifications enable semi-continuous cardiac output estimations and measurement of right ventricular ejection fraction and volumes.

Because of the invasiveness of the PAC and the subsequent risk of complications, other less invasive cardiac output techniques have been developed, including Doppler ultrasound measurement of aortic blood flow, either from a supra-sternal or oesophageal approach, and thoracic bioimpedance which uses an array of electrodes placed on the neck and trunk. The former, in particular, also provides considerable information on left ventricular contractility, pre-load and after-load.

Cardiac output determines oxygen supply. The tissue oxygen delivery is the product of cardiac output and arterial oxygen content ($=$ Hb $\times$ arterial oxygen saturation $\times$ 1.34 $\times$ 10) where 1.34 ml O_2 is carried by 1 g of Hb. However, this does not indicate whether the supply is adequate for the body's needs. Methods of assessing supply adequacy include:

- *Urine output*: as a measure of renal perfusion.
- *Arterial blood gas analysis*: the base deficit is an index of metabolic acid production in excess of the body's capability to clear it. An acute rise is usually due to inadequate tissue perfusion or necrosis resulting in anaerobic metabolism and production of lactic and other acids. In sepsis the causation is more complex and controversial.
- *Arterial lactate*: bedside devices are now available to measure hyperlactacidaemia directly. However, a rise in lactate levels is not specific to excess lactic acid production.

Newer techniques for assessing regional perfusion are being developed, for example *tonometric* measurement of gastric intra-mucosal pH, and tissue PO_2 measured at various sites, but these have yet to attain widespread, routine use.

Respiratory

Pulse oximetry is a ubiquitous tool in the ICU; it provides a painless and continuous estimation of arterial oxygen saturation from a finger or ear pulse and an early warning of arterial desaturation. However, the operator should be aware of potential pitfalls, such as undetected concurrent carboxy-haemoglobinaemia or a misleading result, where peripheral perfusion is poor.

In addition to the metabolic assessment described above, arterial blood gas analysis also provides useful information on arterial oxygen and carbon dioxide tensions. This indicates both the need for, and facilitates management of, inspired oxygen requirements and mechanical ventilation, and assists in the weaning process.

Integral to the ventilator are a variety of monitors which measure, for example, tidal volume, peak inspiratory airways pressure and FiO_2. Other respiratory monitoring devices are available, for example, capnography to measure end-tidal expired PCO_2 and plethysmography to measure flow-volume loops.

Neurological

In neurosurgical ICUs in particular, intra-cranial pressure monitoring via an intra-parenchymal fibre-optic probe or, less commonly, an extra-dural bolt is a relatively routine procedure. It is a useful tool for the detection and management of raised intra-cranial pressure, although the expertise needed to insert these devices precludes most non-specialist units from using them.

Trans-cranial Doppler ultrasonography can measure middle cerebral artery blood flow and provide an indication of either a dilated or constricted cerebral circulation. *Jugular venous bulb oxygen saturation* using a catheter similar to the PAC inserted in a rostral direction from the jugular vein offers similar information to SvO_2 monitoring but is specific for venous drainage from the brain; this provides an indication of the supply–demand relationship of cerebral perfusion. *Continuous electroencephalographic* (EEG) *monitoring* is particularly applicable to patients having prolonged or repeated seizures requiring mechanical ventilation, sedation and/or neuromuscular paralysis.

PRINCIPLES OF MANAGEMENT

Circulatory management

Circulatory management entails attention to both pressure and flow. As mentioned previously, an adequate pressure does not imply a sufficient blood flow. Some low pressure states are associated with hyperdynamic circulation, for example sepsis, but others with low flow, for example cardiogenic shock and hypovolaemia. If any concern exists that flow may be inadequate, as evidenced by organ dysfunction and an increasing metabolic acidosis, early consideration should be given to measurement of cardiac output.

Treatment is guided both by the underlying condition being treated and the findings revealed by monitoring and investigations, for example echocardiography. An arrhythmia will require appropriate pharmacological intervention or, if haemodynamically compromised, cardioversion. Pericardial tamponade will require percutaneous drainage (*pericardiocentesis*), whereas a massive pulmonary embolus may require anticoagulation, and/or thrombolysis or embolectomy. Fluid overload generally occurs in the presence of renal failure and merits vasodilatation, diuresis or renal replacement therapy (e.g., haemofiltration, haemodialysis). Heart failure will generally respond to vasodilator therapy and/or inotropes. It is sound practice to utilize cardiac output monitoring if inotropes are being commenced. Diuretics are generally not indicated in acute heart failure unless the patient also has intra-vascular fluid overload, a rare combination in clinical practice. Indeed, such a patient is usually hypovolaemic on presentation due to sweating, vomiting and fluid redistribution, for example, into the lungs causing pulmonary oedema.

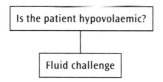

The most common condition requiring haemodynamic manipulation, particularly in the surgical patient, is *hypovolaemia*. This can be due to haemorrhage, inadequate input, excess fluid loss (e.g., diarrhoea, burns) or compartmental redistribution, as seen in sepsis or ileus. *Treatment* includes correction of the precipitating factor in addition to intra-vascular volume repletion. The choice of fluid depends on what is being lost. Blood transfusion will be needed to replace significant blood loss, whereas either colloids or crystalloids are given for salt losses. Standard practice in Europe is to use colloid for rapid intra-vascular volume repletion while crystalloids such as n-saline and 5% glucose are reserved for background fluid replacement. The choice of colloid is controversial; 4.5% albumin is expensive, carries a potential risk of disease transmission and has a relatively short intra-vascular half-life compared to synthetic colloids such as hetastarch (e.g., Hespan, Elohes) or the gelatins (e.g., Gelofusin, Haemaccel).

Deciding how much volume a hypovolaemic patient requires can be difficult, particularly with underlying cardiac disease. This is compounded by the body's own compensatory mechanisms. For example, hypovolaemia will induce sympathetically mediated vasoconstriction; at first, this will maintain (or even elevate) arterial, central venous and pulmonary artery wedge pressures. Only after a certain degree of severity is reached will this reflex be lost, with rapid onset hypotension. Identifying hypovolaemia thus requires adequate monitoring. Fig. 24.1 shows appropriate utilization of the CVP using the 'fluid challenge' principle whereby 200 ml colloid is given rapidly over 5–10 minutes followed by a 5–10-minute equilibration period. The change between baseline CVP and that taken after the equilibration period gives an indication of the position on the pressure–volume curve. No change in CVP is seen in hypovolaemia, whereas additional fluid given to an over-filled circulation will result in a rise in CVP $\geq 3\,mmHg$.

There are pitfalls when using CVP measurements, particularly in cases of ventricular dysynchrony where the left and right hearts may not be working in tandem, for example pulmonary hypertension or isolated left heart failure. In these situations a direct measurement of flow is useful to create a Starling-type curve (Fig. 24.2).

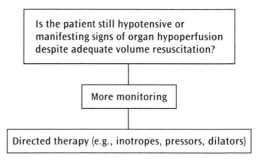

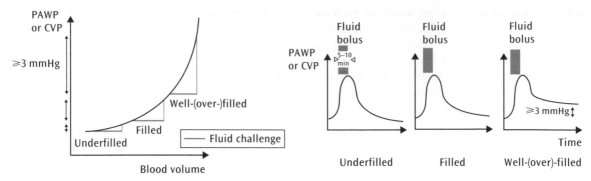

Fig. 24.1 *The fluid challenge. The left-hand panel shows the importance of position on the ventricular end-diastolic pressure (CVP) – blood volume curve; viz. a fluid challenge when underfilled produces little effect on pressure, whereas the same volume given to a well-filled circulation produces a much larger rise in ventricular end-diastolic pressure. The right-hand panel demonstrates how this can be assessed clinically; no rise in central venous (or pulmonary artery wedge) pressure following a fluid challenge is suggestive of underfilling, whereas a rise in pressure ⩾3 mmHg suggests a well-(or over-)filled circulation.*

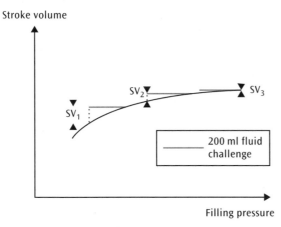

Fig. 24.2 *Starling-type curve for stroke volume optimization. A volume challenge to an underfilled circulation produces a rise in stroke volume; however, the same volume given to a well-(or over-)filled circulation produces no further increase.*

After volume resuscitation, circulatory status may still remain inadequate so pharmacological intervention is required. Knowledge of both pressure and flow is useful to tailor drug therapy appropriately and titrate dosages accurately for optimal effect. As a general rule, drugs with predominant inotropic action (to increase myocardial contractility), such as adrenaline and dobutamine, are useful for low output with or without low pressure states, whereas vasopressors, such as noradrenaline, are used to treat hypotension, usually in the presence of a high cardiac output, vasodilated system. Alternatively, a vasoconstricted circulation will respond to a vasodilating agent (e.g., glyceryl trinitrate, isosorbide dinitrate). Occasionally, drugs are necessary to lower an elevated blood pressure; examples include nitrates, β-blockers and ACE inhibitors.

Failing a prompt and adequate response to fluid optimization and pharmacological interventions, mechanical support devices can be considered. These are particularly pertinent for low output states.

Mechanical circulatory support devices include:

- The *mechanical ventilator* not only improves gas exchange but also rests the heart by removing the work of breathing and reduces ventricular preload through its effects on intra-thoracic pressure.
- The *intra-aortic balloon pump* can be inserted into the descending thoracic aorta via the femoral artery. It inflates in diastole and deflates during systole, thereby augmenting coronary perfusion and reducing left ventricular after-load.
- Specialized cardiac centres may utilize ventricular assist devices.

Respiratory management

The airway must be secured and protected. This is usually achieved by an endotracheal tube placed orally or, occasionally, inserted nasally or via a tracheostomy. A cuff near the tip of the tube is inflated to prevent both air leaks and liquid or solid matter trickling down past the tube into the lungs. This is pertinent in the intubated patient who, at least in the first instance, will usually require sedation and thus often loses the cough reflex.

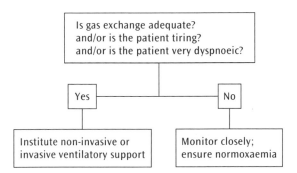

Most critically ill patients will require oxygen in concentrations up to 100%. This can be delivered by face or nasal mask to the patient breathing spontaneously, or via the ventilator. The therapeutic endpoint for additional oxygen administration is to maintain satisfactory arterial oxygen saturations, usually ≥90–95%. Occasionally, lower values may have to be tolerated to reduce the risk of iatrogenic trauma induced by mechanical ventilation.

Augmented breathing can be non-invasive or invasive. Non-invasive techniques include:

- *CPAP (continuous positive airways pressure)*: which consists of the patient breathing a high flow air-oxygen mix via a tight-fitting face (or nasal) mask which is connected to an expiratory valve set to a known pressure, for example 5 cmH$_2$O. CPAP has various benefits such as preventing the lungs from collapsing down to atmospheric pressure at the end of expiration thereby 'splinting' the alveoli open and improving gas exchange.
- *Inspiratory pressure support*: devices including the BromptonPac and the Bird ventilator used by physiotherapists augment the tidal volume of spontaneous breaths to a set pressure. This is particularly useful in the tiring patient.
- *BiPAP*: a combination of CPAP and inspiratory pressure support delivering both inspiratory and/or expiratory support.

Invasive techniques usually involve positive pressure ventilation given by a mechanical ventilator. For volume-controlled ventilation (VCV) a tidal volume is delivered regardless of the inspiratory pressure generated by the ventilator (unless upper pressure cut-off limits are set). For pressure-controlled ventilation (PCV) the ventilator delivers a tidal volume until a pre-set pressure is reached. This limits excessively high pressures from being generated. However, depending on lung compliance (stiffness) and patient position, marked changes in tidal volume may occur.

Basic principles of setting a ventilator

- The tidal volume (for VCV) or pressure (for PCV) is set to deliver a tidal volume around 6–10 ml/kg bodyweight.
- The respiratory rate is set to deliver 12–20 breaths/minute.
- The inspired oxygen concentration is adjusted to produce a satisfactory level of arterial oxygen saturation.
- The PEEP setting is adjusted to deliver 5–10 cmH$_2$O of positive end-expiratory pressure (analogous to CPAP for spontaneous breathing).
- The ratio of inspiratory time to expiratory time (I:E ratio) is usually set at a ratio of 1:2, although this may be longer (e.g., 1:3) when ventilating a patient with bronchospasm and delayed expiration, or shortened ('reversed'), to 1:1 or 2:1 when attempting to deliver larger tidal volumes at lower peak pressures.
- After a period of equilibration (10–15 minutes), an arterial blood sample is taken for blood gas analysis and the ventilator is then adjusted accordingly.

Non-respiratory methods of ventilatory support are occasionally utilized in patients with severe respiratory dysfunction. These are similar to those used in cardiopulmonary bypass; blood is circulated through an extra-corporeal circuit, passing through a membrane where CO$_2$ is removed and O$_2$ added, before being returned to the patient. Unfortunately, this approach has a high complication rate, is limited to specialized centres, and outcome benefits have

protective isolation and aseptic insertion of catheters and drains.

Nutrition is another vital area concerning the critically ill patient. Malnutrition has clearly demonstrable negative effects on the immune response, protein synthesis and muscle breakdown. Prevention of gut villous atrophy and stress ulcer-related bleeding has been demonstrated with enteral nutrition. Ideally, nutrition should be given by the enteral route. This is usually delivered via a (preferably small-bore) nasogastric tube. An oro-gastric tube is inserted if there is a basal skull fracture. Occasionally, the stomach has to be bypassed for reasons of persisting ileus or outlet obstruction. Naso-duodenal or naso-jejunal tube insertion or percutaneous jejunostomy are alternative approaches in this instance.

Reasons for enteral nutrition failure are usually due to either large naso-gastric aspirates, abdominal distension and/or diarrhoea. The latter is rarely due to the feed alone and other causes, for example antibiotics, *Clostridium difficile* infection, should be considered. In the case of large aspirates, various gut motility agents, such as metoclopramide or erythromycin, may be tried. Failure of, or contraindication to, enteral nutrition demands parenteral feeding. This has less direct protective effect on the gut, carries a risk of infection as well as other complications arising from catheter insertion, and is less physiological. Nevertheless, parenteral nutrition is better than no nutrition.

A further aspect to consider is pharmacology. Owing to the large number of drugs and infusions employed, the risk of drug interaction(s) is high, as are side-effects. These may be relatively trivial, for example skin rash, or more serious, such as bone marrow suppression, jaundice or renal failure. Often, co-incident renal and/or hepatic dysfunction will result in altered clearances of the drugs and their metabolites and thus prolonged actions or toxic plasma levels. Compatibility with other drugs in solution and the dilution volumes used are also relevant. It is therefore important to consider a drug complication as a cause of any unexpected development and to monitor blood levels closely (e.g., aminoglycosides, warfarin, aminophylline). The input of an interested and informed pharmacist is invaluable.

Finally, the psychological component should be considered. Intensive care is a stressful environment for aware patients as well as their relatives and friends. Agitation and acute confusional states are frequent accompaniments of critical illness and are also commonly seen on withdrawing agents used for sedation, in particular benzodiazepines. Day–night sleep patterns are often disrupted. Patients so affected may experience frightening hallucinations and nightmares and, in the recovery phase, often become depressed when they begin to appreciate the extent of their illness and become aware of any weakness and incapacity that may persist. Communication, emotional support, encouragement and reassurance are crucial aspects of care, both for patients and their families.

SPECIFIC CONDITIONS

Systemic inflammation/sepsis

Many critically ill patients develop organ dysfunction as a consequence of an exaggerated systemic inflammatory response to the exogenous insult. Whilst infection is the most common insult, many other precipitating factors are recognized, such as severe trauma, major haemorrhage, burns, pancreatitis, smoke inhalation, drug overdose, myocardial infarction, post-surgical procedure, etc. The systemic inflammatory response is manifest clinically as tachycardia, tachypnoea, a raised or lowered body temperature and neutrophilia or neutropenia. In the presence of infection, this is termed *sepsis*.

Definitions

Infection. Microbial phenomenon characterized by an inflammatory response to the presence of microorganisms or the invasion of normally sterile host tissue by those organisms.

Bacteraemia. The presence of viable bacteria in the blood.

Systemic inflammatory response syndrome (SIRS). Two or more of: temperature $> 38°C$ or $< 36°C$; heart rate > 90 bpm; respiratory rate > 20 breaths/minute or $PaCO_2 < 32$ mmHg (4.3 kPa); WBC $> 12,000$ cells/mm^3, < 4000/mm^3 or $> 10\%$ immature forms.

Sepsis. The systemic response to infection. Definition as for SIRS but a result of infection.

Severe sepsis. Sepsis associated with organ dysfunction, hypoperfusion or hypotension. These may include, but are not limited to, lactic acidosis, oliguria or an acute alteration in mental status.

Septic shock. Sepsis with hypotension, despite adequate fluid resuscitation, plus presence of perfusion abnormalities.

The exact pathophysiology underlying SIRS and sepsis has yet to be determined. However, current thinking has the macrophage in a pivotal role, releasing cytokines (e.g., tumor necrosis factor, interleukin-1) which are potent stimulators of other inflammatory systems within the body, for example neutrophils and platelets, endothelium, and the coagulation, contact and fibrinolytic systems. Activation of these cells and systems results in: *release of inflammatory mediators* which produce either vasodilatation or vasoconstriction; *increased capillary permeability*; *plugging of vessels* by aggregated white cells and platelets and *free oxygen radicals and proteases* which result in local tissue damage and fibrosis. Concomitant tissue hypoxia seems to have an additive effect on the degree of the inflammatory response. A response of sufficient severity can result in organ dysfunction or failure which may be single or multiple. There also appear to be intra-cellular abnormalities, for example affecting glycolysis and mitochondrial function, though these have yet to be fully characterized.

Multiple organ dysfunction or failure

Definitions

Multi-organ dysfunction syndrome (MODS). The presence of altered organ function in an acutely ill patient so that homeostasis cannot be maintained without intervention.

Organ dysfunction can result as a consequence of: *inadequate organ perfusion*, for example after cardiogenic shock or major haemorrhage; from *systemic inflammation*, as described above; *direct damage*, for example chest trauma; and as a *complication of therapy*, in particular adverse drug reactions. In a general ICU patient population, the first two are

far more frequent, although in a trauma centre there will be an increased proportion of patients suffering direct organ injury.

Management revolves around *treatment of the underlying cause*, including removal or drainage of pus or necrotic tissue and *organ support*, maintaining biochemical and physiological levels compatible with survival until the patient recovers independent organ function.

Acute respiratory distress syndrome (ARDS)

The acute respiratory distress syndrome (ARDS) is the respiratory component of multiple organ failure arising from systemic inflammation. This abnormality may be the predominant feature of the illness with all other organs functioning relatively normally. It can be caused by direct lung injury or be secondary to distant injury such as infection, trauma or pancreatitis. Histology reveals aggregation and activation of neutrophils and platelets, patchy endothelial and alveolar disruption, interstitial oedema and fibrosis. The acute phase is characterized by increased capillary permeability and the fibroproliferative phase (after 7 days) by a predominant fibrotic reaction. A recent US–European Consensus Conference provided definitions for both ARDS and a milder form of injury termed 'acute lung injury' (*see below*).

Definitions

Acute lung injury (ALI). $PaO_2/FiO_2 \leq 300\,mmHg$ (40 kPa): regardless of level of PEEP; with bilateral infiltrates on chest X-ray; with pulmonary artery wedge pressure $<18\,mmHg$.

Adult respiratory distress syndrome (ARDS). As above but $PaO_2/FiO_2 \leq 200\,mmHg$ (26.7 kPa).

Prognosis depends in part on the underlying insult, the presence of other organ dysfunctions and the age and chronic health of the patient. Predominant single-organ ARDS carries a mortality of 30–50%, although there does appear to have been some improvement over the last few years. Those surviving ARDS often have few (if any) long-term sequelae. Some deterioration in the lung function

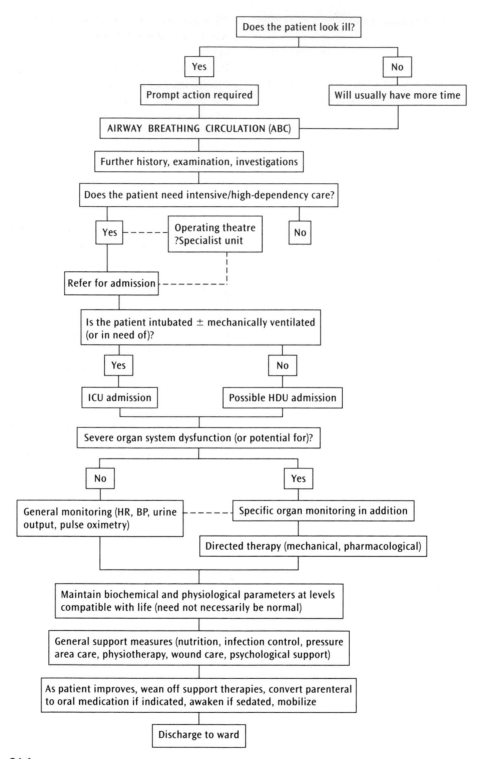

Algorithm 24.1

test is usually detectable but this rarely affects their quality of life.

NEW DIRECTIONS

Intensive care is a rapidly evolving field, both in the understanding of pathophysiological mechanisms and in new therapies, techniques and monitoring devices. This is particularly evident in the area of immunotherapy where a large amount of effort and research is being expended to modulate the inflammatory response to an exogenous insult. Drugs have been developed to block the insult (e.g., endotoxin), to block mediators (e.g., anti-TNF antibody) or to modulate effector cell response (e.g., nitric oxide synthase inhibition). Unfortunately, although trends towards outcome improvement have been found, no single product has yet to show a statistically significant benefit. Deficiencies in trial design, including identification of an appropriate patient group and the timing of treatment, are major contributory factors to these disappointing results. Whether a single agent, or a 'cocktail therapy' of several agents, will prove effective is also open to conjecture.

New modes of ventilatory support are being investigated. These include *surfactant therapy* in adults (this has been shown to be highly effective in neonatal respiratory distress syndrome); *inhaled nitric oxide* which, in some patients, will lower pulmonary hypertension and improve gas exchange by its local vasodilating action; and *'liquid ventilation'* whereby the lungs are actually filled with a perflurocarbon which reduces viscosity, provides surfactant-like properties and improves gas exchange. Devices such as *high frequency oscillation* using an external cuirass are also being studied.

Finally, monitoring technology is also being developed to provide better means of assessing regional perfusion, to measure cardiac output non-invasively, and to measure plasma levels of inflammatory mediators and endotoxin at the bedside.

HIGHLIGHTS

- The sick patient must be promptly recognized and treated
- Hypoxaemia and hypovolaemia are commonplace
- The intensive care unit offers high levels of nursing, monitoring and sophisticated support technology and is a resource to be utilized sooner rather than later

The acute abdomen

PAUL B BOULOS

INTRODUCTION

The *acute abdomen* is the term used to describe conditions that present with a short onset of one or more of the symptoms of abdominal pain, vomiting and diarrhoea, and are life-threatening. The morbidity results from disturbances of the body fluids and sepsis.

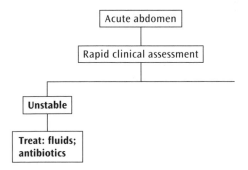

Rational management requires precise diagnosis of the cause, but the threat to life demands that resuscitation is vigorously pursued as the first priority. There are three main types of disturbance of body fluids: blood loss, plasma loss and saline (extracellular fluid) loss. They are distinguished by a brief history and examination. Large volumes of vomiting or diarrhoea produce *saline lack*; generalized peritonitis, strangulation obstruction or septicaemia produce *plasma loss* and a rapid onset of shock indicates *blood loss*. Thus, hypovolaemia is a dominant and abrupt feature in a bleeding viscus, such as a dissecting or ruptured aortic aneurysm, but is progressive in obstruction due to fluid sequestration in dilated intestines and loss by vomiting; or in peritonitis as a result of plasma exudate from the peritoneum combined with splanchnic and systemic vasodilatation by endotoxins. Pyrexia and tachycardia with leucocytosis are indicative of visceral or peritoneal inflammation but are absent in obstruction or in vascular causes unless complicated by perforation of viscus. Clinical evidence of septicaemia should lead to early treatment with antibiotics, even before a diagnosis of the cause has been made. Opiates should be withheld in order not to dampen the symptoms and signs down until the diagnosis is made. Specific treatments are considered in more detail elsewhere.

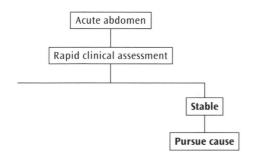

The diagnosis of the cause is simplified by considering: *site* of the pain; *aetiological mechanisms* which determine the *nature of the pain* and *local signs*.

SITE OF PAIN

This is either visceral or parietal. The visceral peritoneum clothing the viscera is poorly supplied with nerves, and *visceral pain* arising therefrom is vague and ill-localized until the pathological process extends to the parietal peritoneum lining the abdominal wall, which is supplied by somatic nerves. *Parietal pain* gives an indication as to the likely organ involved according to its anatomical location within the defined sectors of the abdomen. However, pain may be referred from extra-abdominal sites (*see later*).

Upper abdominal pain may arise from the stomach, duodenum, liver, gall bladder, pancreas and, rarely, the spleen, although the pain may be specifically localized to the region where an individual viscus lies. The kidneys cause pain in the flanks that may radiate to the hypochondria, and should also be considered.

Central abdominal and *para-umbilical pain* usually arise from the small bowel and the aorta.

Lower abdominal pain in the hypogastrium usually arises from the colon or the bladder. In the *right iliac fossa* pain commonly arises from the appendix and the ileo-caecal region. In the *left iliac fossa* pain is usually from the sigmoid colon. The ureter on either side and in females the uterus and either appendage also cause pain in the lower abdomen. However, the pain, as in the upper abdomen is often not confined to a single region but can be diffuse throughout the lower abdomen.

Parietal pain that is from the outset, or has become, generalized throughout the abdomen indicates diffuse irritation of the parietal peritoneum, that is, *generalized peritonitis*. Such patients always present in an unstable condition.

AETIOLOGICAL MECHANISMS

The causes are best categorized according to pathological processes affecting the viscera that present characteristic features and aid in diagnosis and these are:

- *Trauma*: either penetrating or blunt.
- *Inflammation*: as in peptic ulcer, cholecystitis, appendicitis, diverticulitis, salpingitis.
- *Perforation*: which when not due to injury, is a complication of inflammation or ischaemia.
- *Obstruction*: of a luminal viscus includes the biliary tree, the intestines and the ureters.
- *Vascular*: namely aortic dissection or rupture, strangulation and mesenteric thromboembolism.

NATURE OF THE PAIN

This is *intermittent* or *continuous* and with some exceptions helps to differentiate obstruction from inflammation, ischaemia or infarction of a viscus.

Intermittent pain is characteristic of the pain produced by obstruction of a hollow viscus and is probably related to vigorous peristaltic activity in the muscular wall of the viscus proximal to the blockage. It comes in waves when the patient is doubled up and is interspersed with periods of complete remission. This is the pain described as *colic*. However, there are pitfalls in interpretation. In *large bowel obstruction,* a brief and transient colicky pain is followed with continuous pain due to stretching of the seromuscular wall of the colon by rapid gaseous distension. The pain of *obstruction of the biliary tree* is continuous rather than intermittent in the majority of cases, although it is still usually referred to as *biliary colic*. The pain of *obstruction to a ureter* is only intermittent in about half the cases – *renal pain–ureteric colic*.

Constant pain without any period of complete relief is due to inflammation or ischaemia or infarction. It is localized to the area where the involved viscus lies, and is initially vague until the nearby peritoneum is involved. Although continuous, the intensity of the pain may vary in time.

LOCAL SIGNS

Local signs are related to irritation of the peritoneum. The patient is able to point at the *site of the pain* and if this proves to be the site of localized tenderness it is almost certainly the site of diseased viscus. Pain felt when the patient coughs provides further evidence.

Abdominal tenderness is due to parietal irritation or intestinal dilatation as a result of mechanical obstruction or paralytic ileus. Tenderness is elicited by palpation with the forearm horizontal and the hand flat, and pressure is exerted with the pulps, not the tips, of the fingers by flexing the wrist and metacarpo-phalangeal joints.

Guarding is an *involuntary* reflex contraction of the abdominal muscles to palpation and must be carefully distinguished from *voluntary* guarding due to fear, resentment to examination, exposure of the naked abdomen to the cold atmosphere or cold hands, by eliminating these factors during the examination.

Deep palpation followed by a sudden release of the pressure by withdrawal of the palpating hand allows the abdominal musculature to spring back with its underlying peritoneum which when inflamed causes the patient to wince or even cry out in pain (*rebound tenderness* or *Blumberg's sign*). Rebound tenderness does not add more information to that produced by guarding and is very uncomfortable for the patient.

Rigidity is an exaggeration of guarding when the abdominal muscles are contracted all the time, and the abdomen feels hard from the instant the examiner lightly palpates and before deep palpation is exerted.

Percussion delineates any area of dullness due to an inflammatory mass when present from surrounding resonance due to associated gaseous distension as a result of mechanical obstruction or paralytic ileus, and should be carried out gently as it may evoke rebound tenderness.

Auscultation is particularly informative: in mechanical intestinal obstruction the bowel sounds are high-pitched and frequent, whereas in the presence of intra-abdominal sepsis, infarction or ischaemia, the bowel sounds are infrequent or absent because of diminished peristalsis with occasional tinkling sounds due to movement of fluid within dilated loops. Paralytic ileus is a protective mechanism that prevents the spread of intra-peritoneal infection.

ASSESSMENT OF 'ACUTE ABDOMEN'

Although most patients with abdominal symptoms and signs have an intra-abdominal condition, it is a safe policy to rule out the possibility of extra-abdominal causes. This is achieved by obtaining a good history and full examination.

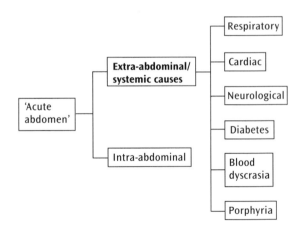

Extra-abdominal causes

Pneumonia and pleurisy, especially at the lung base, give rise to abdominal pain and in the right side can be confused with acute cholecystitis, acute appendicitis or acute pyelonephritis. An increased respiratory rate, pain preventing deep inspiration, a pleural rub or altered breath sounds are suggestive, and a chest X-ray is helpful.

Cardiac ischaemia is characterized by retro-sternal pain radiating as a constricting band across the chest, upwards to the jaw and along the arms, particularly the left arm. However, occasionally it is atypical, is localized in the epigastric region and does not radiate. It should be considered in high-risk patients, that is, smokers and patients with hypertension or a strong family history. An ECG and cardiac enzymes would be necessary.

Pre-herpetic pain of the lower thoracic nerves is localized over the area of innervation. It is associated with marked hyperaesthesia. There are no abdominal symptoms or signs. The herpetic eruption may not appear until 48 hours later. It should be considered in elderly and in immunocompromised patients.

Spinal diseases can be associated with acute abdominal pain. This includes Pott's disease of the spine, secondary carcinomatous deposits, osteoporosis and myelomatosis. The pain is due to compression of the nerve roots and is precipitated by movement. In doubtful cases X-rays or MRI of the spine are the definitive investigations.

Diabetic ketosis can cause severe abdominal pain and vomiting (the *'diabetic abdomen'*). The urine should be tested for sugar in every abdominal emergency.

Blood dyscrasias due to haemophilia or the use of anticoagulants can cause bleeding into the root of the mesentery, the parietes and the retro-peritoneal tissues. The coagulation screen should establish the diagnosis. Anaphylactoid purpuras (e.g., *Henoch–Schönlein*), especially with a recent history of sore throat, measles or smallpox in children and adolescents, cause abdominal colic and melaena because of bleeding into the gut. The platelet count and the bleeding and coagulation times are usually normal. Therefore, the diagnosis may present great difficulty if purpura of the skin or mucous membrane is not present.

Porphyria crisis is characterized by intestinal colic and constipation and can be precipitated by barbiturates. The urine is usually orange in colour and changes to dark red on standing for some hours. The diagnosis should be suspected when intestinal colic is associated with mental or neurological symptoms.

Intra-abdominal causes

A patient with a penetrating or blunt injury usually presents as an emergency and receives instant treatment, as described elsewhere (Chapter 20). However, enquiry should always be made about a history of trauma as a trivial injury that has passed unnoticed or disregarded can be the cause of delayed acute abdominal pain. A rupture of a sub-capsular splenic or liver haematoma should be suspected, especially if the patient shows signs of hypovolaemia. A sub-clinical perforation of the intestine may also present late with peritonitis. A diaphragmatic hernia may not become prominent until some time after the accident. The patient may not complain of any specific symptoms. A CT scan displays the viscera, defines any visceral damage or inflammatory areas and demonstrates free fluid and gas if there is bowel perforation or bleeding into the peritoneal cavity.

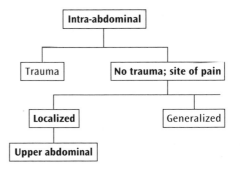

In the absence of history of trauma the patient should be able to describe whether the pain is localized or generalized. Localized pain provides an indication as to the source and associated manifestations aid in determining the underlying condition.

UPPER ABDOMINAL PAIN

Whilst demarcating the upper abdomen into its three zones, the epigastrium, right hypochondrium and left hypochondrium, is the theoretical approach for identifying the source of the pain, it is not always applicable as pain and tenderness often spread across the upper abdomen. This is not surprising as upper abdominal organs may occupy more than one sector. Therefore, although specific conditions are particular to a site, all have to be considered irrespective of site and one relies on other features to distinguish between them.

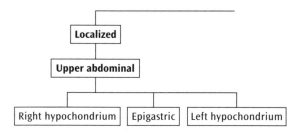

The primary objective is to differentiate between gastroduodenal and pancreatico-hepato-biliary disease. The clinical presentation for individual conditions can be classical but there is usually a marked overlap in symptomatic presentation and physical signs. Jaundice is a leading sign of hepatic or pancreatico-biliary disease. Although diseases of the liver and biliary system are the usual causes of pain in the right hypochondrium, unless the patient is jaundiced or has urinary symptoms the distinction from renal pain–ureteric colic can be difficult.

Management

This starts with non-invasive investigations. The white cell count is non-specific, although the absence of leucocytosis rules out an acute inflammatory or ischaemic process. Estimation of serum amylase is essential in every patient with abdominal pain, as it is with rare exceptions diagnostic of pancreatitis. Deranged liver function tests and bilirubinuria are

suggestive of pancreatico-biliary or hepatic disease. An ultrasound scan is routine. It detects free gas or fluid in the peritoneal cavity and outlines the viscera, in particular defining any abnormality in the liver, biliary system or the pancreas, although it may be normal in hepatitis despite abnormal liver function tests. A chest X-ray demonstrates gas under the diaphragm when perforation of a viscus is suspected. An abdominal X-ray shows the gaseous distribution in the bowel, the presence of a urinary calculus and rarely gallstones.

EPIGASTRIC PAIN

The common specific conditions are gastritis, peptic ulcer, perforated peptic ulcer and acute pancreatitis.

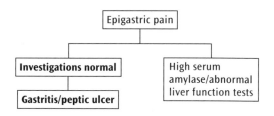

Erosive gastritis and *peptic ulcer disease* are associated with acid hypersecretion, altered composition of mucus and *Helicobacter pylori* infection. These conditions share a common presentation of a history of heartburn, epigastric pain, hunger pain relieved by food and antacids, vomiting, ingestion of aspirin or other non-steroidal anti-inflammatory agents and excessive smoking and alcohol consumption. The patient is apyrexial although the pulse is increased. There is tenderness, guarding and sometimes rigidity, mainly in the epigastrium.

The same history with a sudden and severe onset of localized pain and tenderness with rigidity in the epigastrium suggests a sealed perforated peptic ulcer. The diagnosis is particularly likely if, in the absence of systemic and local signs of peritonitis, there is gas under the diaphragm on a chest X-ray or the ultrasound examination demonstrates free fluid in the para-duodenal area or in the sub-hepatic space with no abnormality in the other viscera.

Management

Erosive gastritis and peptic ulcer disease are suspected on the basis of the clinical picture and normal (or marginally raised) blood count, liver function tests and ultrasound scan. The diagnosis is confirmed by the findings at endoscopy of erosive gastritis or peptic ulcer, and by antral mucosal biopsies subjected to a Campylobacter-like organism (CLO) test which detects the enzyme urease produced by *H. pylori*.

Various regimens of treatment to reduce gastric acid secretion and eliminate *H. pylori* are available, for example a 7-day course of omeprazole 20 mg twice daily, clarithromycin 500 mg twice daily, amoxycillin 1 g twice daily.

When a perforated peptic ulcer is suspected the patient is treated with naso-gastric aspiration, intravenous infusion and antibiotics as well as intravenous H$_2$ antagonists or proton pump inhibitors. Conservative treatment is continued if there is improvement. When there is doubt about the diagnosis it is safer to obtain a water-soluble contrast meal to demonstrate a leak of contrast from the site of the perforation before embarking on an unnecessary laparotomy, although laparoscopy if available is a useful diagnostic and therapeutic modality. After recovery from the acute episode, the diagnosis of peptic ulcer disease is established by endoscopy that is deferred for a few weeks to avoid converting a sealed to an open perforation. Triple therapy is either commenced before endoscopy, or later after the diagnosis is confirmed, since 50% of perforations show associated *H. pylori* infection.

A large perforation usually produces sudden and severe abdominal pain when the patient is pale, anxious, and loath to move, with signs of peritonitis (*see later*), initially as result of chemical irritation when the patient is apyrexial until followed hours later by bacterial peritonitis. Operation as soon as the general condition permits is usually the best course. A duodenal perforation is closed with interrupted sutures reinforced with an omental patch. This treatment is also sufficient in patients with long history suggestive of chronic duodenal ulcer disease as with the advent of triple therapy to eradicate *H. pylori* infection definitive treatment by vagotomy and pyloroplasty or other gastric acid-reducing operations is unnecessary.

A gastric perforation is treated similarly after the ulcer is excised for histological examination to rule out malignancy, although when the perforation is large partial gastrectomy may be required.

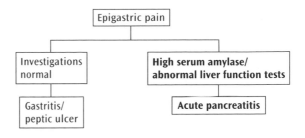

Acute pancreatitis

Acute pancreatitis is an inflammatory condition as a result of autodigestion of the gland by its own enzymes. This is triggered by reflux of duodenal contents into the pancreatic duct caused by a gallstone in the bile duct splinting the sphincter or by protein plugs forming within the pancreatic ducts secondary to altered metabolism of the acinar cells due to high alcohol intake.

Mild to moderate pancreatitis is the usual presentation in the vast majority of cases. It presents with epigastric pain that is constant and severe, radiates to the back and is associated with nausea and vomiting. The diagnosis is suggested by a history of alcoholism, dyspepsia suggestive of gallstones or previous attacks of biliary pain which in 95% of patients are the aetiological factors. The physical signs include pyrexia with tachycardia, upper abdominal tenderness and guarding and diminished or absent bowel sounds. Jaundice may be present due to oedema of the head of the pancreas or a stone in the bile duct.

In severe pancreatitis the picture is more profound. The pancreas undergoes necrosis that extends to the peri-pancreatic tissues. The patient complains of severe abdominal pain that can be diffuse, and is collapsed with a low blood pressure and low urine output, as a result of reduction in plasma volume due to inflammatory exudation into the peritoneal and pleural cavities. There is often evidence of respiratory embarrassment due to complex pulmonary

Table 25.1 *Ranson criteria for grading severity of acute pancreatitis*

Age over 55 years (non-gallstone pancreatitis) or
   70 years (gallstone pancreatitis)
Leucocyte count $> 16 \times 10^9/l$
Haematocrit increase by $> 10\%$
Blood glucose > 10 mmol/l (non-diabetic patient)
Serum LDH > 350 iu/l
SGOT > 250 iu/l
Blood urea > 1.8 mmol/l
Serum calcium < 2.0 mmol/l
Arterial $PaO_2 < 8$ kPa or 60 mmHg

insufficiency. The abdomen shows signs of peritonitis, and in some patients yellowish-brown staining of the flank develops due to tracking of the blood-stained peritoneal exudate through the lumbar triangle (*Grey–Turner sign*).

The severity of pancreatitis is determined by the above features if present and by biochemical changes included in Ranson's criteria (Table 25.1).

A serum amylase level above 100 units confirms the diagnosis, although hyperamylasaemia can occur following gastroduodenal perforation or intestinal ischaemia but does not usually reach such levels. Other laboratory investigations required are a blood count, liver function tests, serum calcium, urea and electrolytes, blood glucose and arterial gases as these are essential parameters employed to measure the severity of the disease and are of prognostic value (*see* Table 25.1).

An ultrasound examination demonstrates pancreatic oedema and stones in the gall bladder or bile duct. Frequently, however, because of gaseous distension the pancreas is not clearly outlined; after a few days any damage in the pancreas is better defined by CT scan. In mild and moderate pancreatitis the pancreas is swollen and oedematous and when severe the pancreas is necrotic. A plain abdominal X-ray is only necessary when in doubt to exclude a perforated peptic ulcer but may show appearances that have been described with acute pancreatitis which include: a sentinel loop of dilated jejunum adjacent to the pancreas due to ileus, distension of the duodenum with an air-fluid level or distension of the transverse colon with collapse of the descending colon – the colon 'cut off' sign.

Management

The patient is maintained on intravenous fluids, restricting oral intake and keeping the stomach empty by naso-gastric aspiration 'to rest the pancreas', analgesia is provided with opiates and the temperature, pulse, blood pressure and urine output are monitored. There is no evidence that antibiotics are of any benefit. Attempts to reduce pancreatic secretion with anticholinergics, glucagon or somatostatin, or to inhibit the pancreatic enzymes with aprotinin (antiprotease) and fresh frozen plasma (as a combined protease inhibitor and volume replacement) have also shown no benefit. In gallstone-associated pancreatitis, endoscopic sphincterotomy is indicated if resolution of an acute attack is slow, otherwise it is deferred until full recovery.

The patient's progress is determined from the improvement in symptoms, in clinical signs and in biochemical indices. A contrast-enhanced CT scan is obtained within a week from onset and is repeated until there are signs of radiological resolution and pancreatic necrosis has been excluded.

A patient may either show complete recovery or deterioration due to progressive pancreatitis and its complications. Patients with severe pancreatitis require resuscitation with intravenous colloids and blood, oxygen therapy if hypoxic and mechanical ventilation if adult respiratory distress syndrome develops, and dialysis if renal function deteriorates. Nutrition is maintained by the parenteral route, although the enteral route is safe via a feeding tube placed distal to the pancreas beyond the duodeno-jejunal flexure in order not to stimulate pancreatic secretion. These patients are treated in the intensive care unit because they are unstable and require monitoring of the cardiovascular, respiratory and renal parameters.

The local complications of acute pancreatitis are necrosis, infection and pseudocysts, and should be suspected if recovery is slow, and the temperature, the white cell count and serum amylase remain raised. A repeated contrast-enhanced CT scan is an important investigation in these patients.

Pancreatic and *peri-pancreatic* necrosis are associated with severe pancreatitis, and if the patient is asymptomatic the necrosis will gradually be reabsorbed, but in up to 40% of patients the necrotic material becomes infected and a pancreatic abscess may develop by the third week from onset of symptoms, when the main features are pain, jaundice and pyrexia.

The role of antibiotics in preventing infected pancreatic necrosis is unclear but antibiotics that penetrate pancreatic tissue and achieve therapeutic levels in pancreatic juice should be selected and these are imipenem, meropenem, ceftazidime, ciprofloxacin, clindamycin and metronidazole.

Percutaneous drainage of an abscess may be sufficient but an open debridement of the necrotic material (*necrosectomy*) is required because of progressive local complications and increased risk of systemic failure.

A *pseudocyst* is a collection of fluid in the lesser sac or other tissue spaces around the pancreas within a wall of fibrous and granulation tissue that may follow pancreatitis or liquefaction of a necrotic area. A pseudocyst should be distinguished from a peri-pancreatic fluid collection that resolves spontaneously. The presence of a cystic fluid collection more than 3 weeks after onset of pancreatitis is diagnostic of pseudocyst. A pseudocyst if symptomatic because of pain or due to obstruction to the gastric outlet or the bile duct is best drained by endoscopic cysto-gastrostomy, placing a stent across the posterior wall of the stomach and the wall of the cyst, than percutaneously as the risk of infection is far less; alternatively, it may be drained by open cysto-gastrostomy or cystojejunostomy.

After successful management, it is crucial that patients with alcohol-associated pancreatitis should abstain from alcohol completely. Those with gallstones are advised to undergo early cholecystectomy during the same admission, in order to avoid the risk of recurrent attacks of pancreatitis. The concern that early operation might expose the patient to greater risk with more difficult dissection as a consequence of peri-pancreatic inflammation is unfounded, particularly in those with mild attacks who can be operated on at any stage of their admission. However, the patient who is recovering from a severe attack should be allowed to settle completely before elective early surgery is undertaken prior to discharge from hospital. Laparoscopic surgery provides minimal access to assess the extent of inflammatory adhesions with the option to delay cholecystectomy rather than embark on a difficult and hazardous dissection in these patients.

If neither of the above causes proves to be responsible, CT scan and endoscopic retrograde cholangio-pancreatography (ERCP) or magnetic resonance cholangio-pancreatography (MRCP) being normal, other aetiological causes should be considered and investigated. They include: hyperlipaedemia; hypercalcaemia; medications, for example azathioprine and 6-mercaptopurine; corticosteroids; viral infections, such as mumps, Coxsackie virus, hepatitis A, B and C; and cytomegalovirus in patients with AIDS. In 10% of patients no definite cause can be identified (*idiopathic*), although some probably have microlithiasis.

PAIN IN THE RIGHT HYPOCHONDRIUM

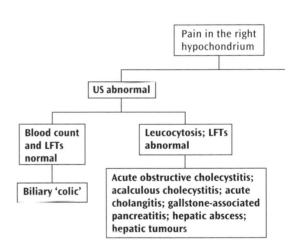

Acute 'biliary colic' is caused by a stone temporarily blocking the cystic duct or Hartmann's pouch or the common bile duct. It presents with a severe attack of continuous pain in the right hypochondrium which radiates round the costal margin to the scapular region and may last several hours. The pain is accompanied by nausea and vomiting. It may subside completely with recurrence weeks or months later, or it may be followed days later by the development of jaundice due to migration of the stone into the bile duct and impaction at its lower end.

Acute obstructive cholecystitis is inflammation of the gall bladder as a result of obstruction at the neck by an impacted stone. The gall bladder wall becomes oedematous and its lumen distended with exudate and infected bile. The stone may become dislodged and fall back into the gall bladder which then drains its contents through the cystic duct with resolution of the inflammation. When the stone remains impacted, the gall bladder fills with pus (empyema of the gall bladder) or develops patchy gangrene in the fundus which, if not contained by adherent omentum to form an inflammatory mass may perforate and lead to biliary peritonitis.

The manifestation of acute obstructive cholecystitis includes pain in the right hypochondrium, nausea and vomiting. The patient is pyrexial and may be jaundiced because of oedema of the bile duct or the presence of ductal stones. There is marked tenderness in the right hypochondrium with a positive Murphy's sign (the patient is asked to take a deep breath while manual pressure is maintained in the right hypochondrium; as the descending diaphragm causes the inflamed gall bladder to impinge against the hand there is sudden cessation of breath). It may be possible to feel the gall bladder if distended, or an inflammatory mass of adherent omentum.

Acute acalculous cholecystitis is a cause of right hypochondrial pain and tenderness in seriously ill patients (e.g., multiple trauma, severe burns and sepsis) requiring intensive care, mechanical ventilation, prolonged opiate analgesia and parenteral nutrition. It is probably a result of stasis in the gall bladder and ischaemia.

Management

In biliary colic the initial inflammation of the gall bladder is chemical. Later, biliary colic may develop into acute obstructive cholecystitis, when the patient shows systemic signs of toxicity, that is, pyrexia, tachycardia and leucocytosis. The urine may contain bilirubin because of an associated obstruction of the biliary system by tissue oedema or a stone. The diagnosis of gallstones is made on ultrasound examination. The scan also defines the thickness of the gall

bladder wall, obstruction at the cystic duct and distension of the gall bladder, or the presence of an inflammatory mass. Ultrasound scan is not reliable in detecting ductal stones unless large or there is ductal dilatation. A plain abdominal X-ray for detection of gallstones is not cost-effective since only 10% of gallstones contain calcium. A lateral view can be employed to distinguish between a stone in the kidney, which lies posterior from a stone in the gall bladder that lies anterior to the vertebral column when the distinction cannot be made on an ultrasound scan. The liver function tests are not usually deranged unless there is infection in the biliary system.

Treatment consists of intravenous analgesia and fluids with restriction of oral intake if the patient is vomiting, and intravenous antibiotics only if there are signs of systemic infection. Patients with empyema are managed by the insertion of a percutaneous tube into the gall bladder under ultrasound guidance (*percutaneous cholecystotomy*) to drain the gall bladder. When such facilities are unavailable urgent open cholecystotomy or, if technically feasible and safe, cholecystectomy is carried out.

Acute cholangitis is infection of the biliary tree due to Gram-negative aerobic bacteria such as *Esherichia coli*. It may be the initial presentation or may complicate biliary colic or acute obstructive cholecystitis when a stone passes into the bile duct. It may complicate acute pancreatitis due to pancreatic oedema. In a patient who previously had a cholecystectomy, a residual ductal stone or an iatrogenic stricture should be suspected.

The patient presents with features similar to those of acute obstructive cholecystitis although usually looks more toxic, has a high fever, rigors and jaundice (*Charcot's triad*). There is also marked tenderness and guarding in the right hypochondrium. The liver function tests are consistent with an obstructive picture. The serum amylase may be elevated due to pancreatitis. Urine analysis shows excessive bilirubin. On ultrasound scan dilatation of the bile ducts is suggestive as the resolution for small stones is not sensitive but the presence of stones in the gallbladder is further evidence of ductal stone obstruction. A CT scan confirms the diagnosis of associated pancreatitis as described already.

In acute cholangitis intravenous antibiotics and urgent ERCP and sphincterotomy with retrieval of the stone and/or stenting of the bile duct for drainage is the primary treatment but if technically unsuccessful, or if the expertise is unavailable, percutaneous trans-hepatic drainage should be attempted. Otherwise, surgical drainage of the biliary system is required.

Following successful treatment of the acute episode elective cholecystectomy is planned. A laparoscopic cholecystectomy can be performed safely within the same admission and not later than 1 week from onset of symptoms, especially in diabetics and immunocompromised patients; otherwise it is deferred for at least 6 weeks.

Similarly, in the presence of an inflammatory mass, early cholecystectomy is difficult and hazardous; time should be allowed for resolution of inflammatory oedema and adhesions, or of associated pancreatitis especially when severe. In patients who had a cholecystotomy the tube drain is not removed unless instillation of dye down the tube shows free drainage into the bile duct; otherwise, if a stone is still impacted in the cystic duct, the tube is left in place and the patient instructed on managing it until elective cholecystectomy can be arranged. Acalculous cholecystitis is managed along the same principles and unless conservative treatment fails cholecystectomy is not deemed necessary except in diabetic and immunocompromised patients.

Unless per-operative cholangiography can be carried out, an ERCP to rule out ductal stones should precede laparoscopic or open cholecystectomy whenever there is ductal dilatation or suspicion of a ductal stone on ultrasonography, disturbed liver function tests with high alkaline phosphatase, a high serum amylase or associated pancreatitis.

What has been discussed represents common presentations but other conditions not encountered as often are described below.

Carcinoma of the gall bladder is associated with gallstones in 90% of cases and the tumour is usually a scirrous or an adenocarcinoma rather than a squamous cell carcinoma which might have been expected to develop in metaplastic epithelium from long-standing irritation by gallstones. Carcinoma of the gall bladder most commonly presents as acute cholecystitis. A few that present with obstructive jaundice and a palpable mass in the right hypochondrium are diagnosed before operation.

At laparoscopy or laparotomy for cholecystitis it is a surprise finding when it is usually advanced because of liver infiltration with secondaries, and therefore incurable. Occasionally, cancer is discovered at pathological examination of the specimen following cholecystectomy for gallstones; the choice between subsequent excision of the liver bed or adjuvant chemotherapy is determined by the extent of tumour infiltration within the gall bladder wall. When the tumour is confined to the mucosa the five-year survival is over 50%, otherwise it is less than 5%.

Hepatic abscesses are commonly in the right lobe, are multiple and are usually pyogenic, caused by a mixture of aerobic and anaerobic bacteria. They complicate a biliary or other intra-abdominal focus of sepsis, although there is no underlying cause in immunocompromised and diabetic patients. An *amoebic abscess* is secondary to intestinal amoebiasis as a result of entamoebae that colonize the liver causing liquefaction necrosis.

The patient presents with fever, lethargy, pain and tenderness in the right hypochondrium. The leucocyte count is increased and the liver function tests are disturbed. The diagnosis can only be established by ultrasound or CT scan of the upper abdomen that also allows access for percutaneous aspiration or drainage. The drained material is purulent in a pyogenic abscess, chocolate-coloured anchovy sauce colour in an amoebic abscess. The causative organism is identified by bacteriological analysis. A pyogenic abscess is treated by percutaneous drainage and systemic antibiotics, such as aminoglycosides, cephalosporins and metronidazole. Small amoebic abscesses respond to metronidazole treatment (800 mg three times daily) for 7–10 days but needle aspiration is required if there is lack of response and the patient is toxic.

Hepatic tumours are usually metastases, although in Africa, China and south-east Asia where hepatitis B is rife, hepatocellular carcinoma complicating cirrhosis is more common. Hepatocellular carcinoma may present with acute pain in the right hypochondrium and tenderness due to bleeding into the tumour, with a short history of anorexia and weight loss. The patient is anaemic. The liver is enlarged and tender and if the tumour has ruptured and is bleeding into the peritoneal cavity, tenderness is more generalized. The diagnosis is suggested by features of chronic liver disease and is confirmed by ultrasound or CT scanning. Embolization of the hepatic artery is the therapeutic option.

Acute hepatitis is due either to infection, usually viral A, B, or C as a consequence of cross infection, blood transfusion, intravenous drug abuse and male homosexuality, or to drugs and alcohol. Anorexia, nausea, malaise and fever with pain and tenderness in the right hypochondrium may precede the development of jaundice.

Deranged liver function tests and a normal biliary system and liver on ultrasound are suggestive, whereupon the case is referred for a medical opinion.

PAIN IN THE LEFT HYPOCHONDRIUM

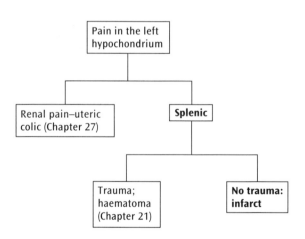

This as the sole symptom is not common and is usually a component of diffuse upper abdominal pain, but when it occurs rare pathological conditions involving the spleen should be differentiated from renal or ureteric pain.

Peri-splenic haematoma is suspected if there is history of a trivial injury and is common in those with splenomegaly, due to infective (bacterial, viral or parasitic) or blood diseases or neoplastic disease of the reticulo-endothelial system. The spleen is palpable either because it is primarily enlarged or displaced by haematoma, and is tender.

The diagnosis is made by CT scan. The blood count and clotting screen are likely to be abnormal, and this requires attention if interventional treatment is planned. Splenectomy, unless detrimental to the course of the underlying disease, is the optimal treatment; otherwise, percutaneous drainage of the haematoma to prevent its expansion and rupture should be considered.

Splenic infarction occurs in patients with massively enlarged spleens due to myeloproliferative disease, or vascular occlusion produced by sickle-cell disease or an embolus complicating bacterial endocarditis. The pain radiates to the shoulder. There is tenderness and guarding and a friction rub may be audible in the left upper quadrant. A CT scan will establish the diagnosis. Sedation and analgesia are sufficient.

CENTRAL ABDOMINAL PAIN

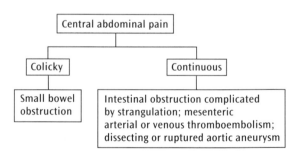

This originates from the small intestine and is usually colicky due to intestinal obstruction. Continuous pain suggests strangulation, or mesenteric arterial or venous thromboembolism (Chapter 26). Aortic dissection or rupture is another cause of pain.

LOWER ABDOMINAL PAIN

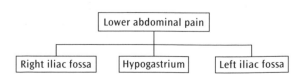

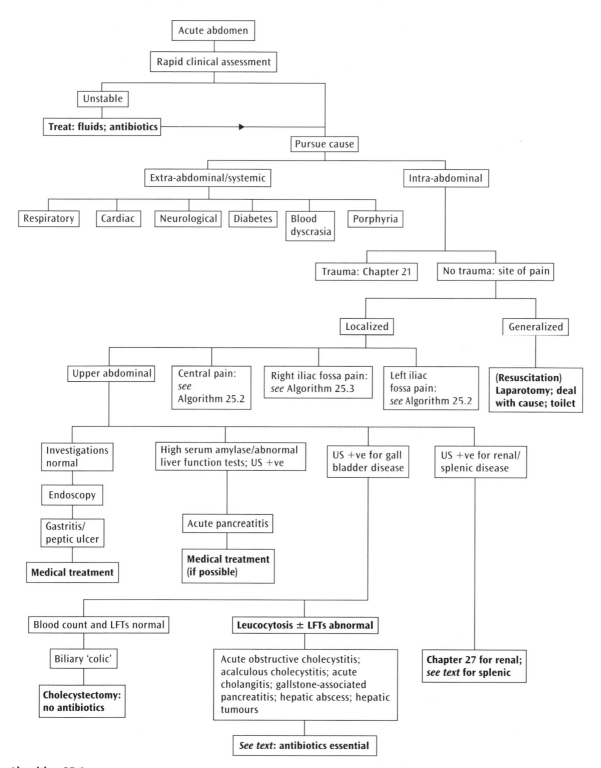

Algorithm 25.1

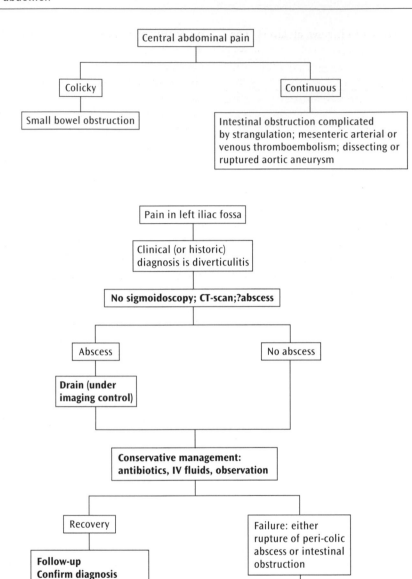

Algorithm 25.2

As in the upper abdomen, the pain may not be confined to a defined quadrant of the lower abdomen and can be diffuse. The most common cause of pain in the right iliac fossa is *acute appendicitis* and in the left iliac fossa is *acute diverticulitis*. Genito-urinary conditions may cause similar symptoms (Chapter 27).

Pain in the right iliac fossa

Acute appendicitis is the usual cause and is the most common surgical emergency in Western countries. It is due to infection secondary to luminal obstruction by a faecolith or impacted faeces. It starts with mucosal inflammation that extends to involve all layers. The lumen becomes distended with necrotic mucosa, exudate and pus. The end-arteries thrombose and the infarcted appendix becomes necrotic or gangrenous. Perforation and peritonitis follow unless the greater omentum walls off the perforation and localizes the spread of infection.

Acute appendicitis is rare before the age of two and its peak incidence is between the ages of 20 and 30, but it may occur at any age. The clinical features are usually typical. The history starts with periumbilical pain due to distension of the appendix and, being visceral in origin, is vague, but when the appendix is obstructed the pain becomes colicky. After a few hours the inflammation in the appendix progresses to involve the parietal peritoneum, when the pain shifts to the right iliac fossa and becomes localized and constant. The patient feels nauseated and may be vomiting.

On examination, the patient is flushed and has tachycardia, a furred tongue and halitosis. Initially, there may be no fever. There is tenderness and guarding on palpation, maximal in the right iliac fossa over McBurney's point (the junction of the upper two-thirds with the lower one-third of the line between the anterior superior iliac spine and the umbilicus). The patient also experiences pain in the same region when coughing. This would not happen were the pain due to a stone in the ureter. The abdominal signs may not be as obvious in the obese patient or when the appendix is retro-caecal. On rectal examination, there is right-sided pelvic tenderness, especially in those with a pelvic abscess. The white cell count is usually, but not always higher than $10 \times 10^9/l$ and plain X-rays are nearly always non-contributory. The urine is always examined for red and pus cells to rule out ureteric colic or urinary tract infection. In difficult cases ultrasonography and CT-scanning are increasingly being employed, and in females laparoscopy is mandatory when there is uncertainty as to the cause of lower abdominal pain.

Management

The treatment of acute appendicitis is appendicectomy. A low skin crease incision (*Lanz*) rather than the higher and more oblique one centred on McBurney's point gives a better cosmetic result. The three musculo-aponeurotic layers: the external oblique, the internal oblique and the transversus abdominis are split along the line of their fibres (this constitutes the '*grid-iron*' incision as the fibres of the external oblique and internal oblique run at right angles to each other). The peritoneum is opened, the appendix is located digitally and delivered into the wound, its blood supply in the mesoappendix is divided between haemostats and ligated. The now mobilized appendix is crushed at its junction with the caecum with a haemostat that is removed and re-applied just distal to the crushed portion; the latter is ligated and the appendix divided and excised. A purse-string suture is placed in the caecum proximal to the appendix base which is inverted and the suture tied. The wound and the pelvis are irrigated with saline to wash out any pus or infected material. Drainage is unnecessary provided adequate peritoneal toilet has been carried out. The peritoneum and the muscle layers are closed. All suture material used is absorbable.

The use of prophylactic antibiotics against anaerobic and aerobic organisms lowers the risk of intra-abdominal sepsis and wound infection. Metronidazole, 1 g (rectally is as effective as intravenously) combined with a cephalosporin is given 2 hours before operation.

Clinical problems before operation

Atypical presentation

Despite careful assessment, sometimes the diagnosis may still not be obvious. There may be no abdominal tenderness if the appendix lies in the pelvis or in the retro-caecal or retro-ileal position. The pelvic lie should produce tenderness on digital pelvic examination, the retro-caecal sometimes produces tenderness in the flank.

In the presence of localized tenderness and guarding, the working diagnosis must be acute appendicitis; in tenderness without guarding or in case of uncertainty for any reason, an ultrasound examination and, in females in particular, laparoscopy can be helpful. If this demonstrates the appendix and changes of acute appendicitis are confirmed, or if the appendix fails to be visualized (and there is no sign of any

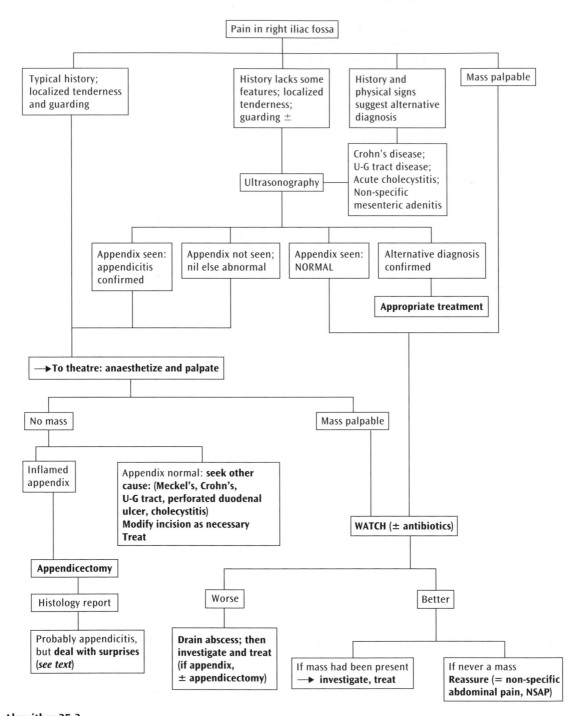

Algorithm 25.3

other abnormality), the decision to proceed to appendicectomy is justifiable. However, if the appendix is seen and is normal and there is no alternative diagnosis, the patient is treated conservatively. A period of observation monitoring the patient's symptoms and signs, the pulse rate and temperature as well as the white cell count, will help to identify *non-specific abdominal pain* that usually improves steadily during observation.

Alternative diagnoses

Other conditions that mimic appendicitis should be considered before a definitive diagnosis is made.

Non-specific mesenteric lymphadenitis is associated with upper respiratory tract infection or sore throat in children. The child usually has a high temperature and the cervical lymph nodes are enlarged. The abdominal signs are less pronounced and the site of tenderness is said to shift when the child turns on to the left side. An ultrasound examination may define the abnormality. It is reasonable to consult with a paediatrician and allow a period of observation.

Constipation may cause colicky abdominal pain and right iliac fossa tenderness and is a cause of confusion. The patient is apyrexial and the white cell count is normal. The rectum is loaded with faeces. A plain film demonstrates faeces in the colon. The diagnosis should be considered with caution: purgatives will stimulate violent peristalsis that will cause perforation and peritonitis if acute appendicitis has been misdiagnosed.

Perforated peptic ulcer may present with pain in the right iliac fossa as a result of duodenal contents tracking down the paracolic gutter to the right iliac fossa. There is usually a history of a *sudden onset of epigastric pain*. This may be overlooked and sometimes patients with appendicitis describe epigastric discomfort from vomiting as pain. If a chest X-ray has been requested and there is gas under the diaphragm, incorrect diagnosis is avoided.

Acute cholecystitis can be confused with acute appendicitis in the pregnant as the appendix is displaced to the upper abdomen with the enlarging uterus. The high frequency of pyelonephritis in pregnancy further complicates the picture. There is a maternal mortality of 20% after the sixth month and a 50% risk of abortion or premature labour

with perforated appendicitis, 30% in non-perforated appendicitis. The history and location of physical signs may not be distinctive unless the patient is jaundiced. Other than urine analysis and liver function tests, ultrasound examination is particularly useful in imaging any abnormality in the kidney or gall bladder and usually outlines the appendix.

Crohn's regional ileitis may cause pain and tenderness in the right iliac fossa indistinguishable from acute appendicitis, but a preceding history of intermittent fever, diarrhoea and weight loss is suggestive. A similar clinical dilemma is the difficulty in making the diagnosis of appendicitis in a patient with known Crohn's disease. The white cell count and the inflammatory markers, that is, ESR and CRP, are not specific, but an ultrasound scan should define thickening of the terminal ileum and may demonstrate an abnormality in the appendix.

Meckel's diverticulitis is usually due to food or foreign body impaction in the diverticulum that is situated in the antimesenteric border of the small intestine 60 cm (2 feet) from the ileocaecal valve and is usually 50 mm (2 inches) in length. It occurs in 2% of the population (the *2's aide memoire*). It is a rare cause of right iliac fossa pain, only likely to be suspected if the patient has previously undergone appendicectomy.

Appendix mass

Omentum and oedematous coils of small intestine wrapped around an inflamed or perforated appendix produce an appendix mass. This is a likely outcome when symptoms of acute appendicitis have been disregarded or masked with antibiotic treatment. The mass appears 48–72 hours after the onset of symptoms and gets more circumscribed over several days. The patient may have few systemic signs. Tenderness over the mass, pyrexia, tachycardia and leucocytosis are variable depending on the time since onset and the degree of inflammation.

Intervention is contraindicated because the adhesions make access to the appendix difficult, and adherent structures are oedematous and friable. There is therefore a risk of bleeding, intra-abdominal sepsis and intestinal fistulae. Since the natural defences have localized the lesion it is illogical to disturb these barriers. Therefore, the standard treatment is conservative. The *Ochsner–Sherren regime* consists of keeping a 4-hourly chart of the pulse rate and temperature; restricting oral intake to fluids only, or completely if the patient is vomiting; intravenous fluids; mild analgesia, avoiding opiates in order not to mask the symptoms and signs; and intravenous antibiotics, usually cephalosporin and metronidazole, but only if there are signs of sepsis. The white cell count is estimated daily.

This policy allows time to investigate the mass as there are other conditions that share the same presentation without necessarily showing any discriminatory features. A *carcinoma of the caecum* should always be considered in high-risk patients. The presence of a palpable hard liver is the only suggestive sign. *Crohn's ileitis* is likely to show other features such as long-term diarrhoea, weight loss and anaemia or the diagnosis is already established and the patient is on medication; however, an inflammatory mass can be the first presentation. *Ileo-caecal tuberculosis* is more likely to be the cause of a mass in the overseas immigrant and in endemic areas than is Crohn's disease, and a history of pulmonary tuberculosis is not a helpful lead as infection is commonly acquired by ingestion of the bovine bacillus. *Carcinoma of the ovary* in elderly females and s*alpingo-oophoritis* in sexually active females are other possibilities. Abdominal examination and bi-manual palpation with digital rectal and vaginal examination differentiates a pelvic visceral mass in females from an intra-abdominal mass. An abdominal ultrasound combined if necessary with endo-vaginal ultrasound or CT scan will further outline the nature of the mass.

During the ensuing days there is in the majority a satisfactory response to treatment shown by improvement in symptoms, normality of pulse and temperature and resolution of the mass. Alternatively, inflammation may progress to suppuration and abscess formation suggested clinically by constant pain, swinging pyrexia above 37.8°C, tachycardia and the mass is larger and more tender. The white cell count rises. Ultrasonography confirms abscess formation and also provides access for percutaneous drainage that is the preferred treatment. If the necessary expertise is not available, open drainage is performed through an incision over the mass.

Following resolution of the inflammatory mass any underlying pathology other than appendicitis must be ruled out before planning for interval appendicectomy. In the young patient, persistent abdominal pain and diarrhoea is suggestive of Crohn's disease, whereas in those more than 50 years old or, if younger, with a strong family history of bowel cancer, a caecal carcinoma must be excluded.

Barium studies and colonoscopy are better deferred for at least 6 weeks since morphological changes due to residual inflammation may distort the results. Once underlying pathology has been ruled out, and at least 6 weeks after complete resolution of the mass, interval appendicectomy can be carried out, although the need for appendicectomy is debatable since nearly 80% of patients are unlikely to have further attacks of appendicitis, presumably because the appendix is replaced with fibrous tissue.

Clinical problems at operation

A palpable mass

Tenderness and guarding in the conscious patient may mask the presence of a mass, which may not become obvious until the patient is anaesthetized. It is therefore always advisable to palpate the right iliac fossa for a mass before making the incision. If present, it is safe to abandon the operation and treat the patient conservatively as explained above. If the mass is only found at exploration, the difficulty is to distinguish between an inflammatory mass due to appendicitis and one due to Crohn's disease or a caecal carcinoma. It is safer not to proceed. The wound is closed. The mass can then be investigated and treated electively.

A doubtful diagnosis of appendicitis: choice of incision

A lower mid-line incision provides better access to the pelvic organs in females, and if necessary it can be readily extended upwards to deal with a perforated duodenal ulcer or other unexpected intra-abdominal pathology. However, it is argued that two small incisions, that is, closing the right iliac fossa incision and making a new one ideally located to deal with the problem found, is better because two small incisions heal more rapidly and with less discomfort than a single long incision which carries a greater risk of infection, wound dehiscence and incisional hernia.

Difficulty in delivering the appendix
Access is improved by cutting the muscle layers in the line of the incision. A retro-caecal appendix requires mobilization of the caecum by dividing the peritoneum along its lateral side. Alternatively, retrograde appendicectomy is performed: the base of the appendix and its blood supply are divided. After the stump has been ligated and invaginated, traction on the caecum allows delivery of the appendix and its removal from base to tip.

A normal ('lily-white') appendix
The terminal ileum, caecum and right fallopian tube and ovary are inspected, and if these are normal at least a 60 cm (2 feet) length of the ileum is delivered into the wound by gentle traction to check whether a Meckel's diverticulum is present. Whether or not an abnormality is found, appendicectomy should still be performed as an appendicectomy scar will lead to confusion should the patient present with symptoms in the future. The normality of the appendix should be established histologically as the appendix may be harbouring a sinister pathology (*see later*). However, if there is no free fluid found in the peritoneal cavity, it is unlikely that serious disease is present.

Pelvic inflammatory disease, ectopic pregnancy, ovarian cyst
Management is discussed in Chapter 27.

A thickened terminal ileum
This is more likely to be acute inflammation with the organism *Yersinia pseudotuberculosis* than Crohn's disease. Thickening of the fat mesentery and fat wrapping are more characteristic of Crohn's disease. The mesenteric nodes are usually enlarged in both conditions. An incision or excision biopsy of a node for histological examination is essential.

Appendicectomy is carried out safely unless the caecum, including the appendicular base, is involved in Crohn's disease, when it is likely that the appendix is also diseased. Ileo-caecal resection is a safer option in a patient with a long history; otherwise, the procedure is abandoned and specific treatment for Crohn's disease is commenced as appendicectomy may result in an enteric fistula.

When Yersinia ileitis is suspected, blood titres are obtained to confirm the diagnosis. It is a self-limiting condition and requires no treatment.

Meckel's diverticulum
When inflamed or perforated, a Meckel's diverticulum is removed with a segment of ileum. If a Meckel's diverticulum is normal, and provided excision can be carried out without additional risk, then this should be done in order to avoid the risk of subsequent complications.

Carcinoma of the caecum
It is always prudent to examine the caecum carefully when appendicectomy is being performed in high-risk patients, that is, those more than 50 years old or with a family history of the condition. When there is an unequivocal tumour mass the Lanz incision is then extended transversely to allow for a right hemicolectomy to be carried out.

Perforated peptic ulcer
The presence of bile-stained fluid when the peritoneum is opened is consistent with a perforated peptic ulcer. A Lanz incision is closed and an upper mid-line incision is carried out and the perforation is treated appropriately.

Solitary caecal diverticulum
This condition is rarely considered in the Western world where diverticular disease, unlike in Asia, is mainly left-sided. Perforation presents with features indistinguishable from acute appendicitis and the diagnosis is made at exploration by the presence of a caecal phlegmon. Treatment is by resection of the caecum with a short segment of adjacent ileum.

Problems after operation

Histological surprise
Carcinoid tumour and adenocarcinoma of the appendix are uncommon but are sometimes reported on histological examination of a normal or inflamed appendix, when further surgery may be required.

Carcinoid tumour (*agentaffinoma*)

This tumour occurs in patients between the ages of 10 and 60 years and nearly 80% are females. The tumour is frequently located at the distal end of the appendix and is readily palpable, or when the appendix is split open it becomes visible lying between the mucosa and the serosa and replacing the muscular layer. Microscopically it consists of spheroidal cells that contain granules that stain with ammoniacal silver stains. Only 4% of carcinoid tumours of the appendix metastasize and produce the *carcinoid syndrome* (cyanosis, flushing, diarrhoea, borborygmi, broncho-spasm, pulmonary and tricuspid stenosis).

Appendicectomy is sufficient treatment unless the caecal wall is involved (i.e., the excision would be incomplete), the tumour is 2 cm or more in size, or involved lymph nodes are found, when a right hemi-colectomy becomes necessary.

Primary carcinoma

Appendicectomy is sufficient if the tumour is in the distal part of the appendix and is within the sub-mucosa, otherwise right hemicolectomy is indi-cated. A mucus-secreting adenocarcinoma produces a malignant mucocoele which, if it ruptures, causes *pseudomyxoma peritonei*. The average five-year sur-vival rate is 60%.

Pain in the left iliac fossa

Sigmoid diverticulitis is the most common cause, although as in the left iliac fossa, genito-urinary conditions should be differentiated (Chapter 27). Sigmoid diverticulitis is inflammation of diverticula which are herniations of colonic mucosa through the circular muscle commonly localized in the sigmoid colon. The local inflammation may extend to involve the peri-colic tissue and may be associated with a micro-perforation that is localized to form a *para-colic abscess.*

This condition should be considered in patients of either sex over the age of 40, or younger in male obese patients, but must not be confused with painful diver-ticular disease due to spastic contractions of the colon not associated with inflammation. Diverticulitis has been likened to left-sided appendicitis. The patient is pyrexial and complains of constant pain, diarrhoea or constipation and occasionally rectal bleeding. The patient may have urinary frequency or dysuria. There is tenderness and guarding in the left and occasionally in the right iliac fossa if the sigmoid colon lies over the mid-line, which may prevent palpation of a sigmoid phlegmon (inflammatory mass) or a para-colic abscess. Rectal examination may reveal a tender mass in the recto-vesical or recto-uterine pouch. Sigmoidoscopy is avoided to prevent the risk of an inflamed diverticulum perforating when insufflating air.

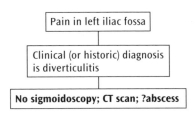

Unless the patient is known to suffer from diver-ticular disease the diagnosis of diverticulitis on first presentation is based on clinical examination, leuco-cytosis and positive blood cultures.

Treatment consists of intravenous antibiotics, usually cephalosporin and metronidazole. If the patient is nauseated or vomiting oral intake is disal-lowed and intravenous fluids are commenced. The pulse and temperature are recorded.

An abdominal CT scan to rule out a para-colic abscess is recommended on presentation if there is rigidity due to localized peritonitis, or later if there is no response to treatment, as antibiotic therapy is ineffective until the abscess is drained. This is best performed percutaneously by siting a drain tube under image control. In a few patients a colo-cutaneous fistula develops after removing the drain or the abscess may drain into the vagina or bladder resulting in a colo-vaginal or colo-vesical fistula.

This management is effective in 75% of patients, but the remaining patients will require surgical inter-vention because of intestinal obstruction due to a combination of acute inflammatory thickening, mus-cle hypertrophy and spasm or because of generalized peritonitis due to rupture of a para-colic abscess or a large perforation complicating diverticulitis. The surgical treatment for obstructive and perforated diverticulitis is the same (Chapter 9).

After recovery from acute diverticulitis the diagnosis, if not already known, is confirmed by colonoscopy or barium enema. This is better delayed for a few weeks as residual inflammation interferes with the performance and the quality of the examination so that the appearances can be confused with a carcinoma, and there is also a risk of perforation.

The general policy is to recommend elective resection of the diseased segment after two attacks of diverticulitis, but only after a single attack in immunocompromised patients, those undergoing organ transplantation and in patients less than 30 years old in whom the disease is believed to be more virulent; when a coincidental carcinoma cannot be excluded; and when diverticulitis is complicated by a fistula.

GENERALIZED PAIN

All the inflammatory conditions described already are usually associated with peritonitis that is localized to the viscus involved and is responsible for the systemic and local signs. With appropriate treatment, localized peritonitis usually resolves. Diffuse inflammation of the peritoneum manifests more pronounced symptoms and signs and is caused by peritonitis.

Peritonitis is divided into three types. The most common is *secondary peritonitis* due to transmigration of intestinal bacteria or escape of intestinal contents into the peritoneal cavity and bacterial contamination caused by many of the morbid conditions that have already been discussed. *Primary peritonitis* is rare and is caused by gonococcal and β-haemolytic streptococcal infection via the fallopian tubes or *Staphylococcus aureus* associated with intra-vaginal tampons in females. Another rare example is primary bacterial peritonitis due to infection of the ascitic fluid in cirrhotic patients. *Chemical peritonitis* is due to extravasation of urine, bile or gastric juice, but before long secondary bacterial peritonitis develops.

Clinical features

The systemic manifestations are due to disturbances of the body fluid compartments and to endotoxaemia.

The patient looks ill and has a pyrexia with rigors and tachycardia. The loss of fluid and electrolytes from vomiting and sequestrated fluid in oedematous intestinal loops and peritoneal exudate as well as insensible loss caused by pyrexia leads to circulatory and renal failure. The patient develops cold, clammy extremities, sunken eyes, a dry tongue, a thready pulse, a drawn and anxious facies, oliguria, and finally lapses into unconsciousness.

The abdominal symptoms are due to diffuse inflammation of the parietal peritoneum and the patient complains of generalized pain, although the pain can be worse in a localised region at the site of the primary source. The pain is severe, constant and aggravated by movement. The patient lies still in the supine position and may draw up the knees to relax the abdominal musculature. When inflammation is under the diaphragm, shoulder tip (*phrenic*) pain may be felt and with pelvic peritonitis patients may complain of urinary symptoms.

On inspection of the abdomen, the abdominal wall movement with respiration is diminished because of reflex spasm of the abdominal muscles. On palpation, there is generalized tenderness, guarding and rigidity. On auscultation, the bowel sounds are infrequent or absent. Rectal examination is essential and may elicit tenderness, boggy swelling in the rectovesical or recto-uterine pouch and tenderness caused by movement of the cervix.

Management

The clinical picture is diagnostic. Generalized peritonitis following abdominal surgery and related to trauma are discussed in Chapters 16 and 21, respectively. The underlying cause is not always easy to determine unless the patient is able to describe antecedent symptoms or specify the site of the pain prior to developing peritonitis. A careful history and an area of maximum tenderness if present may provide a clue as to the cause. This may not seem crucial since irrespective of the cause, laparotomy to drain the infected material and remove the local source (*peritoneal toilet*) is the only treatment; however, pancreatitis and primary peritonitis are better treated conservatively provided the diagnosis can be made with certainty.

Investigations include a white cell count and leucocytosis is usual. Blood cultures may grow organisms that elucidate the source of infection. Urea, electrolytes and plasma proteins may be disturbed and are important baseline measurements. Serum amylase estimation confirms the diagnosis of pancreatitis provided it is remembered that raised values are frequently found following other morbid abdominal conditions (perforated peptic ulcer, strangulated intestine and infarction). A clotting screen is necessary as coagulation is disturbed in septic patients. An X-ray film of the abdomen may reveal free air, or dilated gas-filled loops of bowel with multiple fluid levels. If the patient is too ill for an erect film to demonstrate free air collection under the diaphragm, a lateral decubitus film is as informative. An ultrasound examination of the abdomen or a CT scan identifies free intra-peritoneal fluid or gas and may outline a localized area of inflammation.

Treatment

This consists of resuscitative measures, early correction of the local source of contamination and peritoneal toilet. The patient care starts with nasogastric aspiration, intravenous fluids and/or blood transfusion to replace plasma volume and correct electrolyte imbalance and, in those whose recovery is likely to be prolonged, intravenous feeding is required to correct plasma protein depletion as a result of starvation and loss of protein in the peritoneal exudate. It is important to recognize that depletion of plasma protein can be masked by the loss of extra-cellular fluid (e.g., in vomitus) which artificially raises plasma protein concentration.

Intravenous antibiotics are administered: cephalosporin and metronidazole are given initially until the result of blood or infected material cultures are obtained. Opiate analgesia is allowed when a diagnosis of generalized peritonitis is made. A central venous line and urinary catheterization to monitor fluid replacement should be considered in unstable patients. Once the patient is deemed fit for anaesthesia a laparotomy is carried out.

When the site of origin of the peritonitis is certain, either an upper or lower mid-line incision is made. If the site is uncertain, a short mid-line incision centred at the umbilicus provides access which is then extended either proximally or distally depending on the site of the lesion. When the peritoneal cavity is entered, the nature of any free fluid and examination of the omentum gives an indication as to the cause.

The fluid, which is an outpouring of peritoneal exudates, is initially turbid but as localization occurs around the affected organ, the fluid becomes purulent. A leak from the stomach, duodenum or small intestine is bile stained, it is pure bile when from the gall bladder or the bile ducts, and it is faecal when from the colon. Blood-stained fluid is associated with infarcted bowel or a haemorrhagic lesion, such as acute pancreatitis or a ruptured hepatic tumour, and pure blood is seen with a ruptured aortic aneurysm or spleen.

The greater omentum envelops and becomes adherent to inflamed structures and by tracing the area of adherence, the organ involved and consequently the likely pathology can be determined. Widespread fat necrosis – dull, opaque, yellow-white areas that look like drops of wax – of the omentum and the mesentery is a feature of acute pancreatitis.

Surgical treatment of the individual conditions is carried out as described already. The whole peritoneal cavity is then irrigated liberally with saline until all seropurulent material is removed. Drain tubes are not a substitute for adequate peritoneal lavage and are unnecessary unless extensive dissection has been carried out and excessive ooze is expected, or the viability of a viscus or an anastomosis is in question.

In the presence of significant contamination, particularly faecal, the subcutaneous layer and skin are better not closed but packed with gauze soaked in antiseptic; the wound is subsequently dressed regularly to allow for healing by second intention. Complete closure of the wound increases the risk of wound infection and breakdown and is likely to delay, rather than accelerate, wound healing.

The post-operative management of these patients should take into account morbidity related to persistent toxaemia, paralytic ileus, residual abscesses, bronchopneumonia, electrolyte imbalance and renal failure.

HIGHLIGHTS

- The site and the nature of the pain aids in diagnosis
- Ultrasound and CT scan are useful diagnostic and therapeutic modalities in acute abdominal pain
- Many causes of acute abdominal pain if not identified and treated promptly will lead to generalized peritonitis
- An inflammatory mass is a sign of a defensive barrier and should be treated expectantly
- Peritonitis with the exception of acute pancreatitis and primary peritonitis requires a laparotomy

26

The acute abdomen: intestinal obstruction

PAUL B BOULOS

INTRODUCTION

None of the five questions below is concerned with the cause of the obstruction. Although the underlying cause of the obstruction may influence management, the surgeon's approach depends far more on the answers to the five questions than on the cause.

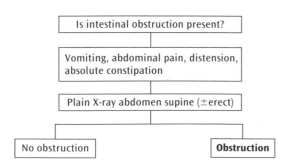

IS OBSTRUCTION PRESENT?

The characteristic features are vomiting, abdominal pain, abdominal distension and absolute constipation, that is, neither faeces nor flatus is passed rectally for longer than the subject and the clinician would consider normal. Intestinal obstruction should be suspected whenever a patient presents with any of these complaints as the full picture may not become clear until later depending on the level and degree of obstruction. Unless complicated by dehydration or strangulation, intestinal obstruction is distinct from other causes of acute abdomen by absence of systemic signs and of abdominal tenderness or guarding. The patient may not look unwell, although uncomfortable because of pain and vomiting, especially when these are severe. Confirmatory evidence is obtained from plain radiographs of the abdomen.

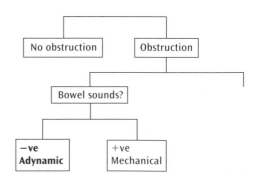

MECHANICAL OR ADYNAMIC?

If vomiting and/or abdominal distension are associated with intermittent abdominal pain and increased bowel sounds, the obstruction is *mechanical*; if there is no pain and the bowel sounds are absent, the obstruction is *adynamic*. A variant of adynamic obstruction is vomiting and/or abdominal distension with pain but absent bowel sounds. This is suggestive of bowel ischaemia from strangulation complicating mechanical obstruction or due to mesenteric arterial or venous occlusion. Intestinal pseudo-obstruction is adynamic obstruction of the large bowel which clinically is only distinguishable from mechanical obstruction by the exclusion of organic disease.

If it is decided that the obstruction is mechanical, the next question is, does the site of obstruction lie in the small or the large bowel?

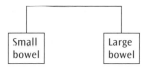

SMALL OR LARGE BOWEL?

Pathophysiology

The manner of onset and the varied symptomatology lie in the pathophysiology, which is related to the level of obstruction. At least 10 l of fluid are secreted into the gastrointestinal tract daily and are mostly absorbed in the ileum and colon. Therefore, acute onset of copious vomiting of bile-stained fluid is a feature of proximal small bowel obstruction. Pain and distension are progressively more pronounced at lower levels of small bowel obstruction because of active intestinal peristalsis and accumulation of intestinal secretions and swallowed air. The vomitus also gradually becomes thicker and foul smelling (*faeculent*). This is small bowel contents altered as a result of bacterial overgrowth and fermentation and should not be confused with the true faecal vomiting usually seen with fistulas between the large bowel and the stomach. The patient may continue to have bowel motions until the distal segment empties, therefore constipation is late to develop.

Large bowel obstruction is less acute in onset. Constipation is the earliest symptom and distension develops rapidly as the capacious colon fills with swallowed air and bowel contents. The abdomen becomes gradually tense but the patient may not feel pain until later when the colonic wall is over-stretched, particularly noticeable in the right iliac fossa where the blind-ended thin-walled caecum may perforate causing localized peritonitis. Vomiting is not a prominent feature since there is little disturbance of re-absorption of water, unless the ileo-caecal valve is incompetent and allows back flow with distension of the small bowel. This decompresses the caecum and delays the progression of colonic dilatation and damage to the caecum.

Clinical features

The progression of symptoms, as already described, the site and the nature of pain are helpful distinguishing parameters. Colicky abdominal pain is more common in small than in large bowel obstruction: in the latter, the pain is dull and is felt in the lower abdomen and the supra-pubic region. The lower the level of obstruction the greater the distension, which is confined to the centre of the abdomen in small bowel obstruction and is in the flanks in large bowel obstruction. The gaseous distension is confirmed by a tympanitic note on percussion. Peristalsis, usually visible in thin patients, coincides with attacks of colic, is accompanied on auscultation with audible or loud sounds, high-pitched or tinkling, and is characteristic of small bowel obstruction. The bowel sounds, unless the small bowel is also obstructed, are usually normal in large bowel obstruction.

Investigation

The mandatory investigation is a plain abdominal X-ray taken with the patient in the erect and the supine positions, although the supine film is usually sufficient. The erect film outlines horizontal levels between gas and fluid contents which are multiple and centrally placed in small bowel obstruction, disposed in a step-ladder pattern (Fig. 26.1).

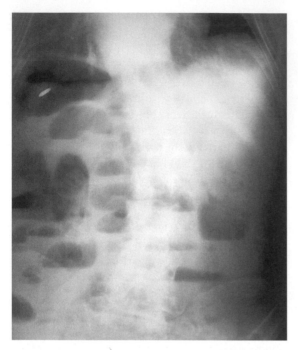

Fig. 26.1 *Plain erect abdominal radiograph of small bowel intestinal obstruction showing the step-ladder patterns. The more the number of fluid levels, the more distal the level of obstruction.*

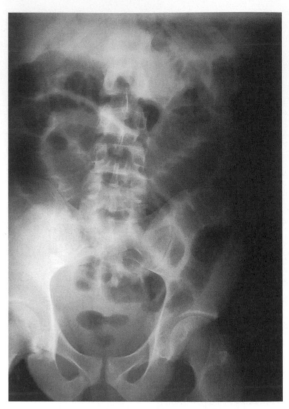

Fig. 26.2 *Plain supine abdominal X-ray of small bowel intestinal obstruction showing gaseous distention. The appearance of parallel soft-tissue lines that cross the lumen completely are features of small bowel obstruction.*

In large bowel obstruction these are fewer and lie in the periphery. The supine film differentiates small from large bowel obstruction by the gaseous outline of the bowel. Dilated jejunum is recognized by its mucosal folds (*valvulae conniventes*) which appear as parallel soft tissue straight lines which completely cross the lumen (Fig. 26.2). The dilated ileum is featureless, whereas in the obstructed colon the haustrations only partially traverse the lumen and draw in the line of the wall (Fig. 26.3). Distension of the caecum is a particularly helpful feature. When the ileo-caecal valve is incompetent, the raised pressure in the obstructed large bowel is transmitted to the small bowel which also appears distended. In the bowel distal to the obstruction there is little or no gas, depending on the level and the degree of obstruction.

Although sigmoid volvulus is rarely seen its radiological appearances must be recognized. A plain abdominal X-ray shows a single grossly dilated sigmoid loop with a characteristic inverted 'U' of bowel gas that occupies the pelvis and reaches the upper abdomen with fluid levels in the two bowel limbs (Fig. 26.4).

A contrast study is unnecessary in small intestinal obstruction as it will not add to the information obtained from a plain film, but a contrast enema is mandatory in large bowel obstruction. Occasionally, in doubtful cases, particularly when the nature of the obstruction cannot be determined, a free flow of the contrast without a hold up distinguishes between adynamic and partial mechanical obstruction. Barium sulphate is avoided as it insipissates within the bowel and converts an incomplete to a complete obstruction. A water-soluble contrast is preferable and should be isotonic as a hypertonic solution causes pulmonary oedema if inhaled.

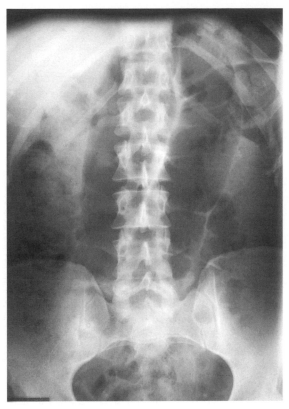

Fig. 26.3 *Plain supine abdominal X-ray of large bowel intestinal obstruction. The haustrations only partially traverse the lumen and distinguish colonic dilatation.*

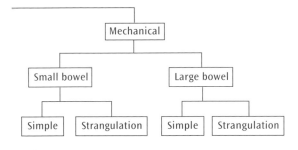

SIMPLE OR STRANGULATION?

Simple obstruction defines a mechanical obstruction to the lumen of the bowel with normal tissue perfusion. Strangulation occurs when, in addition to luminal obstruction, the venous drainage is impeded, when a loop becomes trapped by fibrous bands or adhesions or passes through an omental or mesenteric

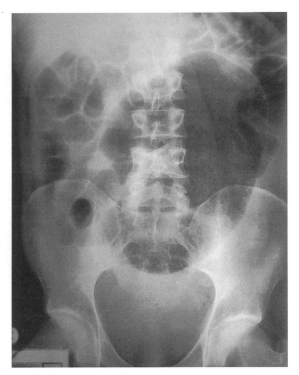

Fig. 26.4 *Plain supine abdominal X-ray of a patient with sigmoid volvulus.*

defect or when a loop twists on its mesentery (*volvulus*). The veins are constricted first because the venous pressure is lower than the arterial, and the resultant high capillary pressure leads to protein-rich transudate into the tissues causing oedema of the bowel wall. Later, the arterial inflow is impeded causing gangrene.

When complicated by strangulation the symptoms and signs of mechanical obstruction are sudden and pronounced. A continuous pain or dull ache persists between the episodes of colic and is localized to the region of the affected bowel. Localized abdominal tenderness does not feature in uncomplicated bowel obstruction, and when present is usually due to distension of the closed loop. However, guarding, absence of bowel sounds and tachycardia are ominous signs of strangulation which should be recognized before bowel necrosis and peritonitis set in.

Strangulation most commonly occurs when small bowel is caught within a hernia (inguinal, femoral umbilical or incisional). The hernia is tense and tender and lacks a cough impulse, but these signs are not necessarily indicative of obstruction as at times a portion of omentum or part of the bowel circumference is contained within the hernial sac while the bowel lumen remains patent (*Richter's hernia*).

Serial haematocrit estimations show a sharper rise with strangulation because sequestration of protein-rich liquid in the bowel and its tissues add an effective plasma loss to the saline loss from vomiting. A raised white cell count is suggestive of bowel ischaemia. On an abdominal X-ray a strangulated loop may appear as a single dilated gas-filled loop.

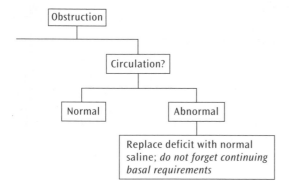

CIRCULATORY DISTURBANCE?

Fluid depletion because of vomiting, diminished oral intake and sequestration of fluid in the small bowel leads to dehydration. This is manifest clinically by dryness of the mouth, loss of skin turgor and elasticity, tachycardia and diminished urine output. In severe cases or when complicated with perforation and peritonitis, peripheral circulatory collapse (shock) develops, the patient is sweaty, cold and clammy, the pulse is feeble or absent and the blood pressure is low or irrecordable. These are clinical observations in a patient with suspected intestinal obstruction.

MANAGEMENT

The essentials are to recognize intestinal obstruction, determine whether it is mechanical or paralytic, decide whether strangulation is present and assess the state of hydration.

Irrespective of the underlying cause, except for a strangulated hernia which demands expedient surgical intervention, the initial management strategy is the same. During evaluation, previous abdominal operations, radiotherapy, intestinal symptoms, altered bowel habit or rectal bleeding, weight loss and a palpable abdominal mass may provide some relevant clues.

The principles of treatment are to decompress the obstructed bowel, replace fluid and electrolyte losses and, in selected cases, to undertake surgical treatment. Decompression is achieved by discontinuing oral intake, inserting a naso-gastric tube and aspirating the gastric contents in order to control nausea and vomiting, remove swallowed air and reduce gaseous distension and the risk of inhalation of gastric contents. The tube is left draining into a bag. The volumes of aspirate are used in estimating the fluid and electrolyte requirements as they need replacing with an equal volume of normal saline and as an indirect measure of recovery as the volumes diminish. The main losses are water, sodium and chloride which are replaced with isotonic saline, and (mostly) 5% dextrose for replacing normal losses through the skin and lungs.

Paralytic ileus

This is a transient cessation of peristalsis, due to handling and exposure of the intestine, that commonly follows abdominal surgery and is then regarded as physiological. The small bowel recovers within hours, followed by the colon in 3–5 days, but the bowel sounds, indicative of resolution of the ileus, are not present until the stomach, which recovers in 2–3 days, allows swallowed air into the small bowel. This is one of the reasons for restricting oral intake in the post-operative days. Other causes of paralytic ileus are intra-abdominal sepsis, retroperitoneal inflammation or haematoma from renal injuries, acute pancreatitis, ruptured abdominal aneurysms and spinal injuries.

Ileus normally resolves within a few days but when it is prolonged, signs of sepsis such as pyrexia, tachycardia, abdominal tenderness and guarding, or a pelvic collection elicited by rectal and/or vaginal examination should be sought. An ultrasound or preferably a CT scan to rule out an intra-abdominal or a pelvic collection is an essential diagnostic and therapeutic tool as it allows guided percutaneous drainage. Opiates inhibit gastric emptying and should be withheld. A high urea and hyperkalaemia may aggravate any disturbance in intestinal motility and should be estimated regularly and corrected. Conservative treatment is continued and intravenous feeding instituted promptly in order to maintain the patient's nutritional status as recovery can be slow.

It is crucial to realize that fibrinous adhesions may precipitate mechanical obstruction in the early post-operative period and this should not be confused with ileus. Clinical differentiation is usually easy to make, but in doubtful cases a water-soluble contrast study can be helpful. Although conservative treatment is frequently successful, re-exploration may be required.

Simple small bowel obstruction

In the absence of signs of strangulation, conservative measures already described are instituted. Deflation of the bowel proximal to the block minimizes the risk of perforation and can also cure some cases. When the obstruction is due to kinking of a loop of bowel by an adhesion or an inflammatory process to some fixed point (e.g., the anterior abdominal wall), distension of the proximal loop increases the kinking and perpetuates the obstruction; deflation of the proximal loop may straighten the bowel, thereby relieving the obstruction. After a suitable period, usually at least 4 hours, on conservative treatment and preferably earlier when the progression of the symptoms and signs is rapid, the patient is reassessed. Unless pain and vomiting are improving, the naso-gastric aspirate is diminishing and the abdomen is less distended, or if on the other hand, there is abdominal tenderness and guarding, a laparotomy is indicated. Otherwise, the patient is reviewed daily and treatment is continued, provided there is demonstrable clinical and radiological improvement. Whilst the decision between continuing with conservative management and surgical

intervention can be difficult, it is safer to err on the side of a laparotomy, particularly if the patient has not had a previous abdominal operation. However, if there is a scar from a previous laparotomy, adhesion obstruction is the most likely cause and the conservative approach often succeeds. A similar approach applies to obstruction from Crohn's disease as is described later.

Laparotomy

A collapsed loop of small bowel is traced proximally to the site of obstruction, which may be outside the wall, in the wall, or within the lumen of the bowel (Table 26.1).

Lesion outside the wall

Fibrous bands and adhesions are divided, bowel trapped in an omental or mesenteric defect is reduced, a volvulus is untwisted and the defect closed. The involved segment of bowel is inspected for direct or ischaemic damage and is resected if not viable (Chapter 10).

Lesion in the wall

This is a stricture more often than a tumour, commonly in the ileum complicating Crohn's or irradiation enteritis. The affected segment of bowel

Table 26.1 *Causes of mechanical obstruction*

Extra-mural
  adhesions, bands
  herniae: external and internal (peritoneal folds)
  volvulus
  compression by tumour, peritoneal and nodal
    deposits
Intra-mural
  inflammatory disease: Crohn's disease
  tumours: carcinomas, lymphomas, etc.
  strictures: post-irradiation
Intra-luminal
  swallowed foreign bodies
  bezoars
  gallstones
  faecal impaction

is resected with immediate restitution of the continuity by end-to-end anastomosis. A primary anastomosis is safe in an obstructed small bowel because of its rich blood supply.

Lesion in the lumen

This can be a swallowed object in the mentally subnormal, a gallstone eroding through the duodenum, known as *gallstone ileus*, or *orange pith* in individuals who previously had a gastrectomy. It may be possible to fragment a soft obstructing object by pinching it from outside or else it is milked distally into the large intestine, although as the ileum narrows large objects are easier to milk proximally into the jejunum and removed through an enterotomy rather than through its site of impaction where the bowel wall can be oedematous and friable.

The proximal bowel, when distended, is decompressed by gently milking the contents in the intestine proximally into the stomach, whence the anaesthetist drains it by aspiration via the naso-gastric tube. Sometimes this may not be sufficient and the contents have to be emptied by suction through an enterotomy, carefully avoiding spillage and contamination. This facilitates closing the abdomen, reduces the risk of vomiting and inhalation, particularly at the time of extubation, and probably lessens the tendency to post-operative ileus. Post-operatively, the naso-gastric tube is left in place until recovery is complete as indicated by minimal aspirates, resolution of abdominal distension, return of normal bowel sounds and passage of flatus and faeces.

Simple large bowel obstruction

There is no place for a conservative approach in mechanical obstruction of the large bowel and early decompression is the first line of treatment. A naso-gastric tube is unnecessary and is ineffective unless there are also clinical or radiological signs of small bowel obstruction. The urgency is even greater when the right iliac fossa is tender, indicative of impending or established caecal perforation. A disposable phosphate enema clears the bowel for a better clinical and radiological interpretation of the

findings. It sometimes relieves the obstruction by dislodging stool at any area of narrowing or in the case of impacted stool in a constipated patient. Digital palpation and sigmoidoscopy should always be carried out and if this fails to identify an obstructing lesion, should be followed with a water-soluble contrast enema in order to locate the site of obstruction and exclude pseudo-obstruction. A free flow of contrast and absence of a colonic pathology favours pseudo-obstruction and avoids an unnecessary laparotomy.

Pseudo-obstruction is a functional obstruction usually encountered in elderly patients with severe associated systemic disorders, for example cardiac, respiratory, renal, hepatic or neurological, who are on a variety of medications. There is no specific treatment other than to treat the primary underlying condition, restrict oral intake and maintain the patient's nutrition by enteral or intravenous feeding until spontaneous resolution. Colonoscopy is often effective in decompressing the colon by sucking out gas and fluid. When not available, this could be attempted by sigmoidoscopy or flatus tube. An urgent caecostomy may be required if the caecum is distended and tender.

When the clinical and radiological appearances are suggestive of a sigmoid volvulus, passing a sigmoidoscope as far as possible successfully decompresses the bowel and relieves the obstruction. A flatus tube inserted through the sigmoidoscope sometimes may aid deflating the colon, and it is left for 24 hours to maintain decompression. If these measures fail then *sigmoid colectomy* is performed, bringing the divided ends of the bowel on to the abdominal wall to form a double-barrelled colostomy, to avoid the risk of a primary anastomosis in dilated, oedematous and unprepared colon.

Resection of the obstructing lesion and restoration of bowel continuity by end-to-end anastomosis is safely carried out in right-sided obstruction, usually due to a carcinoma, but lesions in the left colon, commonly a carcinoma or a diverticular mass in the recto-sigmoid region, require careful planning.

A proximal diverting transverse loop colostomy to decompress the bowel, although the simplest option, leaves behind the primary pathology and carries a higher morbidity and related mortality than resection. It can be considered in the high-risk patient who may not withstand a prolonged anaesthetic, but resection is the favoured approach. A primary anastomosis is usually avoided unless the colon is not grossly dilated or loaded with faeces. Per-operative irrigation of the colon with water through an enterotomy in the terminal ileum or through the appendix stump, the effluent being drained into a container via a large tube placed above the obstructing lesion, cleanses the colon to allow primary anastomosis. However, it prolongs the procedure which is an important consideration in the unfit patient. A proximal colostomy will safeguard against the morbidity of an anastomotic leak in these situations. Alternatively, the proximal end is brought out as a terminal colostomy and the distal stump is closed (*Hartmann's operation*). However, this will entail another laparotomy in the future to restore bowel continuity, usually not before 3 months, and preferably after a longer interval.

Strangulation

The clinical features of small bowel strangulation in a hernia or within the abdominal cavity have already been described. When present, resuscitation and surgical intervention must be prompt before irreversable ischaemic damage to the bowel occurs. In large bowel obstruction, except for sigmoid volvulus and rarely caecal volvulus, dilatation, pain and tenderness in the region of the caecum are indications of a similar urgency.

Circulatory disturbance

No patient should be submitted to a general anaesthetic before the circulatory state is optimized. The repletion of the body fluids should precede the operative management described above. Besides the clinical parameters, essential investigations are haemoglobin, haematocrit (PCV), urea and electrolytes. The haemoglobin and the PCV are elevated because of haemoconcentration. A raised blood urea is the result of diminished renal perfusion due to hypovolaemia. The plasma Na^+ concentration is not reliable as an index of extra-cellular depletion because the extracellular space shrinks but the osmoreceptors maintain normal sodium concentration.

The early recognition of strangulation is sometimes simplified by analysis of the circulatory depletion. In a patient with haemo-concentration due to loss of plasma or saline from the circulation, the proportionate reduction in plasma volume can be indirectly measured from the change of haematocrit value (PCV) assuming that the red cell mass remains constant. When H_1 is the normal haematocrit (decimalwise) and H_2 the observed haematocrit in the hypovolaemic state, the fall in plasma volume (expressed as percentage of original) $= 100 \, [1 - (H_1/(100 - H_1) \times (100 - H_2))/H_2]$. Thus, if $H_1 = 0.45$ and $H_2 = 0.52$, the percentage fall in plasma volume is $100 \, [1 - (0.45/0.55 \times 0.48)/0.52]$ or 24%.

In most cases, a 1% rise in the haematocrit corresponds to a fall in plasma volume of approximately 4%.

The average adult's plasma volume is 3 l. The fall in plasma volume in the example given is, therefore, about 720 ml. This might be a direct loss from the vascular compartment of 720 ml plasma. The same fall in plasma volume from pure loss of saline depleting the whole extra-cellular compartment would be five times this volume (since the extra-cellular compartment is normally about 15 l, that is, five times the plasma volume), thus approaching 4 l.

In the absence of gross dilatation and vomiting, it is more likely that the loss is plasma than saline, and would suggest obstruction with strangulation.

The haematocrit estimation, in providing a measure of the volume and nature of the fluid requirements in a hypovolaemic patient (not from blood loss) is underutilized. Measurements that are essential during fluid replacement in these patients are the pulse and blood pressure, input and output fluid charts, urine output, central venous pressure, particularly in the elderly patient, and regular urea and electrolyte estimations.

PARTICULAR PROBLEMS

Recurrent adhesive small bowel obstruction

Division of adhesions (*enterolysis*) should be avoided even when a patient presents with repeated obstruction, unless an acute episode fails to respond to conservative treatment since adhesions reform. Furthermore, there is risk of inadvertent and unrecognized injury to the bowel which is associated with considerable morbidity due to sepsis and fistula formation. However, it is unavoidable when obstruction occurs at frequent and short intervals, and the patient must be cautioned about these risks. In patients who had a laparotomy for malignancy the possibility that tumour recurrence, usually nodal deposits, rather than adhesions is the cause must be considered and investigated with an abdominal CT scan.

Small bowel obstruction without previous laparotomy

The groins must always be examined since a common cause of small bowel obstruction is a strangulated external hernia. A femoral hernia in particular, unlike an inguinal hernia, rarely causes local symptoms and signs, is usually small and is easily overlooked, especially in obese patients.

Crohn's disease previously diagnosed or when suspected because of a history of abdominal pain, diarrhoea and weight loss prior to the acute presentation, accompanied by leucocytosis and a raised erythrocyte sedimentation rate and C-reactive protein, needs careful management. Intravenous antibiotics and steroids reduce the inflammation and shrink the oedema in the diseased small bowel with resolution of the obstruction. However, this may fail, particularly if the inflammatory markers are not raised because the obstruction then is probably due to a fibrotic stricture more likely in those with chronic disease, and a laparotomy and resection of the diseased segment are indicated.

Intestinal obstruction with an abdominal mass

An abdominal mass, either inflammatory or neoplastic, can cause intestinal obstruction. Unless of substantial size, with gross abdominal distension, it may not be easily palpable. Distinction is made by the presence of systemic and local signs of sepsis, that is, temperature, tachycardia, abdominal tenderness and guarding. A CT scan may show distinctive appearances. A neoplastic lesion is usually a colonic carcinoma, whereas common inflammatory lesions are ileo-caecal Crohn's disease and sigmoid diverticulitis. Initial treatment with antibiotics may diminish the inflammatory process with resolution of the obstruction, whilst intervention is unavoidable when a mass is neoplastic.

Acute bowel ischaemia

This is due to occlusion of the mesenteric vessels, commonly the superior mesenteric artery by a thrombus, or an embolus causing mid-gut ischaemia from the jejunum to the proximal transverse colon, and later infarction and perforation of the bowel. However, when a branch of the main vessel is occluded, the area of infarction is proportionally less. A thrombus readily develops in an already narrowed atherosclerotic vessel. An embolus originates from a left atrial thrombus in atrial fibrillation or from left ventricular wall thrombus following myocardial infarction. Thrombosis of the superior mesenteric vein or its tributaries occasionally occurs in portal hypertension, portal pyaemia, sickle cell disease and women on the pill. Irrespective of whether the occlusion is arterial or venous, haemorrhagic infarction occurs.

Small bowel

Acute bowel ischaemia should always be considered in the elderly with cardiovascular disease and in patients with fibrillation who present with sudden abdominal pain. It can be a difficult diagnosis at its onset when the severity of pain is disproportionate with the abdominal signs which are unremarkable. An abdominal X-ray usually shows no gas in the small intestine. Leucocytosis is suggestive but not diagnostic. When intestinal ischaemia is suspected a laparotomy is the only confirmatory test. It is unwise to wait until there are demonstrable signs. When the abdomen is distended and tender and the bowel sounds are absent, the bowel is already gangrenous.

At laparotomy, when only a short segment is gangrenous it is resected; however, frequently the situation is incurable if extensive resection is involved.

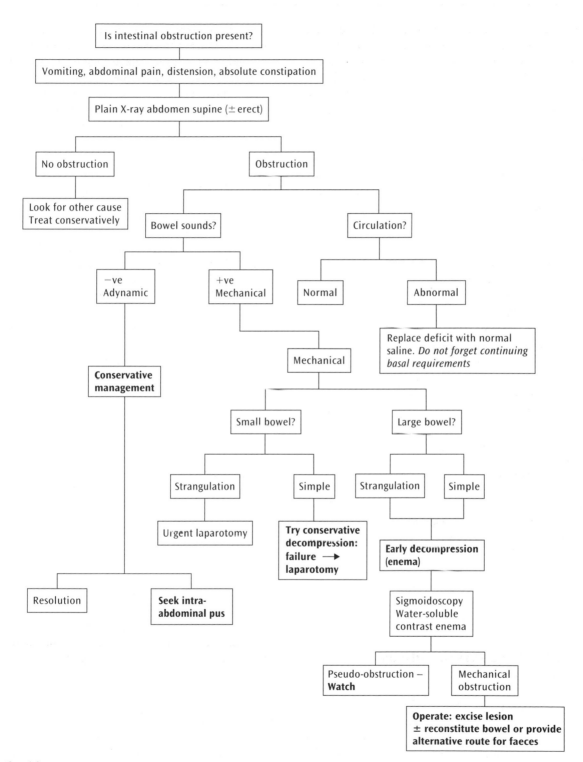

Algorithm 26.1

The ischaemic process can be progressive, hence when a primary anastomosis is carried out its viability is examined at a re-exploratory laparotomy 48–72 hours later. Alternatively, the bowel ends are brought out to the surface as an ileostomy and a mucous fistula. A secondary anastomosis is deferred until later. The plan of operative options depends on the patient's fitness to undergo more than one procedure. When the expertise is available, an attempt is made to improve the mesenteric arterial blood supply by embolectomy or a vascular bypass, although its benefit is debatable. In all cases blood transfusion and anticoagulation are required.

The result of extensive resection in those who survive is the short gut syndrome which carries a morbidity due to malabsorption and failure to thrive, although the availability of home parenteral nutrition has improved survival in these patients.

A variant of small bowel infarction is due to hypoperfusion in patients with chronic hypoxia secondary to pulmonary or heart disease or is a result of vasculitis in patients with connective tissue disease. The mesenteric vessels appear patent and pulsating. The ischaemia is confined and patchy. Resection with primary anastomosis and treatment of the primary cause offer these patients a better outcome.

Large bowel

Inferior mesenteric artery occlusion is less frequent and causes ischaemia in the left colon, especially in the region of the splenic flexure where the blood supply is precarious. The mucosa is particularly vulnerable to the slightest degree of ischaemia. Ulceration and sloughing of the mucosa causes rectal bleeding which is a constant feature in colonic ischaemia and can be the only symptom, without abdominal symptoms or signs. Colonoscopy shows a localized area of ulceration and oedema of the mucosa which heals rapidly once it recovers its blood supply and is not recognizable if the examination is delayed.

With severe ischaemia the full thickness of the bowel wall is involved; there is intra-mural haemorrhage, inflammation and oedema producing a clinical picture indistinguishable from acute diverticulitis or toxic dilatation due to inflammatory bowel disease or infective diarrhoea. The diagnosis can be difficult and is based on the presence of signs of cardiovascular disease, a negative microscopy and culture of the stools. Visualization of the colon by colonoscopy or barium studies can be hazardous and is avoided although a sigmoidoscopy is helpful to rule out pseudomembranous colitis and inflammatory bowel disease.

The tissue ischaemia may progress to infarction and peritonitis, otherwise it is followed by fibrous healing and stricture formation which may require resection.

HIGHLIGHTS

- A suspicion of intestinal obstruction is confirmed on a plain abdominal X-ray
- Barium sulphate should be avoided and a water-soluble contrast is used instead in investigating intestinal obstruction
- A contrast follow-through is rarely necessary in small bowel obstruction but a contrast enema is mandatory in large bowel obstruction to exclude pseudo-obstruction
- Absence of external hernias and abdominal scars and suspicion of strangulation increase the urgency for laparotomy
- Mechanical large bowel obstruction always requires a laparotomy

27

Acute abdomen and the urogenital tract

JULIAN SHAH AND ANTHONY R MUNDY

INTRODUCTION

An acute abdomen due to disorders of the genitourinary tract occurs in these situations:

- Trauma to the trunk.
- Renal pain.
- Bladder pain.
- Gynaecological disorders.
- Lower abdominal peritonitis.
- When gynaecological disorders are found at laparotomy.

TRAUMA

This has been discussed in Chapter 21.

LOIN PAIN – RENAL PAIN–URETERIC COLIC

Renal pain

Renal pain, felt in the thoracolumbar region between the lower ribs, the spine and the iliac crest (the *renal angle*) is caused by renal inflammation or stretching of the renal capsule.

Ureteric colic

Ureteric colic presents with a sudden onset of severe unilateral pain, maximal in the loin but also often radiating to the hypogastrium, groin, labium or scrotum and the upper thigh. Although due to exaggerated ureteric peristalsis, renal 'colic' is in half the cases continuous rather than intermittent and therefore not a typical colicky pain. Most patients are males (M:F 2:1). The patient is restless and writhes in agony, and the pain may be associated with nausea and vomiting. The patient may pass blood in the urine and develop dysuria, frequency and systemic symptoms if obstruction by stone is complicated by infection.

The distinction between renal pain and ureteric colic is, in practice, often blurred. *Renal conditions* can produce colic through blood or pus draining down the ureter, whereas a *calculus* completely blocking the ureter can produce renal pain by distension of the kidney. It is more appropriate to refer to the *renal pain–ureteric colic symptom complex.*

Diagnosis

Urine is collected for dipstick testing which usually confirms the diagnosis, as renal pain–ureteric colic nearly always is associated with microscopic haematuria. A mid-stream specimen of urine (MSU) is sent for microscopical analysis and culture. A sterile pyuria is characteristic of urinary stones, whereas bacteriuria without significant pyuria usually indicates contamination of the urine specimen.

The crucial investigation is an emergency intravenous urogram (IVU). A plain supine abdominal radiograph is followed with an injection of intravenous contrast and further films taken five and 20 minutes later. The plain X-ray is examined for the presence of an opacity in the line of the urinary tract (95% of stones are radio-opaque). Delayed excretion or dilatation indicates the side and site of the obstruction and demonstrates any structural abnormality. If there is no contrast on the side of the pain, delayed films are performed, generally at 1 hour and then at intervals afterwards for 24 hours.

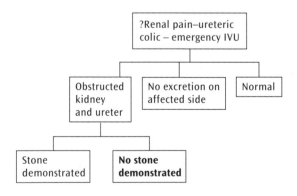

Obstruction without clear evidence of opacity can be due to a radiolucent stone or a blood clot resulting from slow bleeding from a lesion in the kidney or upper ureter. Suggestive features, such as a visible abnormality of the configuration of the pelvicalyceal system or proximal ureter, or frank (as distinct from microscopic) haematuria, require urgent further investigations. A pelvi-ureteric

junction obstruction, a sloughed renal papilla following necrotic changes due to predisposing diseases such as diabetes mellitus and sickle-cell disease, the loin pain/haematuria syndrome and poisoning with certain drugs such as phenacetin may also give symptoms and signs similar to ureteric obstruction.

A diagnostic dilemma can arise if the radiographic evidence of obstruction is limited to lack of excretion on the affected side. The failure of renal excretory function can be due to a renal vein thrombosis or to a unilateral reduction in renal artery flow as a result of asymmetric clot formation in an abdominal aortic aneurysm when renal colic precedes signs of shock due to aortic rupture.

Management of renal pain and colic

The immediate management is pain relief with nonsteroidal anti-inflammatory agents, most effectively achieved with diclofenac, 100 mg suppositories or injection. Rarely, when this is ineffective, pethidine 50–100 mg by intramuscular injection is required.

A normal fluid intake is maintained. There is no indication for increasing fluid intake 'to flush the stone out' because the stone may become wedged more tightly, thereby increasing the degree of obstruction. The temperature is monitored as fever signifies secondary infection which may lead to pyelonephritis or pyonephrosis (*see later*).

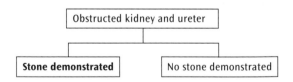

If the stone is less than 5 mm in diameter and is causing dilatation but without complete obstruction, the patient is afebrile and the pain is resolving, the patient can be allowed home and is seen in seven days with a repeat plain abdominal radiograph to assess the position of the stone. Nearly 80% of small stones that are moving down the urinary tract are likely to pass spontaneously within 48 hours. Larger stones, and those that fail to move, especially with evidence of obstruction, should be considered for removal. The indications for abandoning conservative management are persistence of pain, increasing obstruction of the upper urinary tract demonstrated by pelvicalyceal distension on ultrasound scan, and infection characterized by pyrexia, rigors and positive urine cultures. In these circumstances, immediate drainage of the kidney is required by placing a percutaneous nephrostomy tube under imaging control, or else by endoscopic removal of the stone or placement of a stent beside the stone to allow urinary drainage.

Methods of stone removal

The method for removing an impacted stone depends on the size, nature and site of the stone and the availability of expertise and special equipment. Open surgical procedures are rarely used though they may have to be considered if other methods are not available.

Stones in the kidney and in the upper and lower thirds of the ureter can be treated by extra-corporeal shock-wave lithotripsy (ESWL) in some specialized units. The shockwaves are externally generated and focused on the stone with the help of X-rays or ultrasound imaging. For renal stones greater than 2 cm in size, a double pig-tailed ureteric stent is inserted to prevent larger fragments obstructing the ureter and causing colic. Stones that lie over the pelvis or vertebral transverse processes are not suitable as they cannot be localized on fluoroscopy. Therefore, stones in the lower ureter, especially those within a short distance of the ureteric orifice, may have to be retrieved with a basket (*Dormia basket*) passed via a cystoscope or ureteroscope, or alternatively fragmented as described below.

Mid-ureteric stones are treated either by ureteroscopic manipulation into the kidney followed by destruction with shock-wave lithotripsy (*'push–bang'*) or percutaneous removal (*'push–pull'*), or alternatively by fragmenting the stone using a laser fibre or an external source of energy applied by a probe passed along the ureteroscope to the stone (*lithoclast*).

For stones in the renal pelvis which fail to break or are large, direct percutaneous access is obtained under local anaesthesia, using radiological control to place a guide wire into the renal pelvis. The track is dilated to accommodate a nephroscope. The stone is grasped with a forceps, and if large it is fragmented using an ultrasonic lithotrite, and the fragments are extracted. A nephrostomy tube is removed after 48 hours and the track is allowed to close spontaneously.

Open surgery is required when minimal access methods are not available, or correction of an anatomical abnormality which predisposes to stone formation is required, for example pelvi-ureteric obstruction or ureteric stricture, or when the stone is large occupying the pelvis and the collecting system (*staghorn calculus*). For the pelvicalyceal system a nephro- or pyelolithotomy, for the ureter a ureterolithotomy is performed.

When the stone is recovered, either by the patient who has been instructed to sieve the urine or by surgical retrieval, a plain abdominal X-ray (if the stone was radio-opaque) is repeated to ensure that a complete stone has passed, and the stone is sent for biochemical investigation.

Investigation and management of aetiological factors

The chemical nature of the calculus influences management since the patients have a demonstrable metabolic cause. Therefore, every patient should be fully investigated following a first attack by serum analysis of creatinine, urea, electrolytes, calcium and phosphate, urates, proteins and alkaline phosphatase. Blood for serum calcium measurements should be taken after an overnight fast and without a tourniquet. A 24-hour urine is collected for calcium.

Causes of urinary stones:

- Unknown.
- Oxaluria.
- Hypercalciuria, idiopathic or due to raised ionized plasma calcium.
- Cystinuria.
- Urate.
- Phosphate (infection → alkaline).

Cystine stones (2%), although rare, draw attention to an inborn error of the metabolism of cystine. *Urate stones* (8%), like cystine stones, are only relatively insoluble, and recurrences can be reduced by increasing the intake of liquids and alkalinizing the urine using sodium bicarbonate. In hyperuricaemic patients (*gout*) and during chemotherapy for leukaemia, allopurinol is given. Allopurinol inhibits xanthine oxidase, an enzyme involved in the synthesis of uric acid.

Most ureteric calculi consist of *calcium oxalate* (45%), due to *idiopathic hypercalciuria* which is the underlying cause in two-thirds of patients and the sole cause in half of all male stone-formers. The 24-hour urinary output of calcium is high, with normal serum calcium and phosphate levels. Other aetiological factors of calcium oxalate stones are hyperparathyroidism and hyperoxaluria. Oxalate stones may be associated with *hyperoxaluria*, although in most patients there is no demonstrable disorder of oxalate metabolism and dietary restriction does not produce any therapeutic benefit. Increase in the dietary intake of liquids and reduction in dietary calcium may help to reduce the incidence of recurrence in approximately 75% of patients.

Calcium, magnesium ammonium phosphate (triple phosphate) stones, the second most frequent abnormality (15%) are usually associated with urinary tract infection, in particular with Proteus and other urea-splitting organisms that produce ammonia rendering the urine alkaline. These stones are more common in females and usually form within the kidney (staghorn calculus) or in association with abnormalities in the urinary tract such as reflux from the bladder and pelvi-ureteric obstruction.

Mixed calcium oxalate and phosphate stones (15%) and *calcium phosphate stones* (15%) are due to disorders associated with hypercalcaemia and require treatment of the primary cause.

Hyperparathyroidism

This is a rare (2–5%) but important cause of ureteric calculi. *Primary hyperparathyroidism* is commonly due to a parathyroid adenoma or to hyperplasia, and rarely to a parathyroid carcinoma which results in excess production of parathyroid hormone and increased plasma calcium concentration and urinary calcium excretion. Calcium in the plasma is present in ionized form, and in a non-ionized form bound to plasma proteins. Taking the venous sample without stasis and in the fasting, resting state are measures intended to stabilize the plasma protein

concentration and limit the release of calcium from engorged tissues, in order to avoid an erroneous result. The calcium concentration measured, normally 2.25–2.6 mmol/l, must be corrected for deviation in plasma protein concentration from the normal range. Any elevation should be confirmed on two subsequent occasions and, if combined with elevated parathyroid hormone, the diagnosis is almost certain.

Primary hyperparathyroidism may be part of the *multiple endocrine neoplasia* (MEN) syndromes, which may occur sequentially rather than synchronously (*see* Table 27.1).

Secondary hyperparathyroidism is characterized by hyperplasia of the glands secondary to chronic renal failure and impairment of calcium absorption due to failure of the renal parenchyma to convert 25-hydroxycholecalciferol to 1-25 dehydroxycholecalciferol. The output of parathyroid hormone increases, thereby mobilizing bone calcium and reducing urinary excretion in an attempt to maintain normal serum calcium levels; hence serum calcium levels remain low.

Tertiary hyperparathyroidism is a complication of prolonged secondary hyperparathyroidism. The parathyroid hyperplasia fails to regress after treating the underlying cause by renal transplantation. The glands become autonomous and no longer responsive to the negative feed-back stimulus of a rising serum calcium level.

The common clinical features in primary hyperparathyroidism are renal calculi and/or renal

Table 27.1 *Multiple endocrine neoplasia (MEN) syndromes*

MEN I
islet cell tumour of pancreas
pituitary tumour
parathyroid hyperplasia
MEN IIa
phaeochromocytoma
medullary carcinoma of the thyroid
parathyroid adenoma
MEN IIb
phaeochromocytoma
medullary carcinoma of the thyroid
mucosal neuromas and ganglioneuroma

calcification, bone pain and deformity, and pathological fractures due to decalcification and cystic degeneration. The depressive effect of hypercalcaemia on nerve conduction manifests as muscular weakness, anorexia and intestinal atony. Polyuria is not uncommon. Peptic ulcer and acute and chronic pancreatitis are common. Psychiatric disorders may occur.

Other causes of hypercalcaemia (*see below*) should be considered before making a diagnosis of hyperparathyroidism. The cortisone suppression test (150 mg daily for 10 days) restores serum calcium in patients with sarcoidosis, thyrotoxicosis, hypervitaminosis D or bone metastases. The test can be useful when the serum calcium and parathyroid hormone levels are equivocal. The parathyroid glands can be imaged with high-resolution ultrasound, computed tomography (CT) or magnetic resonance imaging (MRI). Dual isotope-scanning using thallium-201 to outline both thyroid and parathyroids, and sodium pertechnetate (^{99m}Tc) or iodine as a subtraction marker for the thyroid, provides useful information.

Causes of hypercalcaemia:

- Hyperparathyroidism.
- Bone metastases.
- Multiple myeloma.
- Paget's disease of bone.
- Sarcoidosis.
- Hypervitaminosis D.
- Milk-alkali syndrome.
- Drugs (thiazides).
- Hyperthyroidism.

Primary hyperparathyroidism is treated surgically. All glands must be identified. An adenoma is present if one of the glands is larger than the others, and it is removed. If no gland is disproportionately enlarged, enough parathyroid tissue is removed to lower the parathyroid hormone level to normal but enough is retained to maintain calcium homeostasis. Repeated examination by frozen section of biopsy material may be required during the operation.

Failure to find an adenoma or hyperplasia entails repeating the investigations. Selective vein catheterization and digital subtraction arteriography are reserved for localizing the parathyroids in patients who have undergone an unsuccessful surgical exploration.

LOIN PAIN – RENAL PAIN–URETERIC COLIC WITH FEVER

Pyelonephritis

This can be an early presentation. Apart from a ureteric calculus, predisposing factors include vesicoureteric reflux; obstruction, either congenital at the pelvi-ureteric junction or acquired, as in urethral strictures; anatomical as in females due to the short length of the urethra and bacterial colonization of the urinary tract; neurogenic bladder dysfunction leading to high intra-vesical pressure and back pressure on the upper urinary tract; and diabetes mellitus.

Loin pain, pyrexia, rigors and dysuria, malaise and anorexia are the classical features. Physical examination often elicits significant tenderness in the costo-vertebral angle.

The most common causative organisms are aerobic Gram-negative bacteria, usually *E. coli*, *Proteus mirabilis* and Klebsiella. They are urea-splitting organisms that release ammonia and render the urine alkaline, leading to the formation of stones. Laboratory findings include a marked leucocytosis, urinalysis showing pyuria, bacteriuria and microscopic haematuria.

An IVU shows an enlarged renal outline and faint nephrogram because of impaired renal concentration, but poor excretion that may not distinctly define obstruction. An ultrasound scan may better define any dilatation of the collecting system due to obstruction, and the presence of renal stones or a renal abscess. Other specialized investigations may be required to identify other causes mentioned above.

The management in the presence of obstruction by a stone has been described earlier. Otherwise, treatment consists of intravenous antibiotic therapy according to the culture and sensitivity until the patient is apyrexial, followed by a 2-week course of oral antibiotics.

Renal abscess

This condition is also characterized by pyrexia, rigors, and loin pain and tenderness. It can complicate pyelonephritis, in which case the patient has a history of urinary tract infection, obstruction or calculus and the abscess involves both cortex and medulla and is multifocal. However, it may also result from haematogenous spread from skin lesions or infection introduced by intravenous drug abuse, when the onset is abrupt and there is no bacteriuria. The common organism in haematogenous spread is *Staphylococcus aureus*. This type of abscess is known as a *renal carbuncle*, and affects the renal cortex.

An abscess is best defined by an ultrasound scan, although a CT or MR scan may be needed to distinguish a renal abscess from a renal tumour. Treatment is by percutaneous drainage under imaging control combined with intravenous therapy; if unsuccessful, open drainage or nephrectomy may be required.

EMERGENCY IVU IS NORMAL

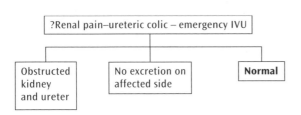

If the IVU is normal other causes must be sought. Ultrasonography of the kidneys is helpful in demonstrating the presence or absence of a pelvicalyceal or ureteric dilatation, stones or other abnormalities such as small tumours or a blood clot that can give rise to renal pain. In the absence of any abnormality it can be assumed that a small calculus may have passed, especially if the urine contained red blood cells.

When the diagnosis of renal pain–ureteric colic cannot be substantiated, other causes must be considered, including acute appendicitis, acute pancreatitis, acute cholecystitis and pelvic inflammatory disease in women. Biliary tract pain is particularly confusing as it may be referred to the thoraco-lumbar region, and especially if the area of abdominal tenderness is more lateral in the sub-costal area than usual.

A posterior duodenal ulcer or pancreatitis can also cause pain in the lumbar region. An aortic aneurysm, particularly if the ureter is compressed, has been already mentioned. Degenerative disease, disc prolapse and infective metastatic malignant disease of the spine may simulate renal pain. Pre-herpetic pain of the lower thoracic roots is associated with hyperaesthesia before the herpetic eruptions appear 36–48 hours later.

The clinical history and findings, with an ultrasound or a CT-scan, should enable the true diagnosis to be reached.

SUPRA-PUBIC – BLADDER PAIN

Pain and tenderness confined to the supra-pubic region are likely to originate in the bladder, especially if there are voiding symptoms, that is, dysuria, frequency, urgency and haematuria. There may be an accompanying low back pain. Pyrexia is infrequent.

The clinical picture is due to an *acute cystitis* with coliform bacteria; it is caused by ascending infection, commonly in the female because of the shortness of the female urethra and colonization of the perineum and vaginal orifice with intestinal flora. Sexual intercourse is also a precipitating factor. Non-infective cystitis may be secondary to radiotherapy and chemotherapy.

A *bladder calculus* can also be an underlying cause for cystitis. Bladder calculi usually arise in the bladder, but a few are renal calculi which have deposited in the bladder and grow in size. Bladder outlet obstruction, foreign bodies and bladder diverticulum are other predisposing factors.

The white cell count may be raised and urinalysis usually shows pyuria and bacteriuria with microhaematuria. Culture of the urine identifies the infecting organism. A bladder calculus shows in a plain X-ray, or as a filling defect on an IVU.

Treatment is with the appropriate antibiotic. Cystoscopy is required if frank haematuria is present and is performed after the infection has been treated, when lithotripsy can also be carried out if a stone is present.

Conditions such as acute appendicitis, diverticulitis and Crohn's disease, and in females pelvic inflammatory disease, can, through local inflammatory adhesions, mimic the symptoms of cystitis.

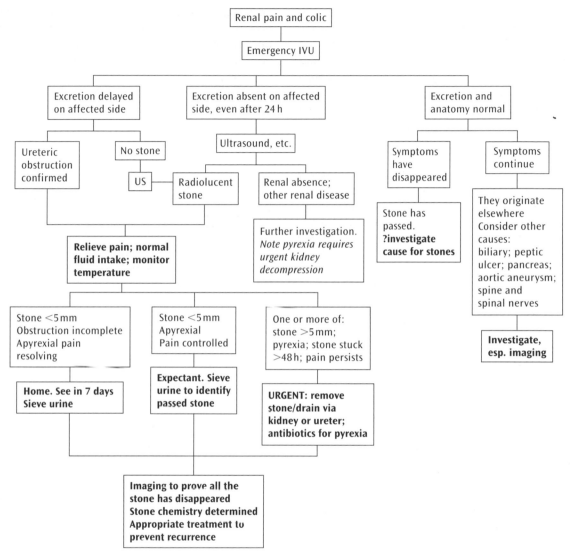

Algorithm 27.1

GYNAECOLOGICAL DISORDERS

Acute abdomen: features suggesting gynaecological origin:

- History of menstrual disturbance.
- Signs: mass on vaginal examination; pus, blood from cervix; tenderness on bi-manual pelvic examination.

- Shock with lower abdominal peritonitis, especially with shoulder-tip pain.

The common gynaecological conditions that present with low acute abdominal pain are acute salpingitis, ruptured ovarian follicle, ectopic pregnancy, twisted ovarian cyst, and torsion or degeneration of a uterine fibroid.

Acute salpingitis

The onset of symptoms usually follows a history of a recent abortion or delivery, an intrauterine device or sexual promiscuity. A vaginal discharge, menstrual irregularity, dysmenorrhoea, dyspareunia and frequency of micturition with burning pain are helpful features. On abdominal examination, maximal tenderness is just above the inguinal ligaments and is usually bilateral. On vaginal examination there is marked adnexal tenderness and moving the cervix from side to side induces pain (*cervical excitation*).

Investigations include the white cell count, a high vaginal swab and urine specimens for microscopy and culture. An ultrasound outlines the abnormality, and if equivocal then a laparoscopy is advised.

Salpingitis is effectively treated with intravenous antibiotics, but infertility is a likely sequel.

Ectopic pregnancy

Tubal pregnancy or tubal abortion causes pain in either iliac fossa. When right-sided, the pain can be mistaken for acute appendicitis. There is a history of a missed period. Very occasionally the patient may remember that the pain commenced on one side; and it is severe. In tubal abortion, intermittent vaginal bleeding may have occurred and the patient may have experienced faintness.

On examination, the pulse may be normal, there is tenderness in one or both iliac fossae or, when there is sufficient blood in the peritoneal cavity, in the whole lower abdomen. The cervix is softer than normal, severe pain is felt when it is moved, and tenderness and/or a mass is palpable in the fornix on the side involved. The signs of intra-peritoneal bleeding may not be obvious until the haemorrhage is considerable, when the clinical signs are unmistakable. At an earlier stage, raising the foot of the bed produces the typical shoulder-tip pain of blood in the peritoneal cavity due to sub-diaphragmatic irritation.

When the patient is in shock a laparotomy is required; otherwise, the diagnosis is based on a positive pregnancy test and ultrasound examination of the pelvis. Laparoscopy confirms the diagnosis and provides therapeutic access with preservation of the tube unless it is unsalvageable. If the facilities or the expertise for laparoscopy are not available, laparotomy is carried out.

Twisted ovarian cyst

This presents with sudden and severe pain and vomiting, symptoms like appendicitis, although the pain is often referred to the loin and is made worse when the patient rolls over. The temperature is normal but the pulse is fast. A tender mobile mass may or may not be palpable on vaginal or pelvic examination.

An ultrasound scan is diagnostic. Laparoscopy confirms the diagnosis and provides access for excision of the cyst or of the ovary itself if unsalvageable, or if there is doubt of malignancy or the patient is post-menopausal. When the facilities or expertise for minimally invasive surgery are not available, laparotomy is performed.

Ruptured ovarian follicle (syn. *mittelschmerz*)

The pain occurs in mid-cycle, commonly in early womanhood. It is acute in onset and can be confused with ectopic pregnancy, but there is no history of a missed period and the sign of a soft cervix is absent. When right-sided the symptoms are like acute appendicitis.

The abdominal signs are not distinctive. An ultrasound shows a normal appendix and normal pelvic viscera and the diagnosis relies on the finding of a ruptured cyst or other cysts and there is usually free fluid in the pouch of Douglas.

Torsion or degeneration of a uterine fibroid

The symptoms and clinical findings are similar to the above. The finding of an enlarged fibroid uterus on vaginal examination is suggestive but it must be remembered that fibroids can be coincidental with other causes of the acute abdomen. The diagnosis is based on an ultrasound scan and laparoscopy.

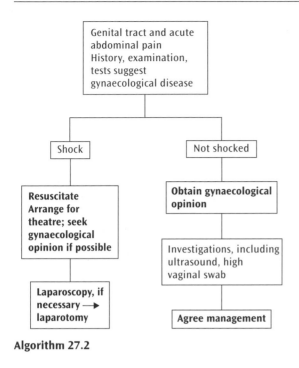

Genital tract and acute
abdominal pain
History, examination,
tests suggest
gynaecological disease

Shock

Not shocked

**Resuscitate
Arrange for
theatre; seek
gynaecological
opinion if possible**

**Obtain gynaecological
opinion**

Investigations, including
ultrasound, high
vaginal swab

**Laparoscopy, if
necessary** →
laparotomy

Agree management

Algorithm 27.2

LOWER ABDOMINAL PERITONITIS AND THE GENITOURINARY TRACT

Lower abdominal pain in the supra-pubic area and the iliac fossae with tenderness and urinary symptoms may occur in association with acute intra-abdominal conditions outside the urinary tract. Voiding symptoms that can be confused with acute cystitis can result from irritation or involvement of the bladder by pelvic sepsis due to acute appendicitis, Crohn's ileitis, acute diverticulitis or sigmoid carcinoma and in women, acute pelvic inflammatory disease.

Careful clinical assessment is a prerequisite. The relevant diagnostic investigations are an ultrasound or CT scan of the pelvis and urine and vaginal fluid microscopy and culture. The management of the above conditions is described in Chapter 25.

MANAGEMENT OF GYNAECOLOGICAL DISEASE FOUND AT LAPAROTOMY

This situation arises when an erroneous diagnosis of acute appendicitis has been made, or in equivocal

cases when an ultrasound or a CT scan are unavailable or the results have been inconclusive. In the latter circumstance, laparoscopy should always precede the laparotomy and the operation should be undertaken with a gynaecologist. Laparoscopic surgery is preferable whenever the expertise is available as it reduces the risk of adhesions associated with open surgery.

Ovarian cyst

In the pre-menopausal woman, ovarian tissue should be conserved if at all possible. One or more small cysts do not in themselves deserve attention. An ovarian cyst can be drained by marsupialization, or enucleation, preserving the ovary and if there is any doubt that the cyst might be malignant, frozen section for histological examination can be helpful. In post-menopausal women conserving the ovary is not as crucial.

Ectopic pregnancy

Blood is drained and the affected tube carefully assessed, with the other pelvic organs. The tube is incised, the pregnancy evacuated and the tube repaired. The tube and ovary should be salvaged whenever possible, unless they have been completely disorganized by the pregnancy. This is a safety measure because of the risk of another ectopic pregnancy in the future that may damage the other tube.

Acute salpingitis

If the abdominal ostia are occluded, incisions are made in the tubes to ensure free drainage into the peritoneum. Pus is squeezed out of the tubes and all exudate collected and the pouch of Douglas cleared out. If a pyosalpinx has formed, the tube is irreparably damaged and should be removed. A tubo-ovarian abscess may also result in complete disorganization of the ovary, and salpingo-oophorectomy is indicated.

HIGHLIGHTS

- Suspicion of renal pain–ureteric colic requires immediate IVU
- Renal tract obstruction with infection requires immediate drainage of kidney
- All confirmed urinary calculi are investigated to determine the cause
- Ultrasound examination and laparoscopy are essential investigations when gynaecological disease is suspected

28

Acute ischaemia of the limbs

M ADISESHIAH

AIMS

1 Identify acute ischaemia of the lower limbs
2 Plan immediate intervention: revascularization or amputation
3 Recognize and prevent the complications that follow revascularization

INTRODUCTION

The limbs, like other organs, are supplied by arteries with collateral or anastomotic branches which maintain the blood supply in the event of occlusion of the main artery. Because the collateral branches are more numerous in the upper than in the lower limbs, acute ischaemia is more commonly seen in the lower limbs, except for ischaemia due to digital artery occlusion which occurs with equal frequency in the hands and feet. However, in acute ischaemia the collateral blood flow does not come into operation and the tissues are rendered anoxic and in danger of irreversible necrosis.

```
            Acute limb ischaemia
           /                    \
Trauma (accidental/        Non-trauma
iatrogenic/self-induced)   (thrombosis/embolism)
```

There are two main settings for acute limb ischaemia, in the *traumatized* and the *non-traumatized* limb. Trauma may be *blunt* (supracondylar fracture, bomb blast and crush injury) or *sharp* injury (knife- or gunshot-induced, iatrogenic causes such as arterial puncture and self-inflicted in intravascular drug abuse). Non-traumatic causes are: *arterial thrombosis* due to atheroma and hypercoagulable states, such as malignancy, polycythaemia rubra vera, thrombocytopenia or leukaemia, and occasionally as a complication of the high-oestrogen contraceptive pill; or *arterial embolism* commonly in patients with atrial fibrillation, recent myocardial infarction, valvular heart disease and prosthetic heart valves. Rare sources of an embolus are an atherosclerotic aorta, an aortic aneurysm or a popliteal artery aneurysm. Emboli usually lodge at branching points where the lumen narrows, at the aortic bifurcation (*saddle embolus*), the common femoral bifurcation and the popliteal trifurcation (Table 28.1).

The history and examination establish the diagnosis and severity of the ischaemia, the possible aetiology and the site of occlusion.

CLINICAL PICTURE

The onset is sudden, sharp, often excruciating pain in the limb, rapid loss of sensation and inability to

Table 28.1 *Causes of acute ischaemia*

Traumatic	Non-traumatic
Blunt	Thrombosis
long bone fractures	atheroma
bomb blast	polycythaemia rubra vera
crush injury	leukaemia
	high-oestrogen
	contraceptive pill
Sharp	Embolism
knife wound	atrial fibrillation
gunshot wound	myocardial infarction
arterial puncture –	valvular heart disease
iatrogenic/	prosthetic heart valves
self-induced	aortic aneurysm
	popliteal artery
	aneurysm

The heart is auscultated for signs of atrial fibrillation and valvular disease. The quality of the pulses is examined, the presence of bruits in the other limb and the major arteries, carotid, subclavian, abdominal aortic and a high blood pressure suggest generalized arteriosclerosis with an acute arterial thrombosis as a cause of acute limb ischaemia. An expansile epigastric pulsation is a sign of an aortic aneurysm, occasionally a source of an arterial embolus.

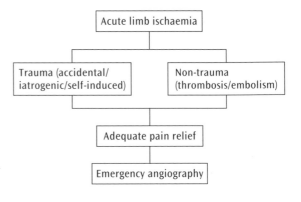

use the limb. The patient invariably seeks help immediately and usually presents within a very short timespan. Although pain and loss of function are features of a traumatized limb, other clinical signs determine the presence of ischaemia due to associated vascular injury.

On examination, the ischaemic limb is pale and cold. Numbness and diminution of sensation in the limb due to nerve ischaemia, and paresis of muscle groups indicative of severe ischaemia, distinguish *acute* ischaemia from *critical* and *chronic* ischaemia (Chapter 13). Mottling and fixed dusky blue discoloration with blistering are signs of irreversible change. When diffuse muscle rigidity develops the limb is unsalvageable.

Examination of the pulses in the affected limb identifies the site of arterial occlusion and the ischaemic part that is usually distal to it. The absence of bilateral femoral pulsations suggests aortic occlusion, whereas loss of the ipsilateral femoral pulse points to an iliac occlusion. Absent popliteal and pedal pulses are diagnostic of a superficial femoral artery occlusion; while this site of occlusion is probably the most common, it is rarely the sole cause of acute ischaemia on its own, possibly because of compensatory collateral blood flow. Normal pulses from femoral to pedal (dorsalis pedis and posterior tibial) level in the presence of acute digital ischaemia is likely to be due to digital artery occlusion from emboli.

MANAGEMENT

Acute ischaemia is a surgical emergency as the outcome is dependent on the promptness of revascularization, and delay leads to considerable morbidity and mortality. An essential consideration in treatment is the relief of pain. Optimal analgesia is achieved with a *long-term epidural* using a local anaesthetic and/or opiate infusion, or a *systemic opiate* combined with a tranquillizer. Anticoagulation with intravenous heparin should be instituted immediately to prevent propagation of the clot. When revascularization is feasible, angiography is essential in order to define the nature and the extent of the occlusion. This can be performed safely in an imaging interventional suite if available, or is undertaken per-operatively. In any event, delay is to be avoided.

When the limb exhibits signs of irreversible damage, it is not salvageable by restoring the circulation. Amputation is a life-saving measure.

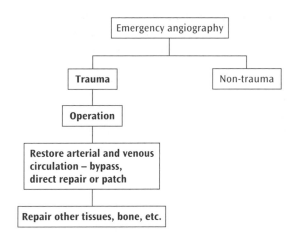

The traumatized limb

Acute ischaemia in the traumatized limb is invariably associated with other injuries. In such instances it is important to allocate priorities. It is a rule that restoration of blood flow takes precedence over all other therapeutic manoeuvres within that limb. It is illogical to perform complex reduction and fixation of a fracture if the limb is at risk of irreversible ischaemic damage! Injuries to nerve, tendon and bone are undertaken after restoration of blood flow during the same anaesthetic if the patient's general condition permits.

The precise procedure is determined by the type and extent of the injury and the findings on angiography. Basic surgical principles must be observed. All devitalized tissue and foreign debris are excised. Blood flow is restored by direct repair of the occluded artery provided that the wall is not contused or that there is no loss of arterial wall, as in the case of a cleanly severed artery. Otherwise, a saphenous or an arm vein bypass is used to bridge the damaged segment. Prosthetic bypass is very much a second choice because the wound is potentially contaminated and this predisposes to graft infection. Attempts should be made to repair veins which are larger than the femoral, although the results are unfavourable because of subsequent occlusion. It is not uncommon to salvage a limb with successful restoration of arterial flow, but disappointingly the limb remains chronically swollen because the venous and lymphatic drainage remains obliterated.

With the advent of endoluminal repair techniques, it is likely that stent-grafts to bridge occluded or bleeding traumatized arteries will be employed. This elegant technique offers the prospect of introducing the stent–prosthesis complex from a site remote from the injured artery under a light general or even local anaesthetic. Its application is obviously only feasible when there is no contamination or an open wound as in the case of blunt traumatic occlusion or rupture of an artery.

The major complications and post-operative care are common both to this situation and to cases due to non-traumatic causes, and are described later.

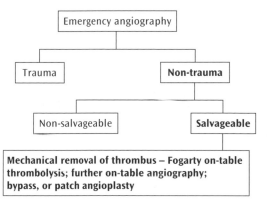

Non-traumatized limb

Spontaneous sudden arterial occlusion is either due to thrombosis or embolism. The onset and the physical signs in the affected limb are indistinguishable between these causes, and it is other aspects in the history and physical examination that will allow a degree of differentiation, which is essentially of theoretical importance only. A history of previous rheumatic fever, or valvular heart disease, recent myocardial infarction and atrial fibrillation suggest embolism, whereas a history of claudication or a blood disorder combined with no obvious source of embolism favours thrombosis. Examination of the other limb provides helpful distinguishing signs; if well-perfused and the pulses are normal then embolus is more likely, whereas abnormal pulses and other signs of atherosclerosis, for example a carotid bruit or hypertension, is suggestive of thrombosis. However, with a saddle embolus in the aorta, signs of poor circulation may be present in both limbs, although more evident on the affected side, and unless recognized may distort the clinical picture. The presence of a pulsatile popliteal aneurysm, when the popliteal pulse is absent on the affected side, favours thrombosis as popliteal aneurysms are frequently bilateral.

Angiography may demonstrate whether thrombosis or embolism is the cause, and certainly demonstrates the site of occlusion and the patency of the distal arteries, features which are relevant in planning revascularization. However, in acute ischaemia the flow in these distal vessels is usually slow and scant so that the angiogram may fail to demonstrate their patency. It is, therefore, necessary to appreciate the limitation of angiography in this situation and proceed to clear the artery of any clots, using a Fogarty embolectomy catheter with caution because the wall of an atherosclerotic vessel is lined by hard calcified plaque and it is easy to traumatize the luminal orifices of the collateral branches, thereby causing more damage. This is usually performed under local anaesthesia, but the patient is prepared for general anaesthesia should it become necessary. Through a groin incision, an arteriotomy is made in the common femoral artery after clamping its branches. A Fogarty balloon catheter is passed proximally and distally, and is withdrawn with the balloon inflated in order to remove the clots, followed by the instillation of a thrombolytic agent such as urokinase or streptokinase for 10 minutes. When the arterial branches are unclamped, backflow bleeding is indicative of a successful embolectomy. Angiography is repeated to ensure the patency of the distal circulation. At this stage it may be possible to decide whether the occlusion is embolic in origin. If it is not, an acute atherosclerotic thrombosis is the problem, for which the treatment is on-table thrombolysis followed by angioplasty or arterial reconstruction, usually a femoro-popliteal or femorotibial bypass. Once the limb is saved, the cardiovascular system is fully investigated for risk of thromboembolism to decide on the need for long-term anticoagulation.

Failure of treatment

Attempts at revascularization sometimes fail, usually due to occlusion of the bypass because of poor run-off distal to the graft or poor inflow proximally from occlusive disease upstream. Poor inflow should be recognized before surgery and is treated by performing proximal balloon angioplasty or other corrective procedure prior to completion of the reconstruction. There is little that can be done, however, to improve the circulation in the distal vessels and this is the most common cause of failure. In the event of failure of the reconstruction, limb necrosis is the inevitable result and amputation becomes necessary.

COMPLICATIONS OF TREATMENT

Reperfusion injury

The reperfusion injury syndrome is a predictable and preventable cause of considerable morbidity and occasional mortality. Acute ischaemia results in degradation of high-energy phosphate bonds in ATP and phosphocreatine to lower energy phosphates, with the release of energy used to sustain anaerobic metabolism in skeletal muscle. If the period of ischaemia is short (as in *tourniquet ischaemia*), the biochemical change is completely reversed on reperfusion without cellular damage. However, prolonged ischaemia causes muscle injury which progresses on reperfusion, resulting in arrhythmias due to hyperkalaemia from leakage of K^+ from the cells, renal failure from myoglobinaemia or respiratory failure due to activated white cells. Patients develop the *myonephropathic metabolic syndrome* and may die as a result.

After reperfusion and with tissue re-oxygenation, the enzyme xanthine dehydrogenase is converted to xanthine oxidase which in turn converts hypoxanthine to xanthine and in the process oxygen free radicals, such as hydroxyl ions and superoxide, are released. These radicals are unstable and react with the lipoprotein of the cell wall in the limb tissues to cause cell lysis, leucocyte activation and the production of leucotrienes causing further cellular damage with the release of K^+ ions, myoglobin and the enzyme creatine kinase.

The peak serum levels of myoglobin occur within 24 hours after reperfusion, and the creatine kinase, which is a larger protein and probably more slowly excreted, peaks at 48 hours. Serial (twice daily) estimations of the serum creatine kinase is of prognostic significance as it is unusual to observe renal or respiratory complications unless the serum creatine kinase level is in excess of 20,000–50,000 per ml.

Although biochemical and sub-clinical reperfusion syndrome frequently occurs unrecognized, acute ischaemia of a massive volume of muscle, as in whole limb ischaemia after iliac or aortic occlusion, leads to sinister complications, namely renal and respiratory failure and local muscle necrosis.

In order to induce diuresis and 'wash out' from the nephrons the myoglobin, which is soluble in an alkaline pH, and also to correct associated metabolic acidosis, mannitol and sodium bicarbonate solutions are administered following successful revascularization. An indwelling urinary catheter is placed to monitor the urine output. There are several biochemical agents that may be tried to thwart the generation of xanthine oxidase or to antagonise the oxygen free radicals. Theoretically, allopurinol would be useful because of its xanthine oxidase inhibition. However, for optimal therapeutic effect it is necessary to achieve measurable cellular levels of the drug, which may not be reached within the period of revascularization. Superoxide dismutase and peroxidase are other promising substances to employ as oxygen species scavengers. In this respect mannitol is also a free radical scavenger and may have a dual role here.

Muscle compartment syndrome

Following ischaemia and reperfusion, muscle swelling within the compartments (a compartment consists of unyielding bone, inter-osseous membranes and an investing layer of deep fascia, and contains muscles, nerves and vessels) raises the pressure above the capillary perfusion pressure, causing further ischaemia and swelling. This is recognized by muscle swelling, weakness, pain and tenderness, especially on passive stretching, and by sensory disturbance. When suspected, encircling bandages and plaster casts are removed and fasciotomy undertaken immediately. Prophylactic muscle compartment fasciotomy limits muscle damage and is especially effective in the anterior tibial compartment where the ankle dorsiflexors are confined in a rigid fibro-osseous compartment. When it is unclear whether the degree of reperfusion injury is severe enough to warrant prophylactic fasciotomy, the compartment pressure, which normally is more than 40 mmHg below the systemic diastolic blood pressure, is easily measured by inserting into the muscle compartment a needle attached to a manometer.

Residual tissue damage

Those parts of the limb with compromised viability prior to treatment will become sharply demarcated following successful revascularization and a digit or several digits may become prominently gangrenous.

The skin and subcutaneous tissues may become demarcated as black scabbed areas which progressively contract over weeks and finally separate leaving well-healed skin and subcutaneous tissues.

Ischaemic nerve damage involving sensory, motor and mixed nerves, causing paraesthesia or anaesthesia over areas of skin, develops rapidly. Foot-drop is usually a consequence of muscle damage in the anterior tibial compartment, but can occur as a result of anterior tibial nerve ischaemia. This is treated with physiotherapy and the use of special footwear to splint the ankle in dorsiflexion. Recovery of nerve function takes place over several months.

Limb swelling after successful revascularization is a consequence of reperfusion injury, lymphatic dysfunction, and occasionally deep venous thrombosis. The swelling may last for a few months. The patient is advised to elevate the foot of the bed to diminish the swelling overnight and to wear graduated compression stockings when ambulant.

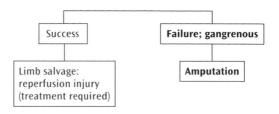

GANGRENOUS LIMB

Delayed or failed revascularization results in gangrene, which implies invasion of the dead ischaemic tissue by saprophytic bacteria. A zone of demarcation between viable and dead tissue is indicated by a band of hyperaemia and hyperaesthesia, and the development of a layer of granulation tissue. Unless painful, or unless the gangrenous tissue becomes secondarily infected with pathogenic organisms and develops into wet gangrene with the risk of spreading infection and septicaemia, amputation is delayed until a sharp demarcation line forms, as this allows maximal recovery of healthy tissue in the salvaged limb.

Amputation should take into account the prosthetic limb and is carried out through healthy tissue, carefully fashioning the muscle and the skin flaps to allow healing and provide a satisfactory stump. In aorto-iliac occlusion, the amputation site is usually above the knee at the lower level of the femur. For more distal occlusion, provided the tissues for at least 12 cm below the knee joint are viable, a below-knee amputation at mid-tibia is usually possible. It is important to judge the correct level for amputation at the outset to avoid re-amputating at a higher level, or needlessly depriving the patient of the knee joint, because if the knee joint can be saved the functional success of a prosthesis is better.

Although prostheses are available to allow through-knee amputation, above knee amputation is preferable as it heals better and the prosthesis is easier to apply. When limb ischaemia is so massive that the necrosis is confluent up to the groin, a disarticulation of the hip and the creation of a posterior buttock flap is the only option.

The cost-effectiveness of a prosthetic limb should be carefully considered because mobility is achieved in only 50% of patients, and within 10 years of amputation 50% are dead.

INTRA-ARTERIAL INJECTION IN DRUG ABUSE

Intra-arterial injection, usually accidental among drug addicts attempting access to the intravenous

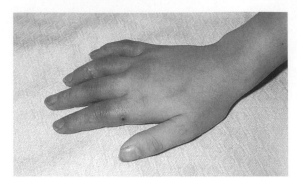

Fig. 28.1 *Pre-gangrenous changes in fingers following inadvertent drug self-injection into the brachial artery whilst attempting intravenous access.*

route, is an alarming cause of acute limb ischaemia in young people. Drugs such as temazepam, heroin and other opiate mixtures, often contaminated with impurities, are injected as a bolus into an artery, usually the femoral or the brachial. The problems posed are similar to those discussed above with two salient features. The pain experienced is excruciating and requires immediate relief, usually by employing regional anaesthesia. The damage or thrombosis is rarely in the large arteries, and the occlusion is always in the smaller arteries of the limb (Fig. 28.1). The anatomical site of arterial occlusion is determined with emergency angiography. Several drugs have been advocated for therapy, including heparin, prostacyclin ana-logues and other vasodilators, and fasciotomy may be required. Counselling and a detoxification programme should be considered for these patients.

Frostbite

This is an uncommon type of thermal injury seen in the inner cities in elderly people and the homeless due to exposure of the limb extremities to freezing temperatures during excessively cold winters (Fig. 28.2). A variable number and extent of the digits and/or the foot or hand undergo irreversible freezing injury. The patient is admitted, gradually warmed, rehydrated and provided with adequate analgesia. In order to achieve maximum conservation of the limb, time is allowed for demarcation to become established.

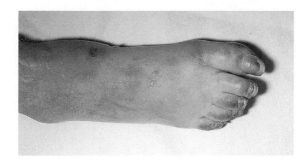

Fig. 28.2 *Frostbite affecting toes following exposure in a homeless patient in deep winter.*

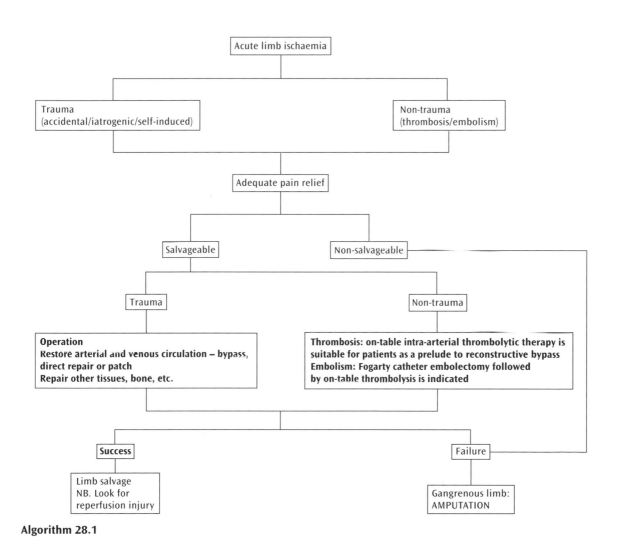

Algorithm 28.1

HIGHLIGHTS

- The physical signs in the affected limb do not distinguish between thrombosis and embolism; the limb is always cold
- Anaesthesia and paralysis of muscles indicate severe ischaemia and differentiate acute from critical and chronic ischaemia
- A limb with fixed blue discoloration, blistering and rigidity of muscles is unsalvageable by revascularization
- Pain relief, anticoagulation and emergency angiography are the mainstay of early management
- In a traumatized limb, repair of damaged arteries takes precedence over repair of other structures
- In thrombosis, on-table intra-arterial thrombolytic therapy is suitable for patients as a prelude to reconstructive bypass
- In embolism, Fogarty catheter embolectomy followed by on-table thrombolysis is indicated
- Failure to recognize and treat the complications of the reperfusion injury syndrome can be fatal
- The cost-effectiveness of prosthetic limbs should be considered carefully

29

Paediatric surgical emergencies

VANESSA M WRIGHT

INTRODUCTION

Many children are brought by their parents for medical advice with a problem perceived by the parent as an emergency, when frequently only an explanation and reassurance are required. Although such consultations in a busy practice may seem inappropriate, taking the time to allay anxiety encourages parents to accept the diagnosis and stops them seeking further urgent opinions. A few cases will, indeed, demand intervention and follow-up by the general practitioner or in an outpatient clinic. In the child under 5 years, the health visitor is informed of the attendance and can ensure further support.

Emergencies in the newborn (the first few days of life) present to specialist units and are not discussed here. This chapter discusses common surgical conditions that affect infants and young children (up to 2 years of age) and older children (up to puberty), conditions with which every clinician should be familiar.

HEAD AND NECK INFECTIONS

AIMS

1 Distinguish lymphadenopathy from lymphadenitis
2 Recognize cervical abscess due to congenital anomalies
3 Understand the management of infection in the head and neck

---

Palpable lymph nodes

Children, especially in the age group 6 months to 3 years, frequently develop palpable cervical lymph nodes (*lymphadenopathy*) after upper respiratory tract infection, otitis media or generalized viraemia. The nodes involved are usually bilateral, commonly in the submandibular region or in the posterior cervical chain, and they are enlarged and mildly tender. With progressive inflammation, the lymph node swelling is painful, restricts neck movement, is tender and hot to touch, and when it suppurates it becomes fluctuant. Most abscesses exhibit the features of acute inflammation but some are 'cold', caused by atypical mycobacteria – avium, intracellulare and scrofulaceum (MAIS).

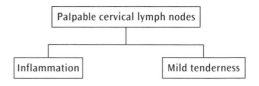

Lymphadenopathy associated with an upper respiratory or ear infection requires no specific treatment, although the underlying infection may require antibiotics. *Lymphadenitis* without abscess formation requires prompt use of antibiotics – the common organisms are *Staphylococcus aureus* and *Streptococcus pyogenes*. A combination of intravenous penicillin and flucloxacillin is the treatment of choice to ensure adequate blood levels. After 48 hours the response to treatment becomes evident. If the signs of inflammation are receding, treatment is continued with oral antibiotics for a further 3–5 days. If the patient remains pyrexial, the overlying skin is still red and shiny, and the mass is unchanged in size or is larger, an abscess should be suspected. Discontinuing the antibiotics and maintaining adequate analgesia for a further 24–48 hours allows the abscess to point onto the skin but this approach is not adopted in the under-3-months-old because of the risk of septicaemia and metastatic staphylococcal osteomyelitis. Incision and drainage can then be carried out easily and effectively, but can be unsuccessful if the abscess is not fully developed because the pus is small in amount, deeply situated and difficult to find. When in doubt, an ultrasound scan examination of the area will decide the size and situation of the abscess. The inflammatory mass may take several weeks to subside completely after treatment (*see* Algorithm 29.1).

Specific sites of cervical inflammation

The site of an abscess in the neck can give an indication as to the cause. An abscess occurring in the mid-line of the neck at the level of the hyoid bone is most likely to arise in a *thyroglossal cyst* (Chapter 2), whereas one at the anterior border of the sterno-mastoid muscle at the junction of its lower and middle thirds is usually an abscess arising in a *branchial fistula* associated with the persistence of the *second branchial cleft*. From the skin opening, the fistula extends upwards through the neck to the tonsillar fossa. A small opening in the skin which may discharge a little mucus is the usual presentation and may not have been recognized prior to the development of inflammation or abscess.

First branchial cleft sinuses are much less common than the second branchial cleft abnormalities and

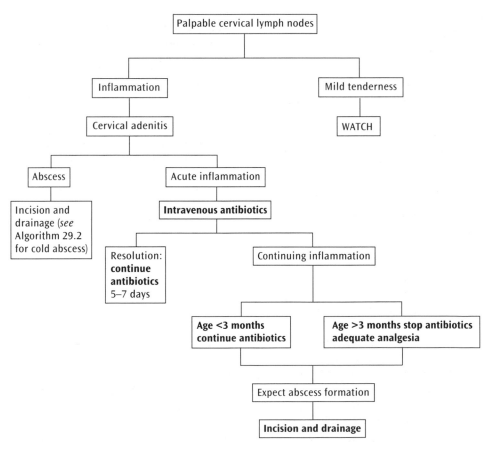

Algorithm 29.1

are the likely aetiology if a child presents with acute inflammation in the submandibular region with an obvious sinus. The sinus tract runs from the skin opening to the external auditory meatus and is closely related to the facial nerve.

Inflammation of the *pre-auricular region* presents with recurrent pain and swelling or abscess, and is associated with a *pre-auricular sinus* which may be visible on careful inspection. The sinus opens at the anterior end of the upper helix of the pinna and the tract, about 1 cm in length, runs downwards and forwards to terminate in a number of small cysts or a single large cyst. The inflammation is usually in the deeper part rather than the cutaneous part of the sinus.

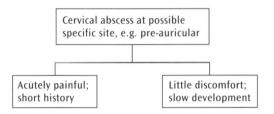

Management is the same in principle for all sites. The treatment for early inflammation is with antibiotics for the common organisms, usually *S. aureus*, except that thyroglossal cysts are often infected by respiratory organisms. An abscess requires incision and drainage. Complete healing cannot be expected because a sinus will persist unless the underlying congenital anomaly is treated; this may involve complicated surgery that should not be undertaken until the infection is completely resolved.

An *atypical mycobacterial abscess* can arise in the pre-auricular lymph nodes. This typically presents as a swelling in front of the ear, although it can occur in other groups of lymph nodes. The overlying skin colour initially is a dull red, then changes to purple colour as pus collects in the subcutaneous tissues. If untreated, the pus eventually discharges through the skin, producing a chronically discharging sinus, until the involved glands are excised. Although all the characteristics of inflammation are present the area is surprisingly non-tender and the overlying skin is not warm which is diagnostic of a 'cold' abscess.

A *cold abscess* is aspirated rather than excised to avoid the development of a chronic sinus, and

pus is sent for microbiological examination, specifically for mycobacteria. If positive for organisms of the MAIS group, excision of the infected nodes is required to eradicate the infection. Unlike human mycobacterial infection, atypical organisms are highly resistant to drug therapy (*see* Algorithm 29.2).

HIGHLIGHTS

- Infection in the neck is due to underlying inflammation in lymph nodes or congenital cysts
- Chronic sinuses complicate infection in congenital cysts and fistulas unless these are excised
- Atypical mycobacterial infection is drug-resistant and is eradicated by excising the infected lymph nodes

---

THE VOMITING INFANT

AIMS

1 Differentiate between vomiting from underlying organic disease and regurgitation from gastro-oesophageal reflux (GOR)
2 Appreciate the significance of bile-stained and non-bile-stained vomiting
3 Recognize the causes of vomiting and its management

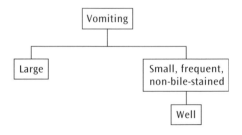

Vomiting as an isolated symptom in a well infant

Many infants vomit after a feed: only about a teaspoonful when the baby burps. The lower

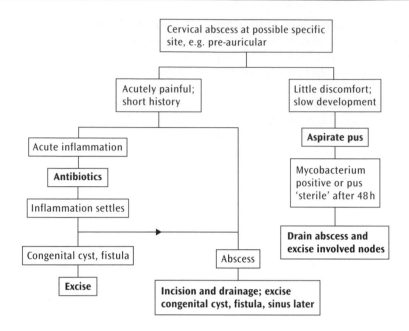

Algorithm 29.2

oesophageal sphincter mechanism in the early months of life is poorly developed and provides little resistance to a liquid feed, particularly when the baby is lying down. In some infants gastro-oesophageal reflux produces larger volume vomits or repeated vomiting between feeds which may worry the mother.

In the majority, despite the vomiting the infant thrives. Giving a smaller volume of feed thickened with one of the agents available, and winding and keeping the baby in an upright position after a feed for an hour or so help to alleviate the problem. With time and the introduction of solids, gastro-oesophageal reflux subsides in the majority of infants.

Vomiting as an isolated symptom associated with failure to gain weight

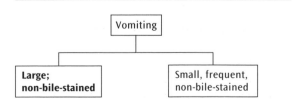

In the infant who is generally well but is vomiting large volumes of feed sufficient to affect weight gain, the cause can be *pyloric stenosis* or *severe gastro-oesophageal reflux*, differentiated by observing the pattern of vomiting.

In *pyloric stenosis* the infant is usually between 3 and 8 weeks of age. The underlying cause is hypertrophy of the circular muscle of the pyloric region. It occurs in one in 400 babies, commonly in male first-born children and in siblings of affected children. After a feed, which is usually taken enthusiastically, a vomit occurs within minutes. At first the vomit is large in volume but not forceful and does not follow every feed, but gradually becomes projectile and more frequent until every feed is vomited. The vomit is milk and is never bile-stained. Initially, the baby simply stops gaining weight but as the vomiting persists dehydration occurs. The baby looks wizened and worried and after a vomit is eager for another feed. Bowel actions become less frequent if the history extends for a week or more and may be described as 'diarrhoea' because the stool is loose and green – but the volume is very small – so-called 'starvation' stools.

The baby with *severe gastro-oesophageal reflux* can bring up large volumes of feed forcefully but vomits between feeds rather than after feeds. Both gastro-oesophageal reflux and pyloric stenosis can cause oesophagitis leading to bleeding. The blood in the vomit is partly digested and has a 'coffee ground' appearance mixed with milk.

There are two important physical signs of pyloric stenosis – visible peristalsis and a palpable pyloric tumour. *Visible peristalsis*, likened to a golf ball rolling from under the left costal margin towards the umbilicus, occurs as the distended, hypertrophied stomach attempts to empty its contents through the obstructing pylorus. It is best seen when the stomach is partly filled and the infant is quiet and relaxed, during or soon after a feed. The pyloric mass or tumour is best palpated by standing on the infant's left side and, using the left middle finger, gently palpating lateral to the right rectus muscle, increasing the depth of palpation gently and moving the finger up and down. Often, a wave of peristalsis intermittently hardens the tumour which is then felt under the finger. A full feed is unnecessary as an overfull stomach will often obscure the pylorus. The object of the 'test feed' should be to calm a fractious baby whilst looking for visible peristalsis and the tumour palpated.

When the diagnosis is not clear, a period of observation on the ward will distinguish between gastro-oesophageal reflux and pyloric stenosis. When the symptoms are suggestive of pyloric stenosis but a tumour is not palpable, an ultrasound of the pylorus may demonstrate either a normal pylorus or an elongated (>17 mm), thickened (>4 mm) pylorus typical of pyloric stenosis. If ultrasound is not available, a barium meal will demonstrate a large stomach, vigorous peristalsis, delayed gastric emptying, and an elongated pylorus with a narrow pyloric canal – the 'string' sign. The hypertrophied stomach is likely to produce significant gastro-oesophageal reflux which radiologically may be interpreted as the primary diagnosis.

An infant with pyloric stenosis or gastro-oesophageal reflux will only become ill if severe dehydration occurs. An infant who is vomiting and unwell is likely to have another cause for the vomiting.

In pyloric stenosis, vomiting results in 'dehydration', that is, extra-cellular depletion, hypokalaemia, hypochloraemia and metabolic alkalosis. The severity of dehydration (Table 29.1) is assessed by clinical parameters and is corrected accordingly.

Table 29.1 *Clinical parameters of severity of dehydration*

	5%	10%
Skin turgor	Loss of turgor	Mottled, prolonged capillary return
Fontanelle	Depressed	Very depressed
Eyes	Sunken	Very sunken
Peripheral pulse	Normal	Poor volume, tachycardia
Mental state	Lethargy	Prostration, unresponsive

Calculation of fluid replacement is $(X/100) \times 1000 \times$ bodyweight (kg), where X is % dehydration. For example, a 3-kg infant who is 5% dehydrated requires $5/100 \times 1000 \times 3 = 150$ ml of fluid to replace losses over a 24-hour period plus normal maintenance requirements of 150 ml/kg per day. Having worked out the water requirements, the potassium and chloride deficits are replaced: in most cases half-normal saline in 5% dextrose with 15 mmol of potassium chloride added to each half-litre usually corrects the fluid and electrolyte deficit within 24 hours, although severe deficits may need 48–72 hours.

The biochemical derangement must be corrected prior to anaesthesia, otherwise the respiratory alkalosis induced by anaesthesia and co-existent metabolic alkalosis may result in the infant failing to breathe post-operatively and necessitate ventilatory support.

The stomach is emptied by naso-gastric aspiration to avoid aspiration per-operatively.

Treatment is by *Ramstedt's pyloromyotomy*, incising through the thickened pyloric muscle along the line of the pylorus and separating the muscle fibres to allow the mucosa to bulge through the incision.

Bile-stained vomiting in the infant

Bile-stained (green, not yellow) vomiting is always suggestive of bowel obstruction, although medical conditions may cause persistent bile-stained vomiting.

The common causes are intussusception and strangulated inguinal hernia. Malrotation associated with a volvulus and Hirschsprung's disease is less common.

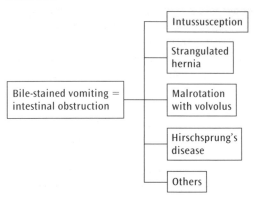

Bile-stained vomiting = intestinal obstruction
- Intussusception
- Strangulated hernia
- Malrotation with volvulus
- Hirschsprung's disease
- Others

Malrotation and volvulus

During early fetal development, the mid-gut develops outside the abdominal cavity in the base of the umbilical cord where it continues to grow and elongate. With increasing abdominal capacity, the bowel returns into the abdominal cavity by a process of rotation which results in the duodenum lying around the head of the pancreas and the duodenojejunal flexure, fixed by the ligament of Treves to the left side of the first lumbar vertebra. The caecum returns to the peritoneal cavity and lies in the subhepatic area, before moving to the right iliac fossa where the fixation of the caecum and ascending colon in the right paracolic gutter results in a broad-based mesentery for the small bowel from the duodenojejunal flexure in the left upper quadrant of the abdomen to the ileo-caecal region in the right lower quadrant. In malrotation (Fig. 29.1) the duodenum fails to form the normal C-shaped curve around the pancreas and with the upper small bowel lying to the right of the vertebral column prevents the caecum from moving to the right. It therefore remains in the mid-line or even to the left. Distinct peritoneal bands bind the caecum to the duodenum and to loops of small bowel – *Ladd's bands*. These bands can produce obstruction by compressing the small bowel against the posterior abdominal wall. However, the most serious problem in malrotation is that the entire mid-gut, instead of being suspended on a

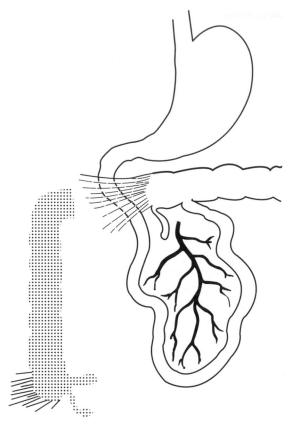

Fig. 29.1 *Malrotation (the stippled area indicates the usual location of the caecum.*

broad well-fixed mesentery, is suspended on a very narrow unfixed mesentery so that the bowel may twist on its axis producing a volvulus, occluding the superior mesenteric vessels and cutting off the blood supply to the whole of the small bowel and the proximal half of the large bowel.

Frequently occurring soon after birth, *volvulus*, although a congenital abnormality, can occur at any time in life. It is to be considered in a healthy neonate or infant with unexplained sudden onset of bile-stained vomiting. A history of a previous episode may be obtained, suggestive of a partial volvulus which had spontaneously resolved. On examination, the abdomen is not distended because the obstruction with volvulus or with Ladd's bands is at the duodenum. The child will gradually show signs of dehydration.

Management

A plain abdominal X-ray taken during the acute episode of bile-stained vomiting usually shows a stomach bubble with a distinct paucity of distal bowel gas. If the X-ray is delayed, or is taken when the symptoms appear to be abating, the change in the X-ray appearance may be dramatic with a normal bowel gas pattern. The definitive diagnosis of malrotation with volvulus is made with a carefully performed barium meal looking at the position of the duodenum. This can be extremely difficult to interpret and a neonate or infant suspected of having a malrotation should be referred to a specialist unit prior to the barium study.

Intravenous fluids are necessary to maintain hydration and correct any dehydration or electrolyte abnormality as a result of vomiting. A naso-gastric tube is passed and left on free drainage with regular aspiration to prevent vomiting and to allow accurate measurement of the gastrointestinal loss which is replaced with normal saline. On confirmation of the diagnosis, a laparotomy is necessary to relieve the obstruction and rearrange the bowel in the abdomen in a non-rotated position – *Ladd's operation*.

Volvulus with gangrenous bowel

The neonate or infant presents with a brief history of bile-stained vomiting containing coffee grounds. The infant is pale and hypotensive. The abdomen is usually distended, and tenderness may be elicited if the infant is responsive enough. The stools may contain frank or altered blood.

The infant should be resuscitated as rapidly as possible, blood cross-matched and urgent arrangements made for transfer to a neonatal intensive care unit for urgent laparotomy to derotate the bowel and resect gangrenous bowel. This complication is frequently fatal or the infant survives with a very short length of bowel and may be dependent on total parenteral nutrition for life.

Hirschsprung's disease

Ganglion cells migrate into the bowel from the neural crest normally in a spiral fashion along the entire length of the bowel to the lower rectum. Failure of this migration results in absence of ganglion cells from the inter-myenteric and the sub-mucous plexuses, usually in the recto-sigmoid region but it can occur at any level; 10% of cases have total aganglionosis of the colon associated with a variable length of aganglionic small bowel, and rarely the condition affects the whole of the gastrointestinal tract. Peristalsis is absent in the aganglionic bowel and the internal sphincter fails to relax, resulting in neonatal intestinal obstruction or severe constipation later in childhood. The bowel proximal to the aganglionic area is dilated, hypertrophied and full of meconium.

The majority of neonates with Hirschsprung's disease are full-term male babies who fail to pass meconium spontaneously in the first 48 hours after birth and are often unwilling to feed, and gradually develop abdominal distension and bile-stained vomiting. Usually these healthy-looking babies are sent home within a few hours of birth and their failure to pass meconium is managed by the administration of a suppository, a rectal examination or the insertion of a thermometer into the rectum. Any such intervention may result in explosive release of air and meconium which is greeted with relief but the true significance of this sign is not appreciated. The cycle of poor feeding, abdominal distension, infrequent stool and bile-stained vomiting continues before the diagnosis becomes apparent.

Management

A contrast enema demonstrates a non-dilated rectum and a dilated proximal colon. The diagnosis is confirmed with a suction rectal biopsy to include the sub-mucosa of the rectum. Haematoxylin and eosin staining, with acetyl cholinesterase staining, reveals an absence of ganglion cells and usually an increase in the cholinesterase-positive (parasympathetic) nerve fibres in the lamina propria of the bowel.

Surgery may be staged with an initial colostomy in gangrenous bowel assessed by frozen section, followed by a 'pull through' of the ganglionic bowel to the anal canal. In appropriate cases, the pull through procedure can be done as the primary definitive operation.

Hirschsprung's enterocolitis

This extremely serious condition occurs in undiagnosed Hirschsprung's disease. The onset is rapid and the neonate or infant presents with pyrexia, gross abdominal distension, septicaemia and hypovolaemia. The introduction of a finger or wide bore tube into the rectum will usually result in the explosive passage of large volumes of foul-smelling grey, gritty, very loose stool.

Urgent resuscitation with intravenous fluids is essential and treatment with broad-spectrum antibiotics against aerobic and anaerobic organisms is commenced.

The bowel is decompressed by defunctioning colostomy.

The unwell infant with vomiting

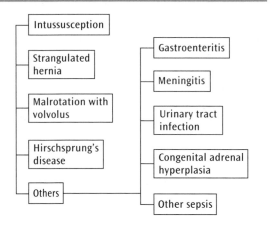

Once intestinal obstruction as a cause of vomiting has been excluded, it is essential to rule out sepsis by obtaining specimens of blood, urine, cerebrospinal fluid, swabs from the nose, the throat, and in a neonate, from the umbilicus for bacteriology. A chest X-ray is required if pneumonia is suspected. If the infant is ill, irritable and lethargic then feeding may be difficult and an intravenous infusion is commenced; if sepsis seems a probable cause, broad-spectrum antibiotics are commenced to cover the more serious bacterial infections until culture results are available.

Other relevant medical conditions that should be considered are briefly described.

Gastroenteritis

Vomiting can precede diarrhoea by several hours. Colic, particularly with campylobacter enteritis, often precedes the passage of stool. The infant is often irritable and pyrexial. The abdomen is frequently distended and generally tender.

Gastroenteritis associated with colic and blood in the stools can be extremely difficult to differentiate from an intussusception. A plain abdominal X-ray if done in gastroenteritis usually shows dilated bowel loops with fluid levels indistinguishable from the picture of a mechanical bowel obstruction. Ultrasonography may be required in order to rule out the possibility of an intussusception.

Urinary tract infection

The infant or child may not exhibit symptoms and signs specific to the urinary tract and the diagnosis is made on investigation of vomiting, with pyrexia, when a urine specimen is examined.

Meningitis

In the baby or infant, meningitis may present with vomiting, irritability and pyrexia without specific features, that is, neck stiffness or a full fontanelle. When in doubt, a lumbar puncture is essential.

Non-specific sepsis

A variety of viral illnesses can cause vomiting usually associated with pyrexia.

Congenital adrenal hyperplasia

This rare cause of vomiting usually occurs in the first two weeks of life and is associated with pallor and hypotension. The acute presentation almost always occurs in boys: there is hyperpigmentation of the nipples, scrotum and penis. Measurement of electrolytes reveals hyponatraemia, hyperkalaemia and often profound hypoglycaemia. This condition is due to an enzyme defect, either 21 α-hydroxylase (>90%) or 11 β-hydroxylase (<10%) is deficient, resulting in disturbance of cortisol and aldosterone synthesis. Urgent resuscitation with normal saline plus glucose is required, with 50 mg of intravenous hydrocortisone. The diagnosis is established by measuring the serum 17-hydroxyprogesterone level which is elevated and the 11-deoxycortisol level, which is low. Ongoing management of the condition by a paediatric endocrinologist is essential.

HIGHLIGHTS

- Vomiting with weight loss should be considered seriously
- Severe gastro-oesophageal reflux should be differentiated from pyloric stenosis
- Bile-stained vomiting suggests intestinal obstruction, commonly due to intussusception, strangulated hernia, volvulus and Hirschsprung's disease
- When intestinal obstruction has been excluded, medical conditions are considered as a cause of vomiting

---

PASSAGE OF FRESH BLOOD IN THE STOOL

AIM

1 Recognize the life-threatening causes of blood in the stool

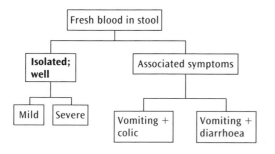

From the early weeks of life throughout childhood, the passage of fresh blood in the stool alarms the child and his parents. The important facts to establish are: first, whether the child is well or ill; and second, the presence of other symptoms, particularly vomiting, diarrhoea, abdominal colic or pain with bowel movement.

A well, otherwise asymptomatic child

Cow's milk protein intolerance usually occurs between 2 and 6 weeks of age. The baby is feeding well and gaining weight. Streaks of fresh blood are noted on the surface of the stool which is loose and may contain more mucus than normal. The underlying cause for the bleeding is a mild colitis, due to a cow's milk protein allergy. Whole cow's milk protein ingested by the mother can cross into the baby through the breast milk. Excluding cow's milk from the mother's diet can be difficult to achieve but will cure the baby. This is a better option than discontinuing breast feeding and introducing an alternative formula that is soya- or casein-based. A paediatrician's opinion should be sought if this diagnosis is suspected.

When the blood is more frequent or is profuse, congenital causes should be considered: Meckel's diverticulum and polyps.

Acute anal fissure. The presence of fresh blood on the surface of the stool in the lavatory or on the toilet paper, associated with the passage of hard stools, is a common cause of rectal bleeding in children of any age. The bowel action is often, but not always, painful.

Examination may reveal a fissure, but an acute tear can heal rapidly and the optimal time to visualize the site of the bleeding is immediately after a bowel action.

Management is to soften the stools with a laxative such as lactulose, to protect and lubricate the anal margin with barrier cream, and to treat constipation by modifying the diet.

Meckel's diverticulum occurs in 2% of the population, is 50 mm (2 inches) in length and usually lies 60 cm (2 feet) proximal to the ileo-caecal junction. It represents the embryological remnant of the

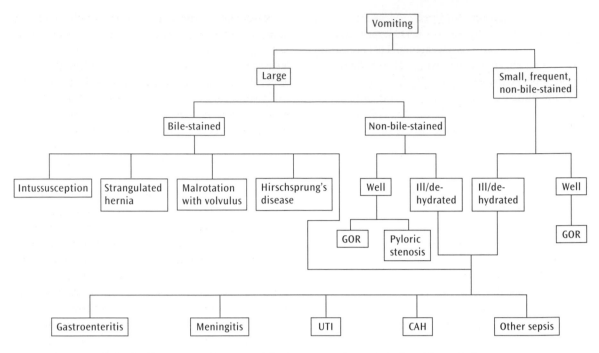

GOR = Gastro-oesophageal reflux; UTI = Urinary tract infection; CAH = Congenital adrenal hyperplasia.

Algorithm 29.3

vitello-intestinal duct. A Meckel's diverticulum may be asymptomatic but sometimes, if lined with parietal cell gastric mucosa, may cause peptic ulceration and bleeding. In children below 2 years it should be considered as a cause of rectal bleeding and may require blood transfusion. In older children, the ectopic gastric mucosa often causes occult bleeding and anaemia. The diagnosis is made by a technetium isotope scan, although a negative scan is not exclusive and a laparotomy may be necessary to confirm the diagnosis and resect the diverticulum.

Polyps. These are usually hamartomas. Juvenile polyps, most commonly seen in infants and children under 10 years old, are nearly always single and 90% occur in the rectum or sigmoid colon. The most common presentation is rectal bleeding followed by prolapse through the anus and occasionally intussusception. Colonoscopy allows snare excision of the polyp and examination of the rest of the colon as 30% of children have multiple polyps.

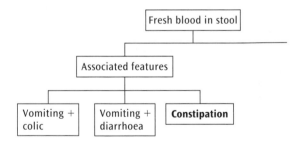

An unwell child with associated symptoms

Vomiting and colic

Intussusception. In an intussusception, commonly in the ileo-caecum, forceful peristalsis precipitated by enlarged Peyer's patches following a viral infection, propel the ileum (the *intussusceptum*) as an invagination into the colon (the *intussuscipiens*) (Fig. 29.2).

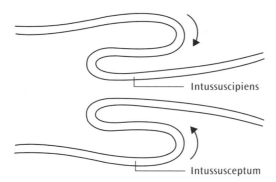

Fig. 29.2 *Intussusception. The intussusception usually consists of ileum invaginating into colon.*

The four layers of the bowel wall produce a sausage-shaped mass. The intussusceptum obstructs the lumen and if not treated it undergoes venous infarction, with mucosal sloughing and the passage of blood and mucus – the *redcurrant jelly stool.*

Intussusception occurs in children aged between 3 and 24 months, with a peak at 5 months. Vomiting is common, initially not bile-stained, and is accompanied by recurrent bouts of severe abdominal pain which rapidly exhaust the child. The lethargy and pallor mimic meningitis or encephalitis and often prompt a lumbar puncture or electroencephalogram. A viral illness confuses the picture when an intussusception follows an episode of gastroenteritis or an upper respiratory tract infection.

At onset, small-volume loose stools may be passed that later contain blood. Profuse diarrhoea associated with vomiting and colic is more likely to be gastroenteritis.

Abdominal distension tends to occur late and makes it difficult to palpate the mass. Localized tenderness and guarding may be elicited overlying the mass.

Blood in the stools is not a feature when the diagnosis is made early, or it may not have been noticed, but on rectal examination characteristic bloody mucus is found, and the intussusception may be palpated in the rectum. Very rarely it may prolapse through the anus and is mistaken for a rectal prolapse.

Delay in establishing a diagnosis of intussusception is common. The triad of colic, 'redcurrant jelly' stools and a palpable abdominal mass is only present in about 50% of children at the time of presentation.

Nevertheless, the diagnosis is usually made on clinical evidence. A plain abdominal X-ray can be confusing because there may be a striking paucity of bowel gas and bowel distension, although sometimes the intussusception shows as a clear soft tissue mass. Not infrequently, there are multiple dilated loops of bowel with fluid levels consistent with bowel obstruction, but not diagnostic of intussusception. An ultrasound scan of the abdomen usually displays the lesion as a 'target' or 'doughnut'.

Where the intussusception has been present for longer than a few hours the child is likely to be dehydrated and a period of resuscitation is essential. Most children are successfully managed non-operatively by *hydrostatic reduction* of the intussusception. This involves instilling into the rectum, under X-ray control at a known pressure, preferably air, or a liquid contrast until the intussusceptum is retrogradely forced through the colon and is completely reduced. The success of this treatment varies from 50% to 95%. Failure of hydrostatic reduction necessitates operative reduction. At operation resection of necrotic or irreducible bowel is necessary in about 10% of cases.

Death from intussusception is almost always the result of delayed diagnosis. A recurrence rate of 5–10% occurs, irrespective of the method of management. If an extensive ileal resection is necessary assessment of vitamin B12 status in later childhood is mandatory.

Vomiting and diarrhoea

Gastroenteritis. The child with gastroenteritis is ill and pyrexial, is vomiting and has abdominal colic and diarrhoea. Gastroenteritis causing bloody diarrhoea is often of a severity requiring admission and intravenous fluids. The typical organisms are campylobacter, shigella and salmonella. It is essential that stools are sent off for microbiology and virology and treatment instituted accordingly. A child with an acute onset of ulcerative colitis may present with indistinguishable symptoms. The failure of symptoms to abate over 48 hours and the absence of positive stool microbiology should raise the suspicion of a non-infective cause. Occasionally, a clotting defect may be revealed during an episode of gastroenteritis and should be suspected if bleeding is significant.

ACUTE ABDOMINAL PAIN – IS IT APPENDICITIS?

Acute abdominal pain in children is common, and a missed appendicitis can be fatal. The keys are a careful history and examination and, in doubt, reassessment every 4–6 hours.

The history is the same as in adults, although it may be difficult to elicit in a child. Vomiting usually follows the onset of pain but may not be a prominent symptom. Nausea is frequent and, in many children, anorexia is striking. An inflamed pelvic appendix by irritating the rectum produces small frequent stools that contain mucus, and if lying against the bladder, causes dysuria and the pain is exacerbated when the bladder is full or during micturition.

A child who is moving freely is unlikely to have an acute abdomen. The child is asked to point with one finger to the site of the pain, and to cough, to blow the abdomen out to touch one's hand held an inch (25 mm) above the abdomen, and to suck the tummy in and 'go very thin', actions which by stretching the peritoneum will increase the pain.

A raised temperature, tachycardia, halitosis and a furred tongue are suggestive signs. Gentle palpation, starting away from the tender spot while distracting the child to prevent voluntary guarding or an exaggerated response to the examination, is performed to elicit tenderness and guarding. Gentle percussion of the abdomen is better used to demonstrate rebound tenderness because sudden lifting of the hand may frighten the child. If the history suggests appendicitis but the abdominal findings are unconvincing, a rectal examination will elicit tenderness on deep digital palpation if the appendix is lying in the pelvis or is retro-caecal.

Management

No investigation is required unless there is doubt about the diagnosis. The main alternative diagnoses are constipation and mesenteric adenitis. The child with constipation is afebrile and systemically well. In mesenteric adenitis the child is pyrexial and may have or is recovering from an upper respiratory tract infection and the cervical lymph nodes are enlarged. Lower urinary tract infection, or occasionally a lower lobe pneumonia should be considered, where the urine analysis and a chest X-ray may be required.

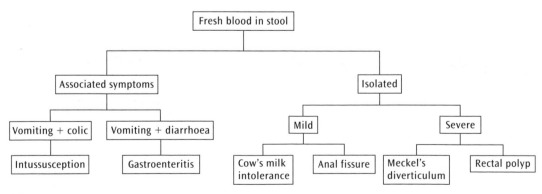

Algorithm 29.4

When the diagnosis is uncertain, *active* observation is planned. This involves the nursing staff observing the child's level of pain and recording the pulse and temperature regularly. The child is reviewed every 4–6 hours for any change or progression in the symptoms and signs. Ensuring appropriate communication with the parents during this period of observation is imperative, particularly if the findings suggest an improvement but the child is still complaining of pain.

The treatment is *appendicectomy*, and if delay is likely then appropriate analgesia, intravenous fluids and antibiotics should be started.

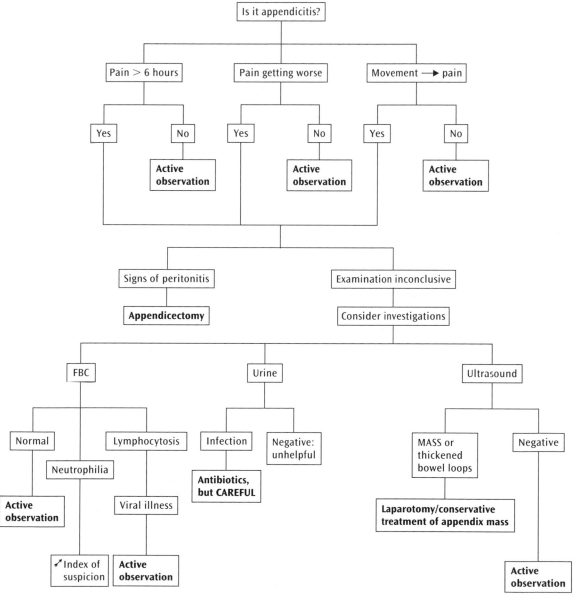

Algorithm 29.5

UMBILICAL HERNIA

Many umbilical hernias develop in the first 2 weeks after birth and increase in size rapidly. Unlike the para-umbilical hernias of adults, these are true hernias through the umbilicus. During episodes of crying and straining, the hernia increases in size and is tense, which alarms the parents who may believe that the hernia is the cause of pain or colic and therefore seek urgent medical advice. On examination, the hernial contents are always easily reducible. Nearly 90 per cent of these hernias undergo spontaneous resolution and disappear by about 4 years of age. In the rare circumstance when the hernia is irreducible, the infant is sedated and left to sleep; on re-examination after an hour the hernia will usually have reduced spontaneously, but if not, and pressure is required to reduce it, a repair is necessary within 48 hours, or as an emergency if the hernia remains irreducible. This rare event occurs when a tiny defect in the umbilical ring allows a capacious hernial sac through – the protrusion looks like a mushroom.

Through a sub-umbilical incision the hernial sac is emptied, ligated and excised and the defect closed.

LUMPS IN THE INGUINO-SCROTAL REGION

These are described in Chapters 10 and 11. The following section details management in infants and children.

Parents noticing such a swelling for the first time are likely to seek urgent medical advice. However, the history and findings may establish that the lump has been present for some time and is asymptomatic.

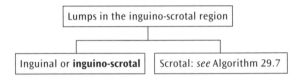

Inguinal/inguino-scrotal lumps

An inguinal or inguino-scrotal swelling is likely to be a *hernia*, and if non-tender, is nearly always easily reducible. This confirms the diagnosis of a hernial sac that extends along the spermatic cord into the scrotum.

A hernia that is irreducible may be confined to the groin but is usually inguino-scrotal. The swelling is tender and is firm or tensely cystic: it extends up to the internal ring, and the cord cannot be felt above the swelling, a feature which differentiates a hernia from a hydrocele. If the presentation is early the symptoms are irritability, reluctance to feed and sometimes vomiting. A baby or infant that seems unhappy may prompt the parent to look for a cause and on removing the nappy the lump is visible, although its significance may not be apparent to the parents. The older child will complain of pain.

When presentation is delayed the infant or child becomes unwell with symptoms and signs of bowel obstruction and the subcutaneous tissues and skin overlying the lump become reddened and indurated. Such a child needs urgent surgery from the outset.

When the hernia is tense and tender on palpation, it is justifiable to attempt reduction by gentle pressure over the lump. A period of sedation and analgesia, with the child lying with the foot of the bed or cot elevated may facilitate reduction. Gallows traction is time-consuming to set up and confers no extra benefit. In the fractious infant, an intramuscular injection of pethidine compound (*Pethco*) may be necessary. The infant is allowed to have at least an hour's sleep and then a further attempt is made to reduce the hernia. With the fingers of both hands, sustained pressure is applied to the lump to reduce the bowel through the external ring, the point where the bowel is likely to be compressed. If the hernia still cannot be reduced, then immediate surgical intervention is required.

Even after successful manual reduction, a hernia should be repaired before the infant is discharged from hospital. In babies and children, the peritoneal sac is excised (*inguinal herniotomy*); unlike in adults, there is no abdominal wall defect to require a repair (*herniorrhaphy*).

An undescended testis (UDT) may present as a lump in the groin, particularly if hydrocele fluid accumulates around the testis or there is an associated hernia. Torsion of an undescended testis usually presents as a tender swelling in the groin associated with redness and oedema of the overlying skin if the history is over 24 hours. The diagnosis can usually be differentiated from an irreducible inguinal hernia by the absence of symptoms of bowel obstruction, but torsion of the testis is frequently associated with vomiting and the differential diagnosis of an irreducible hernia or torsion of an undescended testis may only be made at the time of surgical exploration.

Encysted hydrocele of the spermatic cord can occur quite suddenly and may be quite large. However, it is usually asymptomatic, not particularly tender, usually mobile and clearly related to the spermatic cord. The testis can be palpated below the swelling and is non-tender. If the hydrocele is large and the child thin then the swelling is transilluminable. This is treated by ligating the processus vaginalis if the child is over 2 years of age. Under 2 years the swelling is likely to resolve.

Acute lymphadenitis presents with pyrexia and a tender swelling in the groin with redness of the overlying skin. In a child the pubic tubercle is not easily palpable, but if it is, the mass is lateral to it, whereas the swelling of an irreducible hernia is medial to it. With careful palpation it is usually possible to feel the spermatic cord separately. The perineal region and the lower limb are examined for a likely source of infection which preceded the swelling. An inguinal hernia with redness of the overlying skin is usually associated with symptoms and signs of bowel obstruction. An undescended testis that has undergone torsion is differentiated from inguinal lymphadenitis by the absence of the testis from the scrotum, and the tender mass lies more medially at the external ring, although torsion of an ectopic testis can be mistaken for inguinal lymphadenitis. Inguinal lymphadenitis may respond to a course of flucloxacillin and penicillin. Should an abscess develop, recognized by reddening of the overlying skin and fluctuance, incision and drainage are required.

HIGHLIGHTS

- A child who has had an 'irreducible' hernia manually reduced should not be discharged before the hernia is repaired
- The absence of the testis from the scrotum is a helpful sign when considering lumps in the inguinal region

---

LUMPS CONFINED TO THE SCROTUM

AIMS

1 Define scrotal lumps as non-tender or tender
2 Recognize the common causes and management of scrotal pain

In all these lumps the cord is palpable above the swelling.

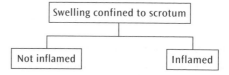

Non-tender lumps

Infantile hydrocele is a swelling confined to the scrotum with a normal spermatic cord palpable. It is transilluminable, and if it is not tense the testis can be palpated and is normal. An infantile hydrocele is fluid contained within the tunica vaginalis. The processus vaginalis is a diverticulum of the peritoneum which protrudes through the internal ring of the inguinal canal and is drawn downwards to the scrotum through the inguinal canal as the testis descends. As the processus elongates it normally becomes obliterated, but this may not be complete at birth and peritoneal fluid tracks down the processus into the space around the testis (*communicating hydrocele*). The hydrocele appears larger during the day and disappears during the night when the child lies flat. Under the age of 2 years, management is conservative since the patent processus will close spontaneously and the fluid in the hydrocele sac resorb. Over the age of 2 years, if a hydrocele persists or suddenly appears, treatment is surgical ligation of the processus vaginalis.

Testicular tumours, although very rare, present as a smooth, tense swelling with a defined upper limit, distinguishable from a hydrocele by the fact that it is not transilluminable.

Tender lumps: the 'acute scrotum'

Torsion of the testis can occur at any age but is most common in early and mid-adolescence. The history is usually of sudden, occasionally of gradual, onset of scrotal or ipsilateral iliac fossa pain, frequently associated with nausea and vomiting. Scrotal oedema and redness develop rapidly and can make examination of the testis and epididymis difficult. However, the testis is usually exquisitely tender and may lie high in the scrotum compared with the unaffected testis. Swelling and tenderness of the spermatic cord is not unusual particularly when the history is of a few hours' duration.

If epididymo-orchitis, resolving torsion of the appendix testis, or idiopathic scrotal oedema as alternative causes of acute scrotum cannot be diagnosed with confidence then surgical exploration of the scrotum is mandatory: a testis twisted for 6 hours

is gangrenous and beyond saving. The starvation policy prior to anaesthesia is ignored, and an experienced anaesthetist is therefore crucial. The opposite hemiscrotum must be explored and the testis fixed as the condition can recur on the contralateral side.

An *appendix testis* refers to vestigial embryological remnants (*hydatid of Morgagni*) attached to the upper pole of the testis or adjacent epididymis which is present in most boys. *Torsion* of these appendages can occur at any age but is most common just before puberty. The presentation can be similar to torsion of the testis with acute onset of scrotal pain, although sometimes the pain is not severe and the boy may not be aware of scrotal redness and swelling which are noted by a parent at bath time. Presentation may be delayed for several days when the symptoms are mild. When presentation is early a small dark spot, more tender than the neighbouring testis, may be visible through the thin scrotal skin. Once scrotal oedema develops, localizing the tenderness to the upper pole of the testis is difficult. The surgical excision of a torted hydatid resolves the symptoms rapidly. With a longer history, torsion of the appendix testis is indistinguishable from torsion of the testis and exploration of the scrotum will be necessary. When symptoms that have been present for several days are subsiding and examination clearly rules out testicular torsion, a waiting policy is reasonable.

Epididymo-orchitis is an important cause of the acute scrotum in infants and often indicates the presence of an underlying urinary tract anomaly. During childhood, epididymo-orchitis is rare but does occur in boys who have had previous urethral surgery, for example hypospadias repair, or have a neurogenic bladder requiring intermittent catheterization. *Mumps orchitis* is extremely rare before puberty. At or after puberty, epididymo-orchitis occurs secondary to reflux of urine up the wider vas. In infancy the parent discovers a red swollen scrotum in a child who is miserable and pyrexial. If examination is carried out before the scrotum becomes oedematous, it may be possible to palpate an indurated enlarged epididymis and a normal testis. The diagnosis is confirmed by the presence of bacteria and pus in the urine. If the urine is clear or the diagnosis of epididymo-orchitis is doubtful, then scrotal exploration is essential to exclude testicular torsion. In the older child with a

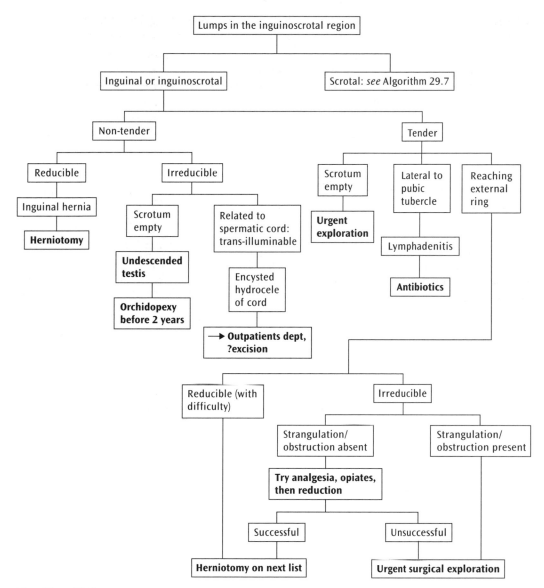

Algorithm 29.6

recognized abnormality of the urinary tract and a definite urinary tract infection, exploration is avoided, but if there is any doubt about the diagnosis exploration should not be delayed. When a diagnosis of epididymo-orchitis is made in a child, antibiotic treatment is commenced and the urinary tract is investigated.

Idiopathic scrotal oedema is the term given to dramatic scrotal swelling and redness that may involve both sides of the scrotum and extend into the perineum, the iliac fossa and the upper thigh. However, the area is not tender and it is usually possible to palpate the testes through the scrotal wall and to confirm their normality. Antibiotics do not help, but itchiness responds to chlorpheniramine maleate (*Piriton*). Idiopathic scrotal oedema is sometimes recurrent; it is the only cause of the acute scrotum that can usually be diagnosed with confidence, thus avoiding surgical exploration. The aetiology is unknown.

Use of Doppler ultrasonography in the acute scrotum

Immediate ultrasonography, by determining the testicular blood flow, can be helpful in establishing a diagnosis of testicular torsion, but if there is strong clinical suspicion of torsion, exploration should not be deferred until this investigation is possible.

HIGHLIGHTS

- An infantile hydrocele may not require treatment as the processus vaginalis will close spontaneously
- A boy with iliac fossa pain and vomiting must have the scrotum examined for testicular torsion
- When the cause of a painful scrotum cannot be identified, exploration is advisable to exclude testicular torsion
- The urinary tract should be investigated for congenital anomalies following epididymo-orchitis

---

BALANITIS AND PARA-PHIMOSIS

AIM

1 Define painful conditions of the foreskin

Balanitis

Inflammation of the foreskin can occur at any age but is more likely to occur in the early years when the foreskin is non-retractile. The foreskin becomes swollen, red, painful and pus may collect between the foreskin and glans in severe cases. Passing urine is painful and acute retention may occur.

Balanitis needs to be distinguished from the generalized ammoniacal dermatitis which involves the perineum and the penis in the child in nappies.

Established balanitis will usually respond to an oral antibiotic, such as trimethoprim, analgesia and salt baths, and when mild may simply require salt

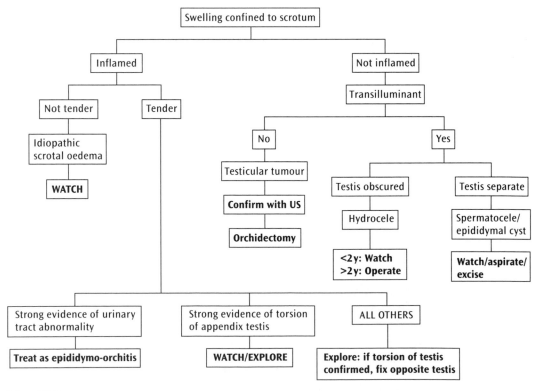

Algorithm 29.7

baths and analgesia. Unless the child is in acute retention, admission is not necessary. Acute retention almost always responds to adequate analgesia and warm baths. Very occasionally, the inflammatory process may extend along the shaft of the penis and on to the skin of the perineum and symphysis pubis, and the child becomes toxic. A swab from the penis and blood cultures are collected before intravenous antibiotics to cover streptococcus and anaerobic organisms are commenced as soon as possible, but resolution is not seen before 12–24 hours, when the child is generally better. This inflammatory process has some of the early features of necrotizing fasciitis and requires careful observation.

An inflamed foreskin may be complicated by stenosis of the preputial orifice (*phimosis*) but a decision on the need for circumcision should be deferred until the inflammation has completely subsided. In the child aged under 6 years the fact that the foreskin does not retract is not pathological and a single episode, or more, of balanitis is not an indication for circumcision.

Paraphimosis

This occurs when the foreskin is fully retracted and is trapped behind the coronal sulcus because the foreskin is tight, making reduction difficult. This promotes swelling of the glans and the lining tissue of the foreskin. It tends to occur in older boys, particularly those who are developmentally delayed.

It is painful and if initial gentle pressure and traction fails to reduce the paraphimosis then the application of a local anaesthetic cream (EMLA) is worth trying and often provides sufficient analgesia to allow sustained pressure on the swollen tissues and traction to effect reduction. If this method is unsuccessful a general anaesthetic is required and very occasionally a dorsal slit may be necessary to allow reduction. Follow-up should be arranged to decide on the need for circumcision.

HIGHLIGHTS

- Balanitis in a child is not an indication for circumcision
- A retracted foreskin should always be reduced to avoid paraphimosis

Index